LUNG DEVELOPMENT

Clinical Physiology Series

Lung Development
Edited by Claude Gaultier, Jacques R. Bourbon, and Martin Post

Flow-Dependent Regulation of Vascular Function
Edited by John A. Bevan, Gabor Kaley, and Gabor M. Rubanyi

Pathophysiology of Hypertension in Blacks
Edited by John C. S. Fray and Janice G. Douglas

Hyperglycemia, Diabetes, and Vascular Disease
Edited by Neil Ruderman, Joseph Williamson, and Michael Brownlee

Endothelin
Edited by Gabor M. Rubanyi

Hypoxia, Metabolic Acidosis, and Circulation
Edited by Allen I. Arieff

Response and Adaptation to Hypoxia: Organ to Organelle
Edited by Sukhamay Lahiri, Neil S. Cherniack, and Robert S. Fitzgerald

Clinical Physiology of Sleep
Edited by Ralph Lydic and Julien F. Biebuyck

High Altitude and Man
Edited by John B. West and Sukhamay Lahiri

LUNG DEVELOPMENT

Edited by

Claude Gaultier

Jacques R. Bourbon

Martin Post

New York Oxford

Published for the American Physiological Society

by Oxford University Press

1999

Oxford University Press

Oxford New York
Athens Auckland Bangkok Bogotá Buenos Aires Calcutta
Cape Town Chennai Dar es Salaam Delhi Florence Hong Kong Istanbul
Karachi Kuala Lumpur Madrid Melbourne Mexico City Mumbai
Nairobi Paris São Paulo Singapore Taipei Tokyo Toronto Warsaw

and associated companies in
Berlin Ibadan

Published for the American Physiological Society by Oxford University Press, Inc.,
198 Madison Avenue, New York, New York 10016
http://www.oup-usa.org

Library of Congress Cataloging-in-Publication Data
Lung development /
edited by Claude Gaultier, Jacques R. Bourbon, Martin Post.
p. cm. — (Clinical physiology series
ISBN 0-19-511278-4.
1. Lungs—Growth. I. Gaultier, C. (Claude) II. Bourbon, Jacques R. III. Post, Martin, 1952– .
IV. American Physiological Society (1887–) V. Series.
[DNLM: 1. Lung—growth & development.
2. Lung—embryology.
3. Lung—physiopathology.
WF 600 L96329 1999] QP121.L838 1999
612.6′40124—dc21 DNLM/DLC for Library of Congress 98-44090

9 8 7 6 5 4 3 2 1

Printed in the United States of America
on acid-free paper

PREFACE

Lung development became a focal point of intensive research when M. E. Avery and J. Mead reported pioneering work on the mechanism of neonatal respiratory distress syndrome (1). During the last two decades there has been an explosive increase in the number of publications on this subject.

Respiratory physiology was the first approach used to investigate the developing lung. P. A. Auld, M. E. Avery, R. C. Bryan, C. D. Cook, K. W. Cross, F. Geubelle, P. Karlberg, L. S. Strang, and others laid the groundwork for an emerging understanding of neonatal lung function during the transition from intrauterine to extrauterine life. Anatomical and morphometrical data were later reported by E. A. Boysen, P. H. Burri, J. L. Emery, S. Engel, L. Reid, W. Thurbeck, J. S. Wiggleworth, E. R. Weibel, and others. All of these studies brought new insights into the processes underlying the development of bronchial, vascular, and alveolar structures. In 1975 and 1980, two reviews summarized knowledge of the relationships between structure and function in the developing lung in health and disease (2, 3).

Cellular biological studies of the lung concentrated initially on surfactant synthesis and metabolism. Investigators such as T. Akino, J. Clements, S. Hawgood, A. Jobe, W. Longmore, F. Possmayer, L. M. G. Van Golde, and J. A. Whitsett worked in this field. In 1991, J. R. Bourbon edited a book on pulmonary surfactant (4), and the following year another book on the same topic written by B. Robertson, L. M. G. Van Golde, and J. J. Batenburg was published (5). Data from the first decade of research on surfactant enabled intensive care physicians, neonatologists, and pediatricians to improve the treatment and survival of patients with respiratory distress syndrome.

Molecular studies of lung development started in the late 1980s and are currently burgeoning. A picture is beginning to form of the complex series of controlled interactions involving genetic influences, hormonal stimulation, and cell-cell interactions that is required for lung development. The role of the time of injury in abnormal development, first emphasized by L. Reid (6), remains important at the molecular level. *Lung Development* provides a comprehensive review of the multiple facets of lung development in health and disease. To meet the challenge of reviewing an ever-changing field, the editors obtained the participation of over 30 international authorities on lung development. Each of these contributors took the standpoint that the developing lung should be understood starting at the bedside and moving toward gene dysfunction. As a result, each chapter brings new insights of clinical relevance into the physiological and pathophysiological processes operative in neonatal and pediatric respiratory disorders. Pediatric pulmonologists, neonatologists, intensive care physicians, obstetricians, and chest surgeons now need to be aware of findings from cellular and molecular as well as from anatomical and physiological studies.

The first four chapters deal with morphogenesis, elastogenesis, maturation of airway epithelial cells, and gene expression in alveolar development. R. Keÿzer and M. Post provide a clear overview of the role of permissive and/or inductive growth factors and the extracellular matrix in lung branching morphogenesis. T. J. Mariani and R. A. Pierce focus on the development of the lung elastic matrix and its significant role in the development and maintenance of normal lung function; they also discuss abnormal elastogenesis in bronchopulmonary dysplasia. D. Gaillard and E. Puchelle provide a comprehensive review of the role of the extracellular matrix and of growth factors in the differentiation and maturation of airway epithelial cells. J. R. Bourbon covers the field of gene expression in pulmonary bronchiolar and alveolar epithelial cells, providing information on the complex mechanisms of gene expression control, including those involving transcription factors and mesenchymal–epithelial interrelationships.

Chapters 5–7 review angiogenesis, pulmonary vasculature, and circulation. P. H. Burri discusses the development of the lung and its vasculature, providing a clear and well-illustrated overview, particularly regarding the pulmonary capillary network, and he emphasizes the deleterious effects of glucocorticoid administration on early postnatal lung development. N. W. Morrell, M. C. M. Weiser, and K. R. Stenmark deal with the mechanisms controlling angiogenesis and vasculogenesis and the development of pulmonary arterial smooth muscle. S. H. Abman, J. P. Kinsella, and J.-C. Mercier describe the role of NO and ET-1 in the developing pulmonary circulation, review the mechanisms implicated in persistent pulmonary hypertension of the newborn, and discuss therapeutic strategies.

Chapters 8–11 cover the developmental aspects of cellular host defense mechanisms, lung epithelial ion transport, cell growth, and tissue repair, as well as the role of bioactive peptides. S. P. Sorokin, R. F. Hoyt, and N. A. F. McNelly describe local defenses provided by resident cells and hematological defenses provided by leukocytes and their products in the neonatal lung. O. Pitkänen and H. O'Brodovich discuss recent work on lung epithelial ion transport and its dysfunction in neonatal lung diseases, including bronchopulmonary dysplasia. A. Clement and J. S. Brody deal with the mechanisms of cell growth and tissue repair in a chapter that supplies a unique overview of abnormal lung development after tissue repair, as in lung fibrosis. M. E. Sunday follows with a comprehensive review of bioactive neuropeptides and lung development.

The last part of the book, Chapters 12–16, centers on the pathophysiology of neonatal and pediatric pulmonary disorders. T. R. Korfhagen and J. A. Whitsett review methods for introducing mutations that affect respiratory function. They concentrate on the SP-B knockout mouse, which provides a model for studying the role of SP-B in lung function and for designing new therapies for surfactant deficiency. M. Kalenga, C. Gaultier, and P. H. Burri review current knowledge on the role of nutrition in lung development, emphasizing alterations produced during the periods characterized by the highest rates of remodeling of the gas exchange compartment. R. Harding and C. Albuquerque cover research on fetal lung hypoplasia and the control of lung expansion in the fetus, discussing congenital diaphragmatic hernia, musculoskeletal and neurological abnormalities, and other causes of lung hypoplasia. R. L. Morton and C. W. White deal with pulmonary antioxidant defense mechanisms and describe the pathogenic events involved in the development of oxygen toxicity in bronchopulmonary dysplasia of premature infants. Finally, S. G. Haworth and A. A. Hislop report their unique experience with lung development after transplantation in immature rats. Their chapter is of obvious clinical relevance because lung transplantation is now a therapeutic option in children with end-stage pulmonary or vascular disease.

C. G.
J. R. B.
M. P.

References

1. Avery, M. E., and J. Mead. Surface properties in relation to atelectasis and hyaline membrane disease. *Am J. Dis. Child.* 97:517–523, 1959.
2. Gaultier, C., and F. Girard. Croissance pulmonaire normale et pathologique: relation structure-fonction. *Bull. Eur. Physiopathol. Resp.* 16:791–842, 1980.
3. Thurlbeck, W. M. Postnatal growth and development of the lung. *Am. Rev. Respir. Dis.* 111:803–844, 1975.
4. Bourbon, J. Pulmonary surfactant: biochemical, functional, regulatory, and clinical concepts. Boca Raton, Fl: CRC Press, Inc., 1991.
5. Robertson, B., L. M. G. Van Golde, and J. J. Batenburg. Pulmonary surfactant from molecular biology to clinical practice. Amsterdam: Elsevier, 1992.
6. Reid, L. The embryology of the lung. In: *Ciba Foundation Symposium: Development of the Lung.* edited by A. V. S. De Reuk and Porter, R. Londres: Churchill, 1967, p. 109–112.

CONTENTS

Contributors

STEVEN H. ABMAN
Pediatric Heart-Lung Center
Department of Pediatrics
University of Colorado School of Medicine
and The Children's Hospital
Denver, Colorado

CHERYL ALBUQUERQUE
Department of Obstetrics and Gynecology
University of California
Davis, California

JACQUES R. BOURBON
INSERM Unité 319
Univerisité Denis Diderot-Paris 7
Paris, France

JEROME S. BRODY
Pulmonary Center
Boston University School of Medicine
Boston, Massachusetts

PETER H. BURRI
Institute of Anatomy
University of Berne
Berne, Switzerland

ANNICK CLEMENT
Department of Pediatric Pulmonology
Trousseau Hospital
St. Antoine Medical School
University of Paris
Paris, France

DOMINIQUE GAILLARD
INSERM Unité 314, IFR 53
Biologie du Développement–Reproduction,
UFR Médecine
Reims, France

CLAUDE GAULTIER
Service de Physiologie-Explorations
Fonctionnelles
Hôpital Robert Debré, Université Paris 7
Paris, France

RICHARD HARDING
Department of Physiology
Monash University
Melbourne, Victoria
Australia

SHELIA G. HAWORTH
Developmental Pharmacology and
Vascular Biology Unit
Institute of Child Health
London, United Kingdom

ALISON A. HISLOP
Developmental Pharmacology and
Vascular Biology Unit
Institute of Child Health
London, United Kingdom

RICHARD F. HOYT, JR.
Department of Anatomy and Neurobiology
Boston University School of Medicine
Boston, Massachusetts

MASENDU KALENGA
Service de Néonatologie
Clinique Saint Vincent
Rocourt, Belgium

RICHARD KEŸZER
Lung Biology Research Program
Hospital for Sick Children
Toronto, Canada

JOHN P. KINSELLA
Section of Neonatology
Department of Pediatrics
University of Colorado School of Medicine
and The Children's Hospital
Denver, Colorado

THOMAS R. KORFHAGEN
Division of Pulmonary Biology
Children's Hospital Research Foundation
Cincinnati, Ohio

THOMAS J. MARIANI
Department of Internal Medicine
Washington University School of Medicine
at Barnes-Jewish Hospital
St. Louis, Missouri

NANCY A. F. MCNELLY
Department of Anatomy and
Neurobiology
Boston University School of Medicine
Boston, Massachusetts

JEAN-CHRISTOPHE MERCIER
Service de Réanimation Pédiatrique
Hôpital Robert Debré
and Laboratoire de Physiologie sur la
Circulation Pulmonaire
Faculté de Médecine Cochin
Paris, France

NICHOLAS W. MORRELL
Developmental Lung Biology
Department of Pediatrics
University of Colorado Health Sciences
Center
Denver, Colorado
and Department of Medicine
Royal Postgraduate Medical School
Hammersmith Hospital
London, United Kingdom

RONALD L. MORTON
Department of Pediatrics
National Jewish Center for Immunology
and Respiratory Medicine
and University of Colorado Health
Sciences Center
Denver, Colorado

HUGH O'BRODOVICH
Medical Research Council Group in
Lung Development
Hospital for Sick Children Research
Institute
Department of Pediatrics
University of Toronto
Toronto, Canada

RICHARD A. PIERCE
Department of Internal Medicine
Washington University School of Medicine
at Barnes-Jewish Hospital
St. Louis, Missouri

OLLI PITKÄNEN
Children's Hospital
University of Helsinki
Helsinki, Finland

MARTIN POST
The Medical Research Council Group in
Lung Development
Hospital for Sick Children Research
Institute
Department of Pediatrics and Physiology
University of Toronto
Toronto, Canada

EDITH PUCHELLE
INSERM Unité 314, IFR 53
Biologie du Développement-Reproduction,
UFR Médecine
Reims, France

SERGEI P. SOROKIN
Department of Anatomy and
Neurobiology
Boston University School of Medicine
Boston, Massachusetts

KURT R. STENMARK
Department of Medicine
Royal Postgraduate Medical School
Hammersmith Hospital
London, United Kingdom

MARY E. SUNDAY
Brigham & Women's Hospital
and Harvard Medical School
Department of Pathology
Boston, Massachusetts

MARY C. M. WEISER
Developmental Lung Biology
Department of Pediatrics
University of Colorado Health Science
Center
Denver, Colorado

CARL W. WHITE
Department of Pediatrics
National Jewish Center for Immunology
and Respiratory Medicine
and University of Colorado Health
Sciences Center
Denver, Colorado

JEFFREY A. WHITSETT
Division of Pulmonary Biology
Children's Hospital Research Foundation
Cincinnati, Ohio

LUNG DEVELOPMENT

chapter 1

LUNG BRANCHING MORPHOGENESIS: ROLE OF GROWTH FACTORS AND EXTRACELLULAR MATRIX

Richard Keijzer and Martin Post

IN the embryonic mouse and rat at 10 and 11.5 days of gestation, respectively, (term mouse = 19 days; term rat = 22 days), the respiratory system develops from paired endodermal buds in the primitive foregut, just proximal to the developing stomach. As the two buds elongate, the primitive tubular foregut tube begins to pinch into two tubes, namely, the dorsal esophagus and the ventral trachea. In the human, however, the lung originates as an out pouch of the ventral wall of the posterior end of the laryngotracheal tube and divides into two bronchial buds at 3–4 weeks of gestation. The origin and fate of the cells forming the lung anlage within the primitive esophagus are unknown. Homeobox-containing genes (*Hox* genes) may play a role in the developmental destination of this particular group of cells in the primitive foregut. *Hox* genes have been implicated in regional conditional specification of morphogenetic progenitor fields, which are defined as regions in an embryo where cells give rise to a morphological structure (30). *Hox* genes are characteristically organized in four clusters on different chromosomes and their 3′ to 5′ position of each gene within a cluster corresponds with their expression along the anterior–posterior axis of the developing body (66, 75). Several *Hox* genes, specifically genes of the 3′ regions of the *Hox* clusters *a* and *b*, have been shown to be expressed in the lung (66). The *Hoxb* cluster is expressed in partially overlapping domains along the anterior–posterior axis of the developing foregut (12, 28, 39, 43,

138). *Hoxb-3, b-4* and *b-5* are expressed more posteriorly in the trachea-esophageal region of the developing foregut whereas *Hoxb-1* and *b-2* expression is more anterior restricted to the branchial arches and the area that develops in the pharynx. *Hoxa* expression has not been studied in the developing lung, but *Hoxa-3* mutants display some minor lung abnormalities (25). In both rat and human, the primary bronchi continue to grow into the splanchnic mesenchyme. Further outgrowths of these buds produce the secondary bronchi. In the mouse, the right lung characteristically has four major lobes (dorsal, caudal, medial, and cranial lobes) whereas the left lung consists of only one small lobe. This arrangement also holds in the rat except the right lung lobes are termed cranial, medial, accessory, and caudal. In the human, the right lung has three lobes whereas the left lung is composed of two lobes (upper, middle, and lower on the right; upper and lower on the left). The early branching of the primary bronchial buds tends to be monopodial. Each secondary bronchus subsequently undergoes progressive dichotomous branching as each branch bifurcates repeatedly into branches (16). This branching process will ultimately yield a functional lung with its very large surface area (size of a soccer field in the human) for gas exchange after birth.

Morphogenesis of many organs, including lung, gut, and mammary gland is controlled by interactions between two tissue layers, epithelium and mesenchyme. The characteristic branching morphogenesis of the bronchial epithelial buds of embryonic lungs has long been known to depend on a specific interaction with bronchial mesenchyme (2, 117). The effect of bronchial mesenchyme on epithelial branching is organ- and species-specific and is temporally regulated (83, 153, 177). In addition, proximal (trachea and main bronchi) and distal (lung bud) mesenchyme differ in their ability to support branching morphogenesis (177). Interestingly, *Hoxb* genes have also been found to be expressed in spatial domains of the developing lung (12). *Hoxb-2* and *b-5* expression is restricted to the distal mesenchyme whereas *Hoxb-3* and *b-4* are found in both proximal and distal mesenchyme. This distinct pattern of regional expression suggests that *Hoxb* genes may be involved in specifying the regional differences in mesenchyme along the anterior–posterior axis of the developing lung (12). As branching proceeds, numerous different cell phenotypes are formed along the anterior–posterior axis of the developing epithelial tubules and associated mesenchymal components, each with different morphologies and patterns of gene expression. This patterning of differentiated lung cells may also be controlled by epithelial–mesenchymal interactions. Tissue recombination studies have recently shown that bronchial mesenchyme grafted into embryonic trachea induces distal epithelial cell differentiation, using surfactant proteins A and C as distal cell markers. (77, 139). Again, this effect is regulated in a temporal and spatial fashion (77, 139). Epithelial differentiation in vitro has also been shown to depend on the quantity of recombined mesenchyme (83). Small quantities of recombined mesenchyme induce a bronchiolar epithelial phenotype whereas larger amounts of grafted mesenchyme result in epithelial differentiation toward a more distal phenotype.

Despite all accumulated evidence that mesenchymal cells are capable of controlling lung branching and epithelial phenotypic expression, the regulatory molecules involved in morphogenic signaling in the lung have yet to be defined. The signals likely include extracellular matrix proteins, cell-associated signaling molecules, and diffusible factors (see reviews 93, 107). This chapter focuses on what is new and relevant to growth factors and extracellular matrix in lung branching morphogenesis.

GROWTH FACTORS AND LUNG BRANCHING

So far, most progress in understanding lung branching morphogenesis has come from studies of early lung explants and lung epithelial cells that can be induced to form rudimentary branched structures in vitro. Recently, several growth factors have been shown to act as inductive signals mediating epithelial–mesenchymal interactions and regulating lung branching morphogenesis.

Epidermal Growth Factor, Transforming Growth Factor Alpha, and Amphiregulin

Epidermal growth factor (EGF), transforming growth factor-alpha (TGF-α), and amphiregulin (AR) are members of the EGF family of growth factors that act through the common EGF receptor (EGFR). All three are expressed in fetal rodent lung (128, 144, 161) and transcripts for EGF and TGF-α have been detected in fetal human lung (118, 160). In the developing mouse, rat and human lung, EGF and TGF-α protein are present in bronchial and bronchiolar epithelium (118, 144, 161, 159), while EGF and TGF-α mRNA expression is mostly localized to the mesenchyme (118, 144), suggesting that both EGF and TGF-α are produced by the mesenchyme and act on the epithelium. However, epithelial cells isolated from fetal rat lung have been shown to synthesize both EGF and TGF-α (161). Amphiregulin is mostly synthesized by lung mesenchymal cells in embryonic mouse lung (128). Their common EGF receptor has mainly been found in fetal mouse (176) and rat (161) lung epithelial cells but also in the mesenchyme surrounding the epithelium. In developing human lung, EGFR has been localized to the epithelium (118, 159). These data are compatible with EGF, TGF-α and AR acting in an autocrine and paracrine fashion. All three proteins influence growth and branching morphogenesis of embryonic murine lung in vitro. Exogenous EGF enhances lung branching and stimulates cellular proliferation of embryonic mouse lung explants (176). Conversely, inhibition of endogenous EGF production with an antisense oligonucleotide directed against EGF precursor mRNA leads to a significant reduction of branching morphogenesis (137). Also, inhibition of EGFR tyrosine kinase activity results in a diminished branching (176). Agarose beads containing EGF induce the formation of supernumerary tracheal buds in embryonic chicken lung similar to that seen in grafting experiments using bronchial mesoderm (45). Transforming growth factor α affects lung branching in vitro via activation of metalloproteinases (41). In embryonic mouse lung explants, antibodies to the AR heparan sulfate binding site inhibit branching whereas exogenous AR stimulates terminal bud formation (128). Retinoic acid may also play an important role in branching morphogenesis (21). It stimulates mouse lung epithelial branching activity via an epithelial–mesenchymal interaction which, in part, involves up-regulation of EGFR expression (135). These data support a role for EGF, TGF-α and AR in the control of lung branching morphogenesis. However, exogenous EGF does not stimulate proliferation of isolated embryonic rat lung epithelial cells (33). Furthermore, genetic ablation of EGFR in mice has led to conflicting interpretations regarding a role of EGF/TGF-α in branching morphogenesis. Mice homozygous for an EGFR null mutation have been reported to die postnatally of respiratory failure which was attributed to lung immaturity (91). In contrast, another null EGFR mutation with a different genetic background did not display any major lung abnormality during development (167). Also, expression of a dominant negative EGF receptor under control of the SP-C promoter does not alter lung morphogenesis in transgenic mice (54). Moreover, mice having EGFR signaling deficiencies, *wa-2/wa-2* mice (37), have normal lung morphology (54). Thus, it appears that EGFR signaling is not essential for lung branching morphogenesis although it is possible that other receptors have replaced EGFR signaling.

Insulin-like Growth Factors

The insulin-like growth factor (IGF) family consists of two related peptides, IGF-I and IGF-II, which interact with two specific IGF receptors. The type 1 IGF receptor transmits most biological responses, such as proliferation and differentiation, while the type 2 IGF/mannose-6-phosphate receptor appears to function in internalizing and transporting IGF-II to the lysozomes (62). Ample evidence suggest that the IGF system has a role in lung development (156). Both IGF-I and IGF-II mRNAs are expressed during lung development (29, 94, 110, 173). In the developing human and rodent lung, transcripts for IGF-I are detected in the mesenchyme (52, 71, 110), while IGF-II mRNA expression is predominantly localized to airway epithelium (110). The IGF peptides have been immunolocalized to early respiratory epithelium in the rat (7) and human (52). During rat lung development, IGF-I expression remains relatively constant whereas that of IGF-II declines with advancing gestation (94). The type 1 IGF receptor is expressed virtually in all cells in the developing lung (110). In contrast, the transcripts for type 2 IGF receptor are mainly found in the mesenchyme (110). Expression of both receptors hardly changes during development (94, 110). These findings are compatible with IGFs, which are synthesized by the mesenchyme, acting on the epithelium via the type 1 IGF receptor during early branching morphogenesis. In contrast to fetal lung fibroblasts (95, 157), however, fetal lung epithelial cells do not respond mitogenically to IGF-I (158). The mitogenic responses might have been modulated by specific IGF binding proteins (IGFBP) as mitogenic effects of IGF in cultured cells have been shown to be markedly increased or inhibited in the presence of IGFBPs (62). Thus, the binding proteins may determine which cell type will respond to an autocrine/paracrine action of the IGF peptides in vivo. To date, six distinct IGFBPs have been characterized (62). Transcripts for IGFBP-2, -3, -4, and -5, but not IGFBP-1 and -6, are present in the developing lung (94, 110). IGFBP-2 is expressed in the distal epithelium throughout development while IGFBP-4 mRNA expression is confined to the mesenchyme. IGFBP-3 and -5 are expressed in many cells and their transcript abundance increase with advancing gestation (94, 110). The function of each IGFBP is unknown, but their spatial and temporal expression patterns suggest a role in controlling IGF action at specific sites during lung development. Genetic studies with transgenic mice argue against a direct role for IGFs in branching morphogenesis. Mice carrying a disrupted IGF-I gene are growth retarded and die at birth from respiratory failure, but no obvious histopathological defect of lung development, besides uninflated lungs, is observed (81). Mice with no functional type I IGF receptor display a similar phenotype (81). Transgenic mice with a disrupted IGF-II gene are small and have small lungs, but no abnormal lung morphology is noted (31). The type 2 IGF receptor is paternally imprinted and mice with a maternally inherited disrupted type 2 IGF receptor gene, which die shortly after birth from heart failure, have abnormal alveoli but no major branching defect (78, 175). In conclusion, although the IGFs may play a role during lung development, they appear not to be a major determinant during early lung morphogenesis.

Fibroblast Growth Factors

Fibroblast growth factors (FGFs) are known to have key roles in embryonic growth and morphogenesis. In *Drosophila*, the FGF system has been shown to play an important role in primary tracheal branching. Loss-of-function of either *breathless* (44, 69), a FGFR gene, or *branchless* (163), a FGF gene, leads to abnormal tracheal branch formation. Fibroblast growth factor 2 is required for mesoderm patterning in *Xenopus laevis* embryo (67) while FGF-4 is essential for postimplantation mouse development (35) and limb pattern formation (98). Four high-affinity FGF receptors have been identified, designated FGFR1–4 (61). Signaling via FGF receptor is required for primary mesoderm induction (3) as well as for later aspects of *Xenopus* development (74). Several members of the FGF family may be involved in controlling lung pattern formation. Basic FGF (FGF-2) is expressed in both epithelial and mesenchymal cells in fetal rat (51) and fetal human (46) lung, while FGFR1 and FGFR2 have been localized to embryonic and fetal lung epithelium (46, 51). Transcripts for FGF-7 (keratinocyte growth factor [KGF]) are detected in embryonic lung mesenchyme at sites of active branching morphogenesis (84, 108). The KGF receptor (KGFR), a FGFR2-IIIb splice variant (32, 92), which has a high affinity for KGF and acidic FGF (FGF-1), is expressed in airway epithelium (100, 108). The mesenchymal–epithelial distribution of KGF and KGFR expression during development has been documented for other branched organs, such as salivary gland, kidney, and mammary gland (116). In addition, appositional expression of KGF and KGFR has also been reported for organs within the gastrointestinal and urogenital systems, whose development are also dependent upon mesenchymal–epithelial interactions (36). Exogenous KGF inhibits rat lung branching morphogenesis in vitro (141) but stimulates proliferation of adult type II pneumocytes in vitro (104) and in vivo

(103). KGF also stimulates the proliferation of isolated epithelial cells from embryonic rat lung (33, 108). Ectopic expression of human KGF in distal lung epithelial cells of transgenic mice using the SP-C promoter resulted in abnormal branching morphogenesis and fetuses failed to survive to term (143). Interpretation regarding the effects of KGF on lung development from the latter experiment is somewhat difficult as KGF is not expressed in lung epithelial cells during normal development. Inhibition of function of KGF with antisense oligonucleotides or neutralizing antibodies has been found to inhibit embryonic lung branching in vitro (108). Surprisingly, mice bearing a null mutation of the KGF gene had no obvious lung abnormalities (48), suggesting that KGF can be replaced by other factors, such as FGF-1 and FGF-10. Fibroblast growth factor 1 is expressed in lung mesenchyme (40) and has been shown to stimulate embryonic epithelial cell proliferation (33, 108). Furthermore, FGF-1, which binds to both splicing variants of FGFR2, KGFR and bek, is crucial for branching of embryonic mouse epithelium in mesenchyme-free culture (99). Fibroblast growth factor 2, which binds to bek, but not to KGFR, did not affect epithelial branching in these cultures, suggesting that the effect of FGF-1 on epithelial branching is mediated via KGFR. The KGFR is the predominant FGFR2 splice variant expressed in embryonic mouse lung (100). Antisense experiments using rat lung explants have suggested that KGFR is more important in regulating epithelial branching morphogenesis than bek (108). A targeted expression of a dominant negative KGFR to the lung epithelium in transgenic mice has been shown to result in dramatically reduced bronchial branching (106). As mentioned earlier homozygous deletions of *breathless*, a FGFR gene, causes abnormal tracheal branch migration in *Drosophila* (44, 69). A newly identified member of the fibroblast growth factor family, designated FGF-10 (181) is highly expressed in the developing lung (8). FGF-10 is closely related to KGF (181). Although FGF-10 and KGF exhibit similar receptor binding properties (60), their signals are transduced in different physiological responses. In vitro, FGF-10 elicits endodermal expansion and bud formation while KGF induces expansion of the endoderm but never progresses to bud formation (8). Taken together, these data indicate that mesenchyme-derived FGF signaling through KGFR is important for branching of lung epithelium (see Fig. 1.1).

Hepatocyte Growth Factor

Another heparin-binding mitogen with motogenic and morphogenic activities is hepatocyte growth factor/scatter factor (HGF/SF). During mouse development, HGF/SF and its receptor, c-*met*, are expressed in different but adjacent tissues, suggesting that they transduce mesenchymal–epithelial signaling (115, 145). Hepatocyte growth factor/scatter factor is produced by fetal lung fibroblasts and stimulates the proliferation of adult type II cells (85, 104, 140). In vitro, exogenous HGF/SF or a neutralizing antibody to HGF/SF has no effect on early branching morphogenesis of mouse lung (141). These data are consistent with genetic ablation experiments. Mouse embryos bearing a null mutation in the HGF/SF gene do not survive beyond E14.5 in utero but show normal branching morphogenesis until that gestational

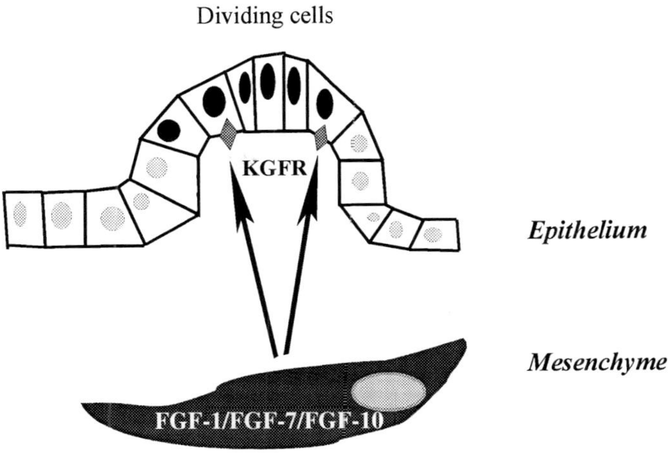

Fig. 1.1. Schematic illustration of fibroblast growth factors (*FGF*) involved in early lung branching morphogenesis. *FGF-1* (acidic FGF), *FGF-7* (keratinocyte growth factor), and FGF-10 are produced and secreted by lung mesenchymal cells. These FGFs bind with high affinity to a splice variant of the FGF receptor-2 (*KGFR*) present on airway epithelial cells stimulating cell growth and branch formation.

time point (127, 171). Also, branching and growth appears normal when lungs of day 14.5 mutant embryos are cultured in vitro (171).

Platelet-derived Growth Factor

Platelet-derived growth factor (PDGF) has been implicated in embryonic development (47, 89). It is a dimeric molecule composed of two distinct but related polypeptides (A and B). The two chains assemble as a heterodimer, PDGF-AB, or as homodimers, PDGF-AA or PDGF-BB (109). Platelet-derived growth factor exerts its effect via specific cell surface receptors (26). Two related transmembrane tyrosine kinase receptors, PDGF α- and β-receptors have been characterized. The α-receptor binds all three isoforms of PDGF whereas the β-receptor binds only PDGF-BB with high affinity (26). Both PDGF homodimers, AA and BB, and both PDGF receptors are present in the early embryonic rat lung (50, 49). At this early stage of lung development, the mesenchyme is enriched in the expression of both receptors (148). In contrast, expression for both PDGF homodimers, AA and BB, is confined to the epithelium of the embryonic lung (50, 148, 149). However, PDGF-AA and -BB transcripts and protein are detected in both tissue layers with advancing gestation (50, 148, 149). Expression in separate but adjacent tissue layers of ligands and receptors for PDGF has been noted in many tissues during development, including mouse lung (102), submandibular salivary gland (102), and placenta (58). The appositional expression of PDGF and its receptors during early lung development is compatible with a role for PDGF in epithelial-to-mesenchymal signaling during branching morphogenesis. The physiological function of PDGF in lung branching morphogenesis has been partly delineated. Translation arrest of endogenous PDGF-BB with antisense oligonucleotide in embryonic rat lung results in smaller lungs but the degree of branching is not affected (149). Similarly, antisense β-receptor oligonucleotides reduce lung size without affecting branching (150). Mice deficient of PDGF-B (79) and β-receptor (146) show no abnormal lung branching phenotype. These results suggest that PDGF-BB is not involved in the regulation of lung branching. Using an antisense strategy, Souza et al. (148) reported that PDGF-AA influences early lung branching morphogenesis. The number of terminal buds of embryonic rat lung explants was significantly reduced in the presence of antisense PDGF-A oligonucleotides. Addition of PDGF-AA, but not PFGF-BB, to the culture system attenuated the inhibitory effect of antisense PDGF-A on early lung branching. Also, antisense PDGF α-receptor oligonucleotides inhibited early lung branching (150). It should be noted that blocking of function of PDGF-A or α-receptor does not completely block branching, indicating that other factors are involved in regulating this morphogenetic process. A null PDGF-A mutant is lethal at two restriction points—one prenatally prior to E10.5, implying a role in early embryonic development, and one postnatally (15). The lung phenotype of PDGF-A null embryos dying prior to day 10.5 was not further investigated and, thus, it is not completely clear whether PDGF-A is involved in the early formation of the lung. The observation that PDGF-A-deficient mice surviving postnatally have normal fetal and early postnatal lung development argues against PDGF-A being a major determinant in lung branching morphogenesis. However, it is possible that the role of PDGF-A is replaced by other non-PDGF factors or maternal leakage of PDGF rescues the early developmental events in the knockout mice. Interestingly, homozygous mice that survive the first bottleneck at E10.5 develop postnatally lung emphysema secondary to the failure of alveologenesis attributed to lack of alveolar myofibroblast differentiation (15). Homozygous mutant mice carrying a targeted disruption in the PDGF α-receptor gene die during embryonic development and exhibit severe developmental defects (147). Most interestingly, the phenotype of the α-receptor mutant mice differs from that of the PDGF-A mutant mice. However, early lung development proceeds normally in the α-receptor null mutants. *Patch* mutant mice which are homozygous for a large deletion of the α-receptor gene (155), also die prenatally prior to E10.5 (101). Heterozygotes, expressing only 50% of the α-receptor on their cells compared with their wild-type littermates, develop normal lungs. Although the genetic data support a role for the PDGF-A/α-receptor axis in embryonic development, further studies such as double mutant knockouts for ligands and receptors are needed to determine whether the PDGF/receptor axis has a regulatory role in lung branching morphogenesis (see Fig. 1.2).

Transforming Growth Factor Beta

Transforming growth factor beta (TGF-β) is a multifunctional peptide that elicits a wide variety of morphogenetic responses in many organs. Several lines of evidence suggest that TGF-β is also important for fetal lung development. All three mammalian TGF-β subtypes (β1, β2, and β3) have been detected in the developing murine

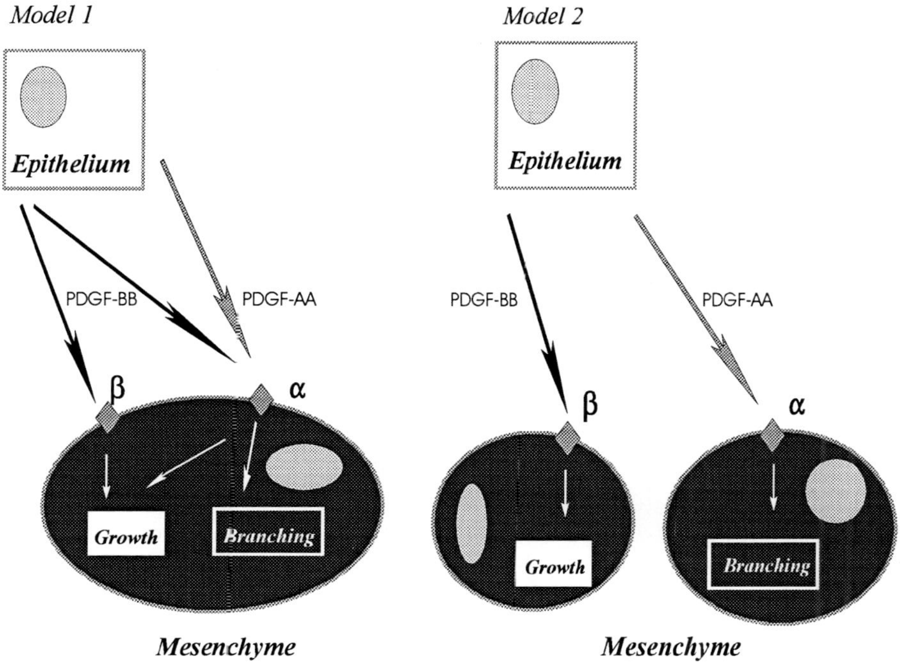

Fig. 1.2. Proposed models for platelet-derived growth factor (*PDGF*) actions during early lung branching. Both PDGF homodimers AA and BB are elaborated by airway epithelial cells and act upon mesenchymal cells via two related tyrosine kinase receptors, PDGF α-receptor (*PDGFR-α*) and β-receptor (*PDGFR-β*). The PDGFR-α binds both isoforms of PDGF, whereas PDGFR-β binds only PDGF-BB. In *model 1*, PDGFR-α and PDGFR-β are localized on the same cell and initiate distinct intracellular transduction pathways that lead to either growth or branching depending on PDGF isoform. In *model 2*, PDGFR-α and PDGFR-β are present on different mesenchymals cells and biological response to PDGF isoforms is likely determined by tissue localization of the cells.

lung (105, 126). TGF-β1 mRNA expression is prominent throughout the mesenchyme while TGF-β2 message is mainly localized to the epithelium of the developing distal airways. The TGF-β3 transcripts are initially found in the tracheal mesenchyme but TGF-β3 signals are visible in the epithelium of the growing bronchioles during the pseudoglandular stage (day 14.5) of murine lung development. Although numerous TGF-β binding proteins have been identified, type I and type II receptors are responsible for most, if not, all biological activities of TGF-βs (5, 86). One type II TGF-β receptor has been identified (80) while two type I TGF-β receptors have been cloned: ALK-5 (38) which has been characterized as a signaling receptor for TGF-β (178), and ALK-1/TSR-I (4), which binds TGF-β and activin in the presence of their respective type II receptor. Both type II TGF-β receptor and ALK-5 are expressed in rat lung mesenchymal cells at late gestation (184, 186) and ALK-1 message and protein have been detected in adult murine lung (164, 180). Transforming growth factor β can exert a variety of biological effects including regulation of extracellular matrix (ECM) production and integrin expression (111). Thus, TGF-β may increase cell–ECM interactions, and by doing so, influence branching morphogenesis (93). A recent study has shown that TGF-β1 co-localizes with collagen I and II, fibronectin, and glycosaminoglycans at the epithelial–mesenchymal interface of clefts of branching lung (56). High dosages of exogenous TGF-β1 inhibit lung branching morphogenesis in vitro (136). The mechanism of inhibition of branching by TGF-β1 is unknown. Transforming growth factor β1 has been suggested to inhibit expression of N-*myc* (136), which has been implicated in lung growth and branching (96, 125). Recent studies have demonstrated that PDGF α-receptor expression in lung fibroblasts is also negatively modulated by TGF-β1 (13). As the PDGF-AA/α-receptor axis may play a role in lung branching morphogenesis in vitro (148, 150), another possibility is that high dosages of TGF-β1 disrupt this axis by adversely influencing α-receptor expression in embryonic mesenchymal cells. Whether TGF-β2 and TGF-β3 have similar effects on N-*myc* or PDGF α-receptor expression as TGF-β1 remains to be elucidated. Studies with transgenic mice have implicated TGF-β in regulating late but not early lung organogenesis. Overexpression of TGF-β1 in lung epithelium of transgenic mice causes a pseudoglandular arrest of lung development (184). However, caution is warranted in extrapolating these data to normal development as TGF-β1 is mainly expressed in the lung mesenchyme of developing lung (105, 126, 174). Surprisingly, inactivation of the mouse TGF-β 1 gene does not affect lung branching (76, 142). Mice lacking TGF-β3 die within several hours after birth and exhibit an arrest in lung development at the late pseudoglandular stage (65). The TGF-β2 null mice exhibit perinatal mortality and a wide range of developmental defects (124). Prenatal lung morphology of the mutant mice appeared to be normal while postnatal lung had collapsed conducting airways. Together, these genetic analyses suggest that none of the TGF-β isoforms play a major biological role in early lung branching morphogenesis. Alternatively, it is possible that redundancy or maternal leakage of TGF-βs rescues the early developmental events in these knockout mice. Analysis of double or triple mutants is now feasible, which may help further understand the requirements of TGF-βs during lung development.

EXTRACELLULAR MATRIX AND LUNG BRANCHING

The extracellular matrix (ECM) plays a complex role in regulating the behavior of cells that contact it, influencing their development, migration, proliferation, and morphology, as well as metabolic functions. In particular, the basement membrane (BM), which separates the epithelium from the surrounding mesenchyme, has been implicated in mediating morphogenetically significant tissue interactions. The epithelial–mesenchymal interface contains laminin, fibronectin, proteoglycans, and collagen as major matrix components.

Collagens

Collagenous proteins are a major constituent of extracellular matrices. In addition to their structural roles, collagens may have numerous developmental and physiological functions (11, 55). There are at least 15 types of collagen. In the adult lung, collagen accounts for 60% of the lung connective tissue protein mass. Collagen types I and III are predominantly associated with mesenchymal connective tissue in the lung. Lung collagen type IV is mainly found in basement membranes. Immunohistochemical studies have observed lung collagen type V close to basement membranes but it may also be associated with the interstitial matrix (27). The amount of collagen has been shown to increase with development (17). Several studies have suggested that collagens play a critical role in lung branching. Branching morphogenesis is affected when lung explants are incubated in the presence of inhibitors of collagen synthesis such as β-aminopropionitrile, a lathyrogen that inhibits extracellular collagen cross-linking, and L-azetidine-2-carboxylic acid, a proline analogue that competes with proline for insertion in the polypeptide chain (151). Since both agents inhibit synthesis of all collagenous proteins, it is not possible to ascribe branching properties to one particular type of collagen. However, branching morphogenesis is not affected in lungs of mutant mouse embryos that do not produce collagen type I (72), suggesting that collagen type I is not essential for lung organogenesis. Collagen type III has been implicated in branching morphogenesis of salivary gland (97) which resembles that of lung branching. The recent observation that collagen type III neither colocalizes with epithelial buds of fetal human lung nor with one of its receptors, α2β1, makes it unlikely that collagen type III plays a significant role in lung branching (172).

Laminin

The laminins are structurally related glycoproteins found mainly in basement membranes. Laminins are large multidomain glycoproteins composed of three polypeptide subunits: α, β and γ (18). Structural isoforms exist for each of these subunits and the association of these isoforms in heterotrimers give rise to different laminins. To date, seven laminins have been identified. Laminins have the ability to self-polymerize and to bind other basement proteins, such as collagen type IV and nidogen (entactin), thereby determining the structure of the basement membrane (168). Laminins stimulate cell adhesion and migration, growth, and morphology, as well as gene expression in a variety of cells (168). Laminin-1, composed of subunits α1, β1, and γ1,which are held together by disulfide bonds in a unique cross-shaped structure (169), appears to be present at all stages of lung development (133). Its expression is low at the onset of lung organogenesis but increases with advancing gestation (134). Laminin α-subunit synthesis is largely confined to lung epithelial cells, whereas β- and γ-subunit expression is seen in many cells (70, 172). In the pseudoglandular period of human lung development, laminin-1 (α1β1γ1) and laminin-2 (α2β1γ1) localize to BM of epithelial buds, laminin-3 (α1β2γ1) more proximally in the tubules, and laminin-5 (α3β3γ2) more widely to all airway epithelia (172). With advancing gestation, laminin-2 disappears and in the bronchi expression shifts from laminin-3 to laminin-1. The role of different laminins in lung branching remains to be determined. Anti-laminin antibodies inhibit branching morphogenesis of murine lung primordia, whereas antibodies to thrombospondin and entactin, two other matrix molecules, show no inhibition of branching (129). However, antibodies to the entactin binding site on the laminin γ-subunit perturbs lung branching (34). The laminin domains involved in cell attachment (cross-intersection of laminin structure and carboxy terminus of α chain) and heparin binding activity (inner globular region of β1 chain) may facilitate lung branching morphogenesis (86, 133). Recent studies suggest that an interaction between laminin and heparan sulfate proteoglycan (HSPG) is critical for the development of epithelial polarization and lumen formation (130, 131). The latter appears to be an essential process for branching morphogenesis as anti-laminin antibodies that block epithelial polarization also inhibit airway development (133). The globular ends of β1 and γ1 chains are important for laminin-laminin assembly and epithelial polarization (132) but the laminin–HSPG interaction is required for lumen development (131). The globular region at the carboxy end of the laminin α-chain has been implicated in alveolar morphogenesis (88). These observations suggest that laminin is a key regulatory matrix component in branching morphogenesis.

Fibronectin

Fibronectin is an adhesive glycoprotein that plays a major role during morphogenesis by promoting cell attachment (119). It consists of two polypeptides of approximately 220 kDa that form a dimer through two disulfide bonds. The fibronectin subunit contains a number of domains with different binding properties. In the developing mouse lung, fibronectin is localized to areas of airway bifurcations (114). Inhibition of ligand binding to the fibronectin receptor with synthetic peptides containing the Arg-Gly-Asp (RGD) sequence diminishes but does not abolish lung branching (112, 113)

SPARC and Tenascin

Since adhesion of cells to the extracellular matrix appears to be critical for lung branching, molecules that disrupt cellular adhesion may also modulate this morphogenic processes. Anti-adhesive properties have been ascribed to several ECM proteins such as SPARC (secreted protein, acidic and rich in cysteine), thrombospondin, and tenascin (123). Both SPARC mRNA and protein are abundant in airway epithelium during early rat lung development (162). A neutralizing anti-SPARC monoclonal antibody diminishes airway branching in rat lung explants (162). Also, treatment of explants with a synthetic SPARC peptide previously shown to have anti-adhesive properties similar to those of intact SPARC inhibits lung branching (162). These findings suggest that SPARC is involved in regulating airway branching. The tenascins are a growing family of extracellular matrix glycoproteins of typical multi domain structure. To date, three members of the family have been described; tenascin-C, tenascin-R, and tenascin-X (23). Tenascin-R seems to be specific for the central and peripheral nervous system, tenascin-X for skeletal and heart structures, and tenascin-C is present in many developing tissues (23). Tenascin-C is often transiently associated with morphogenetic tissue interactions during organogenesis (24), including that of lung (185). Its morphogenic action is contributed to its adhesive-modulating properties (23). Antibodies against tenascin-C inhibit lung branching in vitro (185). In contrast, disruption of the tenascin-C gene in mice does not affect normal lung development (122). The latter finding makes it questionable whether tenascin plays an essential role during lung branching morphogenesis. However, it is possible that the other members of the tenascin family compensate for the loss of tenascin-C.

Proteoglycans

Proteoglycans (PGs) are major components of the basal laminae. The PGs constitute a family of multidomain core proteins to which glycosaminoglycans (GAGs) are attached via *O*-glycosidic linkages to serine residues. GAGs are unbranched carbohydrate chains composed of repeating disaccharide units (uronic acid and hexosamine) carrying a negative charge, except for hyaluronan, which results in their binding to other matrix components, cell adhesion molecules, and growth factors (64, 120, 121). These properties suggest that GAGs may mediate, at least in part, cell adhesion, structural organization, and cell proliferation during fetal lung development. Numerous studies have examined the correlation between GAG synthesis and morphogenic events in several organs, including lung (64, 170). In the chick, hyaluronan is mostly localized in the growing areas of the lung while chondroitin sulfate PGs are deposited in areas of second-order branching (6). The deposition of chondroitin sulfate PGs decreases with advancing gestation in primate lung (61). These studies show that glycosaminoglycan synthesis in vivo alters with development, suggesting that PG/GAGs play a role in organogenesis. Indeed, inhibitors of GAG synthesis such as 6-diazo-5-oxo-L-norleucine and azaserine inhibit branching morphogenesis of cultured embryonic lung rudiments (152). Similarly, β-D-xyloside, which stimulates synthesis of GAG chains but inhibits proteoglycan synthesis, inhibits branching of the embryonic salivary gland (165, 166). The exact mechanism by which PG/GAGs direct branching morphogenesis is unknown. As discussed previously, an interaction between laminin and HSPG is critical for epithelial polarization and lumen formation, which appear to be required for proper lung branching (130, 131, 133). Increasing evidence suggests that PG/GAGs play an important role as modulators of growth factor activities. Several isoforms of FGF bind to high-affinity receptors and are active when bound to specific cell-surface heparan sulfate proteoglycans (68). Similarly, the membrane proteoglycan betaglycan increases the binding of TGF-β to the signaling TGF-β receptor (82). The small interstitial proteoglycans biglycan, decorin, and fibromodulin have been shown to bind TGF-β via their core proteins and to neutralize TGF-β activity (14, 57, 182). These properties suggest that PG/GAG may mediate morphogenetic actions of growth factors, such as FGF and TGF-β, on cell adhesion and cell proliferation during early lung development. Glycosaminoglycan may also directly affect cell proliferation. Heparan sulfate molecules are potent inhibitors of smooth muscle cell growth (9). Additionally, hyaluronic acid inhibits fetal skin fibroblast proliferation but stimulates collagen and noncollagen protein synthesis (87). It has also been suggested that soluble interstitial PGs such as decorin and biglycan may inhibit cell adhesion to fibronectin and collagen by binding to the GAG-binding site of these matrix molecules, thus making it inaccessible to the cell surface PGs (120, 121), such as syndecan, which are able to function as ECM receptors (10).

Integrins

Most cells have multiple mechanisms of attachment to ECM molecules and may interact with two or more distinct regions in the same macromolecule. A family of cell surface proteins, integrins, have been identified that serve as receptors for ECM molecules (1, 59). Integrins are transmembrane glycoproteins that consist of αβ heterodimers. Within a β subfamily, the β subunit can associate with various α subunits. Each heterodimer has its own ligand-binding selectivity, with many integrins binding more than one ligand. Individual cells may vary their adhesive properties by selective expression of integrins and further by modulating the binding properties of integrins (59). Thus, the cell's response to a particular form of an ECM molecule will depend on the number and subunit composition of integrins expressed on its surface and their binding properties. The integrins α1β1 and a2β1 have been shown to function as collagen-binding receptors in fetal rat lung fibroblasts (19). Interestingly, fetal rat lung epithelial cells do not express the α1β1 and α2β1 integrins and do not readily adhere to collagen (19). In the fetal human lung, α2β1 integrin expression is noted in the distal epithelial buds (172, 17). Since no distinct codistribution with one of its ligands, collagen type III, is observed, it is unlikely that this ligand–receptor interaction has an important function during fetal lung morphogenesis (172). The α1 integrin subunit is also not crucial for lung branching as a null mutation in the α1 integrin gene does not result in any loss of viability or obvious phenotype (42). The expression of the fibronectin receptor $\alpha_5\beta_1$ in the developing lung has been reported (114) and inhibition of ligand binding to fibronectin receptor with synthetic peptides containing the RGD sequence affects lung branching morphogenesis in vitro (113, 114). A null α5 mutation leads to embryonic death prior to lung formation (183). As discussed earlier, laminin appears to be a key determinant for regulating lung branching morphogenesis. Several laminin integrins have been identified (90), of which α2β1, α3β1, and α6β1are expressed in the developing human lung (172). The α6β1 integrin colocalizes with laminin-1 in the distal epithelial buds of fetal human lung. With advancing gestation, α2- and α6-subunit expression disappears (172). The α3β1 integrin is highly expressed in distal fetal rat lung epithelial cells and does function as a laminin receptor in these cells (20). This receptor is widely co-distributed with laminin-5 in fetal human lung, which is in line with the capacity of laminin-5 to bind to α3β1 (22). Recently, genetic ablation of the α3 integrin gene has been shown to result in reduced bronchial branching (73). This suggests that the laminin/α3β1 interaction is crucial for lung organogenesis.

SYNOPSIS

The lung originates from two tissue layers, endoderm and mesoderm, and sequential and reciprocal interactions between these tissue layers regulate branching morphogenesis of the lung. During the last decade an increasing amount of molecular data regarding lung organogenesis has accumulated from studies describing the ontogeny of gene expression of molecules, from functional in vitro studies, and from generation of transgenic mice. These studies have implicated several growth factors, particularly in the EGF-, FGF-, PDGF- and TGF-β families, to act as inductive signals mediating epithelial–mesenchymal interactions (see Table 1.1). The growth factors may specify early patterning of lung cells by regulating expression, deposition, and breakdown of extracellular matrix molecules and cell surface receptors. Changes in cell adhesion and matrix remodeling at the epithelial–mesenchymal interface have been found to contribute to lung epithelial branching morphogenesis (see Table 1.2). The mechanism by which ECM components and their receptors are acting on the induction of morphogenesis, in particular, organ- and tissue-specific induction of organ-specific gene expression, remains to be elucidated.

Table 1.1 Overview of In Vitro and In Vivo Assays Implicating Growth Factors in Regulating Enbryonic Lung Branching Morphogenesis

In Vitro Studies			*In Vivo Studies*		
None	*Stimulatory*	*Inhibitory*	*None*	*Stimulatory*	*Inhibitory*
	EGF	EGF^{AS}			
	TGF-α				
		Amhiregulin^{Ab}			
		EGFR^{tyr}	EGFR$^{-/-}$ EGFR^{sign-}		
IGF-1			IGF-1$^{-/-}$		
IGF-2			IGF-2$^{-/-}$		
			Type I IGFR$^{-/-}$		
			Type II IGFR$^{-/-}$		
	FGF-1				
FGF-2					
	FGF-7	FGF-7$^{AS/Ab}$	FGF-7$^{-/-}$		FGF-7^{ect}?
		KGFR^{AS}			KGFR^{dnm}
HGF/SF			HGF/SF		
		PDGF-AA$^{AS/Ab}$	PDGF-AA$^{-/-}$		
		PDGFR-α^{AS}			PDGFR-α$^{-/-}$ (patch)
PDGF-BB^{AS}					?
PDGFR-β^{AS}			PDGFR-β$^{-/-}$		
		TGF-β1	TGF-β1$^{-/-}$		TGF-β1^{ect}? TGF-β$^{-/-}$
			TGF-β2$^{-/-}$		

AS, antisense; Ab, antibody; tyr, tyrphostin; ect, ectopic expression; dnm, dominant-negative mutant; –/–, homozygous deletion mutant; sign-, signaling deficient.

Table 1.2 Overview of In Vitro and In Vivo Assays Implicating Extracellular Matrix Molecules in Regulating Embryonic Lung Branching Morphogenesis

In Vitro Studies			*In Vivo Studies*		
None	*Stimulatory*	*Inhibitory*	*None*	*Stimulatory*	*Inhibitory*
		Collagen synthesis^{inhibition}	Collagen I$^{-/-}$		
			α1 integrin$^{-/-}$		
	Laminin^{matrigel}	Laminin^{Ab}			α3 integrin$^{-/-}$
		Laminin/entactin interaction^{inhibition}			
		Laminin/HSPG interaction^{inhibition}			
Fibronectin		α5 integrin^{RGD}			
		SPARC$^{Ab/peptide}$			
		Tenascin-C^{Ab}	Tenascin C$^{-/-}$		
		Proteoglycan synthesis^{inhibition}			

Ab, antibody; –/–, homozygous deletion mutant.

REFERENCES

1. Albeda, S.M. and C.A. Buck. Integrins and other cell adhesion molecules. *FASEB J.* 4: 2868–2880, 1990.
2. Alescio, T. and A. Cassini. Induction in vitro of tracheal buds by pulmonary mesenchyme grafted on tracheal epithelium. *J. Exp. Zool.* 150: 83–94 1962.
3. Amaya, E., T.J. Musci, and M.W. Kirschner. Expression of a dominant negative mutant of the FGF receptor disrupts mesoderm formation in *Xenopus* embryos. *Cell* 66: 257–270, 1991.
4. Attisano, L., J. Carcamo, F. Ventura, F.M. Weis, J. Massague, and J.Wrana. Identification of human activin and TGF beta type I receptors that form heteromeric kinase complexes with type II receptors. *Cell* 75: 671–680,1993.
5. Attisano, L., J.L. Wrana, F. López-Casillas, and J. Massagué. TGF-beta receptors and actions. *Biochim. Biophys. Acta* 1222: 71–80, 1994.
6. Becchetti, E., R. Evangeliste, G. Stabellini, A. Pagliarini, E. Del Borello, C.Calastrini, and P. Carinci. Developmental heterogeneity of mesenchymal glycosaminoglycan (GAG) distribution in chick embryo lung anlagen. *Am. J. Pathol.* 188: 33–42, 1988.
7. Beck, F., N.J. Samani, J.D. Penschow, B. Thorley, G.W. Tregear, and J.P. Coghlan. Histochemical localization of IGF-I and -II mRNA in the developing rat embryo. *Development* 101: 175–184, 1987.
8. Bullusci, S., Y. Furuta, R. Henderson, G. Winnier, and B.L. Hogan. Involvement of Sonic hedgehog (Shh) in mouse embryonic lung and growth and morphogenesis. *Development* 124: 53–63, 1997.
9. Benitz, W.E., R.T. Kelley, C.M. Anderson, D.E. Lorant, and M. Bernfield. Endothelial

heparan sulfate proteoglycan. I. Inhibitory effects on smooth muscle cell proliferation. *Am. J. Respir. Cell Mol. Biol.* 2: 13–24, 1990.

10. Bernfield, M., R. Kokensky, M. Kato, M.T. Hinkes, J. Spring, R.L. Gallo, and E.J. Lose. Biology of the syndecans: a family of transmembrane heparan sulfate proteoglycans. *Annu. Rev. Cell Biol.* 8: 365–393, 1992.
11. Bienskowski, R.S. Interstitial collagens. In: *The Lung,* edited by R.G. Crystal and J.B. West. New York: Raven Press, p. 381–388, 1991.
12. Bogue, C.W., L.J. Lou, H. Vasavada, C.M. Wilson, and H.C. Jacobs Expression of *Hoxb* genes in the developing mouse foregut and lung. *Am. J. Respir. Cell Mol. Biol.* 15: 163–171, 1996.
13. Bonner, J.C., A. Badgett, P.M. Lindroos, and A.R. Osornio-Vargas.Transforming growth factor beta 1 downregulates the platelet-derived growth factor alpha-receptor subtype on human lung fibroblasts in vitro. *Am. J. Respir. Cell Mol. Biol.* 13: 496–505, 1995.
14. Border, W.A. and E. Ruoslahti. Transforming growth factor-beta in disease: the dark side of tissue repair. *J. Clin. Invest.* 90: 1–7, 1992.
15. Boström, H., K. Willetts, M. Pekny, P. Leveen, P. Lindahl, H. Hedstrand, M. Pekna, M. Hellstrom, S. Gebre-Medhin, M. Schalling, M. Nilsson, S. Kurland, J. Törnell, J.K. Heath, and C. Betsholtz. PDGF-A signaling is a critical event in lung alveolar myofibroblast development and alveogenesis. *Cell* 85: 863–873, 1996.
16. Boyden E.A. Development of the human lung. In: *Practice of Pediatrics* Vol 4, edited by J. Brennemann. Hagerstown, PA: Harper & Row, 1972.
17. Bradley, K., S.D. McConnell, and R.G. Crystal. Lung collagen composition and synthesis. Characterization and changes with age. *J. Biol. Chem* 249: 2674–2683, 1974.
18. Burgeson, R.E., M. Chiquet, R. Deutzmann, P. Ekblom, J. Engel, H.Kleinmann, G.R. Martin, G. Meneguzzi, M. Paulsson, J. Sanes, R. Timpl, K.Tryggvason, Y. Yamada, and P.D. Yurchenco. A new nomenclature for the laminins. *Matrix Biol.* 263: 16536–16544, 1994.
19. Caniggia, I., R. Han, J. Liu, J. Wang, A.K. Tanswell, and M. Post. Differential expression of collagen binding receptors in fetal rat lung cells *Am. J. Physiol. (Lung Cell. Mol. Physiol.)* 268: L136–L143, 1995.
20. Caniggia, I., J. Liu, R. Han, J. Wang, A.K. Tanswell, G. Laurie, and M. Post. Identification of receptors binding fibronectin and laminin on fetal rat lung cells. *Am. J. Physiol. (Lung Cell. Mol. Physiol.)* 270: L459–L468, 1996.
21. Cardoso, W.V., M.C. Williams, S.A. Mitsialis, M. Joyce-Brady, A.K. Rishi,and J.S. Brody. Retinoic acid induces changes in the pattern of airway branching and alters epithelial cell differentiation in the developing lung invitro. *Am. J. Respir. Cell Mol. Biol.* 12: 464–476, 1995.
22. Carter, W., M.C. Ryan, and P.J. Gahr. Epiligrin, a new cell adhesion ligand for integrin alpha3 beta1 in epithelial basement membranes. *Cell* 65: 599–610, 1991.
23. Chiquet-Ehrismann, R. Tenascins, a growing family of extracellular matrix proteins. *Experienta* 51: 853–862, 1995.
24. Chiquet-Ehrismann, R., C. Hagios, and S. Schenk. The complexity in regulating the expression of tenascins. *Bioessays* 17: 873–878, 1995.
25. Chisaka, O. and M.R. Capecchi. Regionally restricted developmental defects resulting from targeted disruption of the mouse homeobox gene *hox-1.5. Nature* 350: 473–479, 1991.
26. Claesson-Welsh, L. Signal transduction by the PDGF receptors. *Prog Growth Factors Res.* 5: 37–54, 1994.

27. Clarke, J.G., C. Kuhn, J.A. McDonald, and R.P. Mecham. Lung connective tissue. *Int. Rev. Connect. Tissue Res.* 10: 249–330, 1983.
28. Conlon, R.A. and J. Rossant. Exogenous retinoic acid rapidly induces anterior ectopic expression of murine *Hox-2* genes in vivo. *Development* 116: 357–368, 1992.
29. Davenport, M.L., A.J. D'Ercole, J.C. Azizkhan, and P.K. Lund. Somatemedin-C/insulin-like growth factor (Sm-c/IGF-I) and insulin-like growth factor II (IGF-II) mRNAs during lung development in the rat. *Exp. Lung Res.* 14: 607–618, 1988.
30. Davidson, E.H. Later embryogenesis: regulatory circuitry in morphogenetic fields. *Development* 118: 665–690, 1993.
31. DeChiara, T.M., A. Efstratiadas, and E.J. Roberstson. A growth-deficiency phenotype in heterozygous mice carrying an insulin-growth factor II gene disrupted by targeting. *Nature* 345: 78–80, 1990.
32. Dell, K.R. and L.T. Williams. A novel form of fibroblast growth factor receptor 2. Alternative splicing of the third immunoglobin-like domain confers ligand binding specificity. *J. Biol. Chem.* 267: 21225–21229, 1992.
33. Deterding, R.R., C.R. Jacoby, and J.M. Shannon. Acidic fibroblast growth factor and keratinocyte growth factor stimulate fetal rat pulmonaryepithelial growth. *Am. J. Physiol.* (*Lung Cell. Mol. Physiol.*) 271: L495–L505, 1996.
34. Ekblom, P., M. Ekblom, L. Fecker, G. Klein, H.-Y. Zhang, Y. Kadoya, M.-L.Chu, U. Mayer, and R. Timpl. Role of mesenchymal nidogen for epithelial morphogenesis in vitro. *Development* 120: 2003–2014, 1994.
35. Feldman, B., W. Poueymirou, V.E. Papaioannou, T.M. DeChiara, and M. Goldfarb. Requirement for FGF-4 for postimplantation mouse development *Science* 267: 246–249, 1995.
36. Finch, P.W., G.R. Cunha, J.S. Rubin, J. Wong, and D. Ron. Pattern of keratinocyte growth factor and keratinocyte growth factor receptor expression during mouse fetal development suggests a role in mediating morphogenetic mesenchymal–epithelial interactions. *Dev. Mech.* 203: 223–240, 1995.
37. Fowler, K.J., F. Walker, W. Alexander, M.L. Hibbs, E.C. Nice, R.M., Bohmer,G.B. Mann, C. Thumwood, R. Maglitto, J.A. Danks, R. Chety, A.W. Burgess, and A.R. Dunn. A mutation in the epidermal growth factorreceptor in waved-2 mice has a profound effect on receptor biochemistry that results in impaired lactation. *Proc. Natl. Acad. Sci. USA* 92: 1465–1469, 1995.
38. Franzén, F., P. Ten Dijke, H. Ichijo, H. Yamashita, P. Schulz, C.-H. Heldin,and K. Miyazono. Cloning of a TGF-β type I receptor that forms aheterodimeric complex with the TGF β type II receptor. *Cell* 75: 681–692, 1993.
39. Frohman, M.A., M. Boyle, and G.R. Martin. Isolation of the mouse *Hox-2,9* gene: analysis of embryonic expression suggests that positional information along the anterior-posterior axis is specified by mesoderm. *Development*110: 589–607, 1990.
40. Fu, Y.-M., P. Spirito, Z.-X. Yu, S. Biro, J. Sasse, J. Lei, V.J. Ferrans, S.E.Epstein, and W. Casscels. Acidic fibroblast growth factor in the developing rat embryo. *J. Cell Biol.* 114: 1261–1273, 1991.
41. Ganser, G.L., G.P. Stricklin, and L.M. Matrisian. EGF and TGFα influence in vitro lung development by the induction of matrix-degrading metalloproteinases. *Int. J. Dev. Biol.* 35: 453–461, 1991.
42. Gardner, H., J. Kreidberg, V. Koteliansky, and R. Jaenishch. Deletion of integrin alpha1 by homologous recombination permits normal murine development but gives rise to a specific deficit in cell adhesion. *Dev. Biol.*175: 301–313, 1996.
43. Gaunt, S.J., R. Krumlauf, and D. Duboule. Mouse homeo-genes within a subfamily, *Hox-*

1,4, -2,6 and -5,1, display similar anteroposterior domains of expression in the embryo, but show stage-and tissue-dependent differences in their regulation. *Development* 107: 131–141, 1989.

44. Glazer, L. and B. Shilo. The *Drosophila* FGF-R homolog is expressed in the embryonic tracheal system and appears to be required for directed tracheal cell extension. *Genes Dev.* 5: 697–705, 1991.
45. Goldin, G.V. and L.A. Opperman. Induction of supernumerary tracheal buds and stimulation of DNA synthesis in the embryonic chick lung and trachea by epidermal growth factor. *J. Embryol. Exp. Morphol.* 60: 235–243, 1980.
46. Gonzalez, A.M., D.J. Hill, A. Logan, P.A. Maher, and A. Baird. Distribution of fibroblast growth factor (FGF)-2 and FGF receptor-1 messenger RNA expression and protein presence in the mid-trimester human fetus. *Pediatr.Res.* 39: 375–385, 1996.
47. Goustin, A.S., C. Betsholtz, S. Pfeifer-Ohlsson, H. Persson, J. Rydnert, M.Bywater, G. Holmgren, C.-H. Heldin, B. Westermark, and R. Ohlson.Coexpression of *sis* and *myc* protooncogenes in developing human placenta suggests autocrine control of trophoblasts. *Cell* 41: 301–312, 1985.
48. Guo, L., L. Degenstein, and E. Fuchs. Keratinocyte growth factor is required for hair development but not for wound healing. *Genes Dev.* 10: 165–175, 1996
49 Han, R.N.N., J. Liu, A.K. Tanswell, and M. Post. Ontogeny of platelet-derived growth factor receptor (PDGFR) in fetal rat lung. *Microsc. Res. Tech.* 26: 381–388, 1993.
50. Han, R.N.N., C. Mawdsley, P. Souza, A.K. Tanswell, and M. Post. Platelet-derived growth factors and growth-related genes in rat lung. III. Immunolocalization during fetal development. *Pediatr. Res.* 31: 323–329, 1992.
51. Han, R.N.N., A.K. Tanswell, and M. Post. Expression of basic fibroblast growth factor and receptor: immunolocalization studies in developing fetal rat lung. *Pediatr. Res.* 31: 435–440, 1992.
52. Han, V.K.M., A.J. D'Ercole, and P.K. Lund. Cellular localization of somatomedin (insulin-like growth factor) messenger RNA in the human fetus. *Science* 236: 1993–197, 1987.
53. Han, V.K.M., D.J. Hill, A. Strain, A.C. Towle, J.M. Lauder, L.E.Underwood, and A.J. D'Ercole. Identification of somatomedin/insulin-like growth factor immunoreactive cells in the human fetus. *Pediatr. Res.* 22: 254–249, 1987.
54. Hardie, W.D., C.B. Kerlakian, M.D. Bruno, K.M. Huelsman, S.E. Wert, S.W.Glasser, J.A. Whitsett, and T.R. Korfhagen. Reversal of lung lesions in transgenic transforming growth factor a mice by expression of mutant epidermal growth factor receptor. *Am. J. Respir. Cell Mol. Biol.* 15: 499–508, 1996.
55. Hay, E.D. *Cell Biology of Extracellular Matrix*, 2nd ed. New York: Plenum Press, 1991.
56. Heine, U.I., E.F. Munoz, K.C. Flanders, A. Roberts, and M.B. Sporn.Colocalization of TGF-β1 and collagen I and III, fibronectin and glycosaminoglycans during lung branching morphogenesis. *Development* 109: 29–36, 1990.
57. Hildebrand, A., M. Romaris, L.M. Rasmussen, D. Heinegard, D.R. Twardzik, W.A. Border, and E. Ruoslahti. Interaction of the small interstitial proteoglycans biglycan, decorin and fibrimodulin with transforming growth factor beta. *Biochem. J.* 302: 527–534, 1994.
58. Holmgren, L., A. Glaser, S. Pfeifer-Ohlsson, and R. Ohlsson. 1991.Angiogenesis during human extraembryonic development involves the spatiotemporal control of PDGF ligand and receptor gene expression. *Development* 113: 749–754, 1991.
59. Hynes, R.O. Integrins: versatility, modulation, and signaling in cell adhesion. *Cell* 69: 11–25, 1992.
60. Igarashi, M., P.W. Finch, S.A. Aaronson. Characterization of recombinant human fibro-

blast growth factor (FGF)-10 reveals functional similarities with keratinocyte growth factor (FGF-7). *J. Biol. Chem.* 273: 13230–13235, 1998.
61. Johnson, D.E. and L.T. Williams, Structural and functional diversity in the FGF receptor multigene family. *Adv. Cancer Res.* 40: 1–41, 1993.
62. Jones, J.I. and D.R. Clemmons. Insulin-like growth factors and their binding proteins: biological actions. *Endocr. Rev.* 16: 3–34, 1995.
63. Juul, S.E., M.G. Kinsella, T.N. Wight, and W.A. Hodson. Alterations in nonhuman primate (*M. Nemestrina*) lung proteoglycans during normal development and acute hyaline membrane disease. *Am. J. Respir. Cell Mol. Biol.* 8: 299–310, 1993.
64. Juul, S.E., T.N. Wight, and V.C. Hascall. Proteoglycans. In: *The Lung,* edited by R.G Crystal and J.B. West, New York: Raven Press, 1991, 413–420.
65. Kaartinen, V., J.W. Voncken, C. Shuler, D. Warburton, D. Bu, N.Heisterkamp, and J. Groffen. Abnormal lung development and cleft palate in mice lacking TGF-β3 indicates defects of epithelial–mesenchymal interaction. *Nat. Genet.* 11: 415–421, 1995.
66. Kappen, C. *Hox* genes in the lung. *Am. J. Respir. Cell Mol. Biol.* 15: 156–162, 1996.
67. Kessler, D.S. and D.A. Melton. Vertebrate embryonic induction: mesodermal and neural patterning. *Science* 266: 596–604, 1994.
68. Klagsburn, M., and A. Baird. A dual receptor system is required for basic fibroblast growth factor activity. *Cell* 67: 229–231, 1991.
69. Klämbt, C., L. Glaser, and B.-Z. Shilo. *breathless,* a *Drosophila* FGF receptor homolog, is essential for the migration of tracheal and specific midline glial cells. *Genes. Dev.* 6: 1668–1678, 1992.
70. Klein, G., M. Ekblom, L. Fecker, R. Timpl, and P. Ekblom. Differential expression of laminin A and B chains during development of embryonic mouse organs. *Development* 110: 823–837, 1990.
71. Klempt, M., A.-M. Hutchins, P.D. Gluckman, and S.J.M. Skinner. IGF binding protein-2 gene expression and location of IGF-I and IGF-II in fetal rat lung. *Development* 115: 765–772, 1992.
72. Kratchowil, K., M. Dziadek, J. Lohler, K. Harbers, and R. Jaenisch. Normal branching morphogenesis in the absence of collagen I. *Dev. Biol.* 117: 596–606, 1986.
73. Kreidberg, J.A., M.J. Donovan, S.L. Goldstein, H. Rennke, K. Shepherd, R.C. Jones, and R. Jaenisch. Alpha 3 beta 1 integrin has a crucial role in kidney and lung organogenesis. *Development* 122: 3537–3547, 1996.
74. Kroll, K.L. and E. Amaya. Transgenic *Xenopus* embryos from sperm nuclear transplantations reveal FGF signaling requirements during gastrulation. *Development* 122: 3173–3183, 1996.
75. Krumlauf, R. *Hox* genes in vertebrate development. *Cell* 78: 191–201, 1994.
76. Kulkarni, A.B., C. Huh, D. Becker, A. Geiser, M. Lyght, K.C. Flanders, A.B.Roberts, M.B. Sporn, J.M. Ward, and S. Karlsson. Transforming growth factor-β1 null mutation in mice causes excessive inflammatory response and early death. *Proc. Natl. Acad. Sci. USA* 90: 770–774, 1993.
77. Kusakabe, M., B.T. Smith, and M. Post. Mesenchymal induction of surfactant protein expression in rat lung epithelium [Abstract]. *Pediatr. Res.* 23: 246A, 1988.
78. Lau, M.M.H., C.E.H. Stewart, Z. Liu, H. Bhatt, P. Rotwein, and C.L. Stewart. Loss of the imprinted IGF2/cation-independent mannose 6-phosphate receptor results in fetal overgrowth and perinatal lethality *Genes Dev.* 8: 2953–2963, 1994.
79. Levéen, P., M. Pekny, S. Gebre-Medhin, B. Swolin, E. Larsson, and C.Betsholtz. Mice defi-

cient for PDGFB show renal, cardiovascular, and hematological abnormalities. *Genes Dev.* 8: 1875–1887, 1994.

80. Lin, Y., X.-F. Wang, E. Ng-Eaton, R.A. Weinberg, and H.F. Lodish.Expression cloning of the TGF-β type II receptor, a functional transmembrane serine/threonine kinase. *Cell* 68: 775–785, 1992.
81. Liu, J.P., J. Baker, A.S. Perkins, E. J. Robertson, and A. Efstratiadis. Mice carrying null mutations of the genes encoding insulin-like growth factor I(IGF-1) and type 1 IGF receptor (Igf1r). *Cell* 75: 59–72, 1993.
82. Lopéz-Casillas, F., J. Wrana, and J. Massagué. Betaglycan presents ligand to the TGF beta signaling receptor. *Cell* 73: 1435–1444, 1993.
83. Masters, J.R.W. Epithelial–mesenchymal interactions during lung development: the effect of mesenchymal mass. *Dev. Biol.* 51: 98–108, 1976.
84. Mason, I.J., F. Fuller-Pace, R. Smith, and C. Dickson. FGF-7 (keratinocyte growth factor) expression during mouse development suggests roles inmyogenesis, forebrain regionalization and epithelial-mesenchymal interactions. *Mech. Dev.* 45: 15–30, 1994.
85. Mason, R.J., C.C. Leslie, K. McCormick-Shannon, R.R. Deterding, T. Nakamura, J.S. Rubin, and J.M. Shannon. Hepatocyte growth factor is a growth factor for rat alveolar type II cells. *Am. J. Respir. Cell Mol. Biol.* 11: 561–567, 1994.
86. Massague, J., L. Attisano, and J.L.Wrana. The TGF-β family and its composite receptors. *Trends Cell Biol.* 4: 172–178, 1994.
87. Mast, B.A., R.F. Diegelmann, T.M. Krummel, and I.K. Cohen. Hyaluronic acid modulates proliferation collagen and protein synthesis of cultured fetal fibroblasts. *Matrix* 13: 441–446, 1993.
88. Matter, M.L. and G.W. Laurie. A novel laminin E8 cell adhesion site required for lung alveolar formation in vitro. *J. Cell. Biol.* 124: 1083–1090,1994.
89. Mercola, M., C. Wang, J. Kelley, C. Brownlee, L. Jackson-Grusby, C. Stiles, and D. Bowen-Pope. Selective expression of PDGF-A and its receptor during early mouse embryogenesis. *Dev. Biol.* 138: 114–122, 1990.
90. Mercurio, A.M. Laminin receptors: achieving specificity through cooperation.*Trends Cell Biol.* 5: 419–423, 1995.
91. Miettinen, P.J., J.E. Berger, J. Meneses, Y. Phung, R.A. Pederson, Z. Werb, and R. Derynck. Epithelial immaturity and multiorgan failure in mice lacking epidermal growth factor receptor. *Nature* 376: 337–341, 1995.
92. Miki, T., D.P. Bottaro, T.P. Fleming, C.L. Smith, W.H. Burgess, A.M. Chan,and S.A. Aaronson. Determination of ligand-binding specificity by alternative splicing: two distinct growth factor receptors encoded by a single gene. *Proc. Natl. Acad. Sci. USA* 89: 246–250, 1992.
93. Minoo, P. and R.J. King. Epithelial–mesenchymal interactions in lungdevelopment. *Annu. Rev. Physiol.* 56: 13–45, 1994.
94. Moats-Staats, B.M., W.A. Price, L. Xu, H.W. Jarvis, and A.D. Stiles.Regulation of the insulin-like growth factor system during normal rat lungdevelopment. *Am. J. Respir. Cell Mol. Biol.* 12: 56–64, 1995.
95. Moats-Staats, B.M., G.Z. Retsch-Bogart, W.A. Price, H.W. Jarvis, A.JD'Ercole, and A.D. Stiles. Insulin-like growth factor-I (IGF-I) antisense oligodeoxynucleotide mediated inhibition of DNA synthesis by WI-38cells: evidence for autocrine actions of IGF-I. *Mol. Endocrinol.* 7: 171–180, 1993.
96. Moens, C.B., A.B. Auerbach, R.A. Conlon, A.L. Joyner, and J. Rossant. A targeted mutation

reveals a role for N-*myc* in branching morphogenesis in the embryonic mouse lung. *Genes Dev.* 6: 691–704, 1992.

97. Nakanishi, Y. and T. Ishii. Epithelial shape change in mouse embryonic submandibular gland: modulation by extracellular matrix components. *Bioessays* 11: 163–167, 1989.
98. Niswander, L., S. Jeffrey, G.R. Martin, and C. Tickle. A positive loop coordinates growth and patterning in the vertebrate limb. *Nature* 371: 609–612.
99. Nogawa, H. and T. Ito. Branching morphogenesis of embryonic mouse lung epithelium in mesenchyme-free culture. *Development* 121: 1015–1022, 1995.
100. Orr-Urtreger, A., M.T. Bedford, T. Burakova, E. Arman, Y. Zimmer, A.Yayon, D. Givol, and P. Lonai. Developmental localization of the splicing alternatives of fibroblast growth factor receptor-2 (FGFR2). *Dev. Biol.* 158: 475–486, 1993.
101. Orr-Urtreger, A., M. Bedford, M.-S. Do, L. Eisenbach, and P. Lonai.Developmental expression of the α receptor for platelet-derived growth factor, which is deleted in the embryonic lethal *Patch* mutation. *Development* 115: 289–303, 1992.
102. Orr-Urtreger, A. and P. Lonai. Platelet-derived growth factor-A and its receptor are expressed in separate, but adjacent cell layers on the mouse embryo. *Development* 115: 1045–1058, 1992.
103. Panos, R.J., PM. Bak, W.S. Simonet, J.S. Rubin, and L.J. Smith. Intratracheal intillation of keratinocyte growth factor decreases hyperoxia-induced mortality in rats. *J. Clin. Invest.* 96: 2026–2033, 1995.
104. Panos, R.J., J.S. Rubin, K.G. Csaky, S.A. Aaronson, and R.J. Mason. Keratinocyte growth factor and hepatocyte growth factor are heparin-binding growth factors for alveolar type II cells in fibroblast-conditioned medium. *J. Clin. Invest.* 92: 969–977, 1993.
105. Pelton, R.W., M.E. Dickinson, H.L. Moses, and B.L. Hogan. In situ hybridization analysis of TGFβ3 RNA expression during mouse development: comparative studies with TGFβ1 and β2. *Development* 110: 609–620, 1990.
106. Peters, K., S. Werner, S. Liao, S. Wert, J.A. Whitsett, and L.T. Williams.Targeted expression of a dominant negative FGF receptor blocks branching morphogenesis and epithelial differentiation of the mouse lung. *EMBO J.* 13: 3296–3301, 1994.
107. Post, M. Tissue interactions. In: *The Lung, Scientific Foundations,* edited by R.G. Crystal, J.B. West, E. Weibel, and P. Barnes. New York: Raven Press, 1996, pp. 1003–1011.
108. Post, M., P. Souza, J. Liu, I. Tseu, J. Wang, and M. Kuliszewski.Keratinocyte growth factor and its receptor are involved in regulating early lung branching. *Development* 122: 3107–3115, 1996.
109. Raines, E.W., D.F. Bowen-Pope, and R. Ross Platelet-derived growth factor. In: *Peptide Growth Factors and Their Receptors I,* edited by M.B. Sporn, and A.B. Roberts. New-York: Springer-Verlag, 1991, pp. 173–262.
110. Retsch-Bogart, G.Z., B.M. Moats-Staats, K. Howard, A.J. D'Ercole, and A.D. Stiles. Cellular localization of messenger RNAs for insulin-like growth factors (IGFs), their receptors and binding proteins during fetal rat lung development. *Am. J. Respir. Cell Mol. Biol.* 14: 61–69, 1996.
111. Roberts, A.B., and M.B. Sporn. The transforming growth factors-βs. In: *Peptide Growth Factors and Their Receptors I,* edited by M.B. Sporn, and A.B. Roberts. New York: Springer-Verlag, 1991, pp. 417–472.
112. Roman, J., E.C. Crough, and J.A. McDonald. Reagents that inhibit fibronectin matrix assembly of cultured cells also inhibit lung branching morphogenesis in vitro. *Chest* 99: 20–21, 1991.

113. Roman, J. and J.A. McDonald. Potential role of RGD-directed integrins in mammalian lung branching morphogenesis. *Development* 112: 551–558 1991.
114. Roman, J. and J.A. McDonald. Expression of fibronectin, the integrin α5, and smooth muscle actin in heart and lung development. *Am. J. Respir. Cell Mol. Biol.* 6: 472–480, 1992.
115. Rosen, E.M., S.K. Nigam, and I.D. Goldberg. Scatter factor and the c-met receptor: a paradigm for mesenchymal/epithelial interaction. *J. Cell. Biol.* 127: 1783–1787, 1994.
116. Rubin, J.S., D.P. Bottaro, M. Chedid, T. Miki, D. Ron, H.-G. Cheon, W.G Taylor, E. Fortney, H. Sakata, P.W. Finch, and W.J. LaRochelle. Keratinocyte growth factor. *Cell Biol. Int.* 5: 399–411, 1995.
117. Rudnick, D. Developmental capacities of the chick lung in chorioallantoic grafts. *J. Exp. Zool.* 66: 125–153, 1933.
118. Ruocco, S., A. Lallemand, J.M. Tournier, and D. Gaillard. Expression and localization of epidermal growth factor, transforming growth factor-α, and localization of their common receptor in fetal human lung development. *Pediatr. Res.* 39: 448–455, 1996.
119. Ruoslahti, E. Fibronectin and its receptor. *Annu. Rev. Biochem.* 57: 375–413, 1988.
120. Ruoslahti, E. Structure and biology of proteoglycans. *Annu. Rev. Cell. Biol.* 4: 229–255, 1988.
121. Ruoslahti, E. Proteoglycans in cell regulations. *J. Biol. Chem.* 264: 13369–13372, 1989.
122. Saga, Y., T. Yagi, Y. Ikawa, T. Sakakura, and S. Aizawa. Mice develop normally without tenascin. *Genes Dev.* 6: 1821–1813, 1992.
123. Sage, E.H. and P. Bornstein. Extracellular proteins that modulate cell-matrix interactions. SPARC, tenascin and thrombospondin. *J. Biol. Chem.* 266: 14831–14834, 1991.
124. Sanford, L.P., I. Ormsby, A.C. Gittenberg-de Groot, H. Sariola, R. Friedman, G.P. Biovin, E.L. Cardell, and T. Doetschman. TGFβ2 knockout mice have multiple developmental defects that are non-overlapping with other TGFβ knockout phenotypes. *Development* 124: 2659–2670, 1997.
125. Sawai, S., A. Shimono, Y. Wakamatsu, C. Palmes, K. Hanaoka, and H. Kondoh. Defects of embryonic organogenesis resulting from targeted disruption of the N-*myc* gene in the mouse. *Development* 117: 1445–1455,1993.
126. Schmid, P., D. Cox, G. Bilbe, R. Maier, and G.K. McMaster. Differential expression of TGFβ1, β2 and β3 genes during mouse embryogenesis. *Development* 111: 117–130, 1991.
127. Schmidt, C., F. Bladt, S. Goedecke, and V. Brinkmann. Scatter factor/hepatocyte growth factor is essential for liver development. *Nature* 373: 699–702, 1995.
128. Schuger, L., G.R. Johnson, K. Gilbride, G.D. Plowman, and R. Mandel. Amphiregulin in lung branching morphogenesis: interaction with heparan sulfate proteoglycan modulates cell proliferation. *Development* 122: 1759–1767, 1996.
129. Schuger, L., S. O'Shea, J. Rheinheimer, and J. Varani. Laminin in lung development: effects of anti-laminin antibody in murine lung morphogenesis. *Dev. Biol.* 137: 26–32, 1990.
130. Schuger, L., S. O'Shea, B.B. Nelson, and J. Varani. Organotypic arrangement of mouse embryonic lung cells on a basement membrane extract: involvement of laminin. *Development* 110: 1091–1099, 1990.
131. Schuger, L., A.P.N. Skubitz, K. Gilbride, R. Mandel, and L. He. Laminin and heparan sulfate proteoglycan mediate epithelial polarization in organotypic cultures of embryonic lung cells: evidence implicating involvement of the inner globular region of laminin β1

chain and the heparan sulfate groups of heparan sulfate proteoglycan. *Dev. Biol.* 179: 264–273,1996.

132. Schuger, L., A.P.N. Skubitz, A. Morenas, and K. Gilbridge. Different laminin domains facilitate lung development by independent mechanism of action *Dev. Biol.* 169: 520–532, 1995.
133. Schuger, L., A.P.N. Skubitz, K.S. O'Shea, J.F. Chang, and J. Varani. Identification of laminin domains involved in branching morphogenesis: effects of anti-laminin monoclonal antibodies on mouse embryonic lung development. *Dev. Biol.* 146: 531–541, 1991.
134. Schuger, L., J. Varani, P.D. Killen, A.P.N. Skubitz, and K. Gilbridge. Laminin expression in the mouse lung increases with development and stimulates spontaneous organotypic rearrangement of mixed lung cells. *Dev. Dyna.* 195: 43–54, 1992.
135. Schuger, L., J. Varani, R. Mitra, and K. Gilbridge. Retinoic acid stimulates mouse lung development by a mechanism involving epithelial–mesenchymal interaction and regulation of epidermal growth factor. *Dev. Biol.* 159: 462–473, 1993.
136. Sera, R., R.W. Pelton, and H.L. Moses. TGFβ 1 inhibits branching morphogenesis and N-*myc* expression in lung bud organ cultures. *Development* 120: 2153–2161, 1994.
137. Seth, R., L. Shum, F. Wu, C.W. Wuenschchell, F.L. Hall, H.C. Slavkin, and D. Warburton. Role of epidermal growth factor expression in early mouse embryo lung branching morphogenesis in culture: antisense oligodeoxynucleotide inhibitory strategy. *Dev. Biol.* 158: 555–559, 1993.
138. Sham, M.H., P. Hunt, S. Nonchev, N. Papalopulu, A. Graham, E. Boncinelli,and R. Krumlauf. Analysis of the murine *hox-2,7* gene: conserved alternative transcripts with differential distributions in the nervous system and the potential for shared regulatory regions. *EMBO J.* 11: 1825-1836, 1992.
139. Shannon, J.M. Induction of alveolar type II cell differentiation in fetal tracheal epithelium by grafted distal lung mesenchyme. *Dev. Biol.* 166: 600–614, 1994.
140. Shiratori, M., G. Michalopoulos, H. Shinozuka, G. Singh, H. Ogasawara, and S.L. Katyal. Hepatocyte growth factor stimulates DNA synthesis in alveolar epithelial type II cells in vitro. *Am. J. Respir. Cell Mol. Biol.* 12: 171–180, 1995.
141. Shiratori, M., E. Oshika, L.P. Ung, G. Singh, H. Shinozuka, D. Warburton, G. Michalopoulos, and S.L. Katyal. Keratinocyte growth factor and embryonic rat lung morphogenesis. *Am. J. Respir. Cell Mol. Biol.* 15: 328–338, 1996.
142. Shull, M.M., I. Ormsby, A.B. Kier, S. Pawloski, R.J. Diebold, M. Yin, R. Allen, C. Sidman, G. Proetzel, D. Calvin, N. Annunziata, and T. Doetschman. Targeted disruption of the mouse transforming growth factor-beta1 gene results in multifocal inflammatory disease. *Nature* 359: 693–699, 1992.
143. Simonet, W.S., M.L. DeRose, N. Bucay, H.Q. Nguyen, L. Wert, T.R. Zhou, A. Ulich, A. Thomason, D.M. Danilenko, and J.A. Whitsett. Pulmonary malformation in transgenic mice expressing human keratinocyte growth factor in the lung. *Proc. Natl. Acad. Sci. USA* 92: 12461–12465, 1995.
144. Snead, M.L., W. Luo, P. Olizer, G. Don-Wheeler, C. Bessem, G.I. Bell, L.B. Rall, and H.C. Slavkin. Localization of epidermal growth factor precursors in tooth and lung during embryonic mouse development. *Dev. Biol.* 134: 420–429, 1989.
145. Sonnenberg, E., D. Meyer, K.M. Weidner, and C. Birchmeier. Scatterfactor/hepatocyte growth factor and its receptor, the c-*met* tyrosine kinase, can mediate a signal exchange between mesenchyme and epithelia during mouse development. *J. Cell Biol.* 123: 223–235, 1993.

146. Soriano, P. Abnormal kidney development and hematological disorders in PDGF β-receptor mutant mice. *Genes Dev.* 8: 1888–1896, 1994.
147. Soriano, P. The PDGF α receptor is required for neural crest cell development and for normal patterning of the somites. *Development* 124: 2691–2700, 1997.
148. Souza, P., M. Kuliszewski, J. Wang, I. Tseu, A.K. Tanswell, and M. Post. PDGF-AA and its receptor direct early lung branching via an epithelial–mesenchymal interaction. *Development* 121: 2559–2567, 1995.
149. Souza, P., L. Sedlackova, M. Kuliszewski, J. Wang, J. Liu, I. Tseu, M. Liu, A.K. Tanswell, and M. Post. Antisense oligodeoxynucleotides targeting PDGF-B mRNA inhibits cell proliferation during embryonic rat lung development. *Development* 120: 2163–2173, 1994.
150. Souza, P., A.K.Tanswell, and M. Post, Different roles for PDGF-α and -β receptors in embryonic lung development. *Am. J. Respir. Cell Mol. Biol.* 15: 551–562, 1996.
151. Spooner, B.S. and J.M. Faubion. Collagen involvement in branching morphogenesis of embryonic lung and salivary gland. *Dev. Biol.* 77: 84–102, 1980.
152. Spooner, B.S., H.A. Thompson-Pletscher, B. Stokes, and K.E. Bassett. Extracellular matrix involvement in epithelial branching morphogenesis. In: *Developmental Biology: A Comprehensive Synthesis, Vol. 3. The Cell Surface in Development and Cancer,* edited by Y.S. Steinberg, New York: Academic Press, 1986, pp. 225–260.
153. Spooner B.S. and N.K. Wessels. Mammalian lung development: interactions in primordium formation and bronchial morphogenesis. *J. Exp. Zool.* 175: 445–454, 1979.
154. Stahlman, M.T., M.E. Gray, and J.A. Whitsett. Expression of thyroid transcription factor-1 (TTF-1) in fetal and neonatal human lung. *J. Histochem. Cytochem.* 44: 673–678, 1996.
155. Stephenson, D.A., M. Mercola, E. Anderson, C. Wang, C.D. Stiles, D.F. Bowen-Pope, and V.M. Chapman. The platelet-derived growth factor alpha subunit gene is deleted in the mouse mutation patch *(Ph)*. *Proc. Natl. Acad. Sci. USA* 88: 6–10, 1991.
156. Stiles, A.D. and J. D'Ercole. The insulin-like growth factors and the lung. *Am. J. Respir. Cell Mol. Biol.* 3: 93–100, 1990.
157. Stiles, A.D. and B.M. Moats-Staats. Production and action of insulin-like growth factor I/somatomedin-C in primary cultures of fetal lung fibroblasts. *Am. J. Respir. Cell Mol. Biol.* 1: 21–26, 1989.
158. Stiles, A.D., B.T. Smith, and M. Post. Recoprocal autocrine and paracrine regulation of growth of mesenchymal and alveolar epithelial cells from fetal lung. *Exp. Lung Res.* 11: 165–177, 1986.
159. Strandjord, T.P., J.G. Clark, D.E. Guralnick, and D.K. Madtes. Immunolocalization of transforming growth factor-α, epidermal growth factor (EGF), and EGF-receptor in normal and injured developing human lung. *Pediatr. Res.* 38: 851–856, 1995.
160. Strandjord, T.P., J.G. Clark, W.A. Hodson, R.A. Schmidt, and D.K. Madtes. Expression of transforming growth factor-α in mid-gestation human fetal lung. *Am. J. Respir. Cell Mol. Biol.* 8: 266–272, 1993.
161. Strandjord, T.P., J.G. Clark, and D.K. Madtes. Expression of TGF-α, EGF, and EGF-receptor in fetal rat lung. *Am. J. Physiol.* (*Lung Cell. Mol. Physid.*) 267: L384–L389, 1994.
162. Strandjord, T.P., E.H. Sage, and J.G. Clark. SPARC participates in the branching morphogenesis of developing fetal rat lung. *Am. J. Respir. Cell Mol. Biol.* 13: 279–287, 1995.
163. Sutherland, D., C. Samakovlis, and M.A. Krasnow. *Branchless* encodes a drosophila FGF homolog that controls tracheal cell migration and the pattern of branching. *Cell* 87: 1091–1101, 1996.

164. ten Dijke, P., H. Ichijo, P. Franzén, P. Schulz, J. Saras, H. Toyoshima, C.-H. Heldin, and K. Miyazono. Activin receptor-like kinases: anovel subclass of cell-surface receptors with predicted serine/threonine kinase activity. *Oncogene* 8: 2879–2887, 1993.
165. Thompson, H.A. and B.S. Spooner. Inhibition of branching morphogenesis and alteration of glycosaminoglycan biosynthesis in salivary glands treated with beta-D-xyloside. *Dev. Biol.* 89: 417–424, 1982.
166. Thompson, H.A. and B.S. Spooner. Proteoglycan and glycosaminoglycan synthesis in embryonic mouse salivary glands: effects of beta-D-xyloside, an inhibitor of branching morphogenesis. *J. Cell Biol.* 96: 1443–1450, 1983.
167. Threadgill, D.W., A.A. Dlugosz, L.A. Hansen, T. Tennenbaum, U. Lichti, D. Yee, C. LaMantia, T. Mourton, K. Herrup, R.C. Harris, J.A. Barnard, S.H.Yuspa, R.J. Coffey, and T. Mjagnuson. Targeted disruption of mouse EGF receptor: effect of genetic background on mutant phenotype. *Science* 269: 230–234, 1995.
168. Timpl, R. and J.C. Brown. The laminins. *Matrix Biol* 14: 275–281, 1994.
169. Timpl, R., M. Rhode, P. Gehron-Robey, S.T. Rennard, J.M. Fiodart, and G.R. Martin. Laminin-A glycoprotein from basement membranes. *J. Biol. Chem.* 254: 9933–9937, 1979.
170. Toole, B.P. Proteoglycans and hyaluronan in morphogenesis and differentiation. In: *Cell Biology of Extracellular Matrix.*, edited by E. Hay. New York: Plenum Press, 1981 p. 259–296.
171. Uehara, Y., O. Minowa, C. Mori, K. Shiota, J. Kuno, T. Noda, and N. Kitamura, Placental defect and embryonic lethality in mice lacking hepatocyte growth factor/scatter factor. *Nature* 373: 702–705, 1995.
172. Virtanen, I., A. Laitinen, T. Tani, P. Pääkkö, L.A. Laitinen, R.E. Burgeson, and V.-P. Lehto. Differential expression of laminins and their integrin receptors in developing and adult human lung. *Am. J. Respir. Cell Mol. Biol.* 15: 184–196, 1996.
173. Wallen, L.D. and V.K.M. Han. Spatial and temporal distribution of insulin-like growth factors I and II during development of rat lung. *Am. J. Physiol. (Lung Cell. Mol. Physiol.)* 267: L531–L542, 1994.
174. Wang, J., M. Kuliszewski, W. Yee, L. Sedlackova, J. Xu, I. Tseu, and M Post. Cloning and characterization of glucocorticoid-induced genes in fetalrat lung fibroblasts: Transforming growth factor β_3. *J. Biol. Chem.* 270: 2722–2728, 1995.
175. Wang, Z., M.R. Fung, D.P. Barlow, and E.F. Wagner. Regulation of embryonic growth and lysosomal targeting by the imprinted IGF2/Mpr gene. *Nature* 372: 464–467, 1994.
176. Warburton, D., R. Seth, L. Shum, P.G. Horcher, F.L. Hall, Z. Werb, and H.C. Slavkin. Epigenetic role of epidermal growth factor expression and signalling in embryonic mouse lung morphogenesis. *Dev. Biol.* 149: 123–133, 1992.
177. Wessels, N.K. Mammalian lung development: interactions in formation and morphogenesis of tracheal buds. *J. Exp. Zool.* 175: 445–460, 1979.
178. Wrana, J.L., L. Attisano, R. Wieser, F. Ventura, and J. Massagué. Mechanism of activation of the TGF-beta receptor. *Nature* 370: 341–347, 1994.
179. Wu, J.E. and S.A. Santoro. Differential expression of integrin α subunits supports distinct roles during lung branching morphogenesis. *Dev. Dyna.* 206: 169–181, 1996.
180. Wu, X., C.E. Robinson, H.W. Fong, J.S. Crabtree, B.R. Rodriquez, B.A. Roe, and J.M. Gimble. Cloning and characterization of the murine activin receptor like kinase-1 (ALK-1) homolog. *Biochem. Biophys. Res. Commun.* 216: 78–83, 1996.
181. Yamasaki, M., A. Miyake, S. Tagashira, N. Itoh. Structure and expression of the rat

mRNA encoding a novel member of the fibroblast growth factor family. *J. Biol. Chem.* 27: 15918–15921, 1996.

182. Yamaguchi, Y., D.M. Mann, and E. Ruoslahti. Negative regulation of transforming growth factor-β by the proteoglycan decorin. *Nature* 346: 281–284, 1990.
183. Yang, J.T., H. Rayburn, and R.O. Hynes. Embryonic mesodermal defects in alpha 5 integrin-deficient mice. *Development* 119: 1093–1095, 1993.
184. Yee, W., J. Wang, J. Liu, I. Tseu, M. Kuliszewski, and M. Post. Glucocorticoid-induced tropoelastin expression in fetal rat lung fibroblasts is mediated via transforming growth-β_3. *Am J. Physiol. (Lung Cell. Mol. Physiol.)* 270: L992–L1001, 1996.
185. Young, S., L.-Y. Chang, and H.P. Erickson. Tenascin-C in rat lung: distribution, ontogeny and role in branching morphogenesis. *Dev. Biol.* 161: 615–625, 1994.
186. Zhao, Y. and S.L. Young. Expression of transforming growth factor-beta type II receptor in rat lung is regulated during development. *Am. J. Physiol. (Lung Cell. Mol. Physiol.)* 269: L419–L426, 1995.
187. Zhou, L., C.R. Dey, S.E. Wert, and J.A. Whitsett. Arrested lung morphogenesis in transgenic mice bearing an SP-C-TGF-β1 chimeric gene *Dev. Biol.* 175: 227–238, 1996.

chapter 2

DEVELOPMENT OF LUNG ELASTIC MATRIX

Thomas J. Mariani and Richard A. Pierce

ELASTIN is the primary elastic vertebrate protein, and is responsible for passive recoil of those compartments of the lung that undergo repeated cycles of expansion and contraction. Thus, alveolar walls, alveolar ducts, conducting airways, pleura, and vascular tissue of the lung all depend on elastic fibers to absorb and store energy upon expansion and then use this energy to return to a smaller volume before the next cycle of ventilation or blood flow.

Tropoelastin, the monomeric, soluble precursor of insoluble elastin, is primarily produced by cells of mesenchymal origin. Together with fibrillar collagens, proteoglycans, and microfibrils, elastic fibers form the interstitial matrix that determines both the architecture and functional properties of elastic tissues such as the lung. In fact, mature (cross-linked) elastin is stable under extremely harsh conditions including high temperature/pressure and high pH.

The single, unique physical property that is conferred by the elastic fiber is recoil. Elastin consists of a very high proportion of hydrophobic amino acids (54). As will be discussed later, regions of hydrophobicity in the protein are bisected by regions that give rise to the cross-links described above. This modular nature is believed to be critically important for the ability of the fiber to undergo many rounds of distention and contraction. Increased hydration of hydrophobic regions of the molecule upon stretch are also thought to account for its biophysical properties (65). Exclusion of hydrophilic water molecules and reassociation of hydrophobic peptidyl residues during recoil leads to an increased state of entropy.

In this chapter, we will discuss the structure of the major components of elastic fibers, as well as recent findings about the interactions between these components.

The spatial and temporal patterns of tropoelastin expression during lung development will be presented, and the factors and mechanisms controlling tropoelastin gene expression will be discussed. New experimental models are being used to test the role of elastin in lung development, and these will also be presented.

ELASTIN AS A DISTINCT COMPONENT OF THE EXTRACELLULAR MATRIX

Elastin has been appreciated as a distinct entity for only about the last 35 years. Before Partridge published his classic comprehensive review on the subject of elastin (46), many believed this extracellular matrix component to be merely a form of collagen. Partridge, his colleagues, and their successors have characterized the unique physical and chemical properties of the elastic fiber, so that today it is appreciated as an integral part of the connective tissues of many organs.

Chemical and Biophysical Properties

The elastic fiber is one of the most durable structures in the human body. Shapiro and colleagues used biochemical techniques to show that humans retain elastin throughout their lifetime (56). This appears to be due, at least in part, to the presence of unique covalent cross-links that occur within and between monomers of elastin in mature elastic fibers. These cross-links are produced from individual lysine residues within soluble monomers of elastin (tropoelastin) and form novel amino acids that are markers for the presence of elastin. The primary cross-link products, desmosine and isodesmosine, can be used to identify and quantify the presence of elastin within tissues (31). The stability of elastin fiber was a useful tool in early attempts to isolate samples for chemical and biochemical evaluation. In fact, mature (cross linked) elastin is stable under extremely harsh conditions including high temperature/pressure and high pH.

Distribution of Elastin

On account of the unique biophysical properties conferred by elastin, it is no surprise that it has a relatively wide distribution throughout the mammalian body. Elastic fibers are found primarily in the lung, vasculature, and skin, but they are also components of the extracellular matrix of other tissues. Of course, elastin occurs in different proportions in various tissues; this is partially dependent on the physical demands of any specific tissue. For instance, insoluble elastin comprises 75% of the dry weight of the bovine nuchal ligament (an elastic ligament found in the neck of grazing ungulates) and 2% of the dry weight of human dermis (44).

Elastin has appeared to play a role in the evolution of the circulatory system, being limited to organisms with a closed circulatory system, yet absent from invertebrates and lower organisms (53). Elastin constitutes a significant proportion of the connective tissue of blood vessels, comprising up to 30% of the dry weight of elastic arteries. In these structures, the primary function of elastin is thought to be the propagation of blood pressure throughout the circulatory system. However, elastin may very well play a significant structural role in blood vessels as elastin pathology has been associated with the development of aneurysms (17) and vascular stenoses (8). In the circulatory system, the major elastic fiber structure is the internal elastic lamella (IEL), which delineates the medial layer of the vessel from the intima. The IEL is a concentric sheet of elastin with individual fibers laying perpendicular to blood flow. Lesser concentric sheets of elastin (lamellae) are found in layers peripheral to the IEL, throughout the vascular media, with the number depending on the thickness and muscularity of the vessel.

Elastic fibers are found in many different compartments of the adult lung; together they (in coordination with collagen fibers) provide a primary force for expiration. Elastin is found in the human dermis, in fibers lying primarily parallel to the surface of the skin. Elastin is found in the human eye; in both the Bruch's membrane and optic nerve head. Elastin is also a major component of elastic cartilage, such as that found in the external ear, and elastic ligaments, such as the ligamentum flava of the vertebral column.

Elastic Fibers

Despite the amorphous appearance of elastic fibers in early electron micrographs, recent work has revealed a surprisingly complex structure. In fact, elastic fibers can be subdivided into two morphologically and chemically distinct entities; elastin and microfibrils. Elastin is an insolubilized polymer made up of soluble tropoelastin monomers. The microfibril is a separate structure that can be found in the absence or presence of polymerized elastin, and it is hypothesized to play roles in both nucleation of fiber formation and maintenance of fiber integrity.

Tropoelastin. Polymerized tropoelastin comprises more than 90% of the mature elastic fiber. Tropoelastin was originally recognized as the precursor to insoluble elastin in swine fed a copper-deficient diet (55). These animals were impaired in their ability to initiate the cross-linking of the tropoelastin monomers and produce insoluble elastin. Tropoelastin has been extensively studied biochemically in numerous species including the rat, mouse, pig, cow, and human. Tropoelastin is now known to be produced as a family of very closely related protein isoforms, of approximately 70 kDa.

The cloning and characterization of the nucleotide sequence of tropoelastin cDNA from multiple species has confirmed previous biochemical inferences regarding the structure of the protein. The coding sequence shows that an extremely high proportion (90%) of the amino acids are nonpolar or uncharged. Although charged residues are scarce, they occur adjacent to one another in hydrophilic "islands" dispersed throughout the protein sequence. These charged sites give rise to cross-linking domains, nestled between domains of extreme hydrophobicity. The result is an elastin precursor with a highly modular structure (Fig. 2.1).

The tropoelastin coding sequence also shows some interesting evolutionary

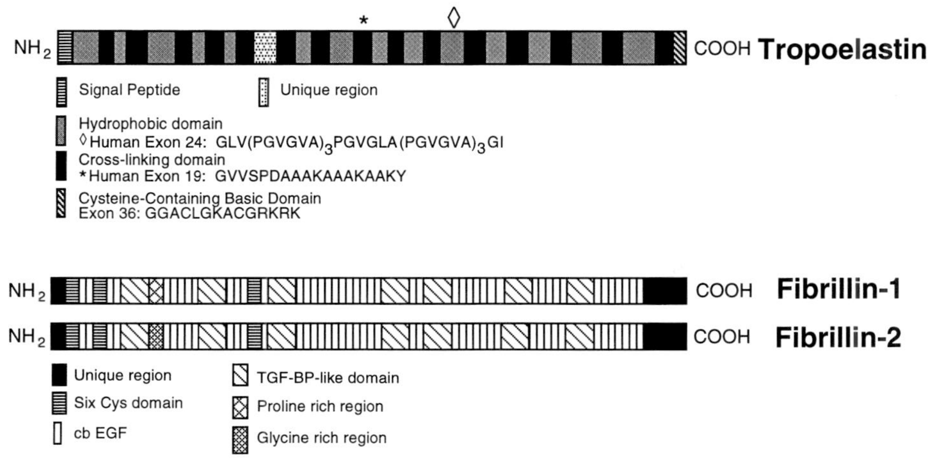

Fig. 2.1 Modular structure of tropoelastin and fibrillins. Tropoelastin monomers consist of a signal peptide, alternating hydrophobic and cross-linking domains, and a cysteine-containing, basic carboxyl terminus. Hydrophobic domains often contain repetitive motifs. The peptide sequence of human tropoelastin exon 24 is given as an example. Cross-linking domains contain polyalanine stretches interrupted by lysine residues, as demonstrated by the peptide sequence of human exon 19. The carboxyl terminus of tropoelastin contains the only two cysteines in the monomer, and a lysine, arginine-rich basic domain. Fibrillins 1 and 2 are modular proteins consisting of stretches of calcium-binding epidermal growth factor-like motifs (*cb EGF*) separated by transforming growth factor β-binding protein-like domains (*TGF-BP*) and domains containing six cysteines. Fibrillin 1 has a proline-rich domain near the amino-terminus, whereas this region is glycine-rich in fibrillin-2.

conservation (2). The tropoelastin sequence in all species analyzed retains a modular structure of alternating hydrophobic and charged cross-linking domains. However, there is divergence in the primary sequence, particularly in the hydrophobic domains. Constraints on the evolution of the hydrophobic domains appear to favor retention of total hydrophobicity rather than sequence. In fact, different species seem to have repeating sequences of different hydrophobic residues. For instance, VPGVG is common in the bovine sequence while IPGVG is common in the rat. Conversely, there seems to have been more strict conservation of the cross-link domains. These regions almost invariably contain a stretch of alanine residues interrupted by two lysines. Alanines are sometimes substituted by other small, nonpolar amino acids. The two lysines are always separated by precisely two or three residues, strongly suggesting structural constraints on these sequences that may be relevant to fibrillogenesis (35).

Cloning of genomic sequences for tropoelastin has yielded further insights (21). Importantly, it has confirmed that the elastin gene is present in a single copy in all mammalian species studied. It has also revealed that the modular structure of the protein is dictated by the structure of the gene. Hydrophobic and cross-linking domains are encoded by separate exons of the gene, which have probably undergone extensive duplication events to produce the more than 30 exons that make up the coding (and untranslated) sequence. The human elastin gene, located on chromosome 7, has 34 exons. Furthermore, genomic sequencing has revealed an unusually high ratio of noncoding to coding bases in the tropoelastin gene, which is nearly 12:1.

As previously indicated, tropoelastin is produced as multiple, closely related isoforms by alternative splicing of a common primary transcript. The coding portions of these alternatively spliced transcripts can differ in regions encoding hydrophobic and/or cross-link domains. Tissue-specific and developmental differences have been noted in the splicing pattern for tropoelastin mRNA (18, 45). However, it remains unclear what role alternative splicing and isoform heterogeneity plays in determining the structure–function relationships of mature elastin fibers (42).

Microfibrils. Over the last 10 years there has been a growing appreciation for a morphologically and biochemically distinct component of the elastic fiber, microfibrils. The association of these "fibrillae" with elastic fibers was first described by Gross and colleagues (16). Biochemically distinct microfibrils (of 10–12 nm diameter) were first recognized as structures that form a covering of mature elastic fibers and within mature fibers. Since the identification of microfibril structures, there has been an appreciation that they can exist both in the presence and absence of an elastic component. In fact, microfibrils occur in nonelastic tissues such as the ciliary zonule of the eye (58). The biochemical similarity between elastic and nonelastic microfibrils has not been completely resolved. During development, the appearance of microfibrils can precede the production of tropoelastin, giving rise to the hypothesis that microfibrils provide a scaffold for the production of elastic fibers (15). The complete function of microfibrils is a source of some debate, however. Naked microfibrils have an intrinsic structure of "beads on a string" (66) and appear to have some endogenous elasticity in the absence of elastin (33, 61). Indeed, on an evolutionary scale, the emergence of microfibrils precedes that of true elastic fibers (51). Speculation exists that naked microfibrils fulfilled the functional role of elastic fibers prior to the evolution of the tropoelastin gene. Furthermore, given that mutations in microfibril proteins are the primary cause of Marfan's syndrome (and congenital contractural arachnadactyly, a closely related syndrome), a structural role for these microfibrils seems likely. The presence of nonelastic microfibrils further suggests a functional role for this structure.

Many researchers have made substantial progress toward the initial identification of the biochemical nature of microfibrils. This work has shown that microfibrils consist of a complex of distinct proteins, many of which have been biochemically and/or genetically characterized. There are at least 12 proteins that have been associated with microfibril structures, which can be divided into families: fibrillins, microfibril-associated glycoproteins (MAGPs), lysyl oxidases (LOs), and others.

The largest and most studied family of microfibril proteins are the fibrillins; fibrillin-1 (fib-1) (32), fibrillin-2 (fib-2) (30), and the closely related, latent transforming growth factor beta (TGF-β)–binding proteins (LTBPs) (40). The fibrillins are large glycoproteins of approximately 350 kDa in size, with a modular structure containing repeating domains of both epidermal growth factor (EGF)-like motifs and "8-cysteine," or TGF-β-binding protein–like motifs (Fig. 2.1). Depending on the tissue, fib-1 or fib-2 is believed to be the major component of microfibrils. Most data support the presence of homopolymers, but fibrillin heteropolymers may also exist. While fib-1 and fib-2 are thought of as integral components of most elastic fibers, the role of the LTBPs (-1, -2, and -3) is less clear. LTBP-2 has been isolated from microfibril-enriched tissue (13) and the structure of LTBPs is similar to that of the fibrillins, containing both EGF-like motifs and "8-cysteine" motifs.

Another family of proteins is the MAGPs, whose original member was thought until recently to be unique (14). MAGP-1 has been immunolocalized to both elastin-associated and nonelastic microfibrils (12). MAGP-1 has been shown to directly interact with tropoelastin monomers (4) and may play a primary role in nucleation of fiber formation. Recently, at least one other closely related protein has been cloned and named MAGP-2 (13).

Lysyl oxidase is the enzyme responsible for modifying the lysine residues in tropoelastin (and collagen). Specifically, lysyl oxidase catalyzes the oxidative deamination of specific peptidyl-lysine residues, via formation of a Schiff-base, producing the reactive α-aminoadipic-D-semialdehyde (referred to as allysine). These modified allysine residues spontaneously form the cross-links necessary for the stability of mature elastin. Although the role of lysyl oxidase is primarily catalytic, this extensively investigated protein has been localized to microfibrils covering elastic fibers (23). Recently, a cDNA encoding a predicted amino acid sequence with a high degree of homology to lysyl oxidase has been cloned (25). A physiological role for this putative lysyl oxidase-like protein has not been established.

Numerous other proteins have been associated with microfibril structures and/or elastic fibers. These proteins include, but are not limited to; the fibulins (52) Big-h3 (MP78/70) (13), emilin (3), AMP/MFAP-1 (19), and MFAP-4 (27). Again, the structural and/or functional roles of these proteins in elastic fiber formation and stability are not clear.

Elastic fiber formation

Relatively little is known of the molecular interactions involved in the coalescence of the multiple proteins (described above) required to build a functional elastic fiber. The requirements for and the coordination of the production of microfibrils is unclear. Similarly, little is known about what guides and aligns tropoelastin monomers in growing fibes. Mecham and co-workers have recently made significant initial strides towards the understanding of these interactions. They have shown that the microfibril component MAGP-1 can directly bind to tropoelastin and may be important in elastin nucleation (4). Furthermore, they have identified favored cross-linking sites within the elastin component of elastic fibers that may provide structural data for monomer configuration and polymer alignment (5). Understanding the molecular mechanisms of elastic fiber production will clearly be one of the most important avenues of future elastin research.

ELASTIN IN THE LUNG

Pierce and Ebert have hypothesized that elastin and collagen form a continuous network of cables that, together, are capable of conferring the structural and functional capacity to the lung (48). The elastic network results from the expression of elastic fiber proteins from numerous cell types throughout the lung. Investigations of the expression of elastin in the lung have focused on tropoelastin, and most of these studies have occurred in the rat and mouse. Expression of tropoelastin in all tissues is subject to very stringent developmental controls. The temporal expression of tropoelastin in the lung closely follows that of other organs—beginning in the fetus, peaking near birth, and declining to absence at maturity. The locations of tropoelastin expression and elastic fiber accumulation, however, are probably more complex in the lung than in any other tissue or organ, making the lung a very useful and interesting subject of study. In this section, we will discuss the induction of tropoelastin expression and the deposition of elastic fibers in the developing lung, using the laboratory rat as an example of mammalian development.

Little or no tropoelastin is expressed in the early lung bud, which in the rat, occurs at approximately day 12. Induction of tropoelastin expression occurs shortly after budding and is first observed in the smooth muscle surrounding developing bronchi and in the developing pulmonary artery (Fig. 2.2). The main trunk of the intralobar pulmonary artery is the primary site of tropoelastin expression during the pseudoglandular stage of lung development, with expression reaching a maximum level by day 15 and continuing through gestation. In the medial layer of the pulmonary vasculature, as in the systemic vasculature, elastic fibers are organized perpendicular to blood flow and form lamellae or concentric sheets around the intima of the vessel. Subsequent, thinner lamellae are found throughout the media, between layers of medial smooth muscle cells (10). These smooth muscle cells are the primary source of tropoelastin production in the vasculature, although early in vasculogenesis, endothelial cells appear to contribute to the production of the IEL.

As development proceeds into the canalicular phase, at approximately day 18 in the rat, the lung begins to lose its glandular appearance. At this time, tropoelastin expression can readily be detected in the developing distal parenchyma. Here, tropoelastin expression specifically colocalizes to branching sites directly adjacent to differentiating epithelium, and is absent in the loose mesenchyme distant from the epithelium (49). The nature of this dichotomy of expression is unclear. Tropoelastin expression in the lung parenchyma steadily increases throughout the canalicular and saccular stages of development, with respect to both the number of expressing cells and the amount expressed per cell.

Parenchymal tropoelastin expression reaches a peak coincident with alveolar-

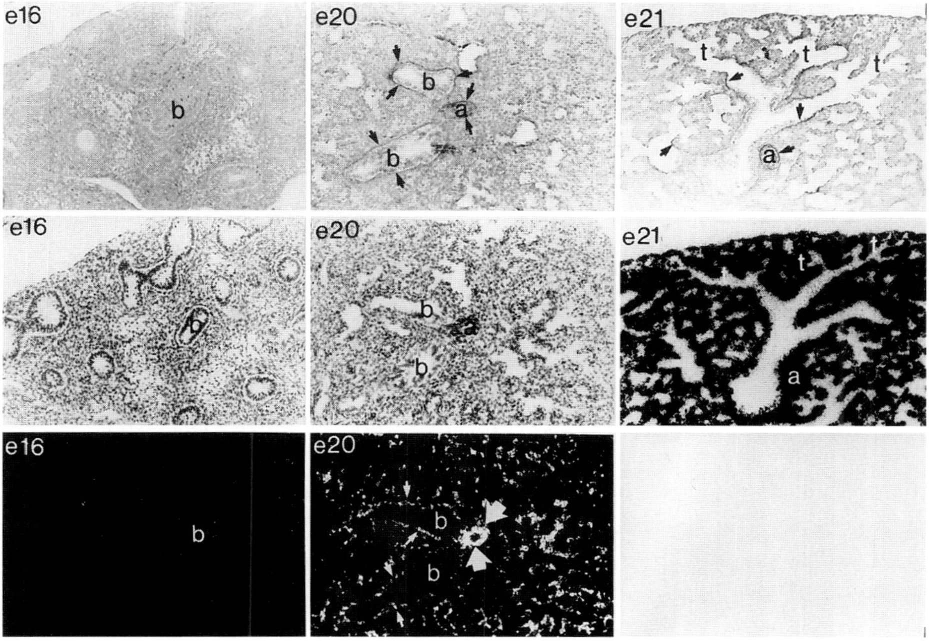

Fig. 2.2 Elastin in the developing rat lung. The *top panels* are sections of fetal rat lung stained with Hart's elastic stain. The *middle* and *bottom panels* are bright- and dark-filed views of sections of the same lungs hybridized in situ for tropoelastin mRNA. At 16 days of gestation, the lung is in the pseudoglandular stage of development, and elastic fibers are not visible. Signal for tropoelastin mRNA (shown as white silver grains in the dark-field view) is minimal, but present in smooth muscle surrounding a bronchiole (*b*). At 20 days of gestation, the lung is in the early saccular stage of development. Elastic fibers (*arrows*) underlay the epithelium of bronchioles (*b*) and are found in concentric lamellae of a branch of the intralobar pulmonary artery (*a*). Signal for tropoelastin mRNA is abundant in the smooth muscle of the pulmonary artery and is found in mesenchyme subjacent to developing airways. At 21 days of gestation, immediately prepartum, the lung is in the saccular stage of development. Terminal airspaces are more complex, and contain flattened epithelium. Elastic fibers (*arrows*) are evident between the cuboidal epithelium of proximal airways and are also found beneath flattened epithelium of the terminal airspaces (*t*). Intense signal for tropoelastin mRNA (black silver grains in the bright-field view) is found throughout the mesenchyme subjacent to epithelium and in the intralobar pulmonary artery.

ization, which occurs in the neonatal rat. At this point, expression is primarily seen at sites of secondary crest formation. These sites are occupied by α-smooth-muscle actin–expressing cells, which are likely responsible for tropoelastin production in the developing lung (41), as they are in adult lung disease (31). In the adult lung, parenchymal elastic fibers are found in morphologically distinct locations within the alveolar wall, concentrated at locations that make up the entrances to individual alveoli (38). Here, the fibers appear to form thin cables that form a ring around the entrance to the alveolus.

In mature conducting airways, elastic fibers are found peripheral to the basement membrane, forming cables parallel to airflow. The size of these cables decreases with decreasing airway diameter and medial thickness. Little is known about the physiological function of these elastic fibers. It appears the smooth muscle cells of the airway media are responsible for the production of tropoelastin in conducting airways during postnatal growth; however, subepithelial fibroblasts abluminal to the smooth-muscle cells may also be responsible. Chondrocytes also appear to contribute to the postnatal production of elastic fibers in the cartilaginous trachea and mainstem bronchi. In the pleura, fine elastic fibers can be seen lying parallel to the surface of the lung. The source of tropoelastin production for these fibers appears to be from mesothelial cells (7).

Very little is known about the temporal and spatial regulation of production of other elastic fiber components. Expression of the fibrillin genes (fib-1 and fib-2) has been observed in the developing lung (68). Fib-2 is produced earlier than fib-1, and appears to be expressed primarily in cuboidal epithelial cells. Fib-1 is expressed later than fib-2, by mesenchymal cells of the parenchyma and vasculature. Other elastic fiber components are reported to be expressed in the lung, but the location and cell population(s) responsible have not been determined.

REGULATION OF LUNG TROPOELASTIN EXPRESSION

There has been a great deal of study looking into the regulation of tropoelastin expression in the lung. Distinct mechanisms of regulation have been elucidated for the developmental induction and cessation of lung elastin expression. Furthermore, endogenous and exogenous signals for the regulation of tropoelastin expression are evolving and being tested.

Transcriptional Initiation

Through comprehensive studies, the transcriptional nature of developmental induction of tropoelastin expression in the lung has been established. Swee et al. (60) have shown that the inception of lung elastogenesis is accompanied by parallel increases in tropoelastin mRNA and pre-mRNA. Pierce et al. (49) further showed that exogenous modulation of elastogenesis in the developing rat lung study using steroids was due to effects on the level of tropoelastin gene transcription.

A great deal of study has gone into the characterization of the promoter for the tropoelastin gene. Although species- and tissue-specific differences exist, some common themes have emerged. The basal promoter of the tropoelastin gene (~0.5 kb) is sufficient for low levels of transcription, while the proximal 5′-flanking region (5 kb) has both positive and negative *cis*-acting regulatory elements. The promoter lacks a TATA box, but contains several putative sites for binding *trans*-acting factors. While the proximal 5′-flanking region may confer some tissue specificity (20), it does not appear to contain all the elements responsible for cell-type and tissue-specific levels of tropoelastin transcription. Furthermore, tropoelastin 5′-flanking sequences invariably confer a relatively low level of transcription in vitro. These data suggest that sequences distant from the basal promoter are necessary for maximal expression and developmental regulation of tropoelastin gene transcription.

Post-transcriptional Repression

In contrast to the transcriptional nature of tropoelastin gene induction in the lung, its developmental cessation occurs at a post-transcriptional level. This can be observed as continued tropoelastin gene transcription in the adult lung, even in the absence of protein production and mRNA accumulation (60). The biological rationale for this method of regulation in a gene subject to such strict temporal regulation is unclear.

The mechanisms responsible for this post-transcriptional repression of tropoelastin expression are beginning to be elucidated. Previous studies have investigated the role of regulation of tropoelastin mRNA stability in response to cytokines and other agents. For instance, mRNA stability contributes to tropoelastin regulation in response to Phorbol myristate acetate (PMA) (43) and TGF-β (24). Some studies have investigated the potential mechanisms for this alteration of mRNA stability and suggest that *cis*-acting sequences responsible for regulating degradation occur within the tropoelastin mRNA sequence (9). Other potential modes of regulating mRNA stability include regulation of polyadenylation site usage and poly-A tail length. Post-transcriptional regulation of gene expression may also take place at the level of pre-mRNA processing/transport or mRNA translation.

Regulation by Soluble Mediators

A great deal of information exists on the regulation of tropoelastin gene expression by numerous types of soluble mediators including cytokines, growth factors, steroids, and vitamins (44). These factors have often been broadly grouped into two categories: inducers and repressors. Interestingly, while repressors can often exert regulatory effects measured on the order of magnitudes, inducers have been restricted to effects of two- to four fold. Therefore, speculation exists as to the necessity of some form of co-stimulation for maximal tropoelastin induction.

The most studied inducers of tropoelastin gene expression are the TGF-β family of peptides. Transforming growth factor β has been shown to be an inducer of tropoelastin expression in many different in vivo and in vitro models. This regulation can take place at transcriptional and post-transcriptional levels. In the lung, TGF-β1 and 3 have been implicated in autocrine regulation of tropoelastin expression (34). Glucocorticoids have been shown to induce tropoelastin expression in the developing lung in a tissue maturation–dependent fashion (49). This regulation may act through effects on fibroblast autocrine TGF-β3 stimulation of tropoelastin expression (67). Other soluble inducers of lung tropoelastin gene expression include insulin-like growth factor (IGF)-1 and retinoids (44).

Repressors of lung tropoelastin expression are more numerous, but there are few studies on their effects in vivo (44). The cytokines interleukin (IL)-1β, TNF-α, and EGF are all potent repressors of tropoelastin expression, as are phorbol esters (approximately tenfold). Basic-FGF, vitamin D3, and ascorbate are also capable of modest repression of tropoelastin expression (approximately threefold).

Regulation by Extracellular Matrix and Stress/Stretch

Many insoluble extracellular stimuli have been shown to have effects on tropoelastin production by various cells. These include static stimuli, such as the extracellular matrix; biophysical stimuli, such as cell deformation in response to stretch; and transient stimuli, such as cell–cell interactions. Although very few of these mechanisms have been thoroughly explored in tropoelastin expression in the lung, their consideration is extremely appropriate.

The effects of cell–matrix interactions on the regulation of cell phenotype and gene expression have become increasingly evident. Coincident with the initial characterization of this hypothesis, Mecham and colleagues observed that an elastin-rich matrix could induce tropoelastin production in pre-elastogenic cells (36). Subsequent experiments on this interaction indicated that elastic matrix could influence the expression of tropoelastin in many different cell types, and at different stages of development (44). This effect appears to be dependent on the three-dimensional nature of elastic matrix, as degraded matrix has no effect. The identification of other matrix effects on tropoelastin expression and the characterization of the mechanisms responsible await further investigation.

Given the structural dependence on matrix-mediated tropoelastin regulation described above and the functional nature of elastic fibers, a regulatory role for mechanical stress or stretch in tropoelastin expression is intriguing. In the terminal air-exchange regions of the lung, elastin accumulates at regions of proposed maximal stress and is produced (primarily) by cells containing stress fibers. Furthermore, maximal expression is induced coincident with the initiation of breathing. Sutcliffe and Davidson have shown changes in smooth-muscle cell elastin production when cells are exposed to static stretching (59). Riley and co-workers have also shown mechanical stress-dependent changes in elastin production from pulmonary artery segments stretched in vitro (64).

The role of cell–cell interactions in the regulation of elastin expression has been appreciated for some time. Mecham et al. (37) reported the identification of a smooth-muscle elastogenic factor (SMEF) that could function in a paracrine fashion to induce elastin production. Others have shown that mechanical stress-dependent changes in elastin expression from pulmonary artery segments is dependent on an intact endothelium (62). More recently, the ability of other cell types to influence tropoelastin expression is receiving renewed attention. In the developing lung, initiation of tropoelastin expression occurs in intimate association with branching morphogenesis and differentiating epithelium (49). This strongly suggests a role for epithelial-derived factors in lung parenchyma elastogenesis. In fact, alveolar epithelial cells are capable of producing factors which regulate lung mesenchymal cell tropoelastin expression (31a). Recent studies have also shown that inflammatory cells are capable of regulating tropoelastin expression in lung cells, albeit through soluble mediators (T. Mariani and R. Pierce, unpublished observations).

ELASTIC FIBER PATHOLOGY IN THE LUNG

Elastogenesis appears to play a significant role in the development and maintenance of normal lung structure and function. Interference with elastin fiber formation by administration of lathyrogens results in severely abnormal alveolar architecture (26). Destruction of lung elastin is responsible for the development of emphysema (22). Recent investigations suggest that altered expression of tropoelastin and/or elastic fiber deposition is associated with many types of developmental defects in lung structure. Furthermore, the re-initiation of tropoelastin expression has been observed in injured adult lung tissue.

Elastic Fibers in Bronchopulmonary Dysplasia

Bronchopulmonary dysplasia (BPD) is a chronic form of lung injury, initiated in infancy, which results in enlarged terminal air spaces and decreased lung function. This disease is commonly associated with hyperoxia resulting from mechanical ventilation. In a recent study by Pierce and co-workers (47), mechanical ventilation of premature lambs was shown to be associated with altered elastogenesis and the development of BPD (Fig. 2.3).

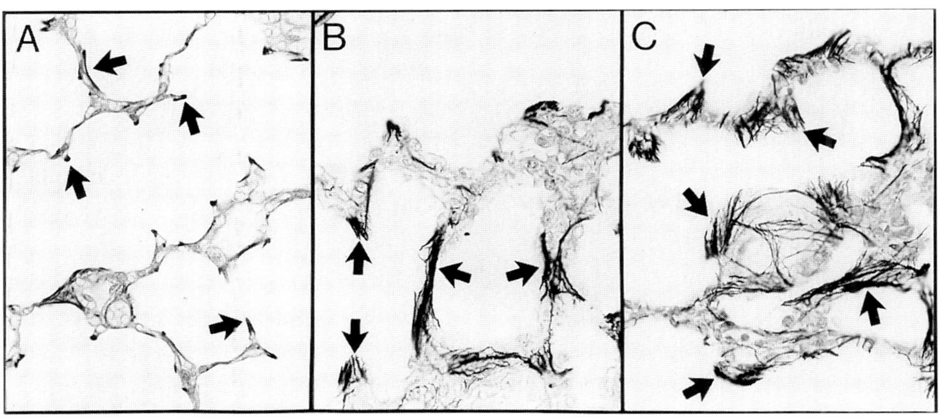

Fig. 2.3 Abnormal alveolarization and excessive elastin deposition in an animal model of bronchopulmonary dysplasia. Preterm lambs at 125 days of gestation (term is 147) were delivered, given surfactant, and ventilated for 3 weeks while maintained on ewe's milk and supplemental nutrition. Ventilation at 40 breaths per minute (*B*) and 20 breaths per minute (C) resulted in diminished alveolar septal development and marked increases in elastic fibers in alveolar walls compared with term control lambs (*A*). Arrows indicate elastic fibers.

Recent studies of mutant strains of mice and genetically engineered animals have further suggested an important role for elastic fibers in normal lung development. Genetic disruption of the gene encoding platelet-derived growth factor (PDGF)-A results in severe developmental lung pathology similar to BPD and loss of alveolar wall elastic fibers (1). The tight-skinned (*tsk*) mouse shows developmental lung defects characteristic of BPD. The genetic mutation responsible for the development of this strain has recently been shown to be in the gene for the elastic fiber component fib-1 (57). Again, this indicates an association between abnormal elastic fibers and lung pathology.

Human Disease and Elastin Pathology

Elastic fiber pathogenesis may be most widely appreciated for two diseases associated with adult mortality: emphysema and Marfan's syndrome. Emphysema is usually an adult-onset lung disease, sometimes associated with a genetic defect of α1-antitrypsin, whose pathology lies in the destruction of alveolar elastic fibers (22). Marfan's syndrome is one of the most common congenital abnormalities, and is manifested as tall stature, due to enhanced long-bone growth, cardiac abnormalities and dissecting aortic aneurysms. The pathology of this disease is derived from primary defects in the elastic fiber protein fibrillin-1 (11). Recently, the vascular disease supravalvular aortic stenosis (SVAS) has been associated with primary defects in the tropoelastin gene (8). Curiously, although Marfan's syndrome and SVAS have obligate alterations in elastic fiber structure (due to the genetic nature of these diseases), neither appears to be associated with pathology in the lung. This may suggest that different biophysical constraints are placed on the elastic fibers in different tissues and/or that the biochemical composition of elastic fibers in different tissues varies considerably.

Reinitiation of Tropoelastin Expression in the Adult Lung

The ability of the adult lung to reinitiate elastogenesis is becoming increasingly noted. In several models of experimental lung disease, increased production of elastin has been reported (6, 29, 39, 50, 62). Recently, we have characterized a silica-induced model of lung fibrosis that includes a significant increase in lung elastin content (31). In this model, the location and cellular populations responsible for tropoelastin expression appear to be identical to those seen in development. Nonetheless, tropoelastin expression in these models of adult lung injury invariably lead to the production of elastic fibers with aberrant morphology.

Koh et al. (28) have shown that elastogenesis occurs during postpneumonectomy lung growth in the adult rat. Importantly, in this model, elastin content (and apparently elastin fiber morphology) remains normal. The basis for this unique, normal elastosis in the adult lung is unclear, but it may be due to a coordinated production of multiple elastic fiber proteins (which may not occur in other injury models). One clue is that no inflammatory response is seen in the pneumonectomy model, whereas inflammation is often seen in the injury models. This compensatory lung growth model, in comparison with other injury models, could provide information that will help to understand the mechanisms of elastic fiber production.

FUTURE DIRECTIONS

There has been incredible growth over the last four decades with respect to the knowledge of the nature of elastin. This time has seen a growing appreciation for the importance of the elastic fiber in the structure and function of many tissues including the lung. Even so, future investigations of the elastic fiber are necessary to answer important questions about human pathologies and basic biological mechanisms. Some of the most important questions needing to be answered include the following: Are elastic fibers from different tissues biochemically different? What are the mechanisms involved in the formation of elastic fibers? What controls the developmental and tissue-specific expression of tropoelastin? How does the regulation of expression of other elastic fiber components compare with tropoelastin? What are the essential signals that drive the development of the elastogenic cell phenotype? Future studies are also essential to an understanding of associations, be they primary or secondary, between abnormal elastic fiber production and diseases such as BPD.

REFERENCES

1. Bostrom, H., K. Willets, M. Pekny, P. Leveen, P. Lindahl, H. Hedstrand, M. Pekna, M. Hellstrom, S. Gebremedhin, M. Schalling, M. Nilsson, S. Kurland, J. Tornell, J.K. Heath, and C. Betscholtz. PDGF-A signalling is a critical event in lung alveolar myofibroblast development and alveogenesis. *Cell* 85: 863-873, 1996.
2. Boyd, C.D., A.M. Christiano, R.A. Pierce, C.A. Stolle, and S.B. Deak. Mammalian tropoelastin multiple domains of the protein define an evolutionarily divergent amino acid sequence. *Matrix* 11: 235–241, 1991.
3. Bressan, G.M., D. Daga-Gordini, A. Colombatti, I. Castellani, V. Marigo, and D. Volpin. Emilin, a component of elastic fibers preferentially located at the elastin-microfibril interface. *J. Biol. Chem.* 121: 201–212, 1993.
4. Brown-Augsberger, P., T. Broekelman, L. Mecham, R. Mercer, M.A. Gibson, E.G. Cleary, W.R. Abrams, J. Rosenbloom, and R.P. Mecham. Microfibril associated glycoprotein binds to the carboxy terminal domain of tropoelastin and is a substrate for transglutaminase. *J Biol. Chem.* 269: 28442–28449, 1994.
5. Brown-Augsberger, P., C. Tisdale, T. Broekelman, C. Sloan, and R.P. Mecham. Identification of an elastin cross-linking domain that joins three peptide chains—possible role in nucleated assembly. *J. Biol. Chem.* 270: 17778–17783, 1995.
6. Cantor, J.O., S. Keller, I. Mandl, and G.M. Turino. Increased synthesis of elastin in amiodorone-induced pulmonary fibrosis. *J. Lab. Clin. Med.* 109: 480–485, 1987.
7. Cantor, J.O., M. Willhite, and B.A. Bray. Synthesis of crosslinked elastin by mesothelial cell culture. *Proc. Soc. Exp. Biol. Med.* 181: 387–391, 1986.
8. Curran M.E., D.L. Atkinson, A.K. Ewart, C.A. Morris, M.F. Leppart, and M.T. Keating. The

elastin gene is disrupted by a translocation associated with supravalvular aortic stenosis. *Cell* 73: 159–168, 1993.

9. Davidson, J.M., M.-C. Zang, O. Zoia, and M.G. Giro. Regulation of elastin synthesis in pathological states. In: *The Molecular Biology and Pathology of Elastic Tissues,* edited by L. Robert. Chichester: Wiley, 1995, p. 81–99.
10. Davis, E.C. Smooth muscle cell to elastic lamina connections in developing mouse aorta role in aortic medial organization. *Lab. Invest.* 68: 89–99, 1993.
11. Dietz, H.C., G.R. Cutting, R.E. Pyeritz, C.L. Maslen, L.Y. Sakai, G.M. Corson, E.G. Puffenberger, A. Hamosh, E.J. Nanthakumar, S.M. Curristan, G. Stetten, D.A. Meyers, and C.A. Francomano. Marfan syndrome caused by a recurrent de novo missense mutation in the fibrillin gene. *Nature* 352: 337–339, 1991.
12. Gibson, M.A. and E.G. Cleary. The immunohistochemical localization of microfibril-associated glycoprotein (MAGP) in elastic and non-elastic tissues. *Immunol. Cell. Biol.* 65: 345–356, 1987.
13. Gibson, M.A., G. Hatzinikolas, J.S. Kumaratilake, L.B. Sandberg, J.K. Nicholl, G.R. Sutherland, and E.G. Cleary. Further characterization of proteins associated with elastic fiber microfibrils including the molecular cloning of MAGP-2 (MP-25). *J. Biol. Chem.* 271: 1096–1103, 1996.
14. Gibson, M.A., L.B. Sandberg, L.E. Grosso, and E.G. Cleary. Complementary DNA cloning establishes microfibril-associated glycoprotein (MAGP) to be a discrete component of the elastin-associated microfibrils. *J. Biol. Chem.* 266: 7596–7601, 1991.
15. Greenlee, T.K.J., R. Ross, and J.L. Hartman. The fine structure of elastic fibers. *J. Cell Biol.* 30: 59–71, 1966.
16. Gross, J. The structure of the elastic tissue as studied by the electron microscope. *J. Exp. Med.* 89: 699–708, 1949.
17. Halloran, B.G. and B.T. Baxter. Pathogenesis of aneurysms. *Semin. Vasc. Surg.* 8: 85–92, 1995.
18. Heim, R.A., R.A. Pierce, S.A. Deak, D.J. Riley, C.D. Boyd, and C.A. Stolle. Alternative splicing of rat tropoelastin mRNA is tissue-specific and developmentally regulated. *Matrix* 11: 359–366, 1991.
19. Horrigan, S.K., C.B. Rich, B.W. Streeten, Z. Li, and J.A. Foster. Characterization of an associated microfibril protein through recombinant DNA techniques. *J. Biol. Chem.* 127: 10087–10095, 1992.
20. Hsu-Wong, S., S.D. Katchman, I. Ledo, M. Wu, J. Khillan, M.M. Bashir, J. Rosenbloom, and J. Uitto. Tissue-specific and developmentally regulated expression of human promoter activity in transgenic mice. *J. Biol. Chem.* 269: 18072–18075, 1994.
21. Indik, Z., H. Yeh, N. Ornstein-Goldstein, and J. Rosenbloom. Structure of the elastin gene and alternative splicing of elastin mRNA. In: *Extracellular Matrix Genes,* edited by L. Sandell and C.D. Boyd. New York: Academic Press, 1990, p. 221–250.
22. Janoff A. Elastases and emphysema. *Am. Rev. Respir. Dis.* 132: 417–433, 1985.
23. Kagan, H.M., C.A. Vaccaro, R.E. Bronson, S.S. Tang, and J.S. Brody. Ultrastructural immunolocalization of lysyl oxidase in vascular connective tissue. *J. Cell Biol.* 103: 1121–1128, 1986.
24. Kähäri, V.-M., D.R. Olsen, R.W. Rhudy, P.A. Carillo, Y.Q. Chen, and J. Uitto. Transforming growth factor-b upregulates elastin gene expression in human skin fibroblast: evidence for posttranscriptional modulation. *Lab. Invest.* 66: 580–588, 1992.
25. Kenyon, K., W.S. Modi, S. Contente, and R.S. Friedman. A novel human cDNA with a pre-

dicted protein similar similar to lysyl oxidase maps to chromosome 15q24-q25. *J. Biol. Chem.* 268: 18435–18437, 1993.

26. Kida, K. and W.M. Thurlbeck. Lack of recovery of lung structure and function after administration of BAPN in the postnatal period. *Am. Rev. Respir. Dis.* 122: 467–473, 1980.
27. Kobayashi, R., Y. Tashima, H. Masuda, T. Shozawa, Y. Numata, K. Miyauchi, and T. Hayakawa. Isolation and characterization of a new 36-kDa microfibril-associated glycoprotein from porcine aorta. *J. Biol. Chem.* 264: 17347–17444, 1989.
28. Koh, D., J. Roby, B. Starcher, R. Senior, and R. Pierce. Postpneumonectomy lung growth: a model of reinitiation of tropoelastin and type I collagen in a normal pattern in adult rat lung. *Am. J. Respir. Cell Mol. Biol.* 15: 611–623, 1996.
29. Last, J.A., T.R. Gelzleichter, K.E. Pinkerton, R.M. Walker, and H. Witschi. A new model of progressive pulmonary fibrosis in rats. *Am. Rev. Respir. Dis.* 148: 487–494, 1993.
30. Lee, B., M. Godfrey, E. Vitale, H. Hori, M. Mattei, M. Sarfarazi, P. Tsipouras, F. Ramirez, and D.W. Hollister. Linkage of Marfan syndrome and a phenotypically related disorder to two different fibrillin genes. *Nature* 352: 330–334, 1991.
31. Mariani, T.J., E. Crouch, J.D. Roby, B. Starcher, and R.A. Pierce. Increased elastin production in experimental granulomatous lung disease. *Am. J. Pathol.* 147: 988–1000, 1995.

31a. Mariani, T.J., S.E. Dunsmore, Q. Li, X. Ye, and R.A. Pierce. Regulation of lung fibroblast tropoelastin expression by alveolar epithelial cells. *Am. J. Physiol. (Lung Cell. Mol. Physiol.)* 18: L47–57, 1993.

32. Maslen, C.L., G.M. Corson, B.K. Maddox, R.W. Glanville and L.Y. Sakai. Partial sequence of a candidate gene for the Marfan syndrome. *Nature* 352: 334–337, 1991.
33. McConnell, C.J., G.M. Wright, and M.E. Demont. The modulus of elasticity of lobster aorta microfibrils. *Experientia* 52: 918–921, 1996.
34. McGowan, S.E. Influences of endogenous and exogenous TGF-β on elastin in rat lung fibroblasts and aortic smooth muscle cells. *Am. J. Physiol. (Lung Cell. Mol. Physiol.)* 263: L257–263, 1992.
35. Mecham, R.P. and J. Heuser. The elastic fiber. In: *Cell Biology of Extracellular Matrix,* edited by E.D. Hay. New York: Plenum Press, 1991, p. 79–109.
36. Mecham, R.P., J.G. Madaras, and R.M. Senior. Extracellular matrix-specific induction of elastogenic differentiation and maintenance of phenotypic stability in bovine ligament fibroblasts. *J. Cell Biol.* 98: 1804–1812, 1984.
37. Mecham, R.P., L.A. Whitehouse, D.S. Wrenn, W.C. Parks, G.L. Griffin, R.M. Senior, E.C. Crouch, K.R. Stenmark, and N.F. Voelkel. Smooth muscle–mediated connective tissue remodeling in pulmonary hypertension. *Science* 237: 423–426, 1987.
38. Mercer, R.R. and J.D. Crapo. Spatial distribution of collagen and elastin fibers in the lungs. *J. Appl. Physiol.* 69: 756–765, 1990.
39. Meyrick, B. and L. Reid. Hypoxia-induced structural changes in the media and adventia of the rat hilar pulmonary artery and their regression. *Am. J. Pathol.* 100: 151–178, 1980.
40. Miyazano, K., U. Hellman, C. Wernstedt, and C. Heldin. Latent high molecular weight complex of transforming growth factor beta 1. *J. Biol. Chem.* 263: 6407–6415, 1988.
41. Noguchi, A., H. Samaha, and D.E. deMello. Tropoelastin gene expression in the rat pulmonary vasculature: a developmental study. *Pediatr. Res.* 31: 280–285, 1992.
42. Parks, W.C. and S.D. Deak. Tropoelastin heterogeneity: implications for protein function and disease. *Am. J. Respir. Cell Mol. Biol.* 2: 399–406, 1990.

43. Parks, W.C., M.E. Kolodziej, and R.A. Pierce. Phorbol ester–mediated downregulation of tropoelastin expression is controlled by a posttranscriptional mechanism. *Biochemistry* 31: 6639–6645, 1992.
44. Parks, W.C., R.A. Pierce, K.A. Lee, and R.P. Mecham. Elastin. In: *Advances in Molecular and Cell Biology*, Vol. 6, edited by H.K. Kleinman. Greenwich, CT: JAI Press, 1993, p. 133-182.
45. Parks, W.C., H. Secrist, L.C. Wu, and R.P. Mecham. Developmental regulation of tropoelastin isoforms. *J. Biol. Chem.* 263: 4416–4423, 1988.
46. Partridge, S.M. Elastin. *Adv. Prot. Chem.* 17: 227–302, 1962.
47. Pierce, R.A., K.A. Albertine, B.C. Starcher, J.F. Bohnsack, B.P. Carlton, and R.D. Bland. Chronic lung injury in preterm lambs: disordered pulmonary elastin deposition. *Am. J. Physiol. (Lung Cell. Mol. Physiol.)* 272: L452–460, 1997.
48. Pierce, J.A. and R.V. Ebert. Fibrosis network of the lung and its change with age. *Thorax* 20: 469–476, 1965.
49. Pierce, R.A., W. Mariencheck, S. Sandefur, E.C. Crouch, and W.C. Parks. Glucocorticoids upregulate tropoelastin expression during late stages of fetal lung development. *Am. J. Physiol. (Lung Cell. Mol. Physiol.)* 268: L491–500, 1995.
50. Raghow, R., S. Lurie, J.M. Seyer, and A.H. Kang. Profiles of steady state levels of messenger RNAs coding for type I procollagen, elastin, and fibronectin in hamster lungs undergoing bleomycin-induced interstitial pulmonary fibrosis. *J. Clin. Invest.* 76: 1733–1739, 1985.
51. Rebermuller, S., T. Spissinger, P. Schuchert, J. Spring, and V. Schmid. An extracellular matrix protein of jellyfish homologous to mammalian fibrillins forms different fibrils depending on the life stage of the animal. *Dev. Biol.* 169: 662–672, 1995.
52. Roark, E.F., D.R. Keene, C.C. Haudenschild, S. Godyna, C.D. Little, and W.S. Argraves. The association of human fibulin-1 with classic fibers. An immunohistological, ultrustructural and run study. *J. Histochem. Cytochem.* 43: 401–411, 1995.
53. Sage, H. and W.R. Gray. Studies on the evolution of elastin. I. Phylogenetic distribution. *Comp. Biochem. Physiol.* 64B: 313, 1979.
54. Sandberg, L.B., N.T. Soskel, and T.B. Wolt. Elastin structure, biosynthesis and relation to disease states. *New Engl. J. Med.* 304: 566–579, 1981.
55. Sandberg, L.B. and T.B. Wolt. Production and isolation of soluble elastin from copper-deficient swine. *Methods Enzymol.* 82: 657–665, 1982.
56. Shapiro, S.D., S.K. Endicott, M.A. Province, J.A. Pierce, and E.J. Campbell. Marked longevity of human lung parenchymal elastic fibers deduced from prevalence of D-aspartate and nuclear weapons-related radiocarbon. *J. Clin. Invest.* 87: 1828–1834, 1991.
57. Siracusa, L.D., R. McGrath, Q. Ma, J.J. Moskow, J. Manne, P.J. Christner, A.M. Buchberg, and S.A. Jimenez. A tandem duplication within the fibrillin 1 gene is associated with the mouse tight skin mutation. *Genome Res.* 6: 300–313, 1996.
58. Streeten, B.W. and P.A. Licari. The zonules and the elastic microfibrillar system in the ciliary body. *Invest. Opthalmol. Vis. Sci.* 21: 130–135, 1983.
59. Sutcliffe, M.C. and J.M. Davidson. Effect of static stretching on elastin production by porcine aortic smooth muscle cells. *Matrix* 10: 148–153, 1990.
60. Swee, M., W.C. Parks, and R.A. Pierce. Developmental regulation of elastin production. Expression of tropoelastin pre-mRNA persists after downregulation of steady-state mRNA levels. *J. Biol. Chem.* 270: 14899–14906, 1995.
61. Thurmond, F.A. and J.A. Trotter. Morphology and biomechanics of the microfibrillar network of sea cucumber dermis. *J. Exp. Biol.* 199: 1817–1828, 1996.

62. Todorovich-Hunter, L., D.J. Johnson, P. Ranger, F.W. Keeley, and M. Rabinovitch. Altered elastin and collagen synthesis associated with progressive pulmonary hypertension induced by monocrotaline, a biochemical and ultrastructural study. *Lab. Invest.* 58: 184–195, 1988.
63. Tozzi, C.A., G.J. Poiani, A.M. Harangozo, C.J. Boyd, and D.J. Riley. Pulmonary vascular endothelial cells modulate stretch-induced DNA and connective tissue synthesis in rat pulmonary artery segments. *Chest* 93: 169S–170S, 1988.
64. Tozzi, C.A., G.J. Poiani, A.M. Harangozo, C.J. Boyd, and D.J. Riley. Pressure-induced connective tissue synthesis in pulmonary artery segments is dependent on intact endothelium. *J. Clin. Invest.* 84: 1005–1012, 1989.
65. Urry, D.W., C.-H. Luan, and S.Q. Peng. Molecular biophysics of elastin structure, function and pathology. In: The Molecular Biology and Pathology of Elastic Tissues, edited by L. Robert. Chichester: Wiley, 1995, p. 4–30.
66. Wright, D.W. and R. Mayne. Vitreous humor of chicken contains two fibrillar systems: an analysis of their structure. *J. Ultrastruct. Mol. Struct. Res.* 100: 224–234, 1988.
67. Yee, W., J. Wang, J. Liu, I. Tseu, M. Kuliszewski, and M. Post. Glucocorticoid-induced tropoelastin expression is mediated via transforming growth factor beta-3. *Am. J. Physiol. (Lung Cell. Mol. Physiol.)* 270: L992–L1001, 1988.
68. Zhang, H., W. Hu, and F. Ramirez. Developmental expression of fibrillin genes suggests heterogeneity of extracellular microfibrils. *J. Cell Biol.* 129: 1165–1176, 1995.

The authors would like to acknowledge the assistance of many long-time colleagues who have directly or indirectly contributed to the information and ideas presented in this review. We also wish to thank Teresa Tolley for superior technical assistance with histological methods. This work was supported by NIH Grants HLR29-54049, HLP01-29594, HL 09179 and an American Heart Association Grant-In-Aid.

chapter 3

DIFFERENTIATION AND MATURATION OF AIRWAY EPITHELIAL CELLS: ROLE OF EXTRACELLULAR MATRIX AND GROWTH FACTORS

Dominique Gaillard and Edith Puchelle

As early as 5 months gestational age (40), the conducting airways are lined with a continuous respiratory epithelium covered by a film of mucus that is continuously cleared by ciliary beating of ciliated cells. The surface epithelium is columnar and pseudostratified along the tracheobronchial tree and includes ciliated, secretory, intermediate, and basal cells (13, 27, 120), as well as neuroendocrine cells (75), terminal processes of nerve fibers (2), and cells involved in the immune response after migration through the epithelial basement membrane (BM) (10). In the largest proximal airways, mucus is partly secreted by the goblet cells lining the lumen but mainly by the mucous and serous cells arranged into acini in the submucosal glands (61). In the distal conducting airways, the thickness of the epithelium decreases. Nonciliated Clara cells represent the only type of secretory cells (13, 140), and the number of ciliated cells decreases.

An understanding of changes in cytodifferentiation patterns and cellular composition of respiratory epithelium during development provides insight into physiological and pathological mechanisms in adults (75). Tracheobronchial epithelium during development displays many similarities with regenerating adult epithelium following injury (40, 65, 101).

The development of the trachea begins by the fourth week postfertilization as a central diverticulum budding from the foregut and lined with epithelium of endodermal origin. This tracheal diverticulum grows caudally, forms the two primary ventrolateral lung buds, and becomes invested by mesenchyme derived from splanchnic mesoderm. The primary hollow endodermal buds and their surrounding mesenchyme divide to form three branches on the right and two on the left of the five-lobed lung. As the bronchial tubes branch dichotomously, the mesenchymal coats condense and differentiate around the growing proximal bronchial tree to form cartilage, muscle, blood and lymphatic vessels, and other connective tissue elements. The numerous blind-ended tubules give the lung a pseudoglandular appearance that is characteristic of the first postembryonic phase. During the pseudoglandular phase, which lasts until up to 16 weeks gestational age, the preacinar branching pattern of the conducting airways is established (18). In the ensuing canalicular phase (17–24 weeks), the vascularization of mesenchyme rapidly increases and the respiratory portion of lung begins to develop. During the last saccular and alveolar phase (over 24 weeks gestational age), the additional respiratory portion of the lung begins to develop and the future respiratory units differentiate.

The mechanisms of cytodifferentiation were examined many years ago through experimental models such as hamsters (82), rats (70), mice (79), rabbits (119) and monkeys (99). However, most of the animals used to study the fetal development have an immature surface epithelium along the airways at birth, whereas the human fetal airway mucosa is functional, with numerous mature cells by 24 weeks of gestation (40). Co-cultures of animal tissues have been very useful for investigating the mechanisms of cytodifferentiation, especially the interaction between epithelial and mesenchymal cells (139). It has been shown that the branching pattern of endodermal lung buds is induced by bronchial mesoderm and its extension appears to be directly proportional to the amount of mesenchyme present in the co-culture (see Chap. 1 for review). The mesenchyme is also necessary for cytodifferentiation and displays a regional identity. The invasion of tracheal mesenchymal cells between the corresponding tracheal epithelium and the inducing bronchial mesenchyme tissue inhibits branching (139), reduces cell proliferation, and favors epithelial cell maturation. The regional specificity of lung mesenchyme likely depends upon homeobox genes (11, 89), which are expressed in a specific spatial and temporal pattern during organogenesis and are involved in specification of regional identity (85). In the mouse, *Hoxb-3, b-4,* and *b-5* genes are highly expressed in the foregut, which gives rise to the tracheal bud, but later on, only *Hoxb-3* and *b-4* are expressed in the mesenchyme of the proximal and distal airways, whereas *Hoxb-2* starts being expressed and *Hoxb-5* continues to be expressed in the mesenchyme of the distal lung buds (11). The results of these co-cultures (139) are now partially explained by the genes of development, especially the *Hoxb* gene (143), which may be involved in specifying the differences between proximal and distal mesenchyme.

In this chapter, we will review the differentiation of respiratory epithelial cells in the conducting airway during human development and the molecules expressed either by the mesenchyme, or by epithelial cells which influence epithelial cell differentiation. A great deal of information is due to new cell culture techniques that represent interesting approaches for studying the mechanisms of cell differentiation. Explant outgrowths of animal or human mature or immature respiratory epithelium can be seeded onto collagen matrix in a culture medium supplemented with growth factors and hormones. This technique is particularly useful for analysing the effects of molecules involved in cell differentiation. Surface respiratory epithelial cells (7, 101) as well as gland cells (59) cultured within three-dimensional collagen lattices are able to form tubular duct–like structures and to undergo morphological changes similar to those observed during development. These three-dimensional culture techniques have been used to investigate the molecular regulation of airway epithelial cell proliferation and differentiation.

DIFFERENTIATION AND MATURATION OF THE SURFACE EPITHELIUM

Until 10 weeks of gestational age, the epithelium remains undifferentiated. Epithelial columnar cells lie on a thin basement membrane and display an ovoid nucleus located in their apical or basal part. These cells express so-called simple cytokeratins, such as cytokeratins 7, 8, 18, and 19 (15). Under an electron microscope, the apical pole of cells, covered with small microvilli, is seen to be swelling out into the lumen and covered by glycocalix (40). The electron-lucent cytoplasm contains a large amount of mature and immature glycogen, many mitochondria, a few microtubules and intermediate microfilaments and occasional centrioles. The cells are polarized and close to the lumen, the lateral plasma membranes are joined together by tight junctions. The differentiation of the epithelium proceeds in a cranial to caudal direction.

Neuroendocrine Cells

Neuroendocrine cells are reported to be the first "mature" cell type to differentiate within primitive airway epithelium, when the 5–8 generations of airways are formed, at 8 weeks (24, 123). These cells are distributed singly or in pairs, close to the basement membrane along the trachea and the main and intrapulmonary bronchi. They are oval, pyramidal, or bottle shaped, metachromatic and weakly argyrophilic (50). Neuron-specific enolase and chromogranin are commonly used as general neuroendocrine markers associated with neurosecretory granules (Fig. 3.1). Their cytoplasm is free of glycogen and shows numerous mitochondria, rough endoplasmic reticulum, Golgi complexes, microtubules, and intermediate filaments. The characteristic dense-cored granules are at first sparse and smaller than those seen in the adult and they are scattered (125). They probably represent granule precursors of the three types of granules found in the adult dense-core granulated cells (24). The cells form dendrite-like processes extending over the BM along long distances, between other epithelial cells.

Serotonin is the first peptide detected in the human airway; it is in single epi-

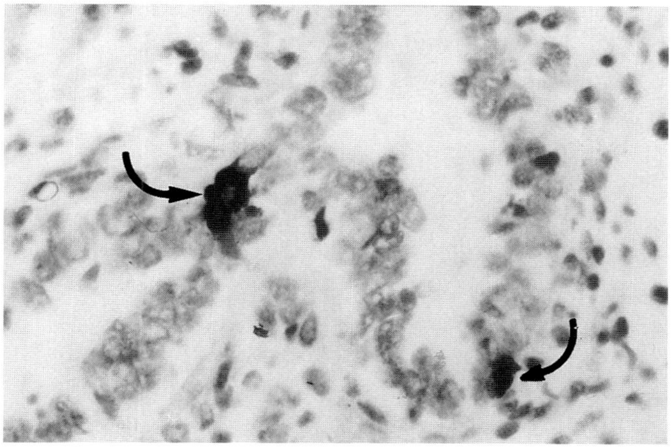

Fig. 3.1 Immunolocalization of chromogranin in a few neuroendocrine cells (*arrow*) scattered in the epithelium of a human bronchus at 15.5 weeks of gestation (×400).

thelial cells at 8, weeks (24). Bombesin and bombesin-like [gastrin-releasing peptide (GRP), a 27 amino acid bombesin homolog] immunoreactivity is found at 10 weeks, at a time when submucosal nerves and ganglia show strong immunoreaction for neuron-specific enolase. The neuroepithelial bodies, first identified by Lauweryns et al. as innervated corpuscles of tall cylindric and argyrophilic cells (74), are apparent by 13–16 weeks. They are preferentially located at airways bifurcations. During the canalicular and alveolar phases of development, the frequency of bombesin and GRP and serotonin-immunoreactivity in dense-core granulated cells increases in neuroepithelial bodies in peripheral airways. The GRP immunoreactivity in lung tissue extracts is at its highest level during the late fetal–neonatal period and decreases during postpartum (25). Bombesin has been found to exhibit potent growth factor–like properties, affecting lung morphogenesis and interfering with smooth muscle cells and neuromodulation (141). The expression of GRP-receptor mRNA is detected in fetal and neonatal human lungs (136), is highest during the canalicular stage of development, and the strongest signal levels are observed in the most peripheral developing bronchial tubes, which represent the sites of the most active lung growth. The lower expression of bombesin in the proximal bronchi suggests that growth stimulation turns off to allow further cellular differentiation. Calcitonin, calcitonin-gene-related peptide (CGRP), and leuenkephalin are detected only late during fetal development and postnatally. Colocalization of bombesin and calcitonin with CGRP is rarely observed in the fetus. The number of most immunoreactive neuroendocrine cells per millimeter bronchiolar or bronchial length decreases during the first years of life (92).

In various pediatric diseases and in experimental models under hypoxia, the number and size of neuroendocrine cells and neuroepithelial bodies increase, suggesting that these structures act as hypoxia-sensitive airway chemoreceptors (25, 92) and peptides are frequently colocalized in the same neuroendocrine cell or even in the same dense-core granule (122).

Ciliated Cells

In unspecialized columnar epithelial cells, a rudimentary primary cilium with a short shaft, including irregular doublets and a basal body without any root, can be identified by electron microscopy. This primary ciliogenesis is transitional and followed by a secondary ciliogenesis that corresponds to the formation of the ciliary border, which is close to that found in the adult (40, 91). Scanning a single area of human fetal surface epithelium at the end of the first trimester shows many undifferentiated epithelial cells, extending longer microvilli with scattered unique flattened primary cilia, and a few mature ciliated cells.

The first ciliated cells appear on the posterior face of the trachea. The secondary ciliogenesis starts around granular cytoplasmic material (deuterosome) located at the apical pole of the surface epithelial cells. This dense material is surrounded by filaments and microtubules which organize themselves into procentrioles, then into centrioles. If the maturation and elongation of procentrioles are synchronous around a single deuterosome, various degrees of differentiation can be seen between the numerous clusters within a single cell and a few centrioles can extend fibers out and form procentrioles. Procentrioles grow, move under the plasma membrane, and rise perpendicularly toward the lumen to form basal corpuscles. Each corpuscle is rapidly covered by electron-dense microfibrillar material to form a ciliary stalk that either develops inside a ciliary vesicle or under the thickened plasma membrane. Between the long and numerous microvilli, the extending microtubules raise the apical plasma membrane and give rise to the ciliary stalk with an axonema that grows rapidly, made up of a pair of central tubules, with nine pairs of peripheral doublets extending two dynein arms. The basal corpuscles are initially low in number and are poorly orientated. They further arrange perpendicularly to the surface when the rootlets grow down and the ciliary beating becomes efficient (146). Compound cilia are observed during the active period of ciliogenesis at mid-gestation (40). The number of mature ciliated cells increases progressively until 24 weeks. From alveolar phase until birth, ciliated cells represent more than 90% of the cells that line the lumen, and the ciliary waves can be observed by scanning electron microscopy (40). The cystic fibrosis transmembrane conductance regulator (CFTR) protein, a cl-channel, is located at the apical domain of ciliated cells by 24 weeks, during the alveolar phase of development (42). The maturation of the ciliated cells occurs much earlier in humans than in animal models (83, 99) and the ratio of ciliated cells to secretory cells is much higher in neonates than in adults. Several cytokeratins—5, 7, 8, 18, 19—can be detected in the columnar cells of human fetal or adult respiratory surface epithelium (15). These intermediate filaments are attached to desmosal plaques that join the lateral cytoplasmic expansions through the narrow apical or large basal intercellular spaces. Ciliated cells form many desmosome attachments with basal cells (27) and other adjacent cells but do not form hemidesmosome attachments with the BM (38).

Secretory Cells

The first secretory cells appear 1 or 2 weeks after the ciliated cell differentiation. They differentiate initially on the ventral surface of the trachea, opposite the cartilaginous rings. These columnar cells are sparse or gathered into small groups and display a central nucleus and thin, poorly stained apical granules through hematoxylin and eosin staining. Goblet-shaped cells with a basally located nucleus are uncommon in fetal mucosa (Fig. 3.2). The secretory cells secrete both neutral and acidic mucins, as shown by coupled Alcian blue pH 2.5–periodic acid Schiff staining (61). The mucins are almost exclusively composed of sulphomucins. The epithelial mucin consists of a filamentous protein core to which oligosaccharide side chains are attached; these play a role in determining the physical and rheological properties of the mucus. Information concerning the glycoconjugates contained within the secretory granules has been provided through the use of lectins (122). The gene expression of human mucin proteins has been investigated using in situ hybridization (5, 35). MUC2, MUC4 and MUC5 have been shown to be expressed in human airways or in mucous secretions (84). The isolation of these cDNAs should provide useful tools for studying mucin synthesis during differentiation. High levels of MUC1 have been reported by 12.5 weeks throughout the airway epithelium, from bronchi to developing distal end sacs, the highest levels being found in larger airways of human fetuses and in bronchioles and alveoli in adults. Very low levels of MUC2 expression have been detected in the fetal respiratory epithelium of large bronchi over 18 weeks of age. In contrast, abundant MUC2 mRNA is detected in epithelial cells of main bronchi and bronchioles in the adult lung (31). It is therefore unlikely that MUC2 mucin plays a key role in early secretory cell differentiation (21).

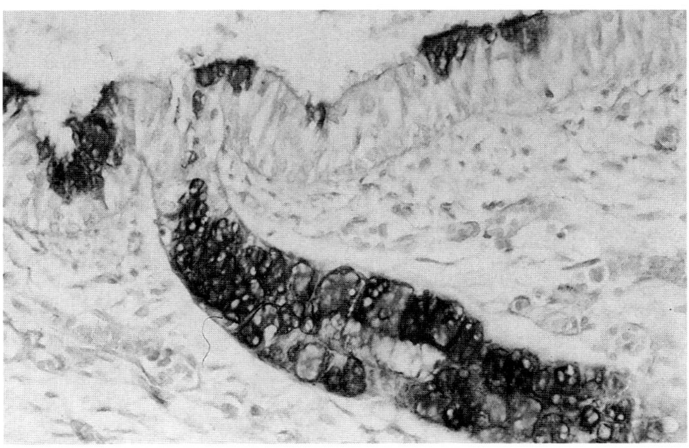

Fig. 3.2 Surface epithelium and developing gland in the trachea at 18 weeks of gestation. Numerous secretions are observed in the apical part of the secretory cells, including a predominance of sulphomucins (*dark secretion*) (high iron diamine/alcian blue, ×250).

At an ultrastructural level, the secretory cells show shorter microvilli and cytoplasm denser under electrons than the ciliated cells and contain fibrillar, electron-lucent material in confluent granules. A few granules are more heterogenous with darker areas. Cells containing electron-dense granules resembling those of rat serous cells are uncommon, but they can be observed in human fetal and small adult bronchi and bronchioles (61). Few cells show lipid vacuoles. Under scanning electron microscope, exocytic secretory granules bulge out of the surface epithelium and are associated with mature ciliated cells and undifferentiated cells: showing short microvilli (Fig. 3.3). Secretory cells contain filaments of cytokeratins 5, 9, 18 and form desmosome attachments with other columnar cells and basal cells.

Secretory cells become increasingly numerous in the surface epithelium during the first half of pregnancy, but from the 19th week on, their number decreases progressively, whereas the ciliated cells continue to differentiate. The decreasing number of secretory cells, associated with the differentiation of ciliated cells, raises the hypothesis that secretory cells may be involved in ciliary maturation and differentiation (40). Ultrastructural images showing ciliogenesis in the apical cytoplasm of secreting cells that already contain mature granules suggest that secretory cells play a role in ciliogenesis (40). The contribution to ciliogenesis of preciliated cells or

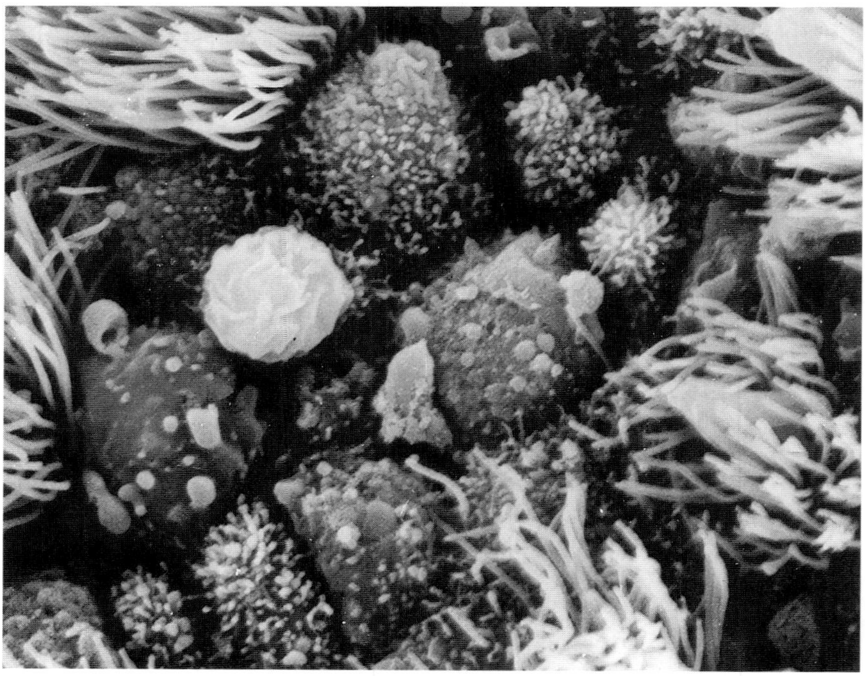

Fig. 3.3 Scanning electron microscopy of human fetal trachea at 16 weeks of gestation showing a few mature ciliated cells, and secretory and undifferentiated cells with short microvilli (×4000).

poorly differentiated cells, previously reported in hamsters, and this has been shown in human fetuses as well (83). This transitional carpet of secretory cells seems to play a role in ciliogenesis and facilitates the protection of the mucous membrane while awaiting the development and secretory functions of the glands, which appear later. The processes of secretory cell differentiation and mucosecretion observed during development are very similar to those observed in altered bronchial epithelium after infection (41).

Clara Cells

Clara cells are columnar secretory cells lining the distal bronchi and the bronchioles, making up about 20% of the cell population of the distal airways in adult humans (37). They are also frequently referred to as nonciliated bronchiolar epithelial cells. Together with ciliated and neuroendocrine cells, Clara cells form a simple and thin epithelium, without basal and goblet cells. Their apical domain bulges into the airway lumen, between the numerous ciliated cells (140). During the period of maturation, these cells protrude slightly into the bronchiolar lumen and their lateral and subluminal plasma membranes are joined by tight junctions. A few scattered and small, electron-dense granules can be observed within an abundant cytoplasmic glycogen (61). Mature cells form dome-like protrusions exhibiting a gradual loss of glycogen in the electron-dense cytoplasm, along with increasing ribosomal content and larger and irregularly shaped electron-dense granules 500–600 nm in diameter, as in adults. Smooth endoplasmic reticulum is generally absent in humans, but it is abundant in rodents.

Most studies on the development and differentiation of Clara cells have been carried out in animal models whose distribution differs from that observed in humans, especially along the proximal airways where Clara cells are numerous in rodents and absent in humans (61, 118). Clara cells secrete a 10 kDa protein (CC10) that can be detected in lung lavage fluid and in amniotic fluid (8, 118). This protein has been used as an immunomarker to study the numerical growth and distribution of Clara cells in human fetuses (6). The first Clara cells were detected by 15 weeks of gestation and were arranged in small clusters of 3 to 5 cells, mainly at the branchings of bronchioles. These cells show large apical projections reaching the airway lumen. The number of clusters increases with age and isolated CC10-reactive cells can be detected at over 22 weeks of age; bronchiolar epithelium includes 11.2% of Clara cells at 24 weeks. In bronchi, Clara cells are less common (5.4% of bronchial epithelium) and are mainly located close to and in the proximal part of the ciliated duct of bronchial glands.

The CC10 protein is the major protein secreted by Clara cells. The degree of sequence identities varies among species (55). A number of functions have been proposed for CC10 protein, although its actual function in humans remain unclear. Clara cells also produce carbohydrate components of pulmonary surfactant, the low-molecular-weight antileucoprotease (61), and two of the major constituent proteins of pulmonary surfactant, the apoproteins A and B (SP-A and SP-B) (85, 143). Human SP-A-immunoreactive nonciliated cells appear along the terminal bronchioles by 29 weeks and increase in number until 39 weeks (33). In larger bronchi, a few positive cells are observed in main and segmental bronchi at 21 weeks of gestational age. Messenger RNAs of the other surfactant proteins, pro-SP-B and SP-C, are detected in bronchi and bronchioles from 15 weeks of gestation. SP-A, SP-B, and SP-C are expressed primarily in distal conducting and terminal airway epithelium of human fetus, well in advance of surfactant lipid synthesis or physiologic requirements for producing pulmonary surfactant at the time of birth [(33, 67); see also Chap. 4].

These nonciliated cells act as progenitor cells for ciliated and Clara cells in the bronchioles (37, 63). Mature Clara cells, however, no longer express SP-C. In developing mouse lung, it was shown that CGRP, CC10, and SP-A were co-expressed in most or all cells of the distal lung epithelium at embryonic days 13–15, and later became restricted to different cell lineages. This transient expression in progenitor cells of gene products characteristic of diverse differentiated cell types may reflect an underlying mechanism of gene regulation that requires further study (143). This is discussed further in Chapter 4.

Basal Cells

During development, basal cells are derived from an undifferentiated columnar epithelium along proximal airways. These cells are the last differentiated cells to appear (83, 99). The number of basal cells present in the airway epithelium is different at various airway levels and in different species (39). It appears to be related to the diameter of the airways and to the height of the epithelium. Basal cells are more numerous in the trachea where the epithelium is pseudostratified and taller than in distal airways, and they are absent in the bronchioles where ciliated and Clara cells make large contact with BM.

The shape of basal cells appears to be more related to the height of the epithelium than to the number of basal cells present in the epithelium. They usually show a cuboidal or triangular shape, but can be flattened, columnar, or pyramidal. Their nucleus occupies a large proportion of the electron-dense cytoplasm containing ribosomes and many mitochondria. During gestation, basal cells express cytokeratins 5, 8, 18, and 19, and progressively lose cytokeratin 18. Cytokeratin 14, usually identified in basal cells of the adult epithelium can only be detected in a few basal cells in human fetuses [Fig. 3.4: (15)], but it is absent (98) or exceptional (15) in normal adult bronchial epithelium. Cytokeratins 10 and 14 are uncommon in normal surface epithelial cells, but they can be observed in basal cells of dysplastic epithelium (98).

Hemidesmosomes are a unique structural characteristic feature of basal cells representing an anatomic marker of these cells. They are attached through an integrin-based mechanism to the underlying basement membrane and stroma (47). The basal cell surface not attached to the basement membrane is smooth or forms in-

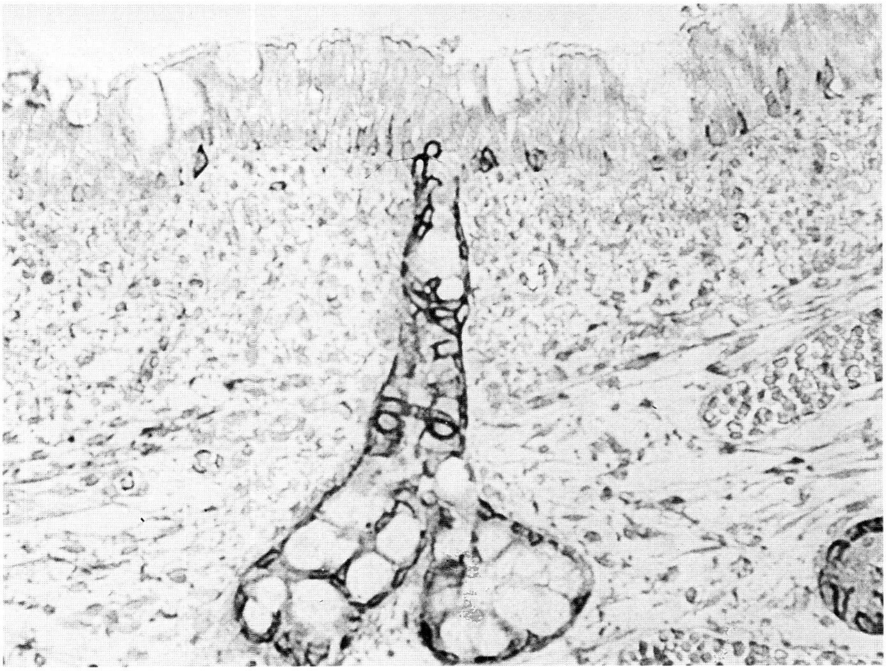

Fig. 3.4 Immunolocalization of cytokeratin 14 in surface human fetal trachea at 20 weeks of gestation. A few basal cells are stained in the surface epithelium as are cells lining the glandular duct and myoepithelial cells in the submucosal glands (×100).

terdigitations with adjacent cells and shows desmosome attachments with adjacent cells (39).

DIFFERENTIATION AND MATURATION OF SUBMUCOSAL GLANDS

The glands begin to develop at the superior and posterior poles of the trachea at the beginning of the 13th week of gestation and appear at the carina level by 14 weeks. In the bronchia, they develop according to a cephalocaudal progression and concentrate in the angles of branching (99). They are never observed in the small bronchi and bronchioles. Each gland develops from an invagination of the surface epithelium where the cells located at the basal part of the epithelium multiply, form a cellular bud that grows into the mesenchyme, then forms a lumen while the cells begin to release a mucosecretion (Fig. 3.2). The underlying extremity of the glands continues to bud and branch out to form mucous tubules and acini (29, 87, 132, 133). The mucous cells, which are polyhedral, possess a basal nucleus and pale cytoplasm and secrete both neutral and acidic mucins. These mucins correspond to the sialomucins and sulphomucins (61). In electron microscopic observations, these glands contain numerous mucous cells with clear, bulky secretory granules that push the nucleus toward the base of the cells. Using immunostaining techniques, markers of serous cells, such as the lysozyme and antileucoprotease, were found through electron microscopy, within the clear granules of the glandular cells as early as 16 weeks of gestation (61). During maturation, the serous cells, which are rich in lysozyme, have a median nucleus and contain dark granules at their apical pole that are sometimes heterogeneous. At the optical level, the first characteristic eosinophilic and pyramidal serous cells appear in the glands of the trachea by 24 weeks, form crescent shapes about the mucous acini, and contain a higher level of enzymes (69). In the peripheral bronchi, the crescent-shaped serous acini are found at the end of gestation and continue to develop during the first 2 years of postnatal life. The proteins secreted by serous cells play an important role in protecting the respiratory tract against bacterial colonization (41). These cells also express CFTR protein in fetuses (42) and in adults (35, 58).

Myoepithelial cells are the third type of cells found in the acini. They appear as spindle or stellar cells located in close contact with the glandular basement membrane. Each myoepithelial cell covers a large surface at the periphery of acini. They show a thin rim of spreading cytoplasm and are difficult to identify without any marker. They can be visualized using immunohistochemistry and antibodies raised against intermediate microfilaments such as cytokeratin 14, which are specifically associated with α-actin filaments. They can be identified during the second trimester of gestation in human fetuses, before the apparition of serous cells; their number is relatively high in the fetus (Fig. 3.4). They play a key role in the release of secretory granules in the glandular lumen. Their role in gland development and glandular cell regeneration remains unknown.

Secretions of the seromucous acini and mucous tubules are released in collecting ducts, where narrow lumens are lined by undifferentiated cuboidal and columnar cells. These cells express cytokeratin 14 (Fig. 3.4) and show a high degree of proliferation. The expression of GRP-R in a few cells of the ducts of submucosal glands in postnatal lungs suggests that this neuroendocrine component may be involved in mucus secretion (136). The collecting ducts are connected to main ducts (ciliated ducts) that open at the surface of the tracheobronchial mucosa. There size increases after birth.

The mechanisms controlling the development and regeneration of acini and ducts are still unclear. Submucosal gland progenitor cells have been identified within the surface airway epithelium in a bronchial xenograft model (34). Recombinant retroviruses applied to this model demonstrated that more than one airway progenitor cell was involved in the initial stages of gland development. Reconstruction experiments in this model showed that 27% of the glands contained more than one duct to the surface airway epithelium and suggested that submucosal glands can communicate through an interactive process of gland morphogenesis. This novel mechanism of gland development could play a key role in glandular remodeling and secretion in airway diseases.

ROLE OF EXTRACELLULAR MATRIX COMPONENTS AND RECEPTORS IN CELL DIFFERENTIATION

Throughout developmental branching morphogenesis, regional specification as well as epithelial cell differentiation of the respiratory tract are dependent on a complex network of interactions among cells and their intermediate filaments, extracellular matrix (ECM) components, and cell surface receptors. The high degree of epithelial cell proliferation progressively decreases when the cells become polarized and begin their differentiation (78). These changes are mediated by integrins and different ECM components in the BM or in the subepithelial mesenchyme (32).

Integrins

Integrins play a critical role in the interactions occurring between cells and the ECM. They may be involved in the mechanisms of signal transduction by affecting the organization of the cellular cytoskeleton through their cytoplasmic domains. Integrins are a large family of heterodimeric transmembrane glycoproteins that were initially identified as receptors for components of the ECM. Through different signaling pathways, they mediate migration, proliferation and cell adhesion, and modulate epithelial cell differentiation (22, 114). Each integrin consists of two noncovalently linked unrelated subunits: one of the 12 known α subunits and one of the 8 known β subunits. Both α and β subunits are transmembrane glycoproteins with large amino-terminal domains, single hydrophobic transmembrane sequences, and carboxy-terminal cytoplasmic domains. The pattern of integrin expression is remarkably similar in most surface epithelia. Integrin receptors link the ECM with the intracellular cytoskeletal network via talin, vinculin, and α actinin. Integrin signaling requires the activation of protein tyrosine kinases and GPT-binding proteins that control cell adhesion as well as formation of the actin cytoskeleton and activation of intracellular signaling cascades (94).

Both α and β chains contribute to the distinct binding specificities of each integrin molecule. The arginine-glycine-aspartate (RGD) sequence on several molecules of the ECM is the binding site recognized by integrins. The binding pattern is complex; several integrins bind more than one ligand and different integrins also bind the same molecule. The β1 chain is most commonly involved in cell adhesion to the BM and connective tissue molecules. In mouse embryos, it has been shown that RGD-dependent integrins, including α3β1, α5β1, and αvβ3, play a role in lung branching morphogenesis (105). One receptor for laminin and collagen (α2 integrin subunit) was only located in epithelial cells at branch tips (142), although other receptors for the same ligands (α3 and α6 integrin subunits) were expressed in the entire epithelium. The subcellular distribution of α3 and α6 subunits in young epithelia became progressively basally restricted with epithelial polarization and maturation. Receptor for fibronectin (α5β1) was predominantly expressed in circumferentially arranged myofibroblasts surrounding the developing proximal airways (105).

The distribution of integrins was recently studied in the very early stages of human lung development during the first trimester. The α2, α5, α6, αv, and β1 subunits were detected in plasma membranes of all epithelial cells budding and branching in the mesenchyme (23). When the undifferentiated cells were polarized, they expressed α3, α6, and β1 subunits on the plasma membrane facing the BM. The membrane redistribution of α3, α6, and β1 integrin subunits suggests that they play a role in cellular polarization and attachment (23, 142). Laminin integrin receptors were studied in human fetuses over 14 weeks of gestation (134). During the late pseudoglandular stage (14–16 weeks), α2 integrin subunit was restricted to epithelial branch tips having a pericellular distribution that was absent in the nearest developing proximal airway epithelium, but immunoreactivity was strong in all bronchial epithelial cells in the larger bronchi. This suggests that this integrin subunit is unlikely to play a role in epithelial cell polarity, but it could have a role in epithelial cell differentiation. The α3 subunit was located in the lateral and basal domains of bronchial epithelium and α6 subunit was confined to the basal aspect of bronchial epithelial cells. The β4 subunit was lacking during that period but was detected in an interrupted and weak manner over 16 weeks in the basal aspect of bronchial cells. The α6β4 integrin, a hemidesmosomal associated protein, may be a marker of basal cells, the last epithelial cells to differentiate. Although the role of these integrins is obvious in cell polarization through their interaction with intracellular cytoskeleton filaments and ECM components, their role in epithelial cell differentiation is still unclear. Only α6β4 integrin was shown to be involved in the assemblage of hemidesmosomes, which are considered specific to basal cells. In the glands, α2, α3, α4, α6, and β1 integrin subunits were expressed in both myoepithelial and secretory epithelial cells while α5, αv, and β4 were only detected in myoepithelial cells (23).

In human adults, collagen and laminin receptors, such as α2β1 and α3β1 integrins are diffusely expressed in all bronchial epithelial cells, with the highest level of expression being in the basal surface of cells (86) and in bronchial smooth muscle (26). One receptor for laminin 5, α6β4 integrin, is principally expressed at the basal surface of basal cells (134) and is concentrated in hemidesmosomes and spatially associated with keratin-containing tonofilaments (47). Receptors for tenascin, such as α9β1 or αvβ5, and receptors for vitronectin are constitutively expressed in basal airway epithelial cells, although these two ligands are distributed below the BM in the subepithelial connective tissue (114). Receptors for fibronectin, such as α5β1 and αvβ6 integrin, are not detected in normal bronchial epithelial cells, but their expression can be induced in vitro or in vivo in patients with bronchial diseases (114, 138). In such conditions, these two integrins are likely to be implied in the regulation of cell proliferation—αvβ6 as a promotor and α5β1 as an inhibitor (3)—but their role in cell differentiation has not been demonstrated.

Basement Membrane Components

The BM can be visualized by electron microscopy as two component layers: the lamina lucida, or lamina rara, and the lamina densa. This BM is separated from the underlying interstitial mesenchyme or connective tissue by a third layer: the lamina fibroreticularis. The BMs are self-assembled from polymers of type IV collagen, laminin, and proteoglycans. The type IV collagen network serves as the scaffold where cross-shaped laminin molecules interact through an entactin bridge and then bind proteoglycan through their glycosaminoglycan components (76). The composition of the pulmonary BM undergoes changes during branching morphogenesis (4, 72, 114) and maturation (1).

Type IV Collagen

The BM is located continuously along the tracheal and proximal bronchial epithelium before 12 weeks of gestation, when the glands are not yet developed. Immunohistochemistry has shown type IV collagen to have a regular and linear distribution along the BM that lines the undifferentiated columnar epithelial cells. During gland formation, the BM is stretched and pushed down into the subepithelial mesenchyme by epithelial cells that proliferate at the basal part of the epithelium and form a glandular bud. At the tips of the buds, the immunoreactivity for type IV collagen is weak and discontinuous (71). This change is very similar to that reported during lung branching morphogenesis. When the bronchial buds elongate and form tubules, the columnar epithelium is lined by type IV collagen. However, collagen α1(IV) and α2(IV) immunofluorescence labeling shows patchy basal distribution and low levels of type IV collagen at branch-tip epithelium (72, 142). In fetal mouse lung, epithelial cells expressing α2β11 integrin also produce type IV collagen and laminin 1 mRNAs. This suggests that α2β1 integrin may be involved in the process of collagen–laminin matrix production or assembly and in the formation of BM at the growing tips (142). Studies of collagen-binding receptors in fetal rat lung cells have produced conflicting results (19). When the receptors were isolated from lung during the pseudoglandular (day 18) or saccular period (day 21), distal epithelial cells expressed α3β1 integrin and α3 mRNA, but not α2β1, these cells did not bind to collagen substrata.

It has been demonstrated that, during fetal rat lung development, high epithelial cell proliferative activity is associated with the degradation of type IV collagen and the presence of metalloproteinases (4, 14). Type IV collagenase (72 kDa metalloproteinase enzyme) is secreted by both epithelial and mesenchymal cells and major gelatinase was produced by fibroblasts. About 80% of the enzymes were present in the active form. The rapid growth of epithelial cells is associated with a high level of cell turnover which permits the reorganization of the tissue. When cell division slows down, epithelial cell polarization and differentiation take place and type IV collagen synthesis increases (4). This BM component is bound to intracellular cytoskeleton filaments through α2β1 and α3β1 integrins (114) and it favors epithelial cell polarization, but its role in ciliated or secretory cell differentiation has not been demonstrated.

Laminin

Laminins are cross-shaped molecules consisting of three disulfide-linked polypeptide subunits (α, β, and γ chains). According to recent nomenclature, several laminins can be identified: laminin 1 (α1-β1-γ1), the major form; laminin 2 (α2-β1-γ1); laminin 3 (α1-β2-γ1); and laminin 5 (α3-β3-γ2). Laminins influence lung development. The addition of anti-laminin antibodies to embryonic lung cultures markedly diminishes tube formation and branching morphogenesis (113). In a mouse model, in situ hybridization techniques have demonstrated expression of β1 and γ1 mRNAs in both mesenchymal cells and epithelial tubules and buds, but α1 mRNA was expressed only in epithelial buds (131, 142). In human fetal lung, mRNAs for laminin have been detected as early as 10 weeks of gestation. Although the degree and the site of expression of the different chains may vary, the mRNA for β1 subunit was expressed in both epithelial and mesenchymal cells, the mRNA for γ1 subunit was only expressed in epithelial cells, and the α1 subunit could not be detected (72).

The immunolocalization of laminin along the BM in the developing lung produced results according to the techniques used. Polyclonal antibodies without any chain specificity showed a continuous and linear immunoreactivity along the BM facing polarized columnar epithelium, irrespective of its degree of differentiation, but focal disruptions of laminin were observed at the tips of the growing buds at 12 weeks of development (72). Using monoclonal antibodies specific to the various chains of laminin, Virtanen et al. (134) recently showed that the distribution of laminin chains forming the BM changed during development. Laminin subunits α1, α3, β3, and γ1 were widely distributed in BM at any age of lung development along bronchial epithelium and at the tips of the growing epithelial buds, regardless of the degree of cell proliferation and differentiation. This suggests that these chains do not play a specific role in epithelial cell polarity and differentiation. The α3 and β3 chains, which are components of laminin 5 (α3-β3-γ2), have been shown to be involved in hemidesmosome attachments in several epithelia (47). Their role in basal cell differentiation has not yet been demonstrated in the respiratory epithelium. The presence of α1 and γ1 laminin subunits and the absence or low expression of α1 and γ1 mRNAs can result from the slow turnover of these subunits in lung tissue, and may be due to mRNAs that are not detected by the techniques used. α2 laminin subunit showed a transient and exclusive expression along growing epithelial buds. This α2 subunit, a component of laminin 2 (α2-β1-γ1), is more likely to be involved in epithelial cell budding and proliferation than in bronchial epithelial cell differentiation.

During the pseudoglandular stage, laminin β1 was detected along the BM of the growing epithelial buds but was absent along the BMs of the developing larger bronchi. Later on, during the canalicular stage and in adults, this β1 subunit was present in all BMs of the epithelium lining bronchi and alveoli. This suggests that this component of laminin 1 (α1-β1-γ1) and laminin 6 (α3-β1-γ1) probably plays no role in cell polarity, but is a good candidate for regulating cell differentiation .

Laminin β2, a component of laminin 3 (α1-β2-γ1) and laminin 7 (α3-β2-γ1), has been shown to be abundant in the BM of the epithelial tubules and of developing larger bronchi during the pseudoglandular stage, but this subunit was not detected later on—neither in BMs of large or distal bronchi of fetuses during the canalicular stage nor in BMs of adult bronchi (134). This suggests a transient role for laminin β2 in the first steps of epithelial cell polarization and maturation in bronchial fetal development and in the shift from laminin 3 or 7 to laminin 1.

Laminin, entactin, and chondroitin sulfate proteoglycan exhibit a comparable distribution in airway BM of postnatal developing and adult rat lungs (111). Entactin is synthesized by mesenchymal cells during development (131). Its functional implication in bronchial development is unknown.

Proteoglycans

Chondroitin and heparan sulfate proteoglycans have been detected in rat airway BMs during development (111). These molecules form the extracellular domain of syndecans, which present a single polypeptide core protein to which the proteoglycans are attached, and a cytoplasmic domain that interacts with the actin cytoskeleton (9). In the developing mouse lung, syndecan was detected on the basolateral and lateral surfaces of epithelial cells and in the underlying mesenchyme during the pseudoglandular stage. During the next canalicular stage, syndecan was localized almost exclusively to the lateral surfaces of the columnar epithelium and absent in the mesenchyme. This change is associated with a reduced size of glycosaminoglycans (12). These structural changes could alter the interaction of cells with the ECM, thereby affecting cellular shape, organization, and differentiation.

Extracellular Matrix Components of the Interstitial Mesenchyme

Interstitial connective tissue consists of fibrillar collagens, elastin fibers, proteoglycans, fibronectin, and tenascin. These last two components are more specific to developmental matrix and play an important role in lung organogenesis. Fibrillar collagens (types I, III, V, and VI) are the major structural components of the connective tissue and are mainly present around large airways. A zone of staining for accumulated type I procollagen has been identified subjacent to the BM in the pseudoglandular and canalicular phase of fetal human lung, although it was not accompanied by a corresponding increase in mRNA expression. This could reflect a local difference in the proteolytic processing of secreted type I procollagen or in the metabolism of liberated amino-terminal epitopes (28). Interstitial collagenase (MMP-1), which degrades type I and III collagens, shows little activity in the lung during fetal life (4). Elastic fibers consist of elastin, an insoluble protein, and microfibrils, including two kinds of proteins: fibrillin and microfibril-associated glycoproteins. Elastin increases during fetal development (112).

Fibronectin

Fibronectin, a dimeric glycoprotein, is abundant in embryonic tissue and plays an important role during morphogenesis and cell migration. In murine lung development, fibronectin and one of its receptors (α5β1) have been localized in the peribronchial mesenchyme and in the areas of airway bifurcation, indicating a possible role in cleft formation (106). In rabbits, fibronectin immunostaining increases throughout fetal development, remains elevated in newborns, and decreases in adults (119). In contrast, fibronectin transcripts appear to be most abundant during the pseudoglandular period, before the maximal fibronectin level is achieved. The accumulation of fibronectin mRNA in mesenchyme of developing lung tissue is probably regulated in a cell-specific manner (119). The role of fibronectin and its specific integrins, such as α5β1 and αvβ6 in bronchial epithelial cell differentiation has not been demonstrated.

Tenascin

Tenascin is an oligomeric glycoprotein that is present in the developing mesenchyme. At least three tenascins (C, X, and R) have been identified (36). They share an amino-terminal domain where subunits connect to form trimers and hexamers, a series of EGF-like domains, fibronectin-like repeats, and a carboxy-terminal fibrinogen domain. In studies of embryonic chick lung, tenascin was localized in the BMs at the tip of epithelial branches, with less labeling occurring toward more proximal, earlier-formed regions of epithelial tubes (68). Tenascin mRNA was restricted to the tips of budding bronchial epithelium and absent in older epithelium and dense mesenchyme. A spatially and temporarily restricted distribution of tenascin-C has also been reported in developing rat lungs (145). A small amount was detected during the pseudoglandular stage and a dramatic accumulation of tenascin protein and mRNA was found in the early postnatal period, with a subsequent reduction. Electron microscopy has shown tenascin-C to be associated with a layer of fibrillar collagen located on the mesenchymal side of the BM. Antibodies against tenascin-C inhibit airway branching, but although this protein is abundant in the subepithelial mesenchyme, its role in airway development is unclear, as mice with a complete lack of tenascin C develop normally (109). In human adults, tenascin is located mainly in the subepithelial mesenchyme around proximal airways and shows weak and patchy staining in distal airways. The α9β1 integrin, the receptor of tenascin, is found predominantly in basal cells of the bronchial epithelium (138).

During development, these subepithelial ECM components are commonly associated with myofibroblast-like cells containing α smooth-muscle actin, which surround the proximal bronchi and are gathered in the clefts between branching tubes (77). Although the role of ECM components and their receptors has been clearly demonstrated in branching morphogenesis during fetal airway development (see Chap. 1), their role in bronchial epithelial cell differentiation remains hypothetical even though they are abundantly distributed in embryonic and fetal lungs. The different subunits of integrins and laminins are still good candidates for influencing epithelial polarization and differentiation. Because few reports have addressed the possible action of ECM components in type II pneumocyte maturation (see Chap. 4), further studies are needed to assess the importance of ECM in both surface and glandular airway epithelium differentiation.

ROLE OF GROWTH FACTORS IN AIRWAY EPITHELIAL CELL DIFFERENTIATION

The process of branching morphogenesis and epithelial cell differentiation in lung development is regulated by epithelial–mesenchymal interaction. A number of growth factors (GF) bind to and are active on ECM and epithelial cells (62, 89). These GFs were first recognized as mitogenic factors for cultured epithelial cells and fibroblasts; they are expressed very early in embryos (45). There is now considerable evidence that these GFs not only regulate cell proliferation but are multifunctional, promoting cell motility, differentiation, ECM synthesis, and epithelial cell maturation (162). Autocrine and paracrine interactions between epithelial cells and mesenchyme control epithelial and mesenchymal cell proliferation and probably cell phenotype. They are associated with ECM and various GF-binding proteins and interact with specific cellular receptors. They are grouped into distinct families on the basis of structural similarities among peptides. Various GFs have been shown to be involved in the process of airway branching and type II pneumocyte maturation (see Chapts. 1 and 4), but little is known about their role in bronchial cell differentiation. Here we will review only the GFs that may regulate the maturation and function of ciliated and secretory cells.

Epidermal Growth Factor and Transforming Growth Factor

Epidermal Growth Factor (EGF) and TGF-α, two members of the EGF family of GFs, have similar biological properties and show a 42% sequence homology. The molecular analysis of murine fetal tissue has demonstrated that TGF-α is more highly expressed than EGF during fetal development. Both TGF-α and EGF mediate their actions through binding to the extracellular domain of a common transmembrane glycoprotein receptor (EGF receptor) with activation of the tyrosine kinase in the intracellular domain. The role of EGF in lung organogenesis was clearly demonstrated in 1980 by Goldin and Opperman (45): grafting agarose pellets containing EGF alongside the embryonic chick tracheal epithelium induced supernumerary tracheal buds. Furthermore, in rat or mouse embryonic lung explants, EGF was shown to stimulate cell proliferation in both mesenchyme and epithelium, resulting in an increased branching activity, or an enlargement of the lung (43, 137). Mice lacking EGF receptor showed epithelial immaturity and multiorgan failure (88).

The TGF-α and EGF mRNAs appear to be confined to the mesenchymal cells, mainly to the dense connective tissue surrounding the large bronchial and vascular structures and the pleura. Through in situ hybridization, mesenchymal cells have been shown to express only low levels of GFs transcripts during the pseudoglandular period, although cell proliferation was active, and the labeling was intense during the following canalicular and alveolar periods (108, 129). Epidermal growth factor, TGF-α and their receptor have been localized by immunohistochemistry in human fetal (Fig. 3.5) and postnatal lung and trachea . At any age, they exhibited a similar distribution in all the cells of the bronchial surface epithelium and in the serous cells

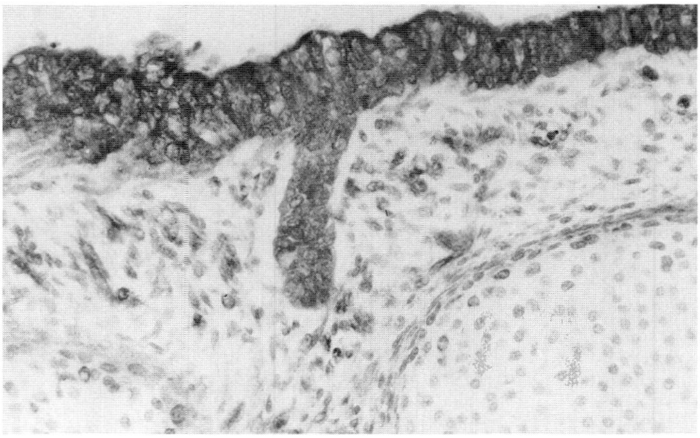

Fig. 3.5 Immunohistochemistry TGF-α reveals in all cells of the surface epithelium and glands of human fetal trachea at 16 weeks of gestation (×250).

of the submucosal glands (64, 108, 124, 128). This suggests that both EGF and TGF-α are mediated mainly by paracrine interactions between epithelial and mesenchymal cells. The colocalization of these GFs and their receptor in bronchial cells during late gestation and postnatal period, when the degree of cell proliferation is very low, suggests that these GFs are also involved in lung maturation. It has been shown that EGF promoted maturation of distal airways and accelerated type II pneumocyte differentiation in the lung of the fetal rhesus monkey (100). Epidermal growth factor also stimulated surfactant production in human lung explants. The lungs of newborn rats with EGF deficiency were small, with abnormal morphology and a decreased iSP-A immunoreactivity in both Clara cells and type II pneumocytes (102). Both EGF and TGF-α increased expression of α2β1 and up-regulated surface levels of α5β1 and αvβ6 integrins (fibronectin and tenascin receptors) in primary cultured human airway epithelial cells (135). They combine with other factors, especially TGF-β, to play a key role in epithelial–mesenchymal interaction.

Injection of EGF into the amniotic fluid of fetal rhesus monkeys during late gestation accelerated the differentiation of tracheal mucus secretory cells and also increased the amount of secretory product released in the airway lumen, but this had no further effect on cell proliferation (126). The reduction in EGF concentration in rat tracheal epithelial cell culture medium resulted in a decrease in the percentage of mucous cells and a high reduction in mucin secretions (49). In addition to a decrease in mucin glycoprotein, the level of MUC5 mRNA was dramatically decreased. Reinduction of MUC5 mRNA by EGF, after EGF deprivation occurred rapidly, suggests that MUC5 synthesis may be directly regulated by EGF. Epidermal growth factor probably has no role in the process of ciliogenesis as rat tracheal epithelial cell cultured on collagen gel–coated membranes at the air–liquid interface showed an increase in the ratio of ciliated cells when EGF and cholera toxin were removed from the media (22).

Insulin-Like Growth Factors I and II

The IGFs are polypeptides with a structural homology with pro-insulin. Both IGF-I and IGF-II mRNAs are expressed in the mesenchyme of human fetal lung throughout gestation, with expression decreasing after the 20th week, especially for IGF-II (48, 53, 54, 73). They are mainly detected in mesenchymal and endothelial cells, which induce cell proliferation and lung maturation through interaction with the specific cell surface type-1 IGF receptor (104). This receptor, as well as the type-2 IGF receptor, which is thought to target IGF-II to lysosomes for degradation (127), are present in human fetal lung (48). They play a major role in lung development; null mutant newborn mice for type-1 IGF receptor gene die from respiratory failure (79). In rats, both IGF receptor mRNAs were found in epithelium and mesenchyme at day 14 of gestation, but only in mesenchyme at day 18, and no type-1 IGF receptor was detectable in adult airways (80, 103). The actions of IGF-I and IGF-II proteins are likely modulated by specific IGF-binding proteins (IGFBPs) whose expression and abundance vary during development (90). These changes, however, are mainly observed in distal airways and influence respiratory and vascular muscle cell development (79). They probably have no incidence in bronchial epithelium differentiation.

Platelet-Derived Growth Factor

Platelet-derived growth factor (PDGF) is a dimeric molecule consisting of A and B peptide chains that can be combined to form three isoforms (PDGF-AA,-AB,-BB). In fetal rats, these proteins are localized in epithelial and mesenchymal cells during the pseudoglandular stage and their level decreases with advancing gestation (52), although PDGF-mRNA levels increase markedly during late canalicular stage (17). The PDGF receptors are made of two subunits, α and β, with three possible combinations (αα, αβ, ββ). These receptors have been detected in epithelial lung cells (20): PDGF-A mRNA is expressed in the epithelial cells of embryonic lungs, while mRNA for PDGF a-receptor is expressed in the mesenchyme. The epithelial–mesenchymal interaction that they mediate induces DNA synthesis and branching morphogenesis (121). Platelet-derived growth factor stimulates epithelial DNA synthesis and endogenous GFs, such as IGF-I, while fibroblasts, which only express PDGF β-receptor, respond with increased glycosaminoglycan synthesis (20). It has been demonstrated that β1 integrin–mediated signaling induces rapid and transient tyrosine phosphorylation of PDGF β-receptors in human fibroblasts (130). This GF seems to be implicated more in fibroblast-mediated tension and mesenchymal function than in direct epithelial differentiation.

Tumor Necrosis Factor α

Tumor necrosis factor α (TNF-α) was first characterized as a protein released by activated macrophages that is able to induce necrosis in tumors through two TNF receptors expressed in a variety of tissues (93). This growth factor and its receptor have been detected in the mesenchyme adjacent to the branching epithelium in mouse fetal lung and during the late pseudoglandular and canalicular stages, in the subepithelial mesenchyme and to a lesser extent, on the apical surface of respiratory epithelium (60). Supplementation of TNF-α in vitro on embryonic lung primordia has a marked dose-dependent stimulatory effect on branching morphogenesis and SP-A expression (60). In normal adult lung, the 55 kDa TNF-α receptor has been detected in alveolar macrophages, bronchioles, and some vessels (116). Tumor necrosis factor α plays a major role in increased air space epithelial permeability during acute lung inflammation, but its role in bronchial differentiation has not yet been reported.

Fibroblast Growth Factors

Fibroblast growth factors (FGFs) form a heparin-binding family characterized by heparin (and heparan) binding activity and a potent angiogenic activity. Acidic FGF (aFGF), basic FGF (bFGF), and keratinocyte growth factor (KGF) have been localized in the lung (110, 117). The FGFs are ubiquitously present in the ECM in inactive, matrix-bound forms that are activated by extracellular proteinases and heparinases. They bind to specific tyrosine kinase receptors: KGFR, the receptor for KGF and aFGF with a similar affinity, and FGFR-2, with high affinity for aFGF and bFGF. The aFGF has been localized in epithelial cells (ciliated airway cells, Clara cells) and interstitial cells in the alveolar septa and colocalized with EGF during postnatal development. (110). Exogenous KGF or aFGF induced inhibition of branching of cultured fetal rat lung primordia and they distorted lung growth, characterized by cystic dilation of lung buds, fluid distension, increased number of type II pneumocytes, and enhanced transcription of the SP-C gene, although they had only a minimal effect on Clara cell differentiation (118). Keratinocyte growth factor had no effect on expression of integrins on cultured airway epithelial cells (135). In vitro, KGF stimulated fluid secretion in type II pneumocytes and inhibited expression of α subunit of epithelial Na^+ channel (α-Enac) mRNA (148). It controls fetal fluid dynamics and ion transport in a CFTR-independent way.

The bFGF has been detected only in hyaluronidase-digested sections and is present in most of the BM associated with alveoli and in airway epithelium. Its distribution in BM is identical to heparan sulfate proteoglycan. Its receptor has been detected in rats as early as day 13, during the pseudoglandular and canalicular stages, especially in the branching areas and in the mesenchymal cells (51). The bFGF appears to be sequestered by ECM and released when necessary. Its transcription in fibroblasts is stimulated by TGF-β and PDGF (46).

Transforming Growth Factor Beta

The TGF-β family includes multifunctional cytokines. Three isoforms, TGF-β-1, TGF-β-2, and TGF-β-3, have been detected in fetal mouse lung (97). The three TGF-β proteins have been localized to the epithelium but higher levels have been detected in the subepithelium of the bronchi and bronchioles and in the smooth-muscle cells of airways and vessels. In human embryos, TGF-β2 transcripts were detected in undifferentiated lung epithelium at day 43, but were confined to epithelial cells at the growing tips by day 57. Transcripts of TGF-β3 were found in bronchial and bronchiolar epithelial cells, as well as in growing epithelial buds (44). Transcripts of TGF-β1 were found predominantly in the mesenchyme.

In human adults, very high levels of mRNA for the three isoforms of TGF-β were found in connective tissue surrounding the epithelium of airways and in muscular walls of vessels (96). The distribution of TGF-β2 and TGF-β3 proteins was ubiquitous in alveolar macrophages, alveolar and bronchial epithelial cells, and smooth-muscle cells. In contrast, TGF-β1 was absent in epithelial cells along normal airways and present in airway epithelial cells from patients with pulmonary fibrosis (66).

TGF-βs act through TGF-β type I, II, and III receptors without protein kinase activity and are involved in lung development. Biological functions reported for TGF-βs are generally those of TGF-β1. Treatment of cultured human tracheobronchial epithelial cells with TGF-β inhibits cell proliferation (62), induces squamous cell differentiation, and stimulates expression of desmosomal proteins (144). Transforming growth factor β plays a key role in ECM deposition. Rat lung epithelial cells exposed to TGF-β synthesized type I, III, and V collagen (30), modulated fibronectin production (107), and regulated biosynthesis of alternative-splicing isoforms of tenascin (147). During lung branching morphogenesis, TGF-β1 was detected at the epithelial–mesenchymal interfaces of stalks and clefts and showed colocalization with ECM components such as type I and III collagen, fibronectin, and glycosaminoglycans (56). TGF-β1 increased expression of virtually all integrins in mesenchymal cells (57) However, TGF-β1 as well as TGF-β2 and TGF-β3 had no effect on surface expression of integrins constitutively expressed on cultured primary human airway epithelial cells, and only increased expression of the αvβ6 integrin, a receptor for fibronectin and tenascin (135). These results differ from those observed in guinea pig tracheal epithelial cells, which increased expression of integrins in response to TGF-β1 (115); this suggests that these effects are species-specific, or alternatively, that the pattern of integrin expression on bronchial epithelial cells can be significantly altered when cells are placed in culture. In addition to the stimulating effect of TGF-β on production of ECM components by lung fibroblasts, TGF-β inhibits production of collagenase and proteolytic enzymes and stimulates production of tissue inhibitors of metalloproteinases, such as plasminogen activator (62).

The interactions among the various GFs are complex. For example, the combination of EGF and TGF-β1 increased levels of α2β1 and decreased expression of α3β1- and α6-containing integrins (136), and TGF-β1 down-regulated the PDGF-α receptor subtype in human lung fibroblasts (16).

CONCLUSION

Airway epithelial cell differentiation is a complex process that is initiated as early as 10 weeks in the human fetus. Genes of development are likely to be involved in epithelial cell differentiation as they are expressed in a temporal and spatial pattern and modulate the expression of growth factors (85). The isolation and identification of airway stem cells could represent an important step in investigating the factors that regulate airway epithelial cell differentiation. Thus far, however, this objective has not been reached (81). Extensive information has been reported concerning epithelial cell differentiation with the interepithelial and the epithelial-mesenchymal interactions through ECM components, integrins, and GFs. However, the current knowledge remains largely descriptive and further studies with new models are needed to draw out the inner mechanisms of differentiation. Intra-amniotic injections may provide a good way to investigate the effects of various molecules on cell maturation, but, compared with humans, most animal models, especially those using rodents, show at birth a differently constituted and immature bronchial epithelium. In the future, human bronchial xenografts (34) and human fetal airways developed in immunodeficient SCID mice (95) will likely be the best way to approach the complex interactions involved in epithelial cell differentiation.

Supported by the Association Française de Lutte contre la Mucoviscidose and by EC-Network (B10-CT 950284).

REFERENCES

1. Adams, J.C. and F.M. Watt. Regulation of development and differentiation by the extracellular matrix. *Development* 117: 1183–1198, 1993.
2. Adriaensen, D. and D.W. Scheuermann. Neuroendocrine cells and nerves of the lung. *Anat. Rec.* 236: 70–85, 1993.
3. Agrez, M., A. Chen, R.I. Cone, R. Pytela, and D. Sheppard. The αvβ6 integrin promotes proliferation of colon carcinoma cells through a unique region of β6 cytoplasmic domain. *J. Cell Biol.* 127: 547–556, 1994.
4. Arden, M.G., M.A. Spearman, and I.Y.R. Adamson. Degradation of type IV collagen during the development of fetal rat lung. *Am. J. Respir. Cell Mol. Biol.* 9: 99–105, 1993.
5. Audie, J.P., A. Janin, N. Porchet, M.C. Copin, B. Gosselin, and J.P. Aubert. Expression of human mucin genes in respiratory, digestive, and reproductive tracts ascertained by in situ hybridization. *J. Histochem. Cytochem.* 41: 1479–1485, 1993.
6. Barth, P.J., M. Wolf, and A. Ramaswamy. Distribution and number of Clara cells in the normal and disturbed development of the human fetal lung. *Pediatr. Pathol.* 14: 637–651, 1994.
7. Benali, R., J.M. Tournier, M. Chevillard, J.M. Zahm, J.M. Klossek, J. Hinnrasky, D. Gaillard, F.X. Maquart, and E. Puchelle. Tubule formation by human surface respiratory epithelial cells cultured in a three-dimensional collagen lattice. *Am. J. Physiol.* 264 (*Lung Cell. Mol. Physiol.* 8): L183–L192, 1993.
8. Bernard, A., N. Thielemans, R. Lauweryns, J.-P. Langhendries, M. Van Lierde, and M.M. Freund. Clara cell protein in human amniotic fluid: a potential marker of fetal lung growth. *Pediatr. Res.* 36: 775–771, 1994.

9. Bernfield, M.R. and S.D. Banerjee. The turnover of basal lamina glycosaminoglycan correlates with epithelial morphogenesis. *Dev. Biol.* 90: 291–305, 1982.
10. Bienenstock, J., I. Johnston, and D.Y. Perey. Bronchial lymphoid tissue II. Functional characteristics. *Lab. Invest.* 28: 693–698, 1973.
11. Bogue, C.W., L.J. Lou, H. Vasavada, C.M. Wilson, and H.C. Jacobs. Expression of *Hoxb* genes in the developing mouse foregut and lung. *Am. J. Respir. Cell Mol. Biol.* 15: 163–171, 1996.
12. Brauker, J.H., M.S. Trautman, and M. Bernfield. Syndecan, a cell surface proteoglycan, exhibits a molecular polymorphism during lung development. *Dev. Biol.* 147: 285–292, 1991.
13. Breeze, R.G. and E.B. Wheldon. The cells of the pulmonary airways. *Am. Rev. Respir. Dis.* 116: 705–777, 1977.
14. Brenner, C.A., R.R. Rappolee, R.A. Pedersen, and Z. Werr. Genes for extracellular matrix degrading metalloproteinases and their inhibitor, TIMP, are expressed during early mammalian development. *Genes Dev.* 3: 848–859, 1989.
15. Broers, J.L.V., L. de Leij, M.K. Rot, A. ter Haar, E.B. Lane, I.M. Leigh, S.S. Wagenaar, G.P. Vooijs, and F.C.S. Ramaekers. Expression of intermediate filament proteins in fetal and adult human lung tissues. *Differentiation* 40: 119–128, 1989
16. Bronner, J.C., A. Badgett, P M. Lindroos, and A.R. Osornio-Vargas. Transforming growth factor β1 downregulates the platelet-derived growth factor a-receptor subtype on human lung fibroblasts in vitro. *Am. J. Respir. Cell Mol. Biol.* 13: 496–505, 1995.
17. Buch, S., C. Jones, J. Liu, R.N.N. Han, A.K. Tanswell, and M. Post. Differential regulation of platelet-derived growth factor genes in fetal rat lung fibroblasts. *Exp. Cell Res.* 211: 142–149, 1994.
18. Bucher, U. and L. Reid. Development of intrasegmental bronchial tree: the pattern of branching and development of cartilage at various stages of intrauterine life. *Thorax* 16: 207-218, 1961.
19. Caniggia, I., R. Han, J. Liu, J. Wang, A. K. Tanswell, and M. Post. Differential expression of collagen-binding receptors in fetal rat lung cells. *Am. J. Physiol.* 268 (*Lung Cell. Mol. Physiol.* 12): L136–L143, 1995.
20. Caniggia, I., J. Liu, R. Han, S. Buch, K. Funa, K. Tanswell, and, M. Post. Fetal lung epithelial cells express receptors for platelet-derived growth factor. *Am. J. Respir. Cell Mol. Biol.* 9: 54–63, 1993.
21. Chambers J.A., M.A. Hollingsworth , A.E.O. Trezise, and A. Harris. Developmental expression of mucin genes *MUC1* and *MUC2*. *J. Cell Sci.* 107: 413–424, 1994.
22. Clark, E.A. and J.S. Brugge. Integrins and signal transduction pathways: the road taken. *Science* 268: 233–239, 1995.
23. Coraux, C., A. Delplanque, J. Hinnrasky, B. Peault, E. Puchelle, and D. Gaillard. Distribution of integrins during fetal development. *J. Histochem. Cytochem.* 46: 803–810, 1998.
24. Cutz, E., J.E. Gillan, and A.C. Bryan. Neuroendocrine cells in the developing human lung: morphologic and functional considerations. *Pediatr. Pulmonol.* I(Suppl.): S1–S29, 1985.
25. Cutz, E., J.E., Gillan, and D.G. Perrin. Pulmonary neuroendocrine cell system: an overview of cell biology and pathology with emphasis on pediatric lung disease. *Perspect. Pediatr. Pathol.* 18: 32–70, 1995.
26. Damjanovich, L., S.M. Albelda, S.A. Mette, and C.A. Buck. Distribution of integrin cell adhesion receptors in normal and malignant lung tissue. *Am. J. Respir. Cell Mol. Biol.* 6: 197–206, 1992.
27. Danel, D.D. Morphological characteristics of human airway structures. In: *Lung Biology*

in Health and Disease. Environmental Impact on the Airways, edited by J. Chretien and D. Dusser. New York: Marcel Dekker, 1996, p. 19–41.

28. Davila, R.M., D. deMello, and E.C. Crouch. Ontogeny of type I procollagen expression during human fetal lung development. *Am. J. Physiol.* 268 (*Lung Cell. Mol. Physiol.* 12): L309–L320, 1995.
29. De Haller, R. Development of mucus-secreting elements. In: *The Anatomy of the Developing Lung*, edited by J. Emery. London: Heinemann Medical Books, 1969, p. 94–115.
30. DiMari, S.J., A.M. Howe, and M.A. Haralson. Effects of transforming growth factor-β on collagen synthesis by fetal rat lung epithelial cells. *Am. J. Respir. Cell Mol. Biol.* 4: 445–462, 1991.
31. Dohrman, A., T. Tsuda, E. Escudier, M. Cardone, B. Jany, J. Gum, Y. Kim, and C. Basbaum. Distribution of lysozyme and mucin (*MUC2* and *MUC3*) mRNA in human bronchus. *Exp. Lung Res.* 20: 367–380, 1994.
32. Dunsmore, S.E., and D.E. Rannels. Extracellular matrix biology in the lung. *Am. J. Physiol.* 270 (*Lung Cell Mol. Physiol.* 14): L3–L27, 1996.
33. Endo, H. and T. Oka. An immunohistochemical study of bronchial cells producing surfactant protein A in the developing human fetal lung. *Early Hum. Dev.* 25: 149–156, 1991.
34. Engelhardt, J.F., H. Schlossberg, J.R. Yankaskas, and L. Dudus. Progenitor cells of the adult human airway involved in submucosal gland development. *Development* 121: 2031–2046, 1995.
35. Engelhardt, J.F., J.R. Yankaskas, S.A. Ernst, Y. Yang, C.R. Marino, R.C. Boucher, J.A. Cohn, and J.M. Wilson. Submucosal glands are the predominant site of CFTR expression in the human bronchus. *Nat. Genet.* 2: 240–247, 1992.
36. Erickson, H.P. Tenascin-C, tenascin-R and tenascin-X: a family of talented proteins in search of functions. *Curr. Opin. Cell Biol.* 5: 869–876, 1993.
37. Evans, M.J., L.J. Cabral-Anderson, and G. Freeman. Role of the Clara cell in renewal of the bronchiolar epithelium. *Lab. Invest.* 38: 648–656, 1978.
38. Evans, M.J., R.A. Cox, S.G. Shami, B. Wilson, and C.G. Plopper. The role of basal cells in attachment of columnar cells to the basal lamina of the trachea. *Am. J. Respir. Cell Mol. Biol.* 1: 463–469, 1989.
39. Evans, M. J. and P.C. Moller. Biology of airway basal cells. *Exp. Cell Res.* 17: 513–531, 1991.
40. Gaillard, D., A.V. Lallemand, A.F. Petit, and E.S. Puchelle. In vivo ciliogenesis in human fetal tracheal epithelium. *Am. J. Anat.* 185: 415–28, 1989.
41. Gaillard D. and M.C. Plotkowski. Changes in airway structure after airway infection. In: *Lung Biology in Health and Disease. Environmental Impact on the Airways*, edited by J. Chretien and D. Dusser. New York: Marcel Dekker, 1996, p. 471–505.
42. Gaillard, D., S. Ruocco, A. Lallemand, W. Dalemans, J. Hinnrasky, and E. Puchelle. Immunohistochemical localization of cystic fibrosis transmembrane conductance regulator in human fetal airway and digestive mucosa. *Pediatr. Res.* 36: 137–143, 1994.
43. Ganser, G.L., G.P. Stricklin, and L.M. Matrisian. EGF and TGF-α influence in vitro lung development by the induction of matrix-degrading metalloproteinases. *Int. J. Dev. Biol.* 35: 453–461, 1991.
44. Gatherer, D., P. Ten Dijke, D.T. Baird, and R.J. Akhurst. Expression of TGFβ isoforms during first trimester human embryogenesis. *Development* 110: 445–460, 1990.
45. Goldin, C.V. and L.A. Opperman. Induction of supernumerary tracheal buds and stimulation of DNA synthesis in the embryonic chick lung and trachea by epidermal growth factor. *J. Embryol. Exp. Morphol.* 60: 235–243, 1980.

46. Goldsmith, K.T., R.B. Gammon, and R.I. Garvier. Modulation of bFGF in lung fibroblasts by TGF-β and PDGF. *Am. J. Physiol.* 261 (*Lung Cell. Mol. Physiol.* 5): L378–L385, 1991.
47. Green, K.J. and J.C.R. Jones. Desmosomes and hemidesmosomes: structure and function of molecular components. *FASEB J.* 10: 871–881, 1996.
48. Grizzard, J.D., A.J. D'Ercole, J.R. Wilkins, B.M. Moats-Staats, and R.W. Williams. Affinity-labeled somatostatin C receptors and binding proteins from the human fetus. *J. Clin. Endocrinol. Metab.* 58: 535–543, 1984.
49. Guzman, K., S.H., Randell, and P. Nettesheim. Epidermal growth factor regulates expression of the mucous phenotype of rat tracheal epithelial cells. *Biochem. Biophys. Res. Commun.* 17: 412–417, 1995.
50. Hage, E. Endocrine cells in the bronchial mucosa of human fetuses. *Acta Pathol. Microbiol. Scand. A* . 80: 225–234, 1972.
51. Han, R.N., J. Liu, A.K. Tanswell, and M. Post. Expression of fibroblast growth factor: immunolocalization studies in developing rat fetal lung. *Pediatr. Res.* 31: 435–440, 1992.
52. Han, R.N.N. , C. Mawdsley, P. Souza, A.K. Tanswell, and M. Post. Platelet-derived growth factor and growth-related genes in rat lung. III. Immunolocalization during fetal development. *Pediatr. Res.* 31: 323–329, 1992.
53. Han, V.K.M., A.J. D'Ercole, and P.K. Lund. Cellular localization of somatomedin (insulin-like growth factor) messenger RNA in the human fetus. *Science* 236: 193–197, 1987.
54. Han, V.K.M., D.J. Hill, A.J. Strain, A.C. Towle, J.M. Lauder, L.E. Underwood, and A.J. D'Ercole. Identification of somatomedin/insulin-like growth factor immunoreactive cells in the human fetus. *Pediatr. Res.* 22: 245–249, 1987.
55. Hashimoto, S., K. Nakagawa, and K. Sueishi. Monkey Clara cell 10 kDa protein CC10): a characterization of the amino acid sequence with an evolutional comparison with humans, rabbits, rats, and mice. *Am. J. Respir. Cell Mol. Biol.* 15: 361–366, 1996.
56. Heine, U.I., E.F. Munoz, K.C. Flanders, A.B. Roberts, and M.B. Sporn. Colocalization of TGF-beta 1 and collagen I and III, fibronectin and glycosaminoglycans during lung branching morphogenesis. *Development* 109: 29–36, 1990.
57. Heino, J., R.A. Ignotz, M.E. Hemler, C. Crouse, and J. Massague. Regulation of cell adhesion receptors by transforming growth factor-beta. Concomitant regulation of integrins that share a common beta 1 subunit. *J. Biol. Chem.* 264: 380–388, 1989.
58. Jacquot, J., E. Puchelle, J. Hinnrasky, C. Fuchey, C. Bettinger, C. Spilmont, N. Bonnet, A. Dieterle, D. Dreyer, A. Pavirani, and W. Dalemans. Localization of the cystic fibrosis transmembrane conductance regulator in airway secretory glands. *Eur. Respir. J.* 6: 169–176, 1993.
59. Jacquot, J., C. Spilmont, H. Burlet, C. Fuchey, A.C. Buisson, J.M. Tournier, D. Gaillard, and E. Puchelle. Glandular-like morphogenesis and secretory activity of human tracheal gland cells in a three-dimensional collagen gel matrix. *J. Cell Physiol.* 161: 407–418, 1994.
60. Jaskoll, T., P.D. Boyer, and M. Melnick. Tumor necrosis factor-α and embryonic mouse lung morphogenesis. *Dev. Dyn.* 201: 137–150, 1994.
61. Jeffery P.K., D. Gaillard, and S. Moret. Human airway secretory cells during development and in mature airway epithelium. *Eur. Respir. J.* 5: 93–104, 1992.
62. Jetten, A.M. Growth and differentiation factors in tracheobronchial epithelium. *Am. J. Physiol.* 260 (*Lung Cell. Mol. Physiol.* 4): L361–L373, 1991.
63. Ji, C.M., C.G. Plopper, and K.E. Pinkerton. Clara cell heterogeneity in differentiation: Correlation with proliferation, ultrastructural composition, and cell position in the rat bronchiole. *Am. J. Respir. Cell Mol. Biol.* 13: 144–151, 1995.
64. Johnson, M.D., M.E. Gray, G. Carpenter, R.B. Pepinsky, and M.T. Stahlman. Ontogeny of

epidermal growth factor receptor and of lipocortin-I in fetal an neonatal human lungs. *Hum. Pathol.* 21: 182–191, 1990

65. Keenan, K.P., J.W. Combs, and E.M. McDowell. Regeneration of hamster tracheal epithelium after mechanical injury. IV. Histochemical, immunocytochemical and ultrastructural studies. *Virchows Arch.* (*Cell Pathol.*) 43: 213–240, 1983.
66. Khalil, N., R.N. O'Connor, K.C. Flanders, and H. Unruh. TGF-β1, but not TGF-β2 or TGF-β3 is differentially present in epithelial cells of advanced pulmonary fibrosis: an immunohistochemical study. *Am. J. Respir. Cell Mol. Biol.* 14: 131–138, 1996.
67. Khoor, A., M.T. Stahlman, M.E. Gray, and J.A. Whitsett. Temporal–spatial distribution of SP-B and SP-C proteins and mRNAs in developing respiratory epithelium. *J. Histochem. Cytochem.* 42: 1187–1199, 1994.
68. Koch, M., B. Wehrle-Haller, S. Baumgartner, J. Spring, D. Brubacher, and M. Chiquet. Epithelial synthesis of tenascin at tips of growing bronchi and graded accumulation in basement membrane and mesenchyme. *Exp. Cell Res.* 194: 297–300, 1991.
69. Kramps J.A., C. Franken, C.J.L.M. Meijer, and J.H. Dijkman. Localization of low molecular weight protease inhibitor in serous secretory cells of the respiratory tract. *J. Histochem. Cytochem.* 29: 712–719, 1981.
70. Kubiak, J., M.M. Mitra, A.R. Steve, J.D. Hunt, P. Davis, and B.R. Pitt. Transforming growth factor-α gene expression in late-gestation fetal rat lung. *Pediatr. Res.* 31: 286–290, 1992.
71. Lallemand, A.V., S.M. Ruocco, and D.A. Gaillard. Expression and immunohistochemical localization of laminin and type IV collagen in developing human fetal tracheal glands. *Int. J. Dev. Biol.* 37: 491–495, 1993.
72. Lallemand, A.V., S.M. Ruocco, and D.A. Gaillard. Synthesis and expression of laminin during human fetal lung development. *Anat. Rec.* 242: 233–241, 1995.
73. Lallemand, A.V., S.M. Ruocco, P.M. Joly, and D.A. Gaillard. In vivo localization of insulin-like growth factor I and II (IGF I and IGF II) gene expression during human lung development. *Int. J. Dev. Biol.* 39: 529–537, 1995.
74. Lauweryns, J.M., M. Cokelaere, and P. Theunymunck. Neuroepithelial bodies in the respiratory mucosa of various mammals. *Z. Zellforsch.* 135: 569–592, 1972.
75. Lauweryns, J.M., V. De Bock, A.A.J. Verhosfstad, and H.W.M. Steinbusch. Immunohistochemical localization of serotonin in intrapulmonary neuroepithelial bodies. *Cell Tissue Res.* 226: 215–223, 1982.
76. Leblond, C.P. and S. Inoue. Structure, composition and assembly of the basement membrane. *Am. J. Anat.* 185: 367–390, 1989.
77. Leslie K.O., J.J. Mitchell, J.L. Woodcock-Mitchell, and R.B. Low. Alpha smooth muscle actin expression in developing and adult human lung. *Differentiation* 44: 143–149, 1990.
78. Lin, C.Q. and M.J. Bissell. Multi-faceted regulation of cell differentiation by extracellular matrix. *FASEB J.* 7: 737–743, 1993.
79. Liu, J.P., J. Baker, A.S. Perkins, E.J. Robertson, and A. Efstratiadis. Mice carrying null mutations of the genes encoding insulin-like growth factor I (IGF-1) and type I IGF receptor (IGF-IR). *Cell* 75: 59–72, 1993.
80. Maitre, B., A. Clement, M.C. Williams, and J. S. Brody. Expression of insulin-like growth factor receptors 1 and 2 in the developing lung and their relation to epithelial cell differentiation. *Am. J. Respir. Cell Mol. Biol.* 13: 262–270, 1995.
81. Mason, R.J., M.C. Williams, H.L. Moses, S. Mohla, and M.A. Berberich. Stem cells in lung development, disease and therapy. *Am. J. Respir. Cell Mol. Biol.* 16: 355–363, 1997.

82. McDowell, E.M., T. Ben, C. Newkirk, S. Chang, and L.M. De Luca. Differentiation of tracheal mucociliary epithelium in primary cell culture recapitulates normal fetal development and regeneration following injury in hamsters. *Am. J. Pathol.* 129: 511–522, 1987.
83. McDowell, E.M., C. Newkirk, and B. Coleman. Development of hamster tracheal epithelium. I. A quantitative morphologic study in the fetus. *Anat. Rec.* 213: 429–447, 1985.
84. Meerzaman, D., P. Charles, E. Daskal, M.H. Polymeropoulos, B.M. Martin and M.C. Rose. Cloning and analysis of cDNA encoding a major airway glycoprotein, human tracheobronchial mucin (MUC5). *J. Biol. Chem.* 269: 12932–12939, 1994.
85. Meneghetti, A., W.V. Cardoso, J.S. Brody, and M.C. Williams. Epithelial marker genes are expressed in cultured embryonic rat lung and in vivo with similar spatial and temporal patterns. *J. Histochem. Cytochem.* 44: 1173–1182, 1996.
86. Mette, S.A., J. Pilewski, C.A. Buck, and S.M. Albelda. Distribution of integrin cell adhesion receptors on normal bronchial epithelial cells and lung cancer cells in vitro and in vivo. *Am. J. Respir. Cell Mol. Biol.* 8: 562–572, 1993.
87. Meyrick, B., J. Sturgess, and L. Reid. Reconstruction of the duct system and secretory tubules of the human bronchial submucosal gland. *Thorax* 24: 729–736, 1969.
88. Miettinen, P.J., J.E. Berger, J. Meneses, Y. Phung, R.A. Pederson, Z. Werb, and R. Derynck. Epithelial immaturity and multiorgan failure in mice lacking epidermal growth factor receptor. *Nature* 376: 337–341, 1995.
89. Minoo, P. and R.J. King. Epithelial–mesenchymal interactions in lung development. *Annu. Rev. Physiol.* 56: 13–45, 1994.
90. Moats-Staats, B.M., W.A. Price, L. Xu, H.W. Jarvis, and A.D. Stiles. Regulation of the insulin-like growth factor system during normal rat lung development. *Am. J. Respir. Cell Mol. Biol.* 12: 56–64, 1995.
91. Moscoso, G., K. Nandra, and M. Driver. Ciliogenesis and ciliation of the respiratory epithelium in the human fetal cartilaginous trachea. *Pathol. Res. Pract.* 184: 161-167, 1989.
92. Nakatani, Y. Pulmonary endocrine cells in infancy and childhood. *Pediatr. Pathol.* 11: 31–48, 1991.
93. Old, L.J. Tumor necrosis factor. *Sci. Am.* 258: 59–75, 1988.
94. Parsons J.T. Integrin-mediated signalling: regulation by protein tyrosine kinase and small GTP-binding proteins. *Curr. Opin. Cell Biol.* 8: 146–152, 1996.
95. Peault, B., R. Tirouvanziam, N.M. Sombardier, S. Chen, M. Perricaudet, and D. Gaillard. Gene transfer to human fetal pulmonary tissue developed in immunodeficient SCID mice. *Hum. Gene Ther.* 5: 1131–1137, 1994.
96. Pelton, R.W., S. Nomura, H.L. Moses, and B.L.M. Hogan. Expression of transforming growth factor beta 2 RNA during murine embryogenesis. *Development* 106: 759–767, 1989.
97. Pelton, R.W., B. Saxena, M. Jones, H.L. Moses, and L.I. Gold. Immunohistochemical localization of TGFβ1, TGFβ2, and TGFβ3 in the mouse embryo: expression patterns suggest multiple roles during embryonic development. *J. Cell Biol.* 115: 1091–1105, 1991.
98. Pendleton, N., G.R. Dixon, J.A. Green, and M.W. Myskow. Expression of markers of differentiation in normal bronchial epithelium and bronchial dysplasia. *J. Pathol.* 178: 146–150, 1996.
99. Plopper, C.G., J.L. Alley, and A.J. Weir. Differentiation of tracheal epithelium during foetal lung maturation in the rhesus monkey *Macaca mulatta*. *Am. J. Anat.* 175: 59–71, 1986.
100. Plopper, C.G., J.A. St Georges, L.C. Read, S.J. Nishio, A.J Weir, L. Edwards, A.F. Tarantal,

K.E. Pinkerton, A. Merrit, J.A. Whitsett, C. George-Nascimento, and D. Styne. Acceleration of alveolar type II cell differentiation in fetal rhesus monkey lung by administration of EGF. *Am. J. Physiol.* 262 (*Lung Cell Mol. Physiol.* 6): L313–L321, 1992.

101. Puchelle, E. and J.M. Zahm. Repair processes of airway epithelium. In: *Lung Biology in Health and Disease. Environmental Impact on the Airways,* edited by J. Chretien and D. Dusser. New York: Marcel Dekker, 1996, p. 157–182.
102. Raaberg, L., E. Nexø, P.E. Jorgensen, S.S. Poulsen, and M. Jakab. Fetal effects of epidermal growth factor deficiency induced in rats by autoantibodies against epidermal growth factor. *Pediatr. Res.* 37: 175–181, 1995.
103. Retsch-Bogart, G.Z., B.M. Moasts-Staats, K. Howard, A.J., D'Ercole, and A.D. Stiles. Cellular localization of messenger RNAs for insulin-like growth factors (IGFs), their receptors and binding proteins during fetal rat lung development. *Am. J. Respir. Cell Mol. Biol.* 14: 61–69, 1996.
104. Retsch-Bogart, G.Z., A.D. Stiles, B. M. Moats-Staats, M. R. Van Scott, R. C. Boucher, and A. J. D'Ercole. Canine tracheal epithelial cells express the type I insulin-like growth factor receptor and proliferate in response to insulin-like growth factor I. *Am. J. Respir. Cell Mol. Biol.* 3: 227-234, 1990.
105. Roman, J., C.W. Little, and J.A. McDonald. Potential role of RGD-binding integrins in mammalian lung branching morphogenesis. *Development* 112: 551–558, 1991.
106. Roman, J. and J.A. McDonald. Expression of fibronectin, the integrin α5 and α-smooth muscle actin in heart and lung development. *Am. J. Respir. Cell Mol. Biol.* 6: 472–480, 1992.
107. Romberg, D.J., J.D. Beckmann, L. Claassen, R.F. Ertl, and S.I. Rennard. Modulation of fibronectin production of bovine bronchial epithelial cells by transforming growth factor-β. *Am. J. Respir. Cell Mol. Biol.* 7: 149–155, 1992.
108. Ruocco, S., A. Lallemand, J.M. Tournier, and D. Gaillard. Expression and localization of epidermal growth factor, transforming growth factor-α, and localization of their common receptor in fetal human lung development. *Pediatr. Res.* 39: 448–454, 1996.
109. Saga, Y., T. Yagi, Y. Ikawa, T. Sakakura, and S. Aizawa. Mice develop normally without tenascin. *Genes Dev.* 6: 1821–1831, 1992.
110. Sannes, P.L., K.K. Burch, and J. Khosla. Immunohistochemical localization of epidermal growth factor and acidic and basic fibroblast growth factors in postnatal developing and adult rat lungs. *Am. J. Respir. Cell Mol. Biol.* 7: 230–237, 1992.
111. Sannes, P.L., K.K. Burch, J. Khosla, K.J. McCarthy, and J.R. Couchman. Immunohistochemical localization of chondroitin sulfate, chondroitin sulfate proteoglycan, heparan sulfate proteoglycan, entactin, and laminin in basement membranes of postnatal developing and adult rat lungs. *Am. J. Respir. Cell Mol. Biol.* 8: 245-251, 1993
112. Schellenberg, J.-C. and G.C. Liggins. Elastin and collagen in the fetal sheep lung. I. Ontogenesis. *Pediatr. Res.* 22: 335–338, 1987.
113. Schuger, L., S. O'Shea, J. Rheinheimer, and J. Varani. Laminin in lung development: effects of anti-laminin antibody in murinelung morphogenesis. *Dev. Biol.* 137: 26–32, 1990.
114. Sheppard D. Epithelial integrins. *BioEssays* 18: 655–660, 1996.
115. Sheppard, D., D.S. Cohen, A. Wang, and M. Busk. Transforming growth factor β differentially regulates expression of integrin subunits in guinea pig airway epithelial cells. *J. Biol. Chem.* 267: 17409–17414, 1992.
116. Shimomoto, H., Y. Hasegawa, Y. Nozaki, N. Takagi, T. Shibagaki, A. Nakao, and K. Shi-

mokata. Expression of tumor necrosis factor receptors in human lung cancer cells and normal lung tissues. *Am. J. Respir. Cell Mol. Biol.* 13: 271-278, 1995.

117. Shiratori, M., E. Oshika, L.P. Ung, G. Singh, H. Shinozuka, D. Warbuton, G. Michalopoulos, and S.L. Katyal. Keratinocyte growth factor and embryonic rat lung morphogenesis. *Am. J. Respir. Cell Mol. Biol.* 15: 328–338, 1996.
118. Singh, G., S.L. Katyal, and M.L. Wong Chong. A quantitative assay for a Clara-cell-specific protein and its application in the study of the development of pulmonary airways in the rat. *Pediatr. Res.* 20: 802–805, 1986.
119. Sinkin, R.A., R.S. Sanders, S. Horowitz, J.N. Finkelstein, and M.B. Lomonaco. Cell-specific expression of fibronectin in adult and developing rabbit lung. *Pediatr. Res.* 37: 189–195, 1995.
120. Söderberg M., S. Hellström, T. Sandström, R. Lundgren, and A. Bergh. Structural characterization of bronchial mucosal biopsies from healthy volunteers: a light and electron microscopical study. *Eur. Respir. J.* 3: 261–266, 1990 .
121. Souza, P., M. Kuliszewski, J. Wang, I. Tseu, A.K. Tanswell, and M. Post. PDGF-AA and its receptor influence early lung branching via an epithelial–mesenchymal interaction. *Development* 121: 2559–2567, 1995.
122. Spicer, S.S., B.A. Schulte, and L.W. Chakrin. Ultrastructural and histochemical observations of respiratory epithelium and gland. *Lung Res.* 4: 137–156, 1983.
123. Stahlman M.T., and M.E. Gray. Ontogeny of neuroendocrine cells in human fetal lung. *Lab. Invest.* 51: 449–463, 1984.
124. Stahlman, M.T., D.N. Orth, and M.E. Gray. Immunocytotechnical localization of epidermal growth factor in the developing human respiratory system and in acute and chronic lung disease in the neonate. *Lab. Invest.* 60: 539–547, 1989.
125. Stahlman, M. and M.E. Gray. Colocalization of peptide hormones in neuroendocrine cells of human fetal and newborn lungs: an electron microscopic study. *Anat. Rec.* 236: 206–212, 1993.
126. St George J.A., L.C. Read, D.L. Cranz, A.F. Tarantal, C. George-Nascimento, and C.G. Plopper. Effect of epidermal growth factor on the fetal development of the tracheobronchial secretory apparatus in rhesus monkey. *Am. J. Respir. Cell Mol. Biol.* 4: 95–101, 1991.
127. Stiles, A. D., and A. J. D'Ercole. The insulin-like growth factors and the lung. *Am. J. Respir. Cell Mol. Biol.* 3: 93-100, 1990.
128. Strandjord, T.P., J.G. Clark, D.E. Guralnick, and D.K. Madtes. Immunolocalization of transforming growth factor α, epidermal growth factor (EGF), and EGF-receptor in normal and injured developing human lung. *Pediatr. Res.* 38: 851–856, 1995.
129. Strandjord, T.P., J.G. Clark, A. Hodson, R.A. Schmidt, and D.K. Madtes. Expression of transforming growth factor-α in mid-gestation human fetal lung. *Am. J. Respir. Cell Mol. Biol.* 8: 266–272, 1993.
130. Sundberg, C. and K. Rubin. Stimulation of β1 integrins on fibroblasts induces PDGF independent tyrosine phosphoryation of PDGF β-receptors. *J. Cell Biol.* 132: 741–752, 1996.
131. Thomas, T. and M. Dziadek. Expression of collagen alpha I(IV), laminin and nidogen genes in the embryonic mouse lung: implications for branching morphogenesis. *Mech. Dev.* 45: 193–201, 1994.
132. Thurlbeck, W.M., B. Benjamin, and L.M. Reid. Development and distribution of mucous glands in the fetal human trachea. *Br. J. Dis. Chest* 55: 54–64, 1961.

133. Tos, M. Development of the tracheal glands in man. *Acta Pathol. Microbiol. Scand.* 185: 1–130, 1966.
134. Virtanen, I., A. Laitinen, T. Taneli, P. Pääkkö, L.A. Laitinen, R.E. Burgeson, and V.-P. Lehto. Differential expression of laminins and their integrin receptors in developing and adult human lung. *Am. J. Respir. Cell Mol. Biol.* 15: 184–196, 1996.
135. Wang, A., Y. Yokosaki, R. Ferrando, J. Balmes, and D. Sheppard. Differential regulation of airway epithelial integrins by growth factors. *Am. J. Respir. Cell Mol. Biol.* 15: 664–672, 1996.
136. Wang, D., H. Yeger, and E. Cutz. Expression of gastrin-releasing peptide receptor gene in developing lung. *Am. J. Respir. Cell Mol. Biol.* 14: 409–416, 1996.
137. Warburton, D., R. Seth, L. Shum, P.G. Horcher, F.L. Hall, Z. Werb, and H.C. Slavkin. Epigenic role of epidermal growth factor expression and signaling in embryonic mouse lung morphogenesis. *Dev. Biol.* 149: 123–133, 1992.
138. Weinacker, A., R. Ferrando, M. Elliott, J. Hogg, J. Balmes, and D. Sheppard. The distribution of integrins $\alpha v\beta 6$ and $\alpha 9\beta 1$ and their ligands, fibronectin and tenascin, in human airways. *Am. J. Respir. Cell Mol. Biol.* 12: 547–557, 1995.
139. Wessells, N.K. Mammalian lung development: interactions in formation and morphogenesis of tracheal buds. *J. Exp. Zool.* 175: 455–466, 1970.
140. Widdicombe, J.G. and R.J. Pack. The Clara cell. *Eur. J. Respir. Dis.* 63: 202–220, 1982.
141. Willey, J.C., J.F. Lechner, and C.C. Harris. Bombesin and the C-terminal tetrapeptide of gastrin-releasing peptide are growth factors for normal human bronchial epithelial cells. *Exp. Cell Res.* 153: 245–248, 1984.
142. Wu J.E., and S.A. Santoro. Differential expression of integrin α subunits supports distinct roles during lung branching morphogenesis. *Dev. Dyn.* 206: 169–181, 1996.
143. Wuenschell, C.W., M.E. Sunday, G. Singh, P. Minoo, H.C. Slavkin, and D. Warburton. Embryonic mouse lung epithelial progenitor cells co-express immunohistochemical markers of diverse mature cell lineages. *J. Histochem. Cytochem.* 44: 113–123, 1996.
144. Yoshida, M., D.J. Romberg, M.G. Illig. H. Takizawa, O. Sacco, J.R. Spurzem, J.H. Sisson, S.I. Rennard, and J.D. Beckmann. Transforming growth factor-β stimulates the expression of desmosomal proteins in bronchial epithelial cells. *Am. J. Respir. Cell Mol. Biol.* 6: 439–445, 1992.
145. Young, S.L., L.-Y. Chang, and H.P. Erickson. Tenascin-C in rat lung: distribution, ontogeny and role in branching morphogenesis. *Dev. Biol.* 161: 615–625, 1994.
146. Zahm, J.M., D. Pierrot, J. Hinnrasky, C. Fuchey, M. Chevillard, D. Gaillard, and E. Puchelle. Functional activity of ciliated outgrowths from cultured human nasal and tracheal epithelia. *Biorheology* 27: 565–569, 1990.
147. Zhao, Y. and S.L. Young. TGF-β regulates expression of tenascin alternative-splicing isoforms in fetal rat lung. *Am. J. Physiol.* (*Lung Cell Mol. Physiol.*) 268: L173–L180, 1995.
148. Zhou, L.R., W. Graeff, P.B. McCray, W.S. Simonet, and J.A. Whitsett. Keratinocyte growth factor stimulates CFTR-independent fluid secretion in the fetal lung in vitro. *Am. J. Physiol.* 271 (*Lung Cell Mol. Physiol.* 15): L987–L994, 1996.

chapter 4

GENE EXPRESSION IN ALVEOLAR DEVELOPMENT

Jacques R. Bourbon

RESPIRATORY epithelium, strictly defined as the epithelium of distal lung that lines walls of respiratory bronchioles and alveoli, is composed of two cell types known as *alveolar type I* and *II cells* or *type I* and *II pneumocytes*. The former is a flat, attenuated, terminally differentiated cell through which air–blood gas exchanges occur. The latter is a cuboidal cell that elaborates and releases all the phospholipid and protein components of pulmonary surfactant (87, 113); it also serves as a progenitor cell for itself and for the type I cell that does not divide (64). Although it belongs to the bronchiolar epithelium at the junction of conducting and respiratory portions of the lung, the nonciliated bronchiolar, or Clara, cell shares features with the type II pneumocyte since, in addition to secretory products proper to this cell type, it also releases some surfactant protein components (87). It also represents the progenitor for itself and for the basal and ciliated cells in the renewal process of the epithelium (64). These cell types, however, represent only a small part of all epithelial lung cell phenotypes. In total, pulmonary epithelium comprises at least 11 differentiated cell types that, to a large extent, determine lung function. To understand phenotypic differentiation in the distal parts of the lung, we need to investigate (*1*) how lung-specific identity is determined, and (*2*), how distal cell lineages are specified relative to those of more proximal parts of the lung, the epithelial cells of conducting airways.

Alveolar and Clara cells differentiate relatively late in gestation, once the bronchial and bronchiolar tree is completed (30). All epithelial cells of the lung derive from a ventral outgrowth of the embryonic endodermal tube. During the earliest phases of lung development, i.e., the embryonic and glandular periods, when branching of the bronchial tree becomes established by dichotomous growing of the anlage (see Chap. 1), epithelial cells remain morphologically undifferentiated and apparently homogeneous. At a definite developmental stage that takes place at the end of the glandular period, the proximal and distal areas of growing tubules become sharply demarcated. Whereas proximal tubules, considered to be the prospective bronchial system (primordial or bronchial tubules), keep the pseudostratified columnar appearance of the primordial epithelium, cells of distal tubules, considered to be the prospective respiratory system (acinar tubules), become cuboidal (170). Functional maturation of the various cell types begins before the completion of the branching process of the bronchiolar and respiratory systems. The precise time when a given cell type or cell type precursor is present is nevertheless in dispute, depending on the nature of the criterion used for investigation: morphological aspects, immunological reactivity, or in situ hybridization.

There is considerable information on diffusible factors capable of modulating (enhancing or decreasing) the expression of lung cell markers. The sequence of molecular events driving pattern formation in the developing lung, i.e., the temporal cascade of gene activation and repression that leads to differential expression characteristic of the various cell phenotypes and to their architectural arrangement, however, remains largely unknown. On the basis of currently available data, only conjectural assumptions can be made with regard to the ultimate mechanisms of cell determination, i.e., to the master genes that specify a pulmonary identity or to the possible morphogens that instruct lung cells to assume proximal- or distal-specific functions. Recently, however, a rapidly increasing number of studies have produced new insights into the molecular mechanisms that confer the ability to express lung-specific genes to alveolar and Clara cells. This chapter reviews the data dealing with distal lung development in this fast evolving field of research. Control mechanisms of growth, morphogenesis, and cell-specific expression of markers are considered, with particular emphasis given to the latter.

ONTOGENY OF DISTAL LUNG MARKERS AND COMMITMENT OF LUNG EPITHELIAL CELLS

Markers of Alveolar Cells and Clara Cells

Alveolar Type II Cell Markers

The alveolar type II cell is the major source of pulmonary surfactant, the proteolipid complex that lines lung alveoli and plays a variety of roles crucial for respiratory function. It presents remarkable and unique biophysical and biological features, including surface tension–lowering capacity, water repellency, anti-edematous activity, and antimicrobial properties. Its major components are lipids, principally phospholipids, that account for as much as 90% of its mass and of which dipalmitoyl-phosphatidylcholine is the most abundant molecule. Another phospholipid, phosphatidylglycerol, appears to be surfactant-specific, as it is virtually absent from animal cells other than alveolar type II cells. The high rate of phospholipid production by type II cells is reflected in the high level of activity of the enzymes involved in their biosynthetic pathway, compared with other cell types. Among the 10% protein components of surfactant, four characteristic proteins, SP-A, -B, -C, and -D, have been described (87). SP-A and SP-D are amphiphilic proteins that belong to the C-type collectin family and are closely related to two seric proteins, mannose-binding protein and conglutinin, respectively. They are active in alveoli as an octadecamer and a dodecamer. Both SP-A and SP-D exhibit a non-phospholipid-linked property of opsonizing microorganisms, which likely facilitates phagocytosis by alveolar macrophages. Furthermore, SP-A, but not SP-D, interacts with surfactant phospholipids and SP-B. The simultaneous presence of SP-A and SP-B is required for the transformation of the content of lamellar bodies, the intracellular storage form of surfactant, into tubular myelin, a three-dimensional square lattice that appears to be a precursor form of the active surfactant film. SP-B and SP-C are much smaller, highly hydrophobic peptides that are closely associated with phospholipids. Their presence appears to be essential for rapid spreading and absorption of surfactant onto the aqueous hypophase lining the alveolar wall. These four proteins are excellent markers of distal lung epithelium. It should be stressed, however, that only SP-C is specific to type II cells, since Clara cells also express SP-A, SP-B, and SP-D genes (91). Their genes, including large upstream promoter regions, have been cloned in several species, allowing one to study transactivation mechanisms of their expression. Attempts to characterize type II cell apical membrane markers have also been made. Characterization and cDNA cloning of an SP-A binding protein considered a type II cell–specific SP-A receptor (165) have been reported.

A major problem in neonatology, respiratory distress syndrome (RDS) of the newborn, is mainly a consequence of pulmonary surfactant deficit; thus thorough knowledge of lung maturation is a prerequisite to efficient prevention of RDS. Prevention of its sequelae, bronchopulmonary dysplasia (BPD), a condition that involves necrotizing bronchiolitis, thickening of septal walls, and fibrosis, also calls for a better understanding of mechanisms governing cell growth, differentiation, and epithelial repair.

Alveolar Type I Cell Markers

The phenotypic transition that type II cells undergo during their transdifferentiation into type I cells includes not only the loss of surfactant component expression but also the acquisition of new membrane markers of the second cell type. This was first illustrated by changes in lectin-binding properties. Lectin ligands, however, have not all been characterized. Whereas *Maclura pomifera* lectin binds to apical surface proteins of type II cells, *Ricinus communis* (reviewed in ref. 113) and *Bauhinia purpurea* (93) lectins specifically label type I cells. Only recently have more specific markers of type I cells begun to be characterized. Antibodies have been raised against apical surface proteins that appear to be type I cell–specific (62). These tools appear to be useful for studying the type II cell–type I cell transition in vitro (55). Similarly, a novel gene encoding for a type I cell protein designated T1α has been described. Interestingly, T1α, which appears to be a transmembrane protein also expressed in the brain and in ciliary epithelia, has been reported to be developmentally regulated (185).

Clara Cell Secretory Protein

A secreted, covalently bound homodimeric protein called the *Clara cell secretory protein* [CCSP; (80)], otherwise designated 10 kDa Clara cell specific protein [CC10; (159)], CC17, RLL (for rat lung lavage), and polychlorinated biphenyl-binding protein, has been described in lung lavage or tissue of various species and localized to vesicles within the Clara cell (12, 159). Its functions are not precisely established, but it displays phospholipase A_2 and proteinase-inhibitory activity (80). It may also act as an immunomodulatory and anti-inflammatory protein similar to its uterine counterpart, uteroglobin (111). Its gene has been cloned in human (186) and rat (147). Along with SP-C, it represents a useful marker for differentiating alveolar type II and Clara cells.

Ontogeny of Surfactant Proteins and CC10 in the Developing Lung

In human pregnancy (term at 40 weeks), the first lamellar bodies appear at about 19–20 weeks. Surfactant amount regularly increases until term. In the rat and rabbit, two species widely used for investigations on lung development, the first lamellar bodies are seen at gestational days 19 and 26 for gestational length of 22 and 31 days, respectively (30). In various species, significant amounts of surfactant-associated proteins have been detected along with the increase in surfactant phospholipids, although their mRNAs could be detected somewhat earlier (30, 148), and the course of phospholipid and protein storage parallels that of development of biophysical properties (65). It has been shown, however, that a low level of expression of surfactant proteins is present much earlier and is not limited to cells destined to become alveolar type II cells. These proteins therefore represent precocious markers of developing pulmonary epithelia, before differentiation of actual type II cells. Thus, SP-A and its mRNA have been evidenced in human tracheal and bronchial epithelium as early as the 13th gestational week (96)—i.e., at least 6 weeks before formation of the first lamellar bodies. SP-A expression in proximal portions ceases when mucociliary differentiation takes place and becomes limited to Clara cells (96). Similarly, in the rat, the mRNAs of SP-A, SP-B, and SP-C have been detected by reverse-transcriptase polymerase chain reaction (RT-PCR) on gestational day 12, the day after the formation of the lung anlage, and were present in all tubules, including the trachea, during the 3 following days (176). In the mouse fetus, immunoreactive pro-SP-B and pro-SP-C have been found in large proximal airways, including main and lobar bronchi, during early lung development, and become restricted to bronchiolar and alveolar epithelial cells in late gestation (195).

CC10 mRNA was first detected in rat lung on gestational day 16 by in situ hybridization and was found to be restricted to bronchial tubules lined with tall columnar cells in which expression appeared to be uniform (167). By gestational day 19, it became limited to secretory epithelial cells lining the bronchi and terminal bronchioles. Ciliated cells and cells lining the prealveolar saccules lacked hybridization signal (167). CC10 transcript increased in abundance during late fetal life and reached adult levels 2 weeks postpartum in this species (82). Surprisingly, in the adult rat, alveolar type II cells appear to express CC10 mRNA (167), which is in contrast with the Clara cell-specific expression of the protein itself, suggesting post-transcriptional control of the message. This overlap could be a peculiarity of the rat, however, since the murine type II cells do not appear to contain CC10 transcripts (179).

An important observation was made through immunocytochemical investigations in the mouse fetus (188): lung epithelial progenitor cells simultaneously express immunohistochemical markers characteristic of different mature cell lineages. Thus, in an early phase spanning from gestational days 13 to 15 (term is 20 days), all epithelial cells of distal airways co-express CC10, SP-A, and calcitonin gene–related peptide (CGRP), a neuropeptide marker of neuroendocrine cells of the bronchiolar system. These markers subsequently seggregate when cell types differentiate from each other. The emergence of staining of the differentiated cell types occurs between days 16 and 18. These temporal expression patterns were recapitulated in serumless organ culture. Consistently, in situ hybridization study revealed SP-C expression throughout the distal epithelium from days 11 to 16 (179). According to Wuenschell et al. (188), the expression of all these gene products in a progenitor cell population may reflect some aspect of an underlying mechanism of developmental gene regulation, rather than early commitment to specific lineages.

Ontogeny of Surfactant in Culture Models

It has been long established that the entire pulmonary anlage can pursue its development in vitro even in the absence of serum (reviewed in ref. 30) This includes branching of the complete bronchial tree and differentiation of ciliated cells in bronchi and bronchioli. Type II cells differentiate at the tips, although actual alveolar sacs do not develop. Type II cell maturation was also observed in cultured fetal lung explants from various species in numerous studies. Starting in the 1960s, a number of experiments (reviewed in ref. 30) using the dissociation-reassociation approach of various epithelia with either homologous or heterologous mesenchyme showed that, even if the presence of mesenchyme was an absolute requirement for bronchial growth and branching, and if the branching pattern was dictated by mesenchyme according to the organ from which it originated, mesenchymes were not able to phenotypically transform epithelial cells that seemed to be already determined. Thus, lung mesenchymal cells appeared to control the degree of differentiation of lung epithelium, but were not able to induce expression of lung epithelial markers in non-pulmonary epithelia.

Although lung mesenchyme does not appear to induce the pulmonary identity of the epithelium, regionalization of the latter appears to be a consequence of regionalization of the mesenchyme. Thus, grafting distal lung mesenchyme onto explanted fetal rat tracheal epithelium induced budding, branching, and alveolar type II cell differentiation in the epithelium. Type II cell differentiation was attested to by the presence of SP-C mRNA (normal tracheal epithelium at the considered stage expressed only SP-A and SP-B mRNAs), lamellar bodies, SP-B and SP-C proteins, and tubular myelin figures, all normally absent in normal tracheal epithelial cells (152). It should be pointed out that the ability of tracheal epithelium to respond to induction by distal mesenchyme was limited in time; day 13–14 tracheal cells were responsive to mesenchyme of the same stage, but day 16 tracheal cells failed to respond. Only distal mesenchyme from the presumptive acinar areas was inductory; mesenchyme of the main bronchus induced at most a barely detectable outpocketting of tracheal epithelium (152). By the same token, distal lung epithelium recombined with tracheal mesenchyme did not branch, but instead formed cysts and differentiated into ciliated and mucous secretory cells (156). Importantly, no lamellar bodies and no SP-C expression were detected with this combination (156). In addition, in another study (38), it was suggested that, depending on the distance of mesenchymal fibroblasts from the epithelium, these fibroblasts could produce different mediators that would promote either epithelial growth or differentiation, the latter being favored by fibroblasts in close proximity to the epithelium and more distant fibroblasts favoring epithelial growth. The phenotypic plasticity of epithelial cells and the role of their local environment was also recently illustrated by results from experiments in which tumor cells from a cell line (MLE 15) were implanted in nude mice. This cell line is derived from lung adenocarcinoma formed in a mouse rendered transgenic for the simian virus 40 early region driven by the SP-C promoter. Whereas cells of this line expressed SP-C but not CC10 in vitro, they expressed both markers in tumor nodules formed in vivo. Both markers were not co-expressed in the same cell, however; SP-C mRNA was detected at the periphery of the tumors in close association with surrounding stromal tissue, and CC10 mRNA was detected in central tumor regions (184). This connects with the existence of direct contact between alveolar type II and stromal cells through focal interruptions of the basement membrane in the normal lung, as this contact is thought to facilitate instruction transfer from the mesenchyme (30). Such contact is not present in bronchiolar cells.

Although adult type II cells cultured on plastic rapidly loose their markers, these markers, including expression of surfactant proteins, are retained when cells are grown on basement membrane matrix material prepared from the murine Engelbreth-Holm-Swarm (EHS) tumor (94, 153). This substratum was therefore used for studying type II cell differentiation in vitro. A first methodological approach consisted of complete enzymic dispersion of cells and removal of fibroblasts by differential adhesion before seeding epithelial cells onto the basement membrane matrix where they formed pseudo-alveolar structures (45, 72). A second method consisted of separating the epithelial rudiment of embryonic rat lung from its surrounding mesenchyme by mild enzyme treatment; successful in vitro development of the entire epithelial tube was obtained through substitution of mesenchymal influence by

EHS basement membrane matrix and a growth factor–enriched medium (60, 130). Branching was observed in the presence of serum and various growth factors in one study using the second model (60), and was in another study obtained in a defined medium in the presence of acidic fibroblast growth factor (FGF-1) (130). In both the dispersed-cell model and the entire rudiment model, full differentiation of type II cells was obtained within a few days, including appearance and accumulation of typical lamellar bodies (45, 60, 72), formation of tubular myelin figures (45), appearance of SP-C mRNA (60, 72), onset of SP-A and SP-B synthesis, a sharp rise in the rate of precursor incorporation in surfactant lipids, and responsiveness to fibroblast-conditioned medium (71, 72). Figure 4.1 illustrates this differentiation capacity of fetal rat lung epithelial cells. With dissociated cells, an increase in the steady state of mRNAs encoding for various enzymes involved in phospholipid synthetic pathway that reproduced normal developmental changes was also observed (71). Scarce ciliated cells also differentiated in this model (71, 72). It should be underscored that the differentiation process was achieved in chemically defined medium devoid of hormones in the first model (45, 71, 72), but not in the second one (60). No evaluation of epithelial differentiation was done in the study of whole rudiment growth in defined medium (130); however, a more recent investigation with the same model indicated poor expression of type II cell markers (40).

Pluripotency of Fetal Lung Epithelial Cells and the Role of Mesenchyme

Taken together, the early expression of surfactant protein genes in undifferentiated lung epithelium, including those areas destined to differentiate into proximal structures that no longer express these markers, and the co-expression in a same progenitor cell of markers subsequently restricted to distinct cell lineages lead to the following conclusions: (*1*) cell commitment to a pulmonary identity is extremely precocious and (*2*) all the information necessary to generate all lung epithelial cell phenotypes is present in the primordial lung bud, including control of the biphasic pattern (common, then specific) of gene expression. The ability of undifferentiated epithelial cells to pursue in vitro the differentiation program of alveolar cells in an autonomous way (at least beyond a definite stage of development) shows that even if an initial mesenchymal induction takes place, it does not need to be maintained. This pulmonary identity may already be imprinted in the initial bud in a potential form, possibly as a consequence of the combined expression of homeotic genes that dictate commitment along the anterior–posterior axis. Regionalization in the capacity of mesenchyme to modulate or reverse epithelial gene expression indicates, however, that the final orientation of a progenitor cell toward a given phenotype among the possible pulmonary cell fates is submitted to mesenchymal control. Presumably, paracrine and/or matricial information compartmentalized along the anterior–posterior axis of the lung orients gene expression in pluripotent epithelial cells. This control is likely to be exerted at the level of differential expression of transcriptional factors, leading in turn to expression of specific epithelial cell markers.

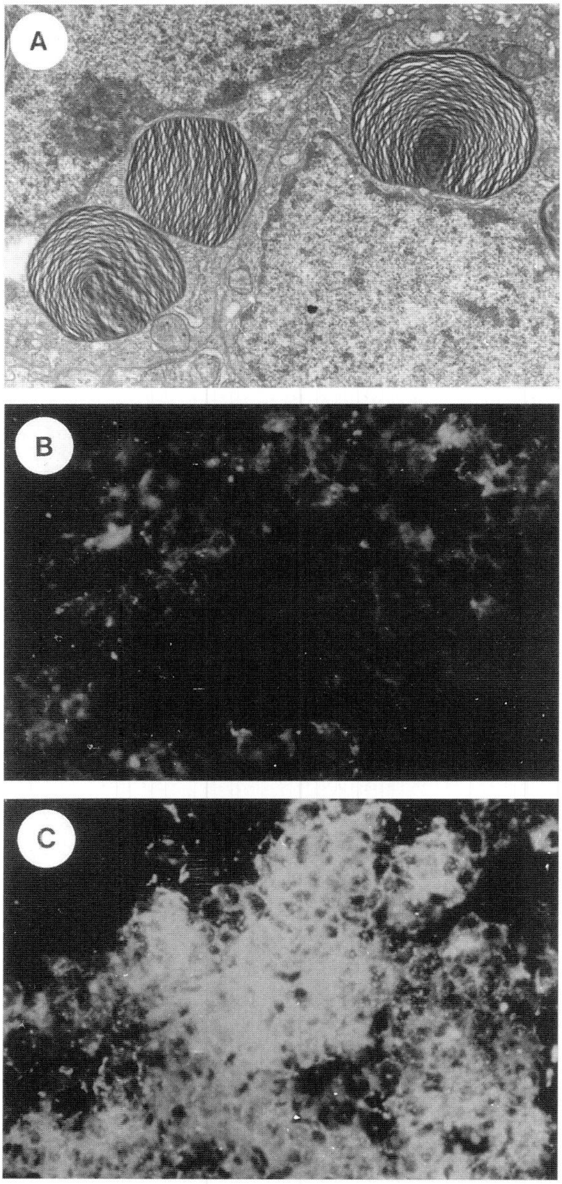

Fig. 4.1 In vitro differentiation of isolated epithelial cells from fetal rat lung. Cells were taken on gestational day 17 and cultured on basement membrane matrix in defined medium. (*A*) Transmission electron microscopy aspect of lamellar bodies formed during a 6-day culture. [Original picture from C. Fraslon.] SP-B immunoreactivity (immunofluorescent-coupled anti SP-B antibody) occurred after 2 days (*B*) and 6 days (*C*) of culture. Note the increase in SP-B content during culture ; immunoreactive SP-B was not detected at culture initiation. [Original pictures from B. Chailley-Heu.]

ROLE OF TRANSCRIPTION FACTORS IN LUNG DEVELOPMENT AND THE CONTROL OF SPECIFIC PROTEIN EXPRESSION

Control of gene expression resides in a combinatorial interaction between gene promoter regions and various nuclear protein ligands known as *transcription factors.* These *trans*-acting factors present characteristic DNA-binding motifs that interact with specific DNA sequences or *cis*-acting elements. Some transcription factors are ubiquitous and are needed for transcription of a number of genes. Tissue, area, or cell-type specificity in expression pattern of other transactivating factors, along with chromatin accessibility to these factors, accounts for restricted expression of cell markers. Analysis of the 5′-flanking regions of marker genes and of the cell-specific nuclear factors that control their transcription may therefore enlighten our understanding of cell differentiation mechanisms. Only these specific transcription factors will be considered here. Transcription factors from three different families, namely thyroid transcription factor 1, hepatocyte nuclear factors-3/forkhead factors, and CCAAT/enhancer binding proteins, have been recently recognized as playing crucial roles in distal lung-specific gene expression and lung developmental processes.

Role of Thyroid Transcription Factor-1

Thyroid transcription factor-1 (TTF-1), otherwise designated *thyroid-specific enhancer-binding protein* (T/EBP) or *Nkx-2.1,* is a homeodomain-containing DNA-binding protein (78) initially described as a transcription factor for thyroid-specific genes (47). It is homologous to the *Drosophila* transcription factor NK-2 and belongs to the NKx class of nuclear factors (53). Homeodomain transcription factors are characterized by a conserved 60 amino acid DNA-binding domain designated the *homeodomain,* which is characterized by a helix-turn-helix motif and is encoded by a 180 nucleotide domain referred to as the *homeobox* (75).

During fetal development, TTF-1 mRNA is present in cell nuclei of the brain, thyroid, and pulmonary epithelium, but is absent from the foregut epithelium prior to the onset of thyroid and lung morphogenesis (53, 105). In the lung and thyroid, TTF-1 is expressed in cells of the primitive lung bud epithelium as well as in subsets of epithelial cells that subsequently differentiate. Interestingly, a gradient establishes along the anterior–posterior axis of these structures, with expression restricted to the distal epithelial tubules and absent from the most proximal segments (105). TTF-1 mRNA is absent from mesenchymal cells (105). It is present in subsets of bronchiolar and alveolar cells in the mature lung (78, 84) and is particularly abundantly expressed in postnatal lung alveolar type II cells (84). Recently, systematic immunohistochemical studies have established more precisely the spatial–temporal changes in TTF-1 protein localization in the developing mouse (195) and human (162) fetal lung. In mouse lung (195), TTF-1 was detected on gestational day 10 in nuclei of main bronchial epithelial cells. From days 12 through 16, it was expressed at high levels in all airways including the trachea, and was particularly prominent in newly formed distal airway tubules. In late gestation, labeling was more intense in type II cells than in cells of conducting airways. In the adult mouse lung, however, type II cells and bronchial or bronchiolar epithelial cells appeared equally stained, which appears to contradict previous mRNA analysis (105). In fetal human lung (162), early detection (11 weeks) was found in undifferentiated columnar epithelial cells. Subsequently, labeling became most prominent in cells at the tip of the developing buds. Close to term, TTF-1 disappeared from proximal columnar epithelium to become restricted to alveolar type II cells, Clara cells, and cells lining bronchioloalveolar portals. It is striking that in both species, TTF-1 distribution overlaps that of SP-A, SP-B, SP-C, and CC10, and decline of TTF-1 from proximal territories coincides with the disappearance of transiently expressed markers such as SP-A or pro-SP-B/C. The persistence of TTF-1 in large airways throughout life in the mouse suggests, however, that other transcription factors could be involved in this regulation. Interestingly, TTF-1 is absent from alveolar type I cells, which implies an arrest of its production during the type II–to–type I transition (162). It should be emphasized that TTF-1 was found in the same study (162) to be deficient in atelectatic areas of the lung in RDS and in collapsed airways in BPD, but was prominent in regenerating tips of terminal airways in the latter condition. Elucidation of mechanisms that regulate TTF-1 gene expression may therefore be important for the treatment of acute and chronic lung disease in infants.

Inhibition of TTF-1 translation through the use of an antisense oligonucleotide in an in vitro model of embryonic mouse lung morphogenesis led to abnormal phenotype, including reduced branching and unorganized hyperplastic epithelium which kept tall columnar immature cells (124). Consistently, inactivation of the TTF-1 gene through homologous recombination in the mouse permitted development until birth but, among other major abnormalities, led to arrested lung development. Fetuses homozygous for the disrupted gene displayed lack of lobar bronchi branching, rudimentary bronchial tree, and absence of bronchioli, alveoli, and lung parenchyma, which were replaced by dilated saccules limited by a columnar epithelium of bronchial type (97). Altogether, these observations point out TTF-1 as having an essential role in the control of lung organogenesis, particularly with regard to epithelial branching growth and development of distal structures, including the ontogenesis of cuboidal cells that serve as progenitors to alveolar epithelial cells.

With regard to expression of lung-specific protein genes, TTF-1 was first demonstrated to control SP-B gene expression. An isolated fragment of the promoter region of the SP-B gene has been shown to contain several sites protected against S1 nuclease by nuclear ligand proteins and to allow strong expression of a reporter gene in a tumoral cell line that expresses SP-B in vitro (28). Two *cis*-acting TTF-1 binding sites have been identified in this DNA sequence, relatively near the start site of transcription (27, 34). A distinct enhancer also mediating TTF-1 transactivation was later found further upstream in the 5′-flanking region of the gene (190). Point mutations in these sites markedly decreased the activity of expression constructs in transfected lung cells in vitro, whereas co-transfection of a reporter gene under the control of the SP-B promoter along with an expression vector of TTF-1 cDNA considerably increased expression of the former (27, 190). TTF-1 was subsequently demonstrated to regulate SP-A (35, 168) and SP-C (95) gene expression. Four distinct TTF-1 responsive fragments were identified in the SP-A promoter and five were found in the SP-C promoter. The same site-specific mutagenesis and co-transfection approaches led to the same conclusions as for SP-B. Three binding sites in the SP-A gene and two in the SP-C gene were shown to be required for TTF-1 activation (35, 95). In SP-A, -B, and -C promoters TTF-1 binds with varying affinity to the different sites, and cooperative binding has been observed at the clustered sites.

TTF-1 has been found to similarly regulate CC10 expression (139, 171). No less than seven TTF-1 binding sites have been identified—five in the distal part of the promoter and two in the proximal part. Deletion and mutational analyses have identified a site located between –282 and –272 base pairs (bp) of the transcription initiation point as the major regulator of CC10 expression. A reporter gene fused to a CC10 promoter fragment containing a mutation in this binding site presented a markedly reduced expression in transgenic mice (139). Co-transfection assays have also demonstrated specific activation by TTF-1 at the level of the most proximal TTF-1 site (171). DNase-I footprint analysis enabled identification of a binding site for a second transactivating factor of the NKx family in the CC10 promoter, namely cardiac muscle–specific homeobox protein (CSX) (139).

Role of Hepatocyte Nuclear Factor 3/Forkhead Factor Family

The hepatocyte nuclear factor 3/forkhead (HNF-3/fkh) factors belong to a wide group of nuclear factors initially discovered in the liver, but subsequently found to be expressed in a number of other tissues. The HNF-3α, β, and γ isoforms were first identified as factors controlling expression of the liver transthyretin and α1-antitrypsin genes (52). Their genes constitute the mammalian counterparts (103) of the homeotic gene *forkhead* in *Drosophila,* thus named because its mutation results in an embryo with a duplicated anterior pole (177). Forkhead factors have been identified in all phyla. This family of DNA-binding proteins is characterized by a conserved 110 amino acid DNA-recognition domain named the *forkhead domain.* This domain presents a characteristic α-helical structure with two wing-like loops resembling the shape of a butterfly, leading to the term the *winged-helix motif* (48). To date, the family includes about 40 identified mammalian members involved in differentiation of various cell lineages. In addition to HNF-3/fkh factors, a number of related factors designated *hepatocyte nuclear factor/forkhead homologues* (HFH) have been identified in rodents (50). The human forkhead-related factors FREAC-1 and -2 expressed in lung are homologous to the murine HFH-8 (136). The human counterpart to the murine HNF-3α has recently been cloned from a pulmonary adenocarcinoma cell line (20).

The adult lung strongly expresses transcripts of HNF-3α and β, HFH-4, and HFH-8, and more weakly expresses HFH-1, HFH-2, HFH-5, and HFH-6 (52, 103). HNF-3γ is not expressed. In situ hybridization experiments have revealed regionalization of expression. For instance, whereas HFH-1 expression is diffuse throughout the organ, HNF-3α and HFH-4 are expressed in Clara cells, but not in type II cells, which by contrast express HFH-8 (50, 52, 81, 103). HFH-8 is also expressed in the pulmonary endothelium and connective fibroblasts of the alveolar sac in the adult lung and in the mesenchyme in the developing lung (135). During development, the expression pattern of HNF-3 family members suggests that they play roles in regional differentiation of the intestinal endoderm and its derivatives, including the lung (8, 127). While HNF-3α expression is sustained in the trachea, HNF-3β, which is expressed in the rat lung bud, disappears from trachea but continues to be expressed, along with HNF-3α, in the growing bronchial tree (21). In the fetal mouse lung, HNF-3β protein, is present at early stages throughout the pulmonary epithelium, including in the trachea. It becomes restricted to epithelial cells of conducting airways and to type II cells in late gestation, and shows a decreased level of expression compared with earlier stages (195). This decrease may provide signals influencing acinar cell differentiation. Similar changes in the temporal–spatial pattern of HNF-3β expression have been found in the developing human lung (163). Interestingly, in infants with BPD, HNF-3β was abundantly expressed in regenerating epithelial cells (163). In the adult lung, HNF-3β mRNA has been found to be expressed in mesenchyme in only one study (49), but HNF-3β protein has been detected in nuclei of epithelial bronchial, bronchiolar, and alveolar (type II) cells in another study (195). Targeted disruption of the HNF-3β gene has been attempted, but because of the early requirement of the gene for node, notochord, and gut tube development, the homozygous genotype is lethal prior to lung budding and the model has not been useful in determining more precisely the role of this gene in lung development (7, 178). Strong expression of HFH-4 has been found in epithelium of bronchiolar tubules but not in more distal tubules destined to generate the alveolar epithelium (81). Thus, the limit of HFH-4 expression coincides precisely with the demarcation between proximal and distal epithelia, which suggests a direct role for HFH-4 in regulating the initial differentiation of airway and alveolar epithelial cells.

A recently described forkhead gene, named *LUN*, is strongly expressed in the lung and more weakly in the small intestine (125). Its forkhead domain is identical to that of HFH-8. This factor has been shown to act as a positive transactivator for the SP-B promoter, which suggests that it may play a role in the determination and maintenance of some cell types in the lung (125).

Transcription factors of the HNF-3/fkh family appear to specify the endodermal lineage and therefore the tissues derived from this embryonic sheet, such as the liver, intestine, thyroid, and lung (8, 127). Organs of endodermal origin posterior to the lung, however, express HNF-3γ, but not TTF-1, which by contrast is expressed in more anterior segments of the body, such as thyroid and brain. Thyroid also expresses Pax-8, which is absent from the lung. A lung-cell identity would therefore be determined by the simultaneous expression of TTF-1, HNF-3α, and HNF-3β in the absence of Pax-8, a pattern found only in lung epithelial cells (27).

A characteristic HNF-3/fkh protein binding site has been shown to be present in the SP-B promoter with a canonic palindromic sequence, TGTTTGT, which is also found in liver-specific gene regulatory regions (27). Point mutation of this binding site eliminated HNF-3 binding and resulted in significantly decreased activity of the transfected SP-B promoter (27). Co-transfection experiments with either HNF-3α or HFH-8 expression vectors and gene constructs that included a fragment of the SP-B promoter have shown that both transcription factors are able to activate reporter gene expression to a similar extent (49). Since SP-B is expressed both in Clara and type II cells, but HNF-3α is restricted to the former and HFH-8 to the latter, it has been proposed that SP-B expression is controlled at the same regulatory sequence by HNF-3α in Clara cells and by HFH-8 in type II cells (49). Although HFH-8 expression during lung development has not been characterized, this suggests a role for this factor in cell differentiation of the developing distal epithelium.

Binding sites for HNF-3 proteins have also been demonstrated in the CC10 promoter (19, 147). In co-transfection experiments with CC10 promoter elements and HNF-3α and β expression vectors in HeLa cells, HNF-3α and HNF-3β have been shown to have opposite effects on CC10 expression: HNF-3α stimulated activity whereas HNF-3β inhibited activity (146). This finding may result, however, from a specificity of HeLa cells, since in another study (21), similar co-transfection in the Clara cell–like NCI-H441 adenocarcinoma cell line led to cooperative action between both factors. More recently, a synergistic activation of the rabbit CC10 promoter was reported for HNF-3α and the ubiquitous transcription factor Sp1 and shown to be absolutely dependent on the integrity of two Sp binding sites (31). Surprisingly, it was shown in the same study that contrary to the rat promoter, the human and rabbit CC10 promoters are not regulated by TTF-1 (31). Figure 4.2 summarizes the

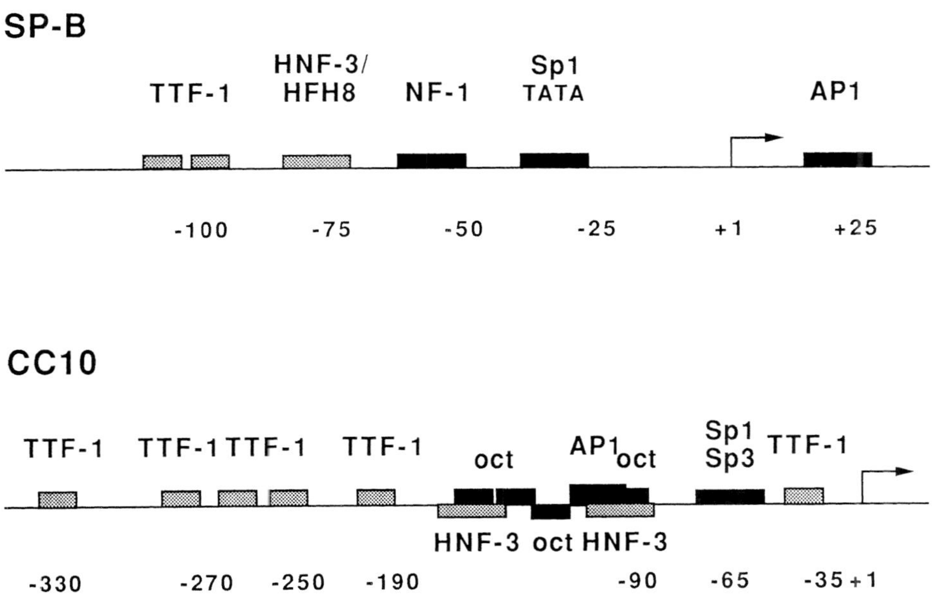

Fig. 4.2 Schematic illustration of the gene promoter region of surfactant protein B (*SP-B*) and of Clara cell protein 10 kDa (*CC10*). *+1* indicates the transcription start site. Ubiquitous transcription factor–binding sites are represented by *black rectangles*. Tissue-specific transcription factor–binding sites are represented by *shaded rectangles*. Drawn from data by Bohinski et al. (28) and Clevidence et al. (49) for SP-B, and from data by Ray et al. (139), Sawaya et al. (147), and Toonen et al. (171) for CC10.

organization of the SP-B and the CC10 gene promoter with localization of ubiquitous and specific transcription factor–binding sites.

In addition to direct effects on lung cell marker genes, HNF-3/fkh factors also transcriptionally control the expression of TTF-1 since, on the one hand, HNF-3β expression precedes that of TTF-1 in lung cells and, on the other hand, HNF-3β and, to a lesser extent, HNF-3α enhance the expression of a TTF-1-reporter construct in MLE cells (85). A hierarchical relationship therefore appears to exist between winged-helix transcription factors and TTF-1.

Role of CCAAT/Enhancer Binding Proteins and Peroxisome Proliferator-Activated Receptor γ

The CCAAT/enhancer binding proteins (C/EBP) are a family of the leucine zipper class of transcription factors that bind to DNA as homo- or heterodimers. The prototype member of the family, C/EBPα, may be involved in the control of type II cell functions. Expression of C/EBPα is restricted to certain tissues and cell types, including the liver, lung, white and brown adipose tissue, and placenta (59). Several genes of enzymes involved in lipid metabolism have been shown to be targets of this transcription factor (59). In the lung, C/EBPα mRNA levels have been found to be substantially enriched in alveolar type II cells, and C/EBPα protein is present in type II cell nuclei (106). Interestingly, C/EBPα is rapidly lost when type II cells are removed from the lung, but similar to surfactant proteins, it is re-expressed when cells are cultured on basement membrane matrix (106). Consistent with a putative role in type II cell differentiation is the fact that C/EBPα mRNA level increases in the developing rat lung between gestational days 18 and 20 (106). Three putative C/EBP-binding sites have been identified in the SP-A gene, one in the 5′ untranscribed region and the others in the first and last introns (160).

Invalidation of the C/EBPα gene in the mouse was reported to result in defects in liver and lung structure and in failure to accumulate lipids in adipocytes (67). The lung of nullizygous mice exhibited disturbed alveolar architecture, with immature appearance and type II cell hyperproliferation. Although no alteration was found in the expression patterns of SP-C, TTF-1, or CC10, these mice displayed respiratory problems and generally died within the first 10 h after birth. Surfactant abnormalities, including an inadequate amount of other surfactant proteins or of surfactant phospholipids, have been assumed but not yet explored. The role of C/EBPα in the control of lipogenetic enzyme expression, especially of fatty acid synthase and acetyl-CoA carboxylase, argues for a role in the synthesis of lipid precursors of surfactant phospholipids by type II cells.

More recently, C/EBPδ messenger RNA has been found to be developmentally regulated in fetal rabbit lung (32). In human fetal lung explants, C/EBPδ expression was induced rapidly during organ culture and increased further by treatment with dexamethasone and cyclic AMP, which, along with its localization primarily in alveolar epithelial cells, suggests a role for this factor in the regulation of type II cell differentiation (32).

Finally, another transcription factor known to be involved in adipogenesis, the nuclear receptor peroxisome proliferator-activated receptor γ (PPARγ), was reported to be expressed in rabbit lung type II cells, to occur coincidentally with SP-A expression during type II cell differentiation, and to be up-regulated by cyclic AMP (121). A role in type II cell differentiation and expression of lipogenic enzymes in this cell type has been postulated for PPARγ (121).

Promoters of Distal Lung-Marker Proteins and Cell Specificity of Expression

SP-A and SP-B Promoters

Analysis of the SP-A promoter function in tissue-specific expression has led to somewhat contradictory findings. It has been reported that a 215 bp fragment of the rat SP-A gene upstream of the transcription start site supports in vitro transcription in the presence of lung nuclear extract but not of liver nuclear extract (102). Consistent with this finding is the fact that the binding profile of nuclear protein extract from the liver or kidney to fragments of the same promoter differed from that of the lung (73, 99). Lung nuclear proteins were found to protect two palindromic sequences in the distal and proximal parts of the promoter (73). Some binding activity was found, however, in nuclear proteins from cardiac and skeletal muscle (73), and from the liver (168) using fragments of the promoter region of different sizes. The transfection of reporter genes coupled with a large portion of the 5′-flanking region of the SP-A gene that included these elements into cells of various origins (including primary cultures of type II cells and cell lines of pulmonary and extrapulmonary origin) led to tissue-specific expression in one study (35) but not in others (6, 160), even if expression was higher in cells of pulmonary origin. These data suggest that regulation of the SP-A gene is complex and that the appropriateness of the different cell systems used should be evaluated carefully. Stuempfle and co-workers (168) have suggested that the lack of in vitro tissue-specific expression of the rat SP-A gene is due to one or more possible factors. Lung-specific DNA–protein complexes identified in various studies may require interaction with other DNA–protein complex(es) to confer tissue specificity to the SP-A gene. A silencer element may be present further upstream or downstream of the region covered by these constructs. The lack of chromatin structure that characterizes transient transcription assays could play a role in the nonspecific transcription. Finally, regulation of the SP-A gene may not be readily discerned via a cell-free transcriptional assay. In addition, it should be pointed out that thus far there has been no report of in vivo transgenic experiments with the SP-A promoter.

In contrast, study of the human SP-B promoter (174) has shown unambiguously that a fragment from −403 to −35 bp was sufficient to confer expression specificity to the Clara cell–like H441 cell line, compared with other cell lines. Moreover, transcriptional control elements were found both 5′ and 3′ of the transcription start site. Promoter activity was strongly and dose-dependently inhibited by phorbol ester, an inhibitor of surfactant protein synthesis. The phorbol-ester response localization does not coincide with a consensus AP1 site (binding site of the Jun-Fos heterodimer) identified in the promoter. It therefore appears possible that novel regulatory sequence binding proteins other than Jun and Fos are involved in this inhibition (174).

Differential Control of SP-C and CC10 Expression

Since SP-C and CC10 are differential markers of alveolar type II cells and bronchiolar Clara cells, respectively, analysis of their promoter sequences and respective regulation processes by transcription factors may produce clues to the compartimentalized expression of regulatory factors that account for the demarcation between bronchiolar and alveolar epithelia. Upon transfection, a small fragment located at –165 to +57 bp of the transcriptional starting point of CC10 has been shown to support expression of a reporter gene exclusively in the Clara cell–like H441 cell line and to elicit expression of a reporter gene in transgenic mice in Clara cells only, suggesting that a Clara cell–specific transcriptional element resides on this fragment (166). Regulation by the ubiquitous transcription factors AP-1 and octamer and by HNF-3/fkh family factors has been accounted for by binding sites in this fragment (147). However, there is no information about specific ligands responsible for differential expression. The presence of the –132 to –76 fragment of the CC10 promoter placed in its normal position, i.e., upstream of its homologous –75 to +37 fragment, is sufficient to allow HNF-3α and HNF-3β to activate reporter gene expression in H441 cells, whereas no reporter gene expression was found when the same fragment was placed upstream of the tyrosine kinase promoter (21). Regulatory elements that control Clara cell–specific expression of CC10 should therefore be investigated in the promoter part extending upstream to the –75 position.

In contrast with CC10 studies, transgenic experiments in mice with chimeric genes that include the 5′-flanking sequence derived from the human SP-C gene have led to lung epithelium–specific but not type II cell–specific expression of the transgene. Indeed, the latter was found to be expressed both in bronchiolar and alveolar cells (76, 179). Expression of the transgene was developmentally regulated, but it did not coincide strictly with either temporal or spatial expression of the SP-C gene. The transgene product was detected early in the development of the primordial lung bud, before the appearance of endogenous SP-C mRNA. Its quantity increased with progressing development, but it disappeared from trachea and main bronchi while its expression was maintained in secondary bronchi and bronchioles. Differentiation of bronchial–bronchiolar epithelium was consistent with the disappearance of SP-C expression and onset of CC10 expression, whereas that of the SP-C chimeric transgene persisted (179). The features of transgene expression nonetheless led to a strategy based on the use of the SP-C promoter for targeting the expression of various transgenes in the developing lung. This approach, however, did not allow the investigators to identify mechanisms responsible for specific SP-C expression in alveolar cells. Because the human SP-C gene was used in transgenic experiments, subtle differences may exist in the *cis*-active elements that would account for the lack of cell-specific expression in the mouse. Alternatively, the authors of this study have proposed that possible differences in the expression of the endogenous and chimeric genes may be related to peculiarities of the human gene being expressed in the mouse. The lack of cell-specific expression may also be explained by a positional effect. In a more recent study (57), microinjection in fertilized eggs of a reporter gene coupled with a smaller human SP-C fragment was reported to lead to expression of the transgene only in alveolar type II cells. Further investigations are therefore required to explore the molecular mechanisms that drive type II cell–specific expression of SP-C.

PUTATIVE MECHANISMS OF ANTERIOR–POSTERIOR SPECIFICATION

In contrast to the rapidly growing body of knowledge about nuclear factors that readily control transcription of distal lung markers at the level of *cis*-acting elements, much less is known about the mechanisms taking place upstream in the cascade of developmental events and that determine cell fate along the anterior–posterior axis of the lung. Currently, putative control factors can only be inferred from indirect arguments such as correlative expression with cell markers or findings from gain- or loss-of-function experiments. Although the list is not limited, possible control factors include the N-*myc* proto-oncogene, homeotic genes, and the retinoic acid–retinoic acid receptor system.

*Role of N-*myc

Transcription factors of the Myc protein family mediate specific responses to signals that regulate cell growth and differentiation during development. Expression of the N-*myc* proto-oncogene appears to be restricted by tissue and stage specificity, in contrast to c-*myc*, which is ubiquitous. During the course of murine lung development, N-*myc* expression has been shown to be greatest during the early phase of branching, and then to decline (83, 129). By in situ hybridization, this expression has been localized to the bronchiolar epithelium, with higher levels occurring in the tips of the developing airways. During the same stages of lung development, *c-myc* expression was found to be restricted to the mesenchyme (83).

Creation of a null mutation in the N-*myc* gene by homologous recombination resulted in death of the homozygous mutant mouse embryos soon after the surge of the lung bud (145, 164). It resulted in the failure of many epithelial structures to develop, including the lung, which showed no sign of branching beyond the main stem bronchi. Culturing explanted lungs from homozygous mutant embryos in a medium containing fetal bovine serum allowed some recovery of bronchial morphogenesis to occur (145), indicating that to some extent, serum components can overcome the lack of N-*myc* expression. The null mutation indicates the probable major importance of N-*myc* in lung development, but it is not useful for evaluating the more specific role of N-*myc* in the development of distal regions. More interesting in this respect are the consequences of an insertional mutation in the N-*myc* locus that did not completely eliminate, but resulted in the formation of, truncated N-*myc* transcripts (126). This "leaky" mutation thus allowed for a 75% reduction in N-*myc* expression through alternative splicing. Homozygous mice developed until term but died at birth of respiratory failure. With the exception of a reduced spleen size, abnormalities were limited to the lung. Whereas the number and distribution of the more proximal bronchi were normal, distal airways and air spaces failed to develop. Along with the highest rate of N-*myc* expression in distal developing airways, this finding is indicative of a major role for N-*myc* in the developmental control of distal lung epithelium. N-*myc* may not be involved in the differentiation of particular cell types, but it may represent an important element in the control of distal lung growth and morphogenesis.

Role of Homeotic Genes

The homeotic *Hox* (mouse) and *HOX* (human) genes are homeodomain-containing genes that share a high degree of homology with the *Drosophila HOM-C* complex. They are expressed during embryonic development and have been shown to regulate pattern formation in specifying anterior–posterior positional information. In vertebrates, 38 *Hox* genes are arranged in four chromosomal clusters designated *a* through *d*. Corresponding genes in the different clusters are called *paralogs* and are numbered 1 through 13. A colinear relation exists between a gene's position in the cluster and its anterior boundary of expression. The combination of expression of different paralogs in various organs forms a *Hox* code that appears to specify regional identity (reviewed in refs. 39 and 92).

Early expression, regionalization, and spatial–temporal developmental regulation of *Hox* genes in the lung argue for an important role for these genes in lung morphogenesis and pattern formation. Twenty *Hox* genes from the four clusters have been found to be expressed in the developing lung—some in both fetal and postnatal lung, others either in fetal or in neonatal lung; no expression of genes located 5′ to paralog group 9 has been detected (reviewed in ref. 39). *Hox* genes appear to be expressed in mesenchyme only (reviewed in ref. 92). Steady-state mRNA levels of *Hoxa-5, Hoxb-5, Hoxb-6,* and *Hoxb-8* are high at early stages and decrease with advancing age in fetal mouse or rat lung (24). By contrast, *Hoxa-2* mRNA levels remain unchanged throughout development (39). Active branching morphogenesis appears to be associated with high levels of expression of several *Hox* genes (reviewed in ref. 39). Thus, *Hoxb-3, b-4,* and *b-5* are highly expressed in the mouse embryonic foregut where the lung buds form (25). Background levels of *Hoxb-6* expression are seen in trachea and proximal lung, while high levels of expression are associated with the distal epithelial forming tubules in the branching lung; these levels become undetectable, however, at late gestation when acinar areas develop (41). The expression of some paralogs is consistent with the principle of co-linearity, and it has been postulated that specific combinations of *Hox* genes may function to specify the developmental fate of distinct regions of the lung through involvement in epithelial–mesenchymal interactions (26). Thus, once the bronchial tree has formed, *Hoxb-3* and *b-4* are expressed in the mesenchyme of the trachea, main-stem bronchi, and distal lung, whereas *Hoxb-2* and *b-5* are expressed only in the mesenchyme of the distal lung buds (26). *Hox* genes in other clusters also appear to be involved in this determination. Elements in the 5′ upstream region of the *Hoxa-4* gene directed a transgene expression with prominent localization in lower lobes in the mouse fetal lung (13). Regulatory elements may therefore control the expression of Hox genes in specific regions of the lung.

Limited information has been gained from mutation disruption of *Hox* gene expression or transgenic overexpression, most likely because of redundancy in the sites of expression. It has nevertheless been reported that *Hoxa-3* mutants die at birth of respiratory failure and have smaller trachea and bronchi with disorganized epithelial cells (46, 110). These results, together with defects in differentiation of endodermal cells in the thyroid, may indicate a role for *Hoxa-3* in specification of endodermally derived cells, including lung epithelial cells. *Hoxa-5* has more recently been shown to be essential for normal organogenesis and function of the respiratory tract (9). In homozygous newborn mutants for this gene, improper tracheal and lung morphogenesis lead to tracheal occlusion and respiratory distress associated with a marked decrease in the production of surfactant proteins and with a reduced TTF-1, HNF-3β, and N-myc gene expression in the pulmonary epithelium (9). Thus, *Hox* gene products appear to control TTF-1 expression, an assumption also supported by the report that the Hoxb-3 protein is an upstream regulator of TTF-1 (77). This hypothesis, however, appears to conflict with the expression of *Hox* genes in mesenchyme and of TTF-1 in epithelium.

Despite the sparse and preliminary character of current data on *Hox* genes , an involvement of *Hox* gene expression in anterior–posterior specification in the developing lung is strongly suggested. Further investigations are needed to determine whether and how a particular *Hox* gene complement specifies the differences between proximal and distal identity of lung mesenchyme—particularly to what degree they affect the expression of factors that may in turn control the expression of epithelial cell markers.

Role of Retinoic Acid and Retinoic Acid Receptors

Retinoic acid (RA) is clearly necessary for the maintenance of mature tracheal-bronchial epithelium. By contrast, its effects on the developing alveolar epithelium have been a matter of debate. Whereas high concentration and/or long-term exposure of in vitro models led to a dramatically altered branching pattern, including total suppression of distal tubules and extension of proximal-like tubules toward the pleural surface (42), and to a decreased amount of surfactant proteins or of their mRNAs (42, 70, 119), low concentration and short-term exposure increased surfactant protein mRNAs (25). It should be stressed that stimulating effects were observed with concentrations in the range of the dissociation constant for in vitro nuclear binding of RA in the lung (10^{-9} M in the rat). Moreover, exogenous retinol and RA enhanced surfactant phospholipid synthesis in vivo and in vitro (69, 70). Several lines of evidence indicate that retinoids are also involved in the control of alveolar morphogenesis. Retinoic acid increased transcription of the elastin gene and elastin synthesis in cultured neonatal rat lung fibroblasts (107), when elastin deposition is a central element in the process of alveolar septation. Furthermore, in vivo postnatal treatment with RA in the rat increased the number of alveoli and prevented the glucocorticoid-induced inhibition of septation (115).

Retinoic acid exerts its effects through binding to a number of different receptors designated RARs α, β, and γ, RXRs α, β, and γ, and their subtypes. These are members of the steroid-thyroid-retinoid nuclear receptor superfamily and form heterodimeric combinations among themselves and other nuclear receptors to transactivate gene expression through site-specific DNA binding. While all-*trans* RA binds specifically to RARs, 9-*cis* RA can bind to both RARs and RXRs. Differential expression of RA receptors has been reported in the different pulmonary structures by in situ hybridization (63). RAR-α and RXR-α/β are ubiquitously expressed in the lung. RAR-β2 mRNA is present in the foregut endodermal precursor of the lung bud. As branching proceeds, it becomes restricted to the trachea and the most proximal bronchi and is not detected in distal lung epithelium. RAR-γ expression is limited to tracheal and bronchial mesenchyme. Whereas the null mutation of a single receptor subtype generally lead to little developmental alteration, double null mutations in RARs α and β result in a variety of abnormalities in many organs, including various lung developmental defects from agenesis to simple growth retardation (118). These abnormalities, however, show little correlation with spatial distribution of RARs in the lung (RXRs are ubiquitous) and provide no information about a role for these receptors in regional specification. Other knockout experiments (reviewed in ref. 39) have not led to any aberrant lung phenotype. Conversely, when the gene of the receptor subtype RAR-β4 was overexpressed in transgenic mice, alveolar hyperplasia and an excess of alveolar type II cells were observed (17), which suggests a role for RA in the control of type II cell differentiation and the involvement of RAR-β4 in the process. A putative RXR responsive element has been found in the third intron of the rat SP-A gene (25), and the SP-B gene has been demonstrated to be transactivated by RAR/RXR heterodimers in the presence of 9-*cis* RA in the H441 adenocarcinoma cell line (189). In the latter study, the RA response element mediating RA stimulation of the human SP-B promoter was identified.

Since the capacity of RA to activate expression of homeotic genes is a fundamental characteristic feature in vertebrate development, the hypothesis that RA's effects on the lung may be mediated through changes in *Hox* gene expression must be considered. Retinoic acid markedly increased *Hoxa-5*, *Hoxb-5*, and *Hoxb-6* mRNA levels in lung explants (24), and that of *Hoxa-5* in lung fibroblasts (18). Retinoic acid also prevented the decrease in *Hoxb-6* and *Sonic hedgehog* expression that spontaneously occurs in cultured whole embryonic lung and reproduces the changes occurring during the course of in vivo development (41). It has been proposed (41) that retinoic acid acts to maintain high levels of expression of pattern-related genes in a fashion characteristic of the immature lung, thus promoting continued formation of proximal lung structures and preventing formation of typical distal lung structures of the mature lung. It should be pointed out, however, that this conclusion was drawn from the results of embryonic lung culture experiments in the presence of high RA concentrations (up to 10^{-5} M).

On the whole, RA appears to be an important element in the control of lung development, including alveolar development and expression of alveolar markers, but its functions are not understood in detail. Current data are still insufficient to determine whether RA is a morphogen along the anterior–posterior axis of the developing lung, as has been shown in other organs. Further investigations are necessary to determine more precisely the local tissue level of retinoids and of cellular binding proteins that sequester retinoids, the distribution of the various RA receptors, and the developmental changes of these parameters. Figure 4.3 summarizes the putative

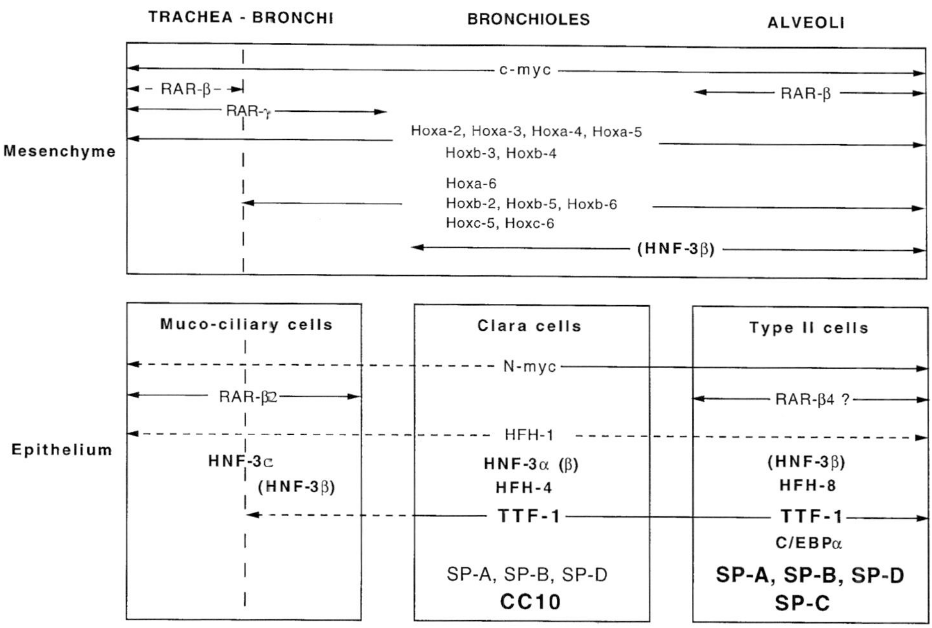

Fig. 4.3 Transcription factors potentially involved in anterior–posterior determination of epithelial cell fate in the developing lung and in Clara cell and alveolar type II cell differentiation. Ubiquitously expressed transcription factors are not shown. Factors are presented vertically in a putative hierarchical order, i.e., retinoic acid receptors (RARs) may control *Hox* gene expression, which may in turn determine expression of cell-specific transcription factors that would finally control cell-specific expression of markers (SP-A, -B, -C, -D, and CC10). For SP-A, -B, -D, *bold characters* indicate that the type II cell is the major source. *Dashed lines* indicate a diffuse weak expression, or, in the instance of TTF-1, contradictory data. *Parentheses* indicate that HNF-3β has been detected in one study but not in another one. Potential mesenchymal influences upon transcription factor expression by epithelium are not included. C/EBPα, CCAAT/enhancer binding protein α; HFH, hepatocyte nuclear factor 3/forkhead homologs; HNF, hepatocyte nuclear factor; TTF, thyroid transcription factor.

factors of anterior–posterior specification and specific transactivating factors of distal lung markers with their possible hierarchical interrelationships.

ROLE OF EXTRACELLULAR MATRIX COMPONENTS

Extracellular matrix is an essential element in the process of branching morphogenesis (see Chap. 1), but it also appears to participate in the control of cell phenotype expression. As stated above, type II cells cultured on tissue culture plastic rapidly flatten and loose their markers. Changes in lectin-binding pattern suggest that they acquire type I cell features (55, 61). Attempts have therefore been made to develop in vitro models supporting type II cell marker expression. The matrix extracted from the murine EHS tumor, which presents features similar to those of the *lamina densa* of basement membrane (98), has emerged as the most favorable substratum for adult (155) and fetal (22) type II cells. The mechanism by which this matrix functions is difficult to interpret, however, because its composition is complex, it includes not only typical basement membrane components but also various growth factors (98). Current evidence suggests that integrins, the cell receptors to matrix components, transmit signals via both the cytoskeleton and second messengers, and that these signals may in turn elicit specific gene expression (2, 89). It appears that formation of close, hollow, alveolar-like structures by type II cells on the EHS matrix and the fact that cells keep a cuboidal shape are crucial factors for sustained expression of their markers (22, 155). The role of cell shape has been illustrated in an investigation that consisted of seeding type II cells onto a collagen gel fixed on a culture dish, then detaching the gel to allow it to float and shrink (154). The cells spread out on fixed collagen, as when cultured directly on plastic, and lost their markers, but when their collagen substratum was detached, they retrieved their cuboidal shape and differentiation markers, including lamellar bodies and surfactant proteins. Further investigation (54) has shown that cells acquire membrane markers of type I cells on attached gels and that this is reversed when the gel is detached. The potential to express type II cell markers therefore appears to be retained in type I cells, and the type II–to–type I cell conversion represents a reversible transdifferentiation process. Since interactions with multiple matrix components are not involved in these elegant experiments, it appears that geometric constraint, which is likely to induce major changes in the cytoskeleton, plays a major role in the control of cell-specific feature expression.

Attempts have been made to explore the role of individual matrix components in growth and differentiation of type II cells. Whereas fibronectin appears to enhance DNA synthesis in isolated type II cells (137), laminin appears to play a role in the preservation of type II cell morphology and function, as cells flattened on an anti-laminin serum-treated EHS matrix (138). Epithelial cells adhere more readily to laminin than fibroblasts, possibly because of higher expression of α_6 integrin subunit and specific expression of α_3 integrin subunit (36, 187). Laminin may play a key role in alveolar morphogenesis, particularly its carboxy-terminal fragment designated *E8,* as an anti-E8 antibody prevented alveolar-like type II cell assembly on EHS matrix (116). A peptide sequence SINNNR in this domain was demonstrated to mediate cation-dependent adhesion of type II cells to the matrix (116). It should be pointed out, however, that type II cells seeded onto purified laminin or fibronectin spread, lose their features, and develop type I cell markers with kinetics similar to those on uncoated plastic (55). This suggests that association with other matrix components is needed for the differentiation and morphogenetic responses to laminin. Collagens have been found to have no effect on DNA or on surfactant phosphatidylcholine synthesis by isolated type II cells (3). Changes in lung glycosaminoglycans that occur in the course of development appear to be temporally related with epithelial differentiation and alveolarization (reviewed in ref. 30). Caniggia et al. (37) have shown that while fibroblasts in close proximity to the epithelium produce and secrete mainly hyaluronan, more distant fibroblasts shift from producing principally heparan sulfate and chondroitin sulfate during the pseudoglandular stage to producing hyaluronan during the canalicular stage of lung development. Because this shift to hyaluronan production occurs simultaneously with the thinning of the alveolar septal wall, the authors suggest that this developmentally regulated glycosaminoglycan production may facilitate epithelial–fibroblast interaction, thus influencing fetal lung growth and cell differentiation.

Little is known about the mechanisms that drive type I cell differentiation in vivo. Type I cells overlie a fused basement membrane that is shared with the vascular endothelium. It had been observed in the developing human lung (104) that cuboidal cells start decreasing in height at focal points where blood vessels contact with the epithelium. Type I cell differentiation is therefore probably induced by endothelial cells. This assumption had not received experimental support until Adamson and Young (4) studied rat lung type II cell behavior on a matrix secreted by a pulmonary vascular endothelial cell line. They observed that after an initial burst of growth, cell proliferation dropped while cells acquired type I cell features, as judged by morphology and *Bauhinia purpurea* lectin binding. These temporal changes reproduce the in vivo process of re-epithelialization that follows type I cell necrosis and denudation of the capillary endothelial basement membrane. Although the components of endothelial basement membrane controlling this process are not yet defined, it is clear that different microdomains must exist in the alveolar basement membrane beneath type I and II cells and that basement membrane produced by endothelial cells provides information first for epithelial proliferation, then for differentiation of type I from type II cells.

ENDOCRINE AND PARACRINE MODULATORS OF GENE EXPRESSION

It is beyond the scope of this chapter to extensively review the role of diffusible factors in the control of alveolar cell development. Only those recent studies relevant to the present purpose are considered here.

Glucocorticoids

Glucocorticoid hormones play crucial roles in architectural maturation of the pulmonary gas-exchange region (reviewed in ref. 114) and in biochemical lung maturation. For architectural maturation, glucocorticoids inhibit epithelial cell growth and alveolar septation and accelerate thinning of the alveolar walls. In neonatal rats, exogenous glucocorticoids induce a precocious termination of the lung developmental process. The clinical relevance of this finding pertains to the use of glucocorticoid hormones in the fetus for accelerating biochemical lung maturation and in the neonate as part of the treatment of RDS and BPD, since the lungs of infants with BPD fail to septate (112). For biochemical maturation, glucocorticoids were historically the first modulators of lung maturation to be recognized. Their key role in the control of lung maturation is well established, and they are known to stimulate in vivo the synthesis of all surfactant components, which has led to their use in the prevention of RDS. Their actions, however, are complex and not always clearly understood at the molecular level.

Insight into the requirement of glucocorticoids for lung development has recently been gained from the gene inactivation approach. One strategy consisted of creating a mammalian model of corticotropin-releasing hormone (CRH) deficiency by targeted mutation in mouse embryonic stem cells (128). This resulted in a markedly atrophic appearance of the zona fasciculata of the adrenal gland, a reduced basal blood level of corticosterone, and impaired corticosterone response to stress. Homozygous CRH-deficient mice born to heterozygous mothers developed normally and exhibited normal viability and fertility. Mating between homozygous animals, however, yielded progeny that died within the first 12 h of life, despite a normal appearance at birth and a normal length of pregnancy. Corticosterone supplementation to pregnant homozygous females resulted in the production of viable litters, demonstrating that maternal corticosteroids in heterozygous pregnant mice are sufficient to compensate for the fetal deficit. Histologic examination of newborn lungs revealed lung dysplasia in the offspring of homozygous mating, including marked hypercellularity, thickened alveolar septae, and paucity of air spaces. SP-B mRNA was reduced to 44% of the wild-type value. Corticosterone treatment completely reversed lung abnormalities. Thus, the study revealed a fetal glucocorticoid requirement for lung maturation, but postnatally, despite marked glucocorticoid deficiency, mice exhibited normal growth, fertility, and longevity, which suggests that the major role of glucocorticoids is during fetal rather postnatal life. In another study (51), the glucocorticoid receptor (GR) gene was disrupted. Similar to the CRH deficiency, homozygous GR-deficient mice developed normally in utero, but died within a few hours after birth because of respiratory failure. Lung development appeared to be impaired from gestational day 15.5, i.e., it arrested in a pseudoglandular state. SP-A, SP-B, and SP-C gene expression did not seem to be markedly impaired, but protein content was not explored. Other abnormalities included blocked adrenergic chromaffin cell development and reduced capacity to activate genes for key gluconeogenic enzymes.

The molecular mechanism of action of glucocorticoids in the control of surfactant synthesis remains imperfectly understood. With regard to the phospholipid moiety of surfactant, an indirect action through stimulated production by the lung fibroblast of a peptide mediator that in turn stimulates phospholipid metabolic pathway was postulated long ago; the putative mediator has not yet been characterized, however (see Chap. 11). Medium conditioned by fibroblasts in the presence of cortisol enhanced the expression of fatty acid–synthesizing enzymes at a pretranslational level in isolated type II cells (11), but this observation was made with type II cells cultured on plastic. In fetal lung explants, dexamethasone did not increase the mRNA level of the rate-limiting enzyme of phosphatidylcholine synthesis, CTP:phosphocholine cytidylyltransferase (68), which supports the concept that the increased activity of this enzyme by glucocorticoids is due to increased fatty acid synthesis.

The actual impact of glucocorticoids on surfactant proteins remains unclear, despite many investigations in this area. Whereas stimulatory effects of glucocorticoids have invariably been observed for SP-B and SP-C gene expression in vivo, in lung explant culture, or in pulmonary adenocarcinoma cell line, SP-A gene expression has been found to be either increased or decreased, or submitted to a biphasic control, i.e., enhanced at low glucocorticoid concentrations and diminished at higher concentrations. Differences among the species, the use of in vivo or in vitro models, the hormonal dose, or length of exposure may account for these conflicting data. Adrenalectomy in the rat showed that glucocorticoids play a minor role in SP gene expression, at least in the adult, and have rather limited translational or post-translational effects (66).

The role of glucocorticoids in the control of SP gene transcription is unclear. Although putative glucocorticoid regulatory elements (GRE) have been evidenced in the 5′-flanking sequence of the SP-A and SP-B genes (102, 180, 181) their role in the regulation of transcription has not been established. No GRE consensus sequence was found in the entire structural SP-A gene in the rabbit (44), despite enhanced transcription of the SP-A gene at all glucocorticoid doses in fetal lung explants of this species (23). When a reporter gene construct including a large portion of the 5′-flanking region of the SP-A gene was transfected in type II cells or in two lung adenocarcinoma cell lines, not only did glucocorticoids fail to increase its transcription but the stimulation of its transcription by cyclic AMP (see below) was unexpectedly antagonized by dexamethasone in a dose-dependent manner (6). Three possible glucocorticoid receptor–binding sites with modest homology to the consensus GRE that appeared to overlap the cAMP-response element (CRE) may account for this inhibition of expression (6). By contrast, evidence for direct stimulation of SP-D expression at the transcriptional level has been demonstrated in transfection experiments with constructs including a large 5′-flanking sequence of the human SP-D gene (142).

Glucocorticoid effects on the developing lung appear to involve interaction with other regulatory factors. Another possible mechanism of inhibited SP-A transcription in lung explants might be through diminished prostaglandin secretion (1). Glucocorticoids also appear to interact with transforming growth factor (TGF) β expression in the developing lung, but conflicting data have been reported. Glucocorticoids were reported by some investigators to down-regulate TGF-β2 and TGF-β3 transcripts in mouse lung (86, 117), whereas others found an induction of TGF-β3 by glucocorticoids in fetal rat lung fibroblasts (175). These contradictory findings, along with the complexity of TGF-β effects on the developing lung (see below), make it difficult to draw conclusions about glucocorticoid-TGF-β interactions. Finally, lung proteins designated A2, B, and D that bind the SP-B promoter at a NF 1 site have been recently characterized. Their cDNAs have been cloned and sequenced; all three proteins are novel (108, 109). Co-transfection of a reporter construct containing 212 bp from the SP-B promoter together with a protein A2 or B expression vector in a lung adenocarcinoma cell line resulted in slightly increased reporter gene expression that was further enhanced by glucocorticoids in the instance of protein B (109). The protein D carboxy-terminal end contains a modified leucine zipper-like DNA-binding motif. Co-transfection with a reporter construct containing 212 bp of the SP-B promoter together with a protein D expression vector led to strongly enhanced reporter gene expression in the presence of dexamethasone only (108). At least for SP-B regulation, glucocorticoid responsiveness appears to involve additional gene transactivating factors that are distinct from the glucocorticoid receptor.

As a whole, glucocorticoids appear to accelerate surfactant accumulation in fetal lung through complex mechanisms that involve cell-specific transcription factors and balanced control of other modulating factors. Moreover, in view of the precocious and marked delay of overall lung development reported in GRH or GR knockout models, it is likely that glucocorticoids play multiple roles and elicit expression of a number of genes other than those of the specific markers of distal lung. The control of some genes may be a prerequisite for expression of the others, thus illustrating the concept of glucocorticoid permissive effect. Clarification of these mechanisms calls for further investigations, especially into the cascade of successive gene activations/inactivations.

Cyclic Adenosine 3′,5′ Monophosphate (cAMP) and cAMP Increasing Agents

Cyclic AMP has been shown to be a potent positive regulator of SP-A gene expression. It markedly increases the transcription rate of the SP-A gene in fetal lung explant culture. Two enhancers have been identified in the 5′-flanking region of the rabbit SP-A gene, whose mutagenesis resulted in a marked reduction in basal and cAMP-stimulated fusion gene expression in transfected type II cells (73). A putative c-AMP response element (CRE) that differs from the consensus CRE by one nucleotide only has been identified in this promoter by the same group and is presumed to mediate transactivation by cAMP of a reporter gene in transfected type II cells grown on extracellular matrix prepared from Madin-Darby canine kidney cells (6). Cyclic AMP did not enhance expression of the reporter gene in type II–related cell lines that do not express SP-A in vitro, despite a relatively high basal rate of transcription in these cells (6). Type II cell–specific transactivator(s) of the CRE or, alternatively, some component of the cAMP response pathway is absent from these cell lines. More recently, mutagenetic study of the SP-A CRE led to the conclusion that this site does not bind classical CRE ligands of the CRE-binding protein/activating transcription factor family, but rather an orphan member of the steroid receptor family (120).

The finding that terbutaline, a β2-adrenergic agonist, increased the accumulation of SP-A in human fetal lung explants (131), suggests a role of catecholamines in the regulation of SP-A expression through β-adrenergic receptors and cAMP. Prostaglandin E_2 synthesis may also promote increased cAMP formation with consequent type II cell differentiation and SP-A gene expression (1).

In comparison, cAMP appears to have more modestly enhancing effects on SP-B and SP-C mRNA levels in rabbit or human lung. Cyclic AMP is nevertheless a stimulating factor of SP-B gene transcription in organ cultures of fetal rabbit lung. Evidence has recently shown that the stimulation of SP-B expression by cAMP is mediated by protein kinase A (PKA)-dependent activation of TTF-1 through the phosphorylation of a site at its NH_2 terminus (191). Consistent with this finding is the fact that a DNA homology search revealed no CRE consensus element within the concerned region of the SP-B promoter, suggesting that the stimulatory effects of PKA were not mediated by direct activation of CRE elements in the SP-B gene (191).

Epidermal Growth Factor and Transforming Growth Factor α

Epidermal growth factor (EGF) has long been recognized as an important control factor of both lung branching growth (see Chap. 1) and lung maturation (reviewed in ref. 30). Location of EGF and TGF-α mRNAs principally in mesenchyme of fetal human lung and of their common receptor (EGF-R) in epithelia suggests their probable role as paracrine mediators of mesenchymal–epithelial interactions (141). Since a high level of TGF-α has been found in fetal lung during the late canalicular and saccular stages when distal lung epithelial cells differentiate and mature (100), this factor may be involved primarily in the corresponding control mechanisms.

Both TGF-α and EGF stimulated type II cell proliferation, and this effect was antagonized by TGF-β (143). Epidermal growth factor also enhanced phosphatidylcholine synthesis in isolated type II cells, particularly when maintained on a basement membrane matrix (69, 43). Since EGF also increased SP-A mRNA and protein in human fetal lung in culture in a dose-dependent fashion (183), EGF and TGF-α both appear to be proliferative and differentiation factors for the alveolar epithelium. Despite this fact, no attempts to further analyze their effects on gene expression have been made.

The EGF-R gene has been invalidated in the mouse (122). Homozygous EGF-R-deficient mice died within the first 8 postnatal days. They exhibited growth retardation and a number of abnormalities, including marked lung abnormalities and breathing problems. Their lungs were condensed, with collapsed alveoli and dilated terminal bronchioles closer to the pleura. Alveolar septa were thicker and more cellular, which is typical of lung immaturity. SP-A and proSP-C immunoreactivity was reduced. This picture resembles that of human neonatal RDS. These findings demonstrate the involvement of EGF-R and therefore of EGF and/or TGF-α in lung development, especially in the morphogenesis and cell maturation of distal areas.

Keratinocyte Growth Factor (Fibroblast Growth Factor 7) and Hepatocyte Growth Factor/Scatter Factor

Both these heparin-binding growth factors have been reported to be present in lung-fibroblast conditioned medium and to synergistically mediate the proliferation-stimulating activity of this medium upon isolated type II cells (133). Keratinocyte growth factor (KGF) has also been shown to be a potent stimulus of type II cell multiplication in vivo through intratracheal administration (173). Again, the restriction of KGF gene expression in mesenchymal tissues and of KGF receptor [KGFR, a fibroblast growth factor receptor (FGFR)-2 splicing variant also designated FGFR2/IIIb] in epithelia (132), as well as the expression of hepatocyte growth factor/scatter factor (HGF/SF) in mesenchymal tissues and of the HGF/SF receptor (c-*met*) in epithelia (161) suggest their implication as mediators of mesenchymal–epithelial interactions in the developing lung. The KGF and KGFR mRNAs have indeed been found to be expressed early in the course of embryonic rat lung development, during the pseudoglandular stage (15, 157), and have been proposed to be involved in the control of early branching morphogenesis (see Chap 1).

With regard to marker expression, it has been shown that exogenous KGF is a potent enhancer of SP-A and SP-B mRNA steady-state levels in isolated type II cells from the adult rat lung (169). In cultured whole embryonic rat lung rudiments, KGF was found to elicit formation of cystic structures filled with fluid and limited by an epithelium that displayed characteristic features of alveolar type II cells, including lamellar bodies and expression of SP-C mRNA (157). This time, the SP-A mRNA was not enhanced, although there was strong stimulation of SP-C mRNA expression. More recently, using cultures of mesenchyme-free embryonic mouse lung epithelium on EHS matrix, it was consistently shown that KGF induced cystic structure formation and a precocious differentiation of type II cells with advanced SP-A and SP-B expression, but SP-C expression seemed to be reduced (40). In type II cells isolated from fetal rat lung during the late gestational period, when surfactant storage takes place, and cultured on the EHS matrix, KGF not only enhanced expression of all three SP-A, SP-B, and SP-C proteins but also stimulated phosphatidylcholine synthesis and storage through the increase of fatty acid synthase gene expression and activity, and the increase of choline phosphate cytidylyltransferase activity (43). Compared with other growth factors, KGF appeared to be the most potent stimulating factor (43). Differences in the models may account for these partially discrepant findings. Nevertheless, taken together, these investigations suggest that KGF is a stimulus of distal lung development and that it plays a role in the differentiation of type II cells. Acidic FGF (FGF-1), which also binds the KGFR, mimicked the effects of

KGF, although at a higher concentration, in three studies (43, 157, 169), but failed to induce type II cell differentiation in the fourth one (40). The HGF/SF neither influenced expression of SP mRNAs (169) nor stimulated phospholipid synthesis (43) nor affected lung morphogenesis in vitro (157), but it was shown to induce formation by LX-1 lung carcinoma cells of pseudo-alveolar structures lined with thin type I–like cells (33). A possible involvement of HGF/SF in the type II–to–type I cell conversion can therefore not be ruled out.

Several genetic manipulations have been made in the mouse to explore the role of KGF and KGFR in lung development. The key role of KGF transduction signal for lung development has been illustrated by lung-targeted expression of a dominant-negative FGFR2 placed under the control of the SP-C promoter for targeting the transgene expression specifically to the lung epithelium (134). Newborn mice expressing the transgene were completely normal, except that instead of having normally developed lungs, they had two unbranched, undifferentiated epithelial tubes that extended from the bifurcation of the trachea down to the diaphragm (see Figure 12.4c). No expression of the endogenous SP-C, chosen as a molecular marker of epithelial differentiation, was detected. Surprisingly, invalidation of the KGF gene (79) led to no obvious abnormality, which suggests that alternative ligands to KGFR, for instance, FGF-1 (40) or FGF-10 (15), play the major role in the KGFR-mediated events of lung morphogenesis. Misexpression of KGF in the lung epithelium of mice rendered transgenic for a human KGF gene fused to the SP-C promoter (158) led to embryonic lethality and to profound disturbance in fetal lung branching, with cystic lungs composed of exaggerated large airways, a deficit in small branching airways, and numerous dilated saccules lined by an immature, columnar epithelium that was unable to produce surfactant proteins B and C despite abundant expression of their genes. Morphological findings are consistent with those obtained with exogenous KGF in embryonic lung cultures (157). The absence of SP-B and SP-C may appear surprising, but the unregulated expression of KGF in epithelial cells that normally do not elaborate it may have profoundly disturbed a regulatory mechanism that implies interaction between distinct cell types in the normal lung. Moreover, the KGF mRNA level has been shown to increase steadily in rat lung during late saccular and early alveolar stages (58, 157). In the transgenic model, the precocious presence of high levels of KGF in the lung bud may therefore have impaired lung development at a stage when the bronchiolar tree is not completed.

More in-depth investigations are necessary to determine the underlying mechanisms that control gene expression, but taken together, these data indicate that KGF and related factors of the FGF family that are acting through the KGFR are important regulatory mediators in lung development. Taking into account the branching effects of FGF-1 (40) and FGF-10 (15), these factors may play a major role in branching morphogenesis, while KGF may control alveolar cell differentiation. Like EGF and TGF-α, KGF is both a mitogenic and differentiation factor of the alveolar epithelium. In this respect, it could become useful for the prevention of RDS through acceleration of lung maturation in utero and for the treatment of epithelial lung injury, including BPD.

Transforming Growth Factor β and Related Substances

Factors of the TGF β family have multiple roles in lung development. Three different TGF-β isoforms are present in mammals, and each has different effects on lung development. TGF-β1 appears to regulate early morphogenesis and extracellular matrix deposition in the developing lung (see Chap. 1). In distal parts of the lung, it inhibits histodifferentiation and the synthesis of SP-A and phospholipids (38, 72, 172, 183). The TGF-β-related Müllerian inhibiting substance, which is responsible for the Müllerian duct regression in the male, has also been reported to inhibit surfactant synthesis and has been proposed to be involved in the delay of lung maturation in males (reviewed in ref. 30). Conversely, TGF-β has been reported to enhance expression of laminin and of α and β subunits of its integrin cell receptors in alveolar epithelial cells, an effect potentially linked to their differentiation process (101). TGF-β1, which inhibited branching morphogenesis in a dose-dependent and reversible manner, also inhibited N-*myc* expression in cultured mouse lung bud (150). It appears, therefore, that reduced levels of N-*myc* resulting from TGF-β1 treatment may have impaired epithelial cell proliferation in lung buds and consequently have affected branching. Expression in the mouse of a TGF-β1 transgene targeted to respiratory epithelial cells by the SP-C promoter led to an arrest of lung development in the pseudoglandular stage (194). Contrary to branching morphogenesis of the bronchial tree, which was only slightly delayed, dilation of terminal buds, thinning of mesenchyme, and epithelial cell differentiation were markedly impaired, including failure to express marker proteins such as CC10 and pro-SP-C also occurred. In addition, the distribution of smooth muscle actin was abnormal, which may account at least in part for the limited expansion of distal leading edges of terminal buds. Consistent with the probable implication of N-*myc* in distal lung morphogenesis is the finding that reduced N-*myc* expression could be involved in these abnormalities. These findings are in keeping with the concept that alveolar epithelial differentiation implies that the inhibition exerted by a TGF-β-like activity produced at early developmental stages by lung mesenchyme is released (172).

Little is known about the role of TGF-β2 in lung development. TGF-β2 knockout mice are born cyanotic, exhibit respiratory distress, and die within minutes (144). Histological examination of the lung did not reveal morphological defects. Collapsed conducting airways were observed, but surfactant was unexplored (144). The role of TGF-β3 is better documented and appears to be crucial. The TGF-β3 null mutant mice exhibited grossly abnormal lung development, including pseudoglandular histology, alveolar hypoplasia, mesenchymal thickening and hypercellularity, and decreased pro-SP-C immunoreactivity (90). This study indicates that this TGF-β isoform is necessary for normal lung development and that, in contrast to TGF-β1, TGF-β3 favors alveolar cytodifferentiation. Transforming growth factor β3 has also been shown to control tropoelastin expression by the fetal lung fibroblast, which is consistent with a possible involvement in alveolarization process (192).

Studies on localization of TGF-β isoforms in the developing lung do not provide much insight into their functions. Through in situ hybridization, TGF-β1 mRNA has been found to be present in both mesenchyme and epithelium (74, 149). While in situ hybridization detected TGF-β2 expression in epithelial cells of the growing tips of developing bronchioles in the human and mouse (74, 123, 149), the immunoreactive peptide was detected in isolated fibroblasts but not in isolated epithelial cells from the developing rat lung (56). TGF-β3 expression appears to be restricted to the columnar epithelial cells of future airways and to be absent in the epithelium of growing end buds or in differentiated alveolar epithelium (123). Since mesenchymal cells express the TGF-β3 gene (123, 149) and contain the immunoreactive peptide (56), this absence from distal lung epithelial cells is consistent with a possible mediation of a mesenchymal–epithelial interaction related to the role of TGF-β3 in alveolar cytodifferentiation.

The TGF-β receptors belong to a superfamily of transmembrane serine-threonine kinases. Three different-sized classes termed types I, II, and III receptors have been identified, although the precise role of each of those in TGF-β signal transduction is not clearly established. Consistent with the involvement of TGF-β in the development of alveolar cells is the finding that the TGF-β receptor type II displays maximal expression in fetal rat lung around birth and is expressed along a proximal-distal gradient. Whereas the cuboidal epithelium of the presumptive alveolar tubes shows intense expression of the receptor, only a low level of expression is detectable in the columnar epithelium of the large proximal conducting airways (193).

Bone morphogenetic protein-4 (BMP-4), a TGF-β-related substance, also appears to play a role in lung morphogenesis and cytodifferentiation (16). The *Bmp-4* gene and the *Sonic hedgehog* (*Shh*) gene, the product of which appears to play a role in *Bmp-4* regulation, have been shown to be expressed at high levels in the distal tips of the growing mouse lung tubules, in contrast with the HNF-3β gene, which is expressed uniformly throughout the epithelium. Moreover, BMP-4 is also present in the mesenchyme adjacent to the most distal epithelium. Its expression declines during late gestation. Overexpression of *Bmp-4* in mice transgenic for a SP-C promoter-*Bmp-4* construct led to abnormal lung development. Transgenic lungs were about half the size of normal lungs and had fewer, greatly distended, epithelial terminal buds separated by abundant mesenchyme. Epithelial cell multiplication was reduced and mesenchymal cell death was enhanced. Whereas the pattern of CC10 expression appeared unchanged, the number of SP-C-expressing cells was greatly diminished. It should be stressed that contrary to normal *Bmp-4* expression, which is limited to the tips of distal lung tubules, the transgene was expressed throughout the distal epithelium. Differences from SP-C- driven TGF-β1 overexpression (194) should be pointed out: whereas TGF-β1 overexpression led to arrested development at the pseudoglandular stage, with a reduced expression of both SP-C and CC-10 but no lung size reduction, *Bmp-4* overexpression led to decreased lung growth and specific reduction in expression of alveolar markers. The factor BMP-4 therefore appears to be associated with growth of the lung epithelial tree, and a down-regulation of its expression may be a prerequisite for alveolar cell differentiation. It is questionable whether BMP-4 is the mediator of the TGF-β-like activity evidenced in previous investigations (172). In a more recent study (14), it was shown that *Shh* overexpression targeted to the mouse lung affected lung growth, with increased mesenchymal and epithelial proliferation and absence of typical alveoli. Type II cells, however, displayed normal ultrastructure, and there was no change in the expression of *Bmp-4*, the KGF gene, or of the specific lung markers CC10 and SP-C. By contrast, the expression of *Ptc*, a murine homologue of the *Drosophila* segment polarity gene *Patched*, was up-regulated in the transgenic mice (14).

Tumor Necrosis Factor α and Interleukins

Although the proinflammatory cytokines, i.e., tumor necrosis factor α and various interleukins, may not have major function in lung developmental processes, they are worth brief mention because of their implication in acute respiratory distress syndrome (ARDS), neonatal RDS, and BPD. Tumor necrosis factor α has indeed been reported to be a potent inhibitor of SP-A, SP-B, and SP-C gene transcription and synthesis (10, 182), which would represent an aggravating factor in RDS and ARDS. A potential role of elevated IL-1 (140) and IL-8 (88) in neonatal RDS has been proposed in the development of BPD, while IL-6 has been assumed to be implicated in excessive alveolar fibroblast proliferation in interstitial lung diseases (151). Therapeutic approaches to these conditions should therefore aim at blockade of the cytokine-mediated inflammatory cascade.

Platelet-Derived Growth Factors

Platelet-derived growth factors (PDGFs) are dimers of two different peptide chains (AA or BB or AB) that interact with two related receptor tyrosine kinases designated PDGF receptor α (PDGFRα) and PDGFRβ. Only PDGFRα binds PDGF-A chains. PDGF-AA is involved in the mesenchymal-epithelial interactions that direct early lung branching (see Chap. 1). The recent production of PDGF-A null mice has provided evidence for the key inductory role that this mediator also plays later in development in the process of alveologenesis (29). The null allele has been shown to be homozygous lethal with two restriction points—one prenatally before embryonic day 10 and one postnatally. In the homozygous mutant mice that survived after birth, fetal and early postnatal lung development appeared to be normal, including the formation of prealveolar saccules, but postnatal alveolarization failed to take place. Emphysematous appearance and large areas of collapsed lung tissue (atelectasis) extended progressively, thus leading to death. The defect in alveologenesis appeared to result from the lack of septal smooth-muscle cells (alveolar myofibroblasts), with subsequent absence of elastin fiber deposition. In addition, PDGFRα-positive cells having the location of putative alveolar myofibroblast progenitors were specifically absent in PDGF-A null mutants. The ontogeny of alveolar myofibroblasts therefore appears to be a prerequisite for alveolar septal formation, most likely because these cells are the source of elastin, and the specification of alveolar myofibroblasts is clearly dependent upon the presence of PDGF-A. Because epithelial cells appear to be the source of PDGF-A, myofibroblast differentiation is likely to be under paracrine control exerted by epithelial cells in close apposition to the mesenchymal cells from which myofibroblasts derive. That differentiation of myofibroblasts is driven through positive direct induction of PDGFRα by PDGF-A appears to be a likely assumption. These remarkable findings illustrate that alveolar development implicates reciprocal action between the epithelium and mesenchyme, an idea that was formerly proposed for lung cell growth (5), and not exclusively one-way mesenchymal influence upon epithelial cell differentiation.

CONCLUSION

The control of gene expression in pulmonary epithelial cells has recently become a field of intensive research. Even if the question of how the fate of lung primordial cells is determined across the developmental process remains largely unanswered, a number of pieces of the puzzle have already been gathered. It appears that when the lung anlage emerges, its epithelial pulmonary identity is already imprinted, likely through positional information. Branching growth and differentiation of the various epithelial cell types are still imperfectly understood processes, but the crucial role of mesenchyme in their control, through actions of diffusible mediators or extracellular matrix components, is firmly established. Transcription factors determining lung-specific marker expression have been identified. Markers of the distal epithelium are early and basically expressed genes, and cell differentiation along an anterior–posterior axis appears as either a repression or reinforcement of their expression in proximal and distal areas, respectively. The same genetic and epigenetic factors control both morphogenesis and lung-specific gene expression. A complex, subtle balance between various mediators with developmentally adjusted changes appears to control morphogenetic and cell maturational events. Multiple approaches are necessary to explore mechanisms more fully. Tumoral or transformed cell lines expressing a particular cell phenotype will certainly be useful. Transgenic models and null mutations have yielded and will continue to produce important new insights (see Chap. 13). It should be pointed out, however, that gene inactivation has led to somewhat disappointing findings in some instances because it sometimes induced little change (e.g., KGF gene), or conversely, the developmental consequences were so dramatic and precocious that no information was provided for the understanding of organ formation (e.g., HNF-3β gene). In this respect, the use of dominant-negative transgenes or conditional gene-expression/inactivation systems, such as Cre-LoxP, would be especially informative. Other strategies, such as differential display RT-PCR using oligo-dT primers and random 5′ oligonucleotides, or investigations of mammalian homologues of genes important for the development of invertebrates (for instance the *Drosophila*'s tubulogenesis driver *trachealess*) may help to identify novel gene expression in the lung. All these approaches, along with investigations of exogenous factors capable of accelerating or facilitating normal processes, should provide the molecular bases for new treatments of various lung diseases.

REFERENCES

1. Acarregui, M.J., J.M. Snyder, M.D. Mitchell, and C.R. Mendelson. Prostaglandins regulate surfactant protein A (SP-A) gene expression in human fetal lung in vitro. *Endocrinology* 90: 1105–1113, 1990.
2. Adams, J.C. and F.M. Watt. Regulation of development and differentiation by the extracellular matrix. *Development* 117: 1183–1198, 1993.
3. Adamson, I.Y.R., G.M. King, and L. Young. Influence of extracellular matrix and collagen components on alveolar type 2 cell morphology and function. *In Vitro Cell. Dev. Biol.* 25: 494–502, 1989.
4. Adamson, I.Y.R. and L. Young. Alveolar type II cell growth on a pulmonary endothelial extracellular matrix. *Am. J. Physiol.* 270 (*Lung Cell. Mol. Physiol.* 14): L1017–L1022, 1996.
5. Adamson, I.Y.R., L. Young, and G.M. King. Reciprocal epithelial:fibroblast interactions in the control of fetal and adult rat lung cells in culture. *Exp. Lung Res.* 17: 821–835, 1991.
6. Alcorn, J.L., E. Gao, Q. Chen, M.E. Smith, R.D. Gerard, and C.R. Mendelson. Genomic elements involved in transcriptional regulation of the rabbit surfactant protein-A gene. *Mol. Endocrinol.* 7: 1072–1085, 1993.
7. Ang, S.L. and J. Rossant. HNF-3β is essential for node and notochord formation in mouse development. *Cell* 78: 561–574, 1994.
8. Ang, S.L., A. Wierda, D. Wong, K.A. Stevens, S. Cascio, J. Rossant, and K.S. Zaret. The formation and maintenance of the definitive endoderm lineage in the mouse: involvement of the HNF3/*forkhead* proteins. *Development* 119: 1301–1315, 1993.
9. Aubin, J., M. Lemieux, M. Trembly, J. Berard, and L. Jeannotte. Early postnatal lethality in Hoxa-5 mutant mice is attributable to respiratory tract defects. *Dev. Biol.* 192: 432–445, 1997.
10. Bachurski, C.J., G.S. Pryhuber, S. Glasser, S.E. Kelly, and J.A. Whitsett.Tumor necrosis factor-α inhibits surfactant protein C gene transcription. *J. Biol. Chem.* 270: 19402–19407, 1995.
11. Batenburg, J.J. and R.H. Elfring. Pre-translational regulation by glucocorticoid of fatty acid and phosphatidylcholine synthesis in type II cells from fetal rat lung. *FEBS Lett.* 307: 164–168, 1992.
12. Bedetti, C.D., J. Singh, G. Singh, S.L. Katyal, and M.L. Wong-Chong. Ultrastructural localization of rat Clara cell 10kD secretory protein by the immunogold technique using polyclonal and monoclonal antibodies. *J. Histochem. Cytochem.* 35: 789–794, 1987.
13. Behringer, R.R., D.A. Crotty, V.M. Tennyson, R.L. Brinster, R.D. Palmiter, and D.J. Wolgemuth. Sequences 5′ of the homeobox of the hox-1,4 gene direct tissue specific expression of *lacZ* during mouse development. *Development* 117: 823–833, 1993.
14. Bellusci, S., Y. Furuta, M.G. Rush, R. Henderson, G. Winnier, and B.L.M. Hogan. Involvement of Sonic hedgehog (*Shh*) in mouse embryonic lung growth and morphogenesis. *Development* 124: 53–63, 1997.
15. Bellusci S., J. Grindley, H. Emoto, N. Itoh, and B.L.M. Hogan. Fibroblast growth factor 10 (FGF 10) and branching morphogenesis in the embryonic mouse lung. *Development* 124: 4867–4878, 1997.
16. Bellusci S., R. Henderson, G. Winnier, T. Oikawa, and B.L.M. Hogan. Evidence from normal expression and targeted overexpression that Bone Morphogenetic Protein-4 (BMP-4) plays a role in mouse embryonic lung morphogenesis. *Development* 122: 1693–1702, 1996.

17. Berard, J., L. Gaboury, M. Landers, Y. de Repentigny, B. Houle, R. Kothary, and W.E.C. Bradley. Hyperplasia and tumors in lung, breast and other tissues in mice carrying a *RAR-β4*-like transgene. *EMBO J.* 13: 5570–5580,1994.
18. Bernacki, S.H., C. Nervi, T.M. Volberg, and A.M. Jetten. Homeobox 1.3 expression: induction by retinoic acid in bronchial fibroblasts. *Am. J. Respir.Cell Mol. Biol.* 7: 3–9, 1992.
19. Bingle, C.D. and J.D. Gitlin. Identification of hepatocyte nuclear factor-3 binding sites in the Clara cell secretory protein gene. *Biochem. J.* 295: 227–232, 1993.
20. Bingle, C.D. and S. Gowan. Molecular cloning of the *forkhead* transcription factor HNF-3α from a human pulmonary adenocarcinoma cell line. *Biochim. Biophys. Acta* 1307: 17–20, 1996.
21. Bingle, C.D., B.P. Hackett, M. Moxley, W. Longmore, and J.D. Gitlin. Role of HNF-3α and HNF-3β in Clara cell secretory protein gene expression in the bronchiolar epithelium. *Biochem. J.* 308: 197–202, 1995.
22. Blau, H., D.E. Guzowski, Z.A. Siddiqi, E.M. Scarpelli, and R.S. Bienkowski. Fetal type 2 pneumocytes form alveolar like structures and maintain long term differentiation on extracellular matrix. *J. Cell. Physiol.* 136: 203–214,1988.
23. Boggaram, V. and C. Mendelson. Transcriptional regulation of the gene encoding the major surfactant protein (SP-A) in rabbit fetal lung. *J. Biol. Chem.* 263: 19060–19065, 1988.
24. Bogue, C.F., I. Gross, H. Vasavada, D.W. Dynia, C.M. Wilson, and H.C. Jacobs. Identification of *Hox* genes in newborn lung and effects of gestational age and retinoic acid on their expression. *Am. J. Physiol.* 266 (*Lung Cell. Mol. Physiol.* 10): L448–L454, 1994.
25. Bogue, C.F., H.C. Jacobs, D.W. Dynia, C.M. Wilson, and I. Gross. Retinoic acid increases surfactant protein mRNA in fetal rat lung in culture. *Am. J. Physiol.* 271 (*Lung Cell. Mol. Physiol.* 15): L862–L868, 1996.
26. Bogue, C.F., L.J. Lou, and H.C. Jacobs. Expression of *Hoxb* genes in the developing mouse foregut and lung. *Am. J. Respir. Cell Mol. Biol.* 15: 163–171, 1996.
27. Bohinski, R.J., R. Di Lauro, and J.A. Whitsett. The lung-specific surfactant protein B gene promoter is a target for thyroid transcription factor 1 and hepatocyte nuclear factor 3, indicating common factors for organ-specific gene expression along the foregut axis. *Mol. Cell. Biol.* 14: 5671–5681, 1994.
28. Bohinski, R.J., J.A. Huffman, J.A. Whitsett, and D.L. Lattier. *Cis*-active elements controlling lung cell-specific expression of human pulmonary surfactant protein B gene. *J. Biol. Chem.* 268: 11160–11166, 1993.
29. Boström, H., K. Willets, M. Pekny, P. Levéen, P. Lindhal, H. Hedstrand, M. Pekna, M. Hellström, S. Gebre-Medhin, M. Schalling, M. Nilsson, S. Kurland, J. Törnell, J.K. Heath, and C. Betscholtz. PDGF-A signaling is a critical event in lung alveolar myofibroblast development and alveogenesis. *Cell* 85: 863–873, 1996.
30. Bourbon, J.R. and C. Fraslon. Developmental aspects of the alveolar epithelium and the pulmonary surfactant system. In: *Pulmonary Surfactant: Biochemical, Functional, Regulatory and Clinical Concepts,* edited by J.R. Bourbon. Boca Raton, FL: CRC Press, 1991, p. 257–324.
31. Braun, H. and G. Suske. Combinatorial action of HNF3 and Sp family transcription factors in the activation of the rabbit uteroglobin/CC10 promoter. *J. Biol. Chem.* 273: 9821–9828, 1998.
32. Breed, D.R., L.R. Margraf, J.L. Alcorn, and C. Mendelson. Transcription factor C/EBPδ in fetal lung: developmental regulation and effects of cyclic adenosine 3′,5′-monophosphate and glucocorticoids. *Endocrinology* 138: 5527–5534, 1997.

33. Brinkman, V., H. Foroutan, M. Sachs, K.M. Weidner, and W. Birchmeier. Hepatocyte growth factor/scatter factor induces a variety of tissue specific morphogenic programs in epithelial cells. *J. Cell Biol.* 131: 1573–1586,1995.
34. Bruno, M.D., R.J. Bohinski, J.E. Carter, K.A. Foss, and J.A. Whitsett. Structure and function of the mouse surfactant protein B gene. *Am. J. Physiol.* 268 (*Lung Cell. Mol. Physiol.* 12): L381–L389, 1995.
35. Bruno, M.D., R.J. Bohinski, K.M. Huelsman, J.A. Whitsett, and T.R. Korfhagen. Lung cell-specific expression of the murine surfactant protein A(SP-A) gene is mediated by interactions between the SP-A promoter and thyroid transcription factor-1. *J. Biol. Chem.* 270: 6531–6536, 1995.
36. Caniggia, I., J. Liu, R. Han, J. Wang, A.K. Tanswell, G. Laurie, and M. Post. Identification of receptors binding fibronectin and laminin on fetal rat lung cells. *Am. J. Physiol.* 270 (*Lung Cell. Mol. Physiol.* 14): L459–L468, 1996.
37. Caniggia, I., K. Tanswell, and M. Post. Temporal and spatial differences in glycosaminoglycan synthesis by fetal lung fibroblasts. *Exp. Cell Res.* 202: 252–258, 1992.
38. Caniggia, I., I. Tseu, R.N. Han, B.T. Smith, A. K. Tanswell, and M. Post. Spatial and temporal differences in fibroblast behavior in fetal rat lung. *Am. J. Physiol.* 261 (*Lung Cell. Mol. Physiol.* 5): L424–L433, 1991.
39. Cardoso, W.V. Transcription factors and pattern formation in the developing lung. *Am. J. Physiol.* 269 (*Lung Cell. Mol. Physiol.* 13): L429–L442, 1995.
40. Cardoso, W.V., A. Itoh, H. Nogawa, I. Mason, and J.S. Brody. FGF-1 and FGF-7 induce distinct patterns of growth and differentiation in embryonic lung epithelium. *Dev. Dyn.* 298: 398–405, 1997.
41. Cardoso, W.V., S.A. Mitsialis, J.S. Brody, and M.C. Williams. Retinoic acid alters the expression of pattern-related genes in the developing lung. *Dev. Dyn.* 207: 47–59, 1996.
42. Cardoso, W.V., M.C. Williams, S.A. Mitsialis, M. Joyce-Brady, A.K. Rishi, and J.S. Brody. Retinoic acid induces changes in the pattern of airway branching and alters epithelial cell differentiation in the developing lung in vitro. *Am. J. Respir. Cell Mol. Biol.* 12: 464–476, 1995.
43. Chelly, N., O.-B. Mouhieddine-Gueddiche, A.-M. Barlier-Mur, B. Chailley-Heu, and J.R. Bourbon. Keratinocyte growth factor enhances maturation of fetal rat lung type II cells. *Am. J. Respir. Cell Mol. Biol.* 20: in press, 1999.
44. Chen, Q., V. Boggaram, and C.R. Mendelson. Rabbit lung surfactant protein A (SP-A) gene: identification of a lung-specific DNAse I hypersensitive site in the 5′-flanking region. *Am. J. Physiol.* 262 (*Lung Cell. Mol. Physiol.* 6): L662–L671, 1992.
45. Chinoy, M.R., M.T. Antonio-Santiago, and E.M. Scarpelli. Maturation of undifferentiated lung epithelial cells into type II cells in vitro: a temporal process that parallels cell differentiation in vivo. *Anat. Rec.* 240: 545–554,1994.
46. Chisaka, O. and M.R. Capecchi. Regionally restricted developmental defects resulting from targeted disruption of the mouse homeobox gene *hox-1,5*. *Nature* 350: 473–479, 1991.
47. Civitareale, D., R. Lonigro, A.J. Sinclair, and R. Di Lauro. A thyroid-specific nuclear protein essential for tissue expression of the thyroglobulin promoter. *EMBO J.* 8: 2537–2542, 1989.
48. Clark, K.L., E.D. Halay, E. Lai, and K.S. Burley. Co-crystal structure of the HNF-3/fork head DNA recognition motif resembles histone H5. *Nature* 364: 412–420, 1993.
49. Clevidence, D.E., D.G. Overdier, R.S. Peterson, A. Porcella, H. Ye, K.E. Paulson, and

R.H. Costa. Members of the HNF-3/forkhead family of transcription factors exhibit distinct cellular expression patterns in lung and regulate the surfactant protein B promoter. *Dev. Biol.* 166: 195–209,1994.

50. Clevidence, D.E., D.G. Overdier, W. Tao, X. Qian, L. Pani, E. Lai, and R.H. Costa. Identification of nine tissue-specific transcription factors of the hepatocyte nuclear factor 3/forkhead DNA-binding domain family. *Proc. Natl. Acad. Sci. USA* 90: 3948–3952, 1993.
51. Cole, T.J., J.A. Blendy, A.P. Monaghan, K. Krieglstein, W. Schmid, A. Aguzzi, G. Fantuzzi, E. Hummler, K. Unsicker, and G. Schütz. Targeted disruption of the glucocorticoid receptor gene blocks chromaffin cell development and severely retards lung maturation. *Genes Dev.* 9: 1608–1621, 1995.
52. Costa, R.H., D.R. Grayson, and J.E. Darnell, Jr. Multiple hepatocyte-enriched nuclear factors function in the regulation of transthyretin and α1-antitrypsin. *Mol. Cell. Biol.* 9: 1415–1425, 1989.
53. Damante, G. and R. Di Lauro. Thyroid specific gene expression. *Biochim. Biophys. Acta* 1218: 255–266, 1994.
54. Danto, S.I., J.M. Shannon, Z. Borok, S.M. Zabski, and D.E. Crandall Reversible transdifferentiation of alveolar epithelial cells. *Am. J. Respir. Cell Mol. Biol.* 12: 497–502, 1995.
55. Danto, S.I., S.M. Zabski, and E.D. Crandall. Reactivity of alveolar epithelial cells in primary culture with type I cell monoclonal antibodies. *Am. J. Respir. Cell Mol. Biol.* 6: 296–306, 1992.
56. De Bortoli, C., B. Chailley-Heu, and J.R. Bourbon. Production of transforming growth factor (TGF) β by fetal lung cells. *Biol. Cell* 84: 215–218, 1995.
57. Degryse, E., M.M. De Santi, M. Dietrich, D. Ali Hadj, J.-F. Spetz, D. Villeval, and G. Lungarella. A human SP-C promoter fragment targets a1-proteinase inhibitor gene expression to lung alveolar type II cells in transgenic mice. *Transgenic Res.* 5: 139–143, 1996.
58. Dekowski, S.A., M. Pajeau, and R.J. Panos. Keratinocyte growth factor and keratinocyte growth factor mRNA content in late gestation fetal and neonatal rat lung. *Pediatr. Res.* 39: 56A, 1996.
59. De Simone, V. and R. Cortese. Transcription factors and liver-specific genes. *Biochim. Byophys. Acta* 1132: 119–126, 1992.
60. Deterding, R.R. and J.M. Shannon. Proliferation and differentiation of fetal rat pulmonary epithelium in the absence of mesenchyme. *J. Clin. Invest.* 95: 2963–2972, 1995.
61. Dobbs, L.G., M.C. Williams, and A.E. Brandt. Changes in biochemical characteristics and pattern of lectin binding of alveolar type II cells with time in culture. *Biochim. Biophys. Acta* 846: 155–166, 1985.
62. Dobbs, L.G., M.C. Williams, and R. Gonzalez. Monoclonal antibodies to apical surfaces of rat alveolar type I cells bind to surfaces of cultured, but not freshly isolated, type II cells. *Biochim. Biophys. Acta* 970: 146–156,1988.
63. Dollé, P., E. Ruberte, P. Leroy, G. Morriss-Kay, and P. Chambon. Retinoic acid receptors and cellular retinoid binding proteins. I. A systematic study of their differential pattern of transcription during mouse organogenesis. *Development* 110: 1133–1151, 1990.
64. Evans, M.J. and S.G. Shami. Lung cell kinetics. In: *Lung Cell Biology*, Vol. 41, edited by D. Massaro. New York Marcel Dekker, 1989, p. 1–36.
65. Farrell, P.M., J.R. Bourbon, R.H. Notter, L. Marin, L. Nogee, and J.A. Whitsett. Relationships among surfactant fraction lipids, proteins and biophysical properties in the developing lung. *Biochim. Biovhys. Acta* 1044: 84–90, 1990.

66. Fisher, J.H., F. McCormack, S.S. Park, T. Stelzner, J.M. Shannon, and T. Hofmann. In vivo regulation of surfactant by glucocorticoids. *Am. J. Respir. Cell Mol. Biol.* 5: 63–70, 1991.

67. Flodby, P., C. Barlow, H. Kylefjord, L. Ährlund-Richert, and K.G. Xanthopoulos. Increased hepatic cell proliferation and lung abnormalities in mice deficient in CCAAT/enhancer binding protein α. *J. Biol. Chem.* 271: 24753–24780, 1996.

68. Fraslon, C. and J.J. Batenburg. Pre-translational regulation of lipid synthesizing enzymes and surfactant proteins in fetal rat lung in explant culture. *FEBS Lett.* 325: 285–290, 1993.

69. Fraslon, C. and J.R. Bourbon. Comparison of effects of epidermal and insulin-like growth factors, gastrin-releasing peptide and retinoic acid on fetal lung cell growth and maturation in vitro. *Biochim. Biophys. Acta* 1123: 65–75, 1992.

70. Fraslon, C. and J.R. Bourbon. Retinoids control surfactant phospholipid biosynthesis in fetal rat lung. *Am. J. Physiol.* 266 (*Lung Cell. Mol. Physiol.* 10): L705–L712, 1993.

71. Fraslon, C., B. Chailley-Heu, J.J. Batenburg, R. Elfring, and J.R. Bourbon. Ontogeny of surfactant proteins and lipid-synthesizng enzymes in cultured fetal lung epithelial cells. *Am. J. Physiol.* 267 (*Lung Cell. Mol. Physiol.* 11): L375–L383, 1994.

72. Fraslon, C., T. Lacaze-Masmonteil, V. Zupan, B. Chailley-Heu, and J.R. Bourbon. Fetal rat lung type II cell differentiation in serum-free isolated cell culture: modulation and inhibition. *Am. J. Physiol.* 264 (*Lung Cell. Mol. Physiol.* 8): L504–L516, 1993.

73. Gao, E., J.L. Alcorn, and C.R. Mendelson. Identification of enhancers in the 5′-flanking region of the rabbit surfactant protein A (SP-A) gene and characterization of their binding proteins. *J. Biol. Chem.* 268: 19697–19709, 1993.

74. Gatherer, D., P.T. Dijke, D.T. Baird, and R.J. Arkhurst. Expression of TGF-β isoforms during first trimester human embryogenesis. *Development* 110: 445–460, 1990.

75. Gehring, W.J., M. Affolter, and T. Bürglin. Homeodomain proteins. *Annu. Rev. Biochem.* 63: 487–526, 1994.

76. Glasser, S.W., T.R. Korfhagen, S.E. Wert, M.D. Bruno, K.M. McWilliams, D.K. Vorbroker, and J.A. Whitsett. Genetic element from human surfactant protein SP-C gene confers bronchiolar-alveolar cell specificity in transgenic mice. *Am. J. Physiol.* 261 *(Lung Cell. Mol. Physiol.* 5*)*: L349–L356, 1991.

77. Guazzi, S., R. Lonigro, L. Pinotello, E. Bonicelli, R. DiLauro, and F. Mavilio. The thyroid transcription factor-1 is a candidate target for regulation by Hox proteins. *EMBO J.* 13: 3339–3347, 1994.

78. Guazzi, S., M. Price, M. De Felice, G. Damante, M.-G. Mattei, and R. DiLauro. Thyroid nuclear factor 1 (TTF-1) contains a homeodomain and displays a novel DNA binding specificity. *EMBO J.* 9: 3631–3639, 1990.

79. Guo, L., L. Degenstein, and E. Fuchs. Keratinocyte growth factor is required for hair development but not for wound healing. *Genes Dev.* 10: 165–175,1996.

80. Gupta, R.P., S.E. Patton, A.M. Jetten, and G.E.R. Hook. Purification, characterization and proteinase activity of a Clara-cell secretory protein from the pulmonary extracellular lining of rabbits. *Biochem. J.* 248: 337–344, 1987.

81. Hackett, B.P., S.L. Brody, M. Liang, I.D. Zeitz, L.A. Bruns, and J.D. Gitlin. Primary structure of hepatocyte nuclear factor/forkhead factor homologue 4 and characterization of gene expression in the respiratory and reproductive epithelium. *Proc. Natl. Acad. Sci. USA* 92: 4249–4253, 1995.

82. Hackett, B.P., N. Shimizu, and J.D. Gitlin. Clara cell secretory protein gene expression in bronchiolar epithelium. *Am. J. Physiol.* 262 *(Lung Cell. Mol. Physiol.* 6*)*: L399–L404, 1992.

83. Hirning, U., P. Schmid, W.A. Schultz, G. Rettenberger, and H. Hameister. A comparative

analysis of N-*myc* and c-*myc* expression and cellular proliferation in mouse organogenesis. *Mech. Dev.* 33: 119–126, 1991.

84. Ikeda, K., J.C. Clark, J.R. Shaw-White, M.T. Stahlman, C. Bouteil, and J.A.Whitsett. Gene structure and expression of human TTF-1 in respiratory epithelial cells. *J. Biol. Chem.* 270: 8108–8114, 1995.
85. Ikeda, K., J.R. Shaw-White, S. Wert, and J.A. Whitsett. Hepatocyte nuclear factor 3 activates transcription of thyroid transcription factor 1 in respiratory epithelial cells. *Mol. Cell. Biol.* 16: 3626–3636, 1996.
86. Jaskoll, T., H.A. Choy, and M. Melnick. The glucocorticoid-glucocorticoid receptor signal transduction pathway, transforming growth factor-β, and embryonic mouse lung development in vivo. *Pediatr. Res.* 39: 749–759,1996.
87. Johansson, J., T. Curstedt, and B. Robertson. The proteins of the surfactant system. *Eur. Respir. J.* 7: 372–391, 1994.
88. Jones, C.A., R.G. Cayabyab, K.Y.C. Kwong, C. Stotts, B. Wong, H. Hamsdan, P. Minoo, and R. de Lemos. Undetectable interleukin (IL)-10 and persistent IL-8 expression early in hyaline membrane disease: a possible developmental basis for the predisposition to chronic lung inflammation in preterm newborns. *Pediatr. Res.* 39: 966–975, 1996.
89. Juliano, R.L. and S. Haskill. Signal transduction from the extracellular matrix. *J. Cell Biol.* 120: 577–585, 1993.
90. Kaartinen, V., J.W. Voncken, C. Shuler, D. Warburton, D. Bu, N. Heisterkamp, and J. Groffen. Abnormal lung development and cleft palate in mice lacking TGF-β3 indicates defects of epithelial mesenchymal interaction. *Nat. Genet.* 11: 415–421, 1995.
91. Kalina, M., R.J. Mason, and J.M. Shannon. Surfactant protein C is expressed in alveolar type II cells but not in Clara cells of rat lung. *Am. J. Respir. Cell Mol. Biol.* 6: 594–600, 1992.
92. Kappen, C. *Hox* genes in the lung. *Am. J. Respir. Cell Mol. Biol.* 15: 156-162, 1996.
93. Kasper, M., D. Schuh, and M. Muller. *Bauhinia purpurea* lectin (BPA) binding of rat type I pneumocytes: alveolar epithelial alterations after radiation-induced lung injury. *Exp. Toxicol. Pathol.* 46: 361–367, 1994.
94. Kawada, H., J.M. Shannon, and R.J. Mason. Improved maintenance of adult rat type II cell differentiation in vitro: effect of serum-free hormonally defined medium and a reconstituted basement membrane. *Am. J. Respir. Cell Mol. Biol.* 3: 33–43, 1990.
95. Kelly, S.E., C.J. Bachurski, M.S. Burhans, and S.W. Glasser. Transcription of the lung-specific surfactant protein C gene is mediated by thyroid transcription factor 1. *J. Biol. Chem.* 271: 6881–6888. 1996.
96. Khoor, A., M.E. Gray, W.M. Hull, J.A. Whitsett, and M.T. Stahlman.Developmental expression of SP-A and SP-A mRNA in the proximal and distal respiratory epithelium in the human fetus and newborn. *J. Histochem. Cytochem.* 41: 1311–1319, 1993.
97. Kimura, S., Y. Hara, T. Pineau, P. Fernandez-Salguero, C.H. Fox, J.M.Ward, and F.J. Gonzalez. The T/ebp null mouse: thyroid-specific enhancer-binding protein is essential for the organogenesis of the thyroid, lung, ventral forebrain, and pituitary. *Genes Dev.* 10: 60–69, 1996.
98. Kleinman, H.K., M.L. McGarvey, J.R. Hassell, V.L. Star, F.B. Cannon,G.W. Laurie, and G.R. Martin. Basement membrane complexes with biological activity. *Biochem. USA* 28: 312–318, 1986.
99. Kouretas, D., A.M. Karinch, A. Rishi, K. Melchers, and J. Floros. Conservation analysis of rat and human SP-A gene identifies 5′ flanking sequences of rat SP-A that bind rat lung nuclear proteins. *Exp. Lung Res.* 19: 485–503, 1993.

100. Kubiak, J., M.M. Mitra, R. Steve, J.D. Hunt, P. Davies, and B.R. Pitt. Transforming growth factor-α gene expression in late-gestation fetal rat lung. *Pediatr. Res.* 31: 286–290, 1992.

101. Kumar, N.M., S.L. Sigurdson, D. Sheppard, and J.S. Lwebuga-Mukasa. Differential modulation of integrin receptor and extracellular matrix laminin by transforming growth factor-β1 in rat alveolar epithelial cells. *Exp. Cell Res.* 221: 385–394, 1995.

102. Lacaze-Masmonteil, T., C. Fraslon, J. Bourbon, M. Raymondjean, and A. Khan. Characterization of the rat pulmonary surfactant protein A promoter. *Eur. J. Biochem.* 206: 613–623, 1992.

103. Lai, E., V.R. Prezioso, W. Tao, W. Chen, and J.E. Darnell, Jr. Hepatocyte nuclear factor 3A belongs to a gene family in mammals that is homologous to the *Drosophila* homeotic gene *fork head*. *Genes Dev.* 5: 416–427, 1991.

104. Langston, C., K. Kida, M. Reed, and W.M. Thurlbeck. Human lung growth in late gestation and in the neonate. *Am. Rev. Respir. Dis.* 129: 607–613, 1984.

105. Lazzaro, D., M. Price, M. De Felice, and R. Di Lauro. The transcription factor TTF-1 is expressed at the onset of thyroid and lung morphogenesis and in restricted regions of the foetal brain. *Development* 113: 1093–1104, 1991.

106. Li, F., E. Rosenberg, C.I. Smith, K. Notarfrancesco, S.R. Reisher, H. Shuman, and S.I. Feinstein. Correlation of expression of transcription factor C/EBPα and surfactant protein genes in lung cells. *Am. J. Physiol.* 269 (*Lung Cell. Mol. Physiol.* 13): L241–L247, 1995.

107. Liu, R., C.S. Harvey, and S.E. McGowan. Retinoic acid increases elastin in neonatal rat lung fibroblast cultures. *Am. J. Physiol.* 265 (*Lung Cell. Mol. Physiol.* 9): L430–L437, 1993.

108. Luzi, P., M. Anceschi, and D.S. Strayer. Glucocorticoid responsiveness conferred by a cloned DNA binding protein. *Receptor* 5: 93–103, 1995.

109. Luzi, P. and D.S. Strayer. Binding proteins that amplify surfactant protein B gene expression: isolation and characterization. *Biochem. Biophys. Res.Commun.* 208: 153–160, 1995.

110. Manley, N.R. and M.R. Capecchi. The role of Hoxa-3 in the thymus and thyroid development. *Development* 121: 1989–2003, 1995.

111. Mantile, G., L. Miele, E. Cordella-Miele, G. Singh, S.L. Katyal, and A.B. Mukherjee. Human Clara cell 10-kDa protein is the counterpart of rabbit uteroglobin. *J. Biol. Chem.* 25: 20343–20351, 1993.

112. Margraf, L.R., J.R. Tomashefski, Jr, M.C. Bruce, and B.B. Dahms. Morphometric analysis of the lung in bronchopulmonary dysplasia. *Am. Rev. Respir. Dis.* 143: 391–400, 1991.

113. Marin, L. The type II pneumocyte. In: *Pulmonary Surfactant: Biochemical, Functional, Regulatory and Clinical Concepts,* edited by J.R. Bourbon, Boca Raton, FL: CRC Press, 1991, p.15–36.

114. Massaro, G.D. and D. Massaro. Formation of pulmonary alveoli and gas-exchange surface area: quantitation and regulation. *Annu. Rev. Physiol.* 58: 73–92, 1996.

115. Massaro, G.D. and D. Massaro. Postnatal treatment with retinoic acid increases the number of pulmonary alveoli in rats. *Am. J. Physiol.* 270 (*Lung Cell. Mol. Physiol.* 14): L305–L310, 1996.

116. Matter, M.L. and G.W. Laurie. A novel laminin E8 cell adhesion site required for lung alveolar formation in vitro. *J. Cell Biol.* 124: 1083–1090,1994.

117. Melnick, M., H.A. Choy, and T. Jaskoll. Glucocorticoids, tumor necrosis factor-α, and epidermal growth factor regulation of pulmonary morphogenesis: a multivariate in vitro analysis of their related actions. *Dev. Dyn.* 205: 365–378, 1996.

118. Mendelsohn, C., D. Lohnes, D. Decimo, T. Lufkin, M. LeMeur, P. Chambon, and M. Mark. Function of retinoic acid receptors (RARs) during development. II. Multiple abnormalities at various stages of organogenesis in *RAR* double mutants. *Development* 120: 2749–2771, 1994.
119. Metzler, M.D. and J.M. Snyder. Retinoic acid differentially regulates expression of surfactant-associated proteins in human lung. *Endocrinology* 133: 1990–1998, 1993.
120. Michael, L.F., J.L. Alcorn, E. Gao, and C.R. Mendelson. Characterization of the cyclic adenosine 3′-5′-monophosphate response element of the rabbit surfactant protein-A gene: evidence for transactivators distinct from CREB/ATF family members. *Mol. Endocrinol.* 10: 159–170, 1996.
121. Michael, L.F., M.A. Lazar, and C.R. Mendelson. Peroxisome proliferator-activated receptor γ1 expression is induced during cyclic adenosine monophosphate-stimulated differentiation of alveolar type II pneumonocytes. *Endocrinology* 138: 3695–3703, 1997.
122. Miettinen, P.J., J.E. Berger, J. Meneses, Y. Phung, R.A. Pedersen, Z. Werb, and R. Derynck. Epithelial immaturity and multiorgan failure in mice lacking epidermal growth factor receptor. *Nature* 376: 337–341, 1995.
123. Millan, F.A., F. Denhez, P. Kondaiah, and R.J. Arkhurst. Embryonic gene expression patterns of TGF-β1, β2 and β3 suggest different developmental functions in vivo. *Development* 111: 131–144, 1991.
124. Minoo, P., H. Hamdam, D. Bu, D. Warburton, P. Stepanik, and R. de Lemos. TTF-1 regulates lung epithelial morphogenesis. *Dev. Biol.* 172: 694–698,1995.
125. Miura, N., H. Kakinuma, M. Sato, N. Aiba, K. Terada, and N. Sugiyama. Mouse forkhead (winged helix) gene *LUN* encodes a transactivator that acts in the lung. *Genomics* 50: 346–356, 1998.
126. Moens, C.B., A.B. Auerbach, R.A. Conlon, A.L. Joyner, and J. Rossant. A targeted mutation reveals a role for N-*myc* in the embryonic mouse lung. *Genes Dev.* 6: 691–704, 1992.
127. Monaghan, A.P., K.H. Kaestner, E. Grau, and G. Schütz. Postimplantation expression patterns indicate a role for the mouse *fork head*/HNF-3 α, β and γ genes in determination of the definitive endoderm, chordamesoderm and neurectoderm. *Development* 119: 567–578, 1993.
128. Muglia, L., L. Jacobson, P. Dikkes, and J.A. Majzoub. Corticotropin-releasing hormone deficiency reveals major fetal but not adult glucocorticoid need. *Nature* 373: 427–432, 1995.
129. Murgrauer, G., F.W. Alt, and P. Ekblom. N-*myc* proto-oncogene expression during organogenesis in the developing mouse as revealed by in situ hybridization. *J. Cell Biol.* 107: 1325–1335, 1988.
130. Nogawa, H. and T. Ito. Branching morphogenesis of embryonic mouse lung epithelium in mesenchyme-free culture. *Development* 121: 1015–1022,1995.
131. Odom, M.J., J. Snyder and C. Mendelson. Adenosine 3′, 5′-monophosphate analogs and β-adrenergic agonists induce the synthesis of the major surfactant apoprotein in human fetal lung in vitro. *Endocrinology* 1212: 1155–1163, 1987.
132. Orr-Urtreger, A., M.T Bedford, T. Burakova, E. Arman, Y. Zimmer, A. Yayon, D. Givol, and P. Lonai. Developmental localization of the splicing alternatives of fibroblast growth factor receptor-2 (FGFR2). *Dev. Biol.* 158:475–486, 1993.
133. Panos, R.J., J.S. Rubin, S.A. Aaronson, and R.J. Mason. Keratinocyte growth factor and hepatocyte growth factor/scatter factor are heparin-binding growth factors for

alveolar type II cells in fibroblast-conditioned medium. *J. Clin. Invest.* 92: 969–977, 1993.

134. Peters, K., S. Werner, X. Liao, S. Wert, J. Whitsett, and L. Williams. Targeted expression of a dominant negative FGF receptor blocks branching morphogenesis and epithelial differentiation of the mouse lung. *EMBO J.* 13: 3296–3301, 1994.

135. Peterson, R.L., L. Lim, H.G. Ye, H.P. Zhou, D.G. Overdier, and R.H. Costa. The winged helix transcriptional factor HFH-8 is expressed in the mesoderm of the primitive streak stage of mouse embryos and its cellular derivatives. *Mech. Dev.* 69: 53–69, 1997.

136. Pierrou, S., M. Hellqvist, L. Samuelsson, S. Enerbäck, and P. Carlsson. Cloning and characterization of seven human forkhead proteins: binding site specificity and DNA binding. *EMBO J.* 13: 5002–5012, 1994.

137. Rannels, S.R., C. Stinson Fisher, L.J. Heuser, and D.E. Rannels. Culture of type II pneumocytes on a type II-cell derived fibronectin-rich matrix. *Am. J. Physiol.* 253 (*Cell Physiol.* 22): C759–C765, 1987.

138. Rannels, S.R., J.A. Yarnell, C. Stinson Fisher, J.P. Fabisiak, and D.E. Rannels. Role of laminin in maintenance of type II pneumocyte morphology and function. *Am. J. Physiol.* 253 (*Cell Physiol.* 22): C835–C845, 1987.

139. Ray, M.K., C.-Y. Chen, R.J. Schwartz, and F.J. De Mayo. Transcriptional regulation of a mouse Clara cell-specific protein (mCC10) gene by the NKx transcription factor family members thyroid transcription factor 1 and cardiac muscle-specific homeobox protein (CSX). *Mol. Cell. Biol.* 16: 2056-2064, 1996.

140. Rindfleisch, M.S., J.D. Hasday, V. Taciak, K. Broderick, and R.M. Viscardi. Potential role of interleukin-1 in the development of bronchopulmonary dysplasia. *J. Interferon Cytokine Res.* 16: 365–373, 1996.

141. Ruocco, S., A. Lallemand, J.M. Tournier, and D. Gaillard. Expression and localization of epidermal growth factor, transforming growth factor-α, and localization of their common receptor in fetal human lung development. *Pediatr. Res.* 39: 448–455, 1996.

142. Rust, K., L. Bingle, W. Mariencheck, A. Persson, and E.C. Crouch. Characterization of the human surfactant protein D promoter: transcriptional regulation of SP-D gene expression by glucocorticoids. *Am. J. Respir. Cell Mol. Biol.* 14: 121–130, 1996.

143. Ryan, R.M., M.M. Mineo-Kuhn, C.M. Kramer, and J.N. Finkelstein. Growth factors alter neonatal type II alveolar epithelial cell proliferation. *Am. J. Physiol.* 266 (*Lung Cell. Mol. Physiol.* 10): L17–L22, 1994.

144. Sanford, L.P., I. Ormsby, A.C. Gittenberg-de Groot, H. Sariola, R. Friedman, G.P. Boivin, E.L. Cardell, and T. Doetschman. TGFβ2 knockout mice have multiple developmental defects that are non-overlapping with other TGFβ knockout phenotypes. *Development* 124: 2659–2670, 1997.

145. Sawai, S., A. Shimono, Y. Wakamatsu, C. Palmes, K. Hanaoka, and H. Kondoh. Defects of embryonic organogenesis resulting from targeted disruption of the N-*myc* gene in the mouse. *Development* 117: 1445–1455, 1993.

146. Sawaya, P.L. and D.S. Luse. Two members of the HNF-3 family have opposite effects on a lung transcriptional element; HNF-3α stimulates and HNF-3β inhibits activity of region I from Clara cell secretory protein (CCSP) promoter. *J. Biol. Chem.* 268: 22211–22216, 1994.

147. Sawaya, P.L., B.R. Stripp, J.A. Whitsett, and D.S. Luse. The lung-specific CC10 gene is regulated by transcription factors from the AP-1, octamer, and hepatocyte nuclear factor 3 families. *Mol. Cell. Biol.* 13: 3860–3871, 1993.

148. Schellase, D.E., P.A. Emrie, J.H. Fisher, and J.M. Shannon. Ontogeny of surfactant apoproteins in the rat. *Pediatr. Res.* 26: 167–174, 1989.
149. Schmid, P., D. Cox, G. Bilbe, R. Maier, and G.K. McMaster. Differential expression of TGF β1, β2 and β3 genes during mouse embryogenesis. *Development* 111: 117–130, 1991.
150. Serra, R., R.W. Pelton, and H.L. Moses. TGFβ1 inhibits branching morphogenesis and N-*myc* expression in lung bud organ cultures *Development* 120: 2153–2161, 1994.
151. Shahar, I., E. Fireman, M. Topilsky, J. Grief, S. Kivity, Z. Spirer, and S. Ben Efraim. Effect of IL-6 on alveolar fibroblast proliferation in interstitial lung diseases. *Clin. Immunol. Immunopathol.* 79: 244–251, 1996.
152. Shannon, J.M. Induction of alveolar type II cell differentiation in fetal tracheal epithelium by grafted distal lung mesenchyme. *Dev. Biol.* 166: 600–614, 1994.
153. Shannon, J.M., P.A. Emrie, J.H. Fisher, Y. Kuroki, S.D. Jennings, and R.J. Mason. Effect of a reconstituted basement membrane on expression of surfactant apoproteins in cultured adult rat alveolar type II cells. *Am. J. Respir. Cell Mol. Biol.* 2: 183–192, 1990.
154. Shannon, J.M., S.D. Jennings, and L.D. Nielsen. Modulation of alveolar type II cell differentiated function in vitro. *Am. J. Physiol.* 262 (*Lung Cell. Mol Physiol.* 6): L427–L436, 1992.
155. Shannon, J.M., R.J. Mason, and S.D. Jennings. Functional differentiation of alveolar type II epithelial cell in vitro: effects of cell shape, cell-matrix interaction and cell-cell interactions. *Biochim. Biophys. Acta* 931: 143–156,1987.
156. Shannon, J.M., L.D. Nielsen, S.A. Gebb, and S.H. Randell. Mesenchyme specifies epithelial differentiation in reciprocal recombinants of embryonic lung and trachea. *Dev. Dyn.* 212: 482–494, 1998.
157. Shiratori, M., E. Oshika, L.P. Ung, G. Singh, H. Shinozuka, D. Warburton, G. Michalopoulos, and S.L. Katyal. Keratinocyte growth factor and embryonic rat lung morphogenesis. *Am. J. Respir. Cell Mol. Biol.* 15: 328–338, 1996.
158. Simonet, W.S., M.L. DeRose, N. Bucay, H.Q. Nguyen, S.E. Wert, L. Zhou, T.R. Ulich, A. Thomason, D.M. Danilenko, and J.A. Whitsett. Pulmonary malformation in transgenic mice expressing human keratinocyte growth factor in the lung. *Proc. Natl. Acad. Sci. USA* 92: 12461–12465, 1995.
159. Singh, G., J. Singh, S.L. Katyal, W.E. Brown, J.A. Kramps, I.L. Paradis, J.H. Dauber, T.A. MacPherson, and N. Squeglia. Identification, cellular localization, isolation, and characterization of human Cara cell-specific 10 KD protein. *J. Histochem. Cytochem.* 36: 73–80, 1988.
160. Smith, C.I., E. Rosenberg, S.R. Reisher, F. Li, P. Kefalides, A.B. Fisher, and S.I. Feinstein. Sequence of rat surfactant protein A gene and functional mapping of its upstream region. *Am. J. Physiol.* 269 (*Lung Cell. Mol. Physiol.* 13): L603–L612, 1995.
161. Sonnenberg, E., D. Meyer, K.M. Weidner, and C. Birchmeier. Scatter factor/hepatocyte growth factor and its receptor, the c-*met* tyrosine kinase, can mediate a signal exchange between mesenchyme and epithelia during mouse development. *J. Cell Biol.* 123: 223–235, 1993.
162. Stahlman, M.T., M.E. Gray, and J.A. Whitsett. Expression of thyroid transcription factor-1 (TTF-1) in fetal and neonatal human lung. *J. Histochem. Cytochem.* 44: 673–678, 1996.
163. Stahlman, M.T., M.E. Gray, and J.A. Whitsett. Temporal-spatial distribution of hepatocyte nuclear factor-3β in developing human lung and other foregut derivatives. *Histochem. Cytochem.* 46: 955–962, 1998.

164. Stanton, B.R., A.S. Perkins, L. Tessarollo, D.A. Sassoon, and L.F. Parada. Loss of N-*myc* function results in embryonic lethality and failure of the epithelial component of the embryo to develop. *Genes Dev.* 6: 2235–2247,1992.

165. Strayer, D.S., S. Yang, and H.H. Jerng. Surfactant protein A–binding proteins. Characterization and structures. *J. Biol. Chem.* 268: 18679–18684, 1993.

166. Stripp, B.R., P.L. Sawaya, D.S. Luse, K.A. Wikenheiser, S.E. Wert, J.A. Huffman, D.L. Lattier, G. Singh, S.L. Katyal, and J.A. Whitsett. *Cis*-acting elements that confer lung epithelial cell expression of the CC_{10} gene. *J. Biol. Chem.* 267: 14703–14712, 1992.

167. Strum, J.M., R.S. Compton, S.L. Katyal, and G. Singh. The regulated expression of mRNA for Clara cell protein in the developing airways of the rat, as revealed by in situ hybridization. *Tissue Cell* 24: 461–474, 1992.

168. Stuempfle, K.J., M. Koptides, P.G. Quinn, and J. Floros. In vitro analysis of rat surfactant protein A gene expression. *Am. J. Physiol.* 270 (*Lung Cell. Mol. Physiol.* 14): L504–L516, 1996.

169. Sugahara, K., J.S. Rubin, R.J. Mason, E.L. Aronsen, and J.M. Shannon. Keratinocyte growth factor increases mRNAs for SP-A and SP-B in adult rat alveolar type II cells in culture. *Am. J. Physiol.* 269 (*Lung Cell. Mol. Physiol.* 13): L344–L350, 1995.

170. Ten Have-Opbroek, A.A.W. The development of the lungs in mammals: an analysis of concepts and findings. *Am. J. Anat.* 162: 201–219, 1981.

171. Toonen, R.F.G., S. Gowan, and C.D. Bingle. The lung enriched transcription factor TTF-1 and the ubiquitously expressed proteins Sp-1 and Sp-3 interact with elements located in the minimal promoter of the rat Clara cell secretory protein gene. *Biochem. J.* 316: 467–473, 1996.

172. Torday, J.S. and S. Kourembanas. Fetal rat lung fibroblasts produce a TGF β homolog that blocks alveolar type II cell maturation. *Dev. Biol.* 139: 35–41, 1990.

173. Ulich, T.R., E.S. Yi, K. Longmuir, S. Yin, R. Blitz, C. F. Morris, R. Housley, and G.F. Pierce. Keratinocyte growth factor is a growth factor for type II pneumocytes in vivo. *J. Clin. Invest.* 93: 1298–1306, 1994.

174. Venkatesh, V.C., B.C. Planer, M. Schwartz, J.N. Vanderbilt, R.T. White, and P.L. Ballard. Characterization of the promoter of human pulmonary surfactant protein B gene. *Am. J. Physiol.* 268 (*Lung Cell. Mol. Physiol.* 12): L674–L682, 1995.

175. Wang, J., M. Kuliszewski, W. Yee, L. Sedlackova, J. Xu, I. Tseu, and M. Post. Cloning and characterization of glucocorticoid-induced genes in fetal rat lung fibroblasts: transforming growth factor β_3. *J. Biol. Chem.* 270: 2722–2728, 1995.

176. Wang, J., P. Souza, M. Kuliszewski, A.K. Tanswell, and M. Post. Expression of surfactant proteins in embryonic rat lung. *Am. J. Respir. Cell Mol. Biol.* 10: 222–229, 1994.

177. Weigel, D., G. Jurgens, F. Kuttner, E. Seifert, and H. Jäckle. The homeotic gene *fork head* encodes a nuclear protein and is expressed in the terminal regions of the *Drosophila* embryo. *Cell* 57: 645–658, 1989.

178. Weinstein, D.C., A. Ruiz i Altaba, W.S. Chen, P. Hoodless, V.R. Prezioso,T.M. Jessell, and J.E. Darnell. The winged-helix transcription factor *HNF-3β* is required for notochord development in the mouse embryo. *Cell* 78:575–585, 1994.

179. Wert, S.E., S.W. Glasser, T.R. Korfhagen, and J.A. Whittsett. Transcriptional elements from the human SP-C gene direct expression in the primordial respiratory epithelium of transgenic mice. *Dev. Biol.* 156: 426–443, 1993.

180. White, R.T., D. Damm, J. Miller, K. Spratt, J. Schilling, S. Hawgood, B. Benson, and

B. Cordell. Isolation and characterization of the human pulmonary surfactant apoprotein gene. *Nature* 317: 361–363, 1985.

181. Whitsett, J.A. and J.E. Baatz. Hydrophobic surfactant proteins SP-B and SP-C: molecular biology, structure and function. In: *Pulmonary Surfactant, from Molecular Biology to Clinical Practice,* edited by B. Robertson, L.M.G. van Golde, and J.J. Batenburg. Amsterdam: Elsevier, 1992, p. 55–75.

182. Whitsett, J.A., J.C. Clark, J.R. Wispé, and G.S. Pryhuber. Effects of TNF-α and phorbol ester on human surfactant protein and MnSOD gene transcription in vitro. *Am. J. Physiol.* 262 (*Lung Cell. Mol. Physiol.* 6): L688–L693, 1992.

183. Whitsett, J.A., T.E. Weaver, M.A. Lieberman, J.C. Clark, and C. Daugherty. Differential effects of epidermal growth factor and transforming growth factor-β on synthesis of Mr = 35,000 surfactant-associated protein in fetal lung. *J. Biol. Chem.* 262: 7908–7913, 1987.

184. Wikenheiser, K.A. and J.A. Whitsett. Tumor progression and cellular differentiation of pulmonary adenocarcinomas in SV40 large T transgenic mice. *Am. J. Respir. Cell Mol. Biol.* 16: 713–723, 1997.

185. Williams, M.C., Y.-X. Cao, A. Hinds, A.K. Rishi, and A. Wetterwald. T1α protein is developmentally regulated and expressed by alveolar type I cells, choroid plexus, and ciliary epithelia of adult rats. *Am. J. Respir. Cell Mol. Biol.* 14: 577–585, 1996.

186. Wolf, M., J. Klug, R. Hackenberg, M. Gessler, K.-H. Grzeschik, M. Beato, and G. Suske. Human CC10, the homologue of rabbit uteroglobin: genomic cloning, chromosomal localization and expression in endometrial cell lines. *Hum. Mol. Genet.* 1: 371–378, 1992.

187. Wu, J.E. and S.A. Santoro. Differential expression of integrin α subunits supports distinct roles during lung branching morphogenesis. *Dev. Dyn.* 206: 169–181, 1996.

188. Wuenschell, C.W., M.E. Sunday, G. Singh, P. Minoo, H.C. Slavkin, and D. Warburton. Embryonic mouse lung epithelial progenitor cells co-express immunohistochemical markers of diverse mature cell lineages. *J. Histochem. Cytochem.* 44: 112–123, 1996.

189. Yan, C., M. Ghaffari, J.A. Whitsett, X. Zeng, Z. Sever, and S. Lin. Retinoic acid receptor activation of SP-B gene transcription in respiratory epithelial cells. *Am. J. Physiol.* 275 (*Lung Cell. Mol. Physiol.* 19): L239–L246, 1998.

190. Yan, C., Z. Sever, and J.A. Whitsett. Upstream enhancer activity in the human surfactant protein B gene is mediated by thyroid transcription factor 1. *J. Biol. Chem.* 270: 24852–24857, 1995.

191. Yan, C. and J.A. Whitsett. Protein kinase A activation of the surfactant protein B gene is mediated by phosphorylation of thyroid transcription factor 1. *J. Biol. Chem.* 272: 17327–17332, 1997.

192. Yee, W., J. Wang, J. Liu, I. Tseu, M. Kuliszewski, and M. Post. Glucocorticoid-induced tropoelastin expression is mediated via transforming growth factor-β_3. *Am. J. Physiol.* 270 (*Lung Cell. Mol. Physiol.* 14): L992–L1001, 1996.

193. Zhao, Y. and S.L. Young. Expression of transforming growth factor-β type II receptor in rat lung is regulated during development. *Am. J. Physiol.* 269 (*Lung Cell. Mol. Physiol.* 13): L419–L426, 1995.

194. Zhou, L., C.R. Dey, S.E. Wert, and J.A. Whitsett. Arrested lung morphogenesis in transgenic mice bearing an SP-C-TGF-β1 chimeric gene *Dev. Biol.* 175: 227–238, 1996.

195. Zhou, L., L. Lim, R.H. Costa, and J.A. Whitsett. Thyroid transcription factor-1, hepatocyte nuclear factor-3β, surfactant protein B, C, and Clara cell secretory protein in developing mouse lung. *J. Histochem. Cytochem.* 44:1183–1193, 1996.

chapter 5

LUNG DEVELOPMENT AND PULMONARY ANGIOGENESIS

Peter H. Burri

TWO structural factors are of fundamental importance to successful gas-exchange function of the lung: the gas-exchange surface area and the thickness of the air–blood barrier in the pulmonary parenchyma. Both these factors depend on the dimensions and morphology of the lung capillary network; its total volume, the density of its meshes, and its three-dimensional structure greatly affect the gas–loading and transport function of the blood.

After a brief description of the normal structure of the lung, the development of the lung will be presented, with special emphasis given to the changes in lung vasculature at each stage of development. Two special sections will address the zone concept of lung development and the structural development of the capillary system respectively. Finally, we will discuss how the lung capillary network keeps pace with the growth of the organ and how some risk factors interfere with postnatal lung development and growth.

MORPHOLOGY OF THE LUNG

The Gas-Exchange Region or Lung Parenchyma

Three compartments—air, blood, and tissue—compose the gas-exchange region. The tissue compartment functions as a framework for two dynamic and continuously moving components, air and blood. It has the double function of not only keeping the air and blood separated but also of allowing intimate contact between them to ensure rapid uptake of O_2 and release of CO_2. Therefore, the lung parenchyma provides a large internal surface area for gas exchange and resembles a sponge in structure and consistency. It consists of the respiratory bronchioles, alveolar ducts, and alveoli. These air spaces are delineated by a delicate tissue framework, the interalveolar septa, which are covered on both sides by a thin squamous epithelium and contain a dense capillary network interwoven with a skeleton of connective tissue fibers (Fig. 5.1). In addition to a few free cells, the cellular elements of the septal interstitium are myofibroblastic cells (37) of at least two phenotypes [see review by Mc Gowan and Torday; (55)]. These cells are responsible on the one hand for the formation and maintenance of the fibrous skeleton, and on the other hand for the regulation of the compliance of the interstitial space as the cells can contract (85). They have been described as being coupled by gap junctions and are assumed to behave like a functional syncytium (4). Because they strut together the epithelial covers of the interalveolar walls (Fig. 5.2), the myfibroblastic cells can prevent the accumulation of fluid in the septum. It also appears that they have an important metabolic function related to surfactant synthesis in alveolar type II cells (55). The lung capillaries are lined with a continuous endothelium, which, except for the nuclear region, is kept extremely thin over wide areas (typical range: 0.05–0.25 m), where the only

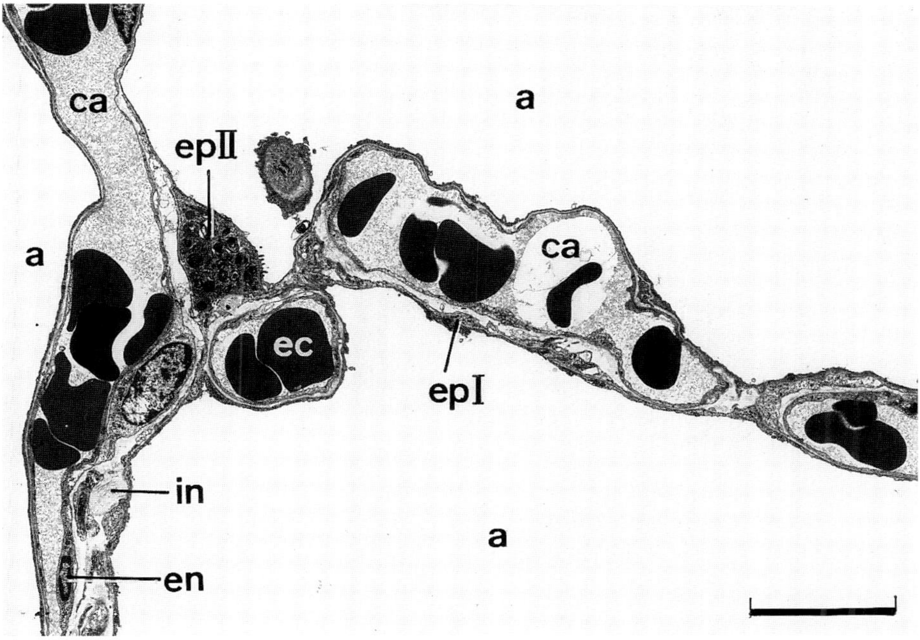

Fig. 5.1 Electron micrograph of mature interalveolar septum of adult human lung. Notice the central position of a single capillary layer interwoven with connective tissue fibers. *a*, alveolar space; *ca*, capillary; *ec*, erythrocyte; *en*, endothelium; *epI*, type I epithelial cell; epII, type II epithelial cell; in, interstitium. Bar = 10 μm.

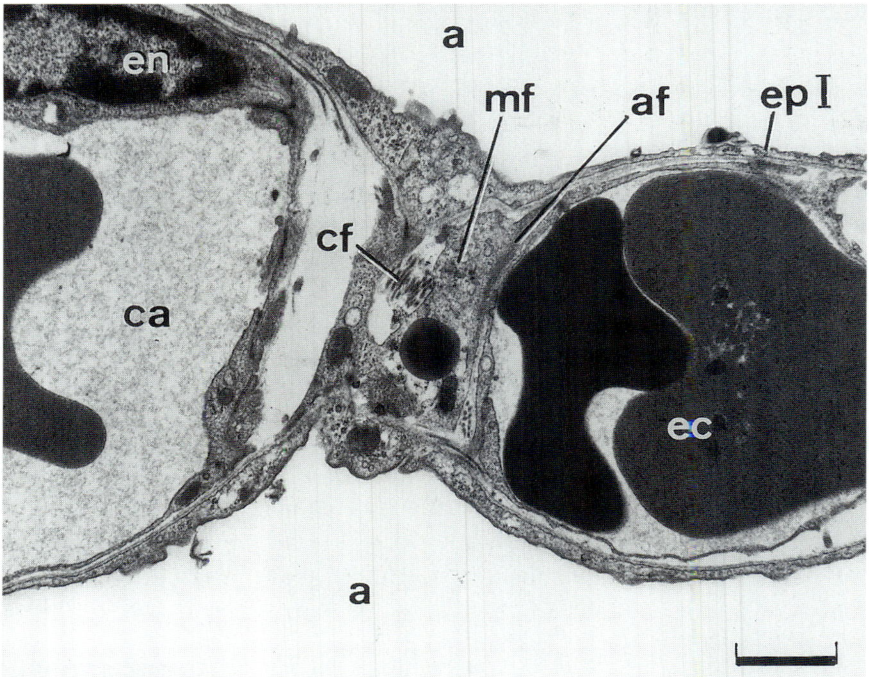

Fig. 5.2 Electron micrograph showing cytoplasmic extension of myofibroblast typically positioned in a tissue pillar between two capillaries. The cell struts together the two epithelial layers. *a*, alveolar space; *af*, actin filaments; *ca*, capillary; *cf*, collagen fibrils; *ec*, erythrocyte; *en*, endothelium; *epI*, type I epithelial cell; *mf*, myofibroblast. Bar = 1 μm.

organelles present are micropinocytotic vesicles. Despite this paucity of organellar content, lung endothelial cells assume numerous metabolic functions, particularly with regard to vasoactive agents in the blood circulation (34, 54). Because of their exquisite and strategically unique positioning in the circulatory system (the lung is the only organ of the body which "sees" practically the entire blood volume with each circulatory cycle), the pulmonary endothelial cells can monitor and influence the concentration of various molecules in the blood. The lung capillaries are partially wrapped by pericytes and their thin cytoplasmic processes, cells whose precise function is still not yet known. The epithelial cover on both sides of the interalveolar wall is composed mainly of two cell types: the squamous type I epithelium covering 93% of the total alveolar surface and the type II epithelial cells or granular pneumocytes that produce the surfactant and have important functions in fluid transport (33, 53). A third cell type, the alveolar brush cell, has thus far only been demonstrated in the rat lung where it is assumed to have a receptor function (44), since nerve fibers were found in its vicinity. In the human lung, similar cells have been observed only in the conductive airways, but they have also been described in other gut-derived organs (44, 59).

Type I cells have cytoplasmic extensions, or "plates," reaching far from the cell body, thus producing the picture of non-nucleated plates under the light microscope. Their complex topological configuration may be the reason why these cells do not divide. Type II cells, in addition to exhibiting surfactant secretory activity, are considered the stem cells of the pulmonary epithelium (46). When the inner lung surface is damaged they proliferate, covering the epithelial defects and subsequently transforming into type I cells.

At the air–tissue interface, the surfactant, a liquid-lining layer, has the ability to reduce the surface tension and to smooth out cell surface irregularities. It also prevents the delicate parenchymal tissue from drying out and provides an adequate environment for the alveolar macrophages patroling the inner lung surface.

The Airway Tree

In order to carry out pulmonary gas exchange, the lungs must be continuously replenished with oxygen through a branching system of tubes called the *airway tree*. Functionally, the airways consists of three segments: the purely conducting airways located proximally, the uttermost periphery, where there is diffusion only, and in between these areas, a region of transition where both functions, gas transport and gas exchange, coexist.

In the human lung, the conducting airways extend from the trachea (generation 0 of the airway tree) to the terminal bronchioles, which represent small tubes of 0.7–1 mm in diameter and correspond on average to the 16th dichotomous division of the airway tree (84). From here to the periphery the gas-exchange function becomes increasingly more important, as the airway tubes have an increasing number of outpouchings, or alveoli, in their walls where the tissue interface between air and blood is very thin.

On average, starting from the terminal bronchiole toward the periphery, there are three generations of respiratory bronchioles and three generations of alveolar ducts, followed by the alveolar sacs at generation 23 (84). Alveoli, the sites of gas exchange, are thus found on average over the length of seven airway generations; these minute air chambers provide the lung with an internal air tissue interface of about 140 m^2.

The Blood Vessels

The lung possesses two vascular systems: a low-pressure pulmonary system and a high-pressure bronchial system. While the former is responsible for the O_2 supply of the organism (thus it is called *vasa publica*), the latter assumes the maintenance of the walls of the bronchial tree and of the large pulmonary vessels (*vasa privata*).

With the exception of a few branches, arteries usually end several generations proximal to the terminal bronchioles by splitting into capillaries around the walls of bronchioles and vessels that also supply adjacent alveolar walls (70). From there the blood is naturally drained into small collecting veins of the pulmonary circulation.

The structure and development of the two circulatory systems are completely different. Pulmonary arteries develop early along with the bronchial tree. They also branch with it and are thin walled in accordance with the low pressure they are exposed to. The bronchial vessels develop late and their walls are typically systemic, i.e., they are comparable to other arteries of corresponding size in the body. Although the two vascular systems of the lung develop separately, they are interconnected at many levels—arterial, capillary, and venous.

Whereas the existing arterioarterial bronchopulmonary connections are negligible with respect to their functional significance, the bronchial blood drains largely into the pulmonary veins. This situation is responsible for the normal admixture of some venous blood to the arterialized output of the lung.

DEVELOPMENT OF THE LUNG AND ITS VASCULATURE

Embryonic Period

The stages of lung development and their respective timing are listed in Table 5.1. The embryonic stage, which lasts from week 3 to about week 7, is the period during which the various organ systems are laid down in the body. The lung appears around fetal day 26 as a ventral diverticulum of the foregut, which is then separated in a caudocranial direction from the prospective esophagus by the laryngotracheal grooves. The resulting bud then divides and grows into the surrounding mes-

Table 5.1 Overview of the Stages of Lung Development

Period	*Stage*	*Duration*	*Characteristics*
Embryonic	Embryonic	26th day to 7 weeks	Organogenesis; formation of major airways
Fetal	Pseudoglandular	5 to 17 weeks	Formation of bronchial tree and large portions of prospective respitory parenchyma; birth of the acinus
	Canalicular	16 to 26 weeks	Formation of last generations of prospective lung periphery; epithelial differentiation; formation of air-blood barrier and appearance of surfactant
	Saccular or terminal sac	24 to 38 weeks	Expansion of air spaces
Postnatal	Alveolar	36 weeks/birth to 1–2 years	Alveolization by septation
	Microvascular maturation	Birth to 2–3 years	Remodeling of interalveolar septa and restructuring and maturation of capillary bed

enchyme, giving rise to the left and right lungs. Through rapid growth and further dichotomous divisions the sprouting tubules produce the future airway tree by forming its eventual branching pattern: the lobar airways are present at day 37, the segmental branches at day 41, and the future subsegmental branches by day 48.

During this early period of organ formation the embryo is extremely tiny, the embryonic disc measuring only 3–6 mm in length. The distance between heart and lung is in the range of microns, and although the heart has started to beat at around day 20, the vascular system is still rudimentary. Development of the lung vasculature is closely linked to development of the heart and primitive systemic blood vessels. The heart expels the blood into the paired cranial ventral aortae which are connected through the aortic arches to the dorsal aortae. Six pairs of arches are distinguished in vertebrate vascular development (Fig. 5.3). They are never present, however, all at the same time and their individual fate and significance to the adult vascular system differ widely. Whereas the first and second pairs rapidly regress and

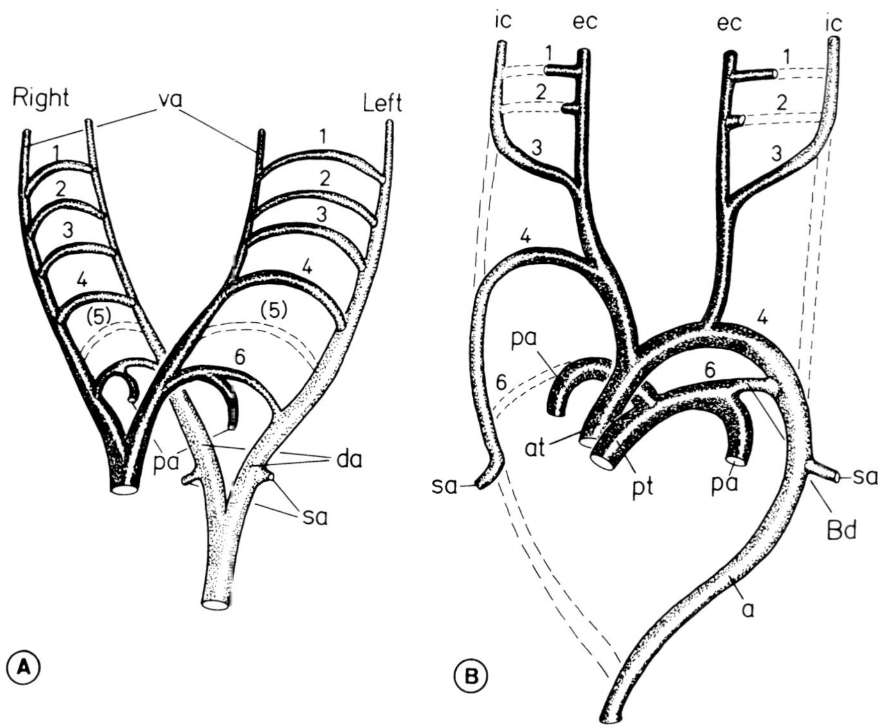

Fig. 5.3 Idealized diagram of arterial tree development showing origin and fate of pulmonary arteries. (*A*) Paired ventral and dorsal aortae are interconnected by six pairs of aortic arches (1–6). (*B*) Fate of the arches: Filled areas represent preserved segments (dark = derived from ventral, light = derived from dorsal vessels); dashed lines represent eliminated segments. *a*, aorta; *Bd*, Botallo's duct; *da*, dorsal aortae; *ec*, external carotid artery; *ic*, internal carotid artery; *pa*, pulmonary artery; *pt*, pulmonary trunk; *sa*, subclavian artery; *va*, ventral aortae. [From Burri (18), with permission.]

disappear, the fifth is never apparent in human development. The third pair connects the external carotid to the internal carotid artery. The fourth pair is also maintained and gives rise to the definitive aortic arch on the left hand side and to the brachiocephalic trunk and part of the subclavian artery on the right hand side. The sixth pair is linked to the development of the pulmonary vessels. The pulmonary arteries branch off from the proximal parts of the arches and join the freshly formed lung buds where they form a vascular plexus in the surrounding mesenchyme. The distal portions of the sixth aortic arches have distinctly different fates, depending whether it is the left or right. On the right, the distal (or dorsal) portion joining the right dorsal aorta regresses and disappears. On the left, the distal part is maintained and gives rise to Botallo's duct connecting the pulmonary artery to the definitive aortic arch. In their proximal portions the sixth aortic arches separate from the aortic trunk and form a common pulmonary trunk emerging from the right ventricle of the heart, which by then has evolved into its definitive configuration with paired atria and ventricles.

While this happens on the arterial side, a tiny bud develops from the sinoatrial portion of the heart. This bud grows in dorsal direction, divides, and connects to the pulmonary plexus, which is already linked to vessels around the trachea and esophagus. With the expansion of the cardiac atria, the single pulmonary vein is taken up into the right atrium. The integration does not stop there; two further successive branches of the original lung vein are finally absorbed into the left atrium. At the end of this process four separate lung veins open into the left atrium.

Fetal Period

Following the embryonic period of organogenesis, the fetal period proper extends from about the fifth week to birth. Fetal lung development progresses through three consecutive but partially overlapping stages: the pseudoglandular, the canalicular, and the saccular stage. Classification of these stages is based purely on morphological criteria. Since during lung development there are no abrupt structural changes and because there may be differences in speed of development between cranial and caudal lung lobes (40, 42), transitions between stages cannot be sharply defined.

Pseudoglandular Stage (week 5 to week 17)

At the beginning of this stage, the lung resembles a tiny primitive gland; at its end, the future acini become visible with prospective lung tissue incompletely delineated by slender connective tissue septa radiating into the lung from the pleura. During this stage, the epithelial buds undergo multiple dichotomous branchings at their tips. While analysis of the factors governing early pulmonary development is still in its infancy, our knowledge of these factors should progress rapidly through the use of immmunohistochemical, immunocytochemical, and molecular biological techniques (15, 56, 92). Transgenic animals represent another promising source for improving our understanding of these developmental events (46, 88). Today, the close and intense interaction between the endodermally derived tubules and the mesenchyme of mesodermal origin occurring during early and later stages of lung development is, however, well assessed (1, 69, 76).

On the basis of work by Bucher and Reid (14) and by Boyden (11), the pseudoglandular stage is usually defined as the stage of formation of the conductive airway tree down to the terminal bronchioles, the latter being capped by a small cluster of saccules. Ten Have Opbroek (78) provided early evidence through immunohistochemical techniques that the epithelial cells at the periphery of the airway tree in mice were precursors to the later alveolar epithelium.

According to more recent morphological and morphometric findings it appears that in the rat lung, for instance, the quantity of prospective gas-exchange tissues present at the end of the pseudoglandular stage has been grossly underestimated (20, 62). The quantitative data on the pulmonary epithelium indicate that half of the parenchymal epithelial cell mass present during the saccular stage before birth (day 23) was already present on day 20 in the late pseudoglandular stage. In the rat, the pseudoglandular stage extends over most of the fetal period, up to 3 to 4 days before birth—a situation very much different from human lung development. Nevertheless, the work of Kitaoka and co-workers (41) indicates that the human pseudoglandular lung periphery also contains large portions of the future gas-exchanging parenchyma. The authors counted the number of end segments in samples of three human lungs and calculated that 20 generations of air spaces were present at the end of the pseudoglandular stage and 22 generations in the canalicular stage. Since the adult human lung contains on average 24 generations of airways, the authors concluded that the end pseudoglandular human lung already contained all the airway divisions down to the level of alveolar ducts.

During this stage, the airways are lined proximally by a high columnar epithelium, which decreases in height to cuboidal cells in the periphery. At week 13 of gestation, basal, ciliated, nonciliated, and goblet cells are present in the epithelium, while mucous glands can already be found in the mucosal layer. All these structures, as is true also for cartilage and smooth-muscle cells, show a proximal-to-distal pattern of differentiation, i.e., they appear first in the prospective trachea, extending from there to the periphery. Beautiful investigations by confocal microscopy have demonstrated that the airways are surrounded by an extensive network of nerve fibers already during early stages of development (86).

The arterial tree develops in close synchrony to the bronchial tree. As a rule, arterial branches accompany the airway branches (the so-called conventional arteries), but in addition, smaller vessels, the supernumerary arteries, branch in between, supplying regions along the airways. While there are little data on vascular development before gestational week 12, it is known that around week 14 the main arterial pathways are present along the airways together with the supernumerary branches (31). This means that conventional and supernumerary branches develop simultaneously at every given level.

The veins behave quite differently. They run interaxially in mesenchymal septa delineating segments and subsegments. Positioning of the veins has been carefully modeled by Verbeken and co-workers (82), who showed that venous branches run systematically in connective tissue septa extending in a plane between each generation of dichotomous airway branching. Obviously, the veins depart from this rule in the central lung portions, where the larger branches join the arteries and airways to reach the pulmonary hilum. From currently available data, it appears that up to five-sixths of the entire pulmonary airway and arterial and venous tree is preformed at the end of the pseudoglandular stage. For reasons of exponential increase (2^n) and growth proper, this holds for the number of generations only, not for the number of branches, total length or total volume of these structures. Their increase is enormous with the last divisions.

Canalicular Stage (Week 16 to Week 26)

Although, much more of the prospective gas-exchange apparatus than what has been mapped out thus far is present at the end of the pseudoglandular stage, the transition to the canalicular stage is marked by the fact that the future gas-exchange tissue becomes discernible by light microscopy. Boyden, who carefully analyzed airway development by means of wax reconstructions, stated that the "birth of the acinus" represented the landmark for the transition between the pseudoglandular and the canalicular stage (11).

The canalicular stage represents a very important period because of 2 developmental steps, easily detectable by light microscopy, that are relevant to future lung function: the differentiation of the pulmonary epithelium into type 2 cells, which allows for secretion of surfactant, and into type 1 cells, which contributes to formation of the first areas having a thin air–blood barrier. After these steps, a prematurely born baby gets the first chance to survive. It is evident, however, that without the additional changes that occur during capillary development, these epithelial differentiation steps would remain functionally irrelevant. Indeed, this stage is marked by a tremendous increase in capillarization of the primitive interstitium. This latter process originally gave this stage its name: the lung tissue becomes "canalized" by capillaries. In a process to be discussed later, the capillaries come to lie in close apposition to the epithelium. Where this happens, the epithelial barrier thins out, forming the eventual air–blood barrier. Not only do the thin, type I epithelial cells appear during this stage but the cuboidal epithelium gives rise to type II cells, which start to accumulate lamellar bodies containing components of the surfactant material. Soon after this differentiation step, surface active material appears in the lung liquid, which is actively secreted by type II cells. In contrast to most species, in which surfactant appears late in gestation (at about 80%–85% of total gestation duration), it is already present at about 60% of gestational time in the human fetus. There is good evidence that these structural changes in the epithelium are the result of epithelial–mesenchymal interactions, which play an important role throughout lung development (1, 10, 29, 69, 72, 75, 76).

Interestingly, according to Mercurio and Rhodin (57, 58), who performed three-dimensional reconstruction studies on differentiating air-space epithelium, the cuboidal, glycogen-filled epithelial cells start differentiation by degrading their glycogen content. They then show a few small lamellar bodies before transforming into typical type II cells or before beginning to produce thin cytoplasmic extensions. This observation makes it less surprising that in the mature lung, type II cells are considered the stem cells of both type II and type I cells.

While the cellular and structural differentiations represent important steps for future lung function, it is evident that further growth of the preacinar, but especially of prospective parenchymal structures, represents a predominant issue during the canalicular stage and the following saccular stage. The tubules not only grow in length but also widen to structures called *canaliculi*, giving the lung an increasingly "spongy" appearance. We must also assume that a few more peripheral airway generations are added to the airway tree by the time of birth, but no precise data are available about this. Indirect evidence for the continuing dichotomous branching process is the finding that a cuboidal, undifferentiated epithelium can still be found at the outer periphery of the human lung at 1 month after birth (90). Arteries and veins closely follow both the growth of preacinar airways as well as the expansion and branching pattern of the prospective lung parenchyma.

In summary, the canalicular stage is characterized by expansion of the airway tree and massive organ growth, and by differentiation of the air space epithelium into type II cells, which are responsible for surfactant production, and into type I cells, which form thin air–blood barriers.

Saccular Stage (week 24 to birth)

According to Boyden (11), three more air-space generations are to be formed during this stage. These would correspond to future alveolar ducts and alveolar sacs. In light of findings by Kitaoka and co-workers (41), however, we expect this number to be lower.

During the saccular stage, the lung gains its alveolar appearance, even though there are no alveoli present yet. The peripheral air spaces expand in length and width, and at the expense of the intervening mesenchyme, they become saccules, a term that is, in fact, not adequate. The "saccules," as seen in light microscopic lung sections, correspond either to ducts or to true saccules. Furthermore, if a sac gives rise to two new sacs by dichotomous branching, it transforms itself into a duct. We have therefore recommended that these structures be called *transitory air spaces* (18), which takes into account the fact that the air spaces reach their definitive status only after alveolization, when the ducts become alveolar ducts and the terminal sacs become alveolar sacs. The interstitium in between the air spaces contains the capillary network and numerous interstitial cells, but only a delicate network of collagen fibers. During the course of this stage, a network of elastic fibers is deposited throughout the interstitium, which lays the foundation for alveolar formation. In 1936, Dubreuil and co-workers (26) observed that the elastic material was laid down where the future interalveolar walls would be formed. This temporal coincidence has since been verified experimentally (16, 83).

Having adapted to the growth of the lung parenchyma, the arterial pathway increases in length and diameter. Measurements on arteriograms of human lungs at various fetal ages show that the diameter of an artery depends mainly on its distance from the pathway's end. This means that, irrespective of lung size, the diameter of an arterial branch is more or less constant at a given distance from the end of the arterial tree (32). Arterial growth is faster centrally than in the periphery and conventional arteries usually grow more than supernumerary ones. Obviously, central vessels have to grow faster because distally the number of additional branches increases exponentially.

Whereas the structure of the arteries along the axial pathway in later fetal life already corresponds to the adult structure with elastic, muscular, and partially muscular walls, the intrapulmonary veins (depending on their diameter) have very little or no smooth muscle during much of the fetal period. During the saccular stage they begin to develop a circular muscle layer and to resemble the mature vessels.

The Zone Concept of Fetal Lung Development

Figure 5.4 illustrates the zone concept as established in the rat lung (20), this is also likely valid for the human lung. In the developing lung we can distinguish four morphologically distinct zones.

Zone I is morphologically characterized by a lighter staining in light- and electron-microscopic sections. It contains a loose network of mesenchymal cells and capillaries and forms a mantle of undifferentiated tissue around the lung core composed of zones II to IV. Proximally it also contains the dividing end tips of the airway tubules. Zone I represents the main region of organ growth. Here, in most peripheral lung portions, the cells multiply, engendering a massive gain in organ volume and, importantly, the epithelial tubules divide dichotomously. Zone I does not increase in thickness, however, because in its proximal part the cells are continuously differentiating into more mature forms and concomitantly enter zone II. The few capillaries present form a wide and scarce three-dimensional network (Fig. 5.4 A). Because zone I acts as a cambial layer whose function obviously runs out during the saccular stage, it is no longer present towards the end of this stage.

Zone II corresponds to a region densely packed with cells; it therefore appears darker in most light-microscopic stainings. It occupies the more central lung portions and corresponds to the future gas-exchanging compartment (Fig. 5.4 B). During development, zone II shows the largest increase in volume. It grows continuously at the periphery, where cells differentiate at the border between zones I and II, and shift from zone I into zone II. In the central portions of zone II, a smaller amount of cells further differentiate and shift into zone III.

Zones III and IV represent the prospective nonparenchymal structures of the lung, i.e., the conducting airways and the larger blood vessels. In zone III, airways and blood vessels are ensheathed by smooth-muscle cell precursors; in zone IV, they are additionally enveloped by a layer of adventitial cells. During development, zones III and IV grow peripherad—zone III by differentiation of mesenchymal cells into smooth-muscle cell precursors at the border between zones II and III, and zone IV by differentiation of adventitial cells at the border between zones III and IV (Fig. 5.4 C and D).

Thus, it becomes evident from this description that the lung develops in a centrifugal manner. In the outermost lung periphery a mantle of undifferentiated mesenchyme continuously adds more mass to the lung. This allows each zone to grow toward the periphery by recruiting cells from the next outer zone. This means that a primitive mesenchymal cell of zone I can become an interstitial cell in zone IV, III, or

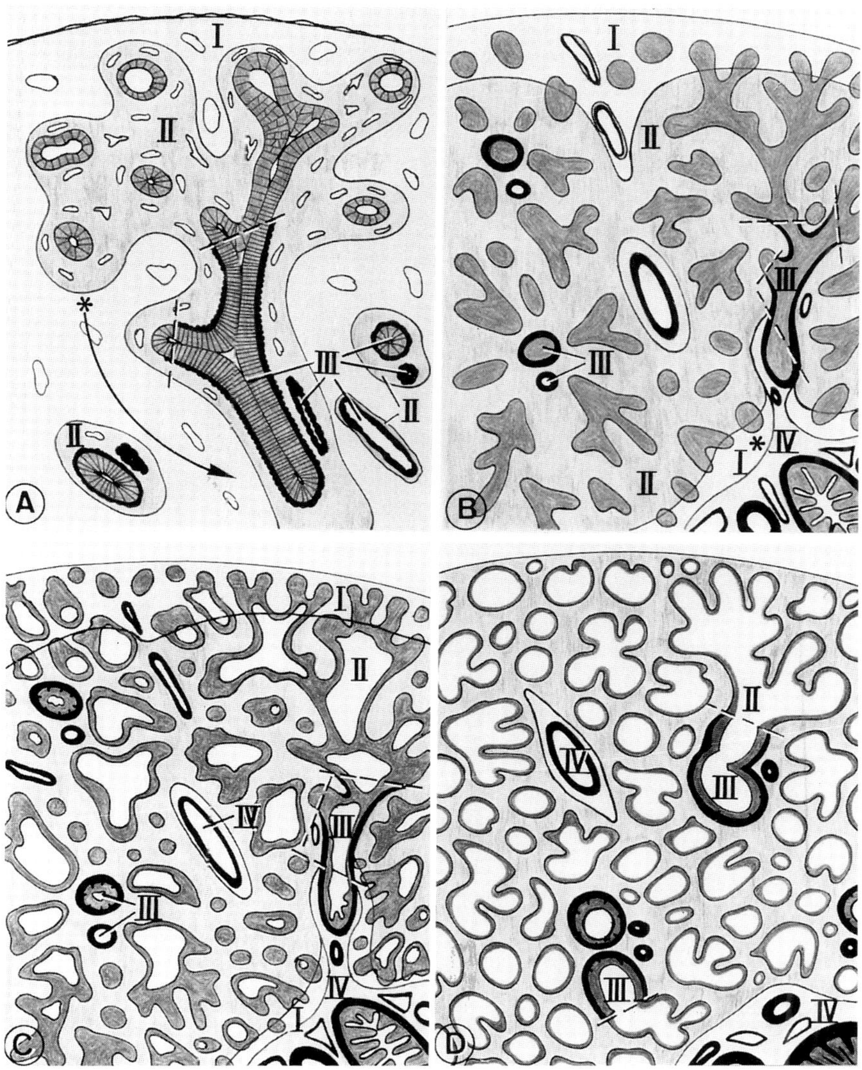

Fig. 5.4 Schematic representation of zone concept. For explanations, see text.

II, the latter being by far the most frequent situation. By analogy, zone I epithelial and endothelial cells can undergo the same zonal shifts.

The developmental mechanism described above, however, should not be misunderstood. The mitoses in zone I and the shifting of cells from one zone into the next proximal one do not account for total lung growth. Zone I is needed to continuously produce the mantle of undifferentiated tissue permitting the sprouting growth of the airway tree. The differentiation processes between zones determine the type of airway produced and indirectly determine the proper number of generations in each type of airway. But, evidently, each zone and each airway or vessel generation also grows in itself, once it is formed.

Developmental Alterations in Capillary Network Structure

During the fetal period of lung development, important alterations in the three-dimensional architecture of the capillary network prepare the foundation for alveolization of the lung. Figure 5.5 illustrates how the intersaccular septa get their double capillary networks, a structure representing the prerequisite for alveolar formation. The pulmonary capillary system arises as a small plexus around the budding

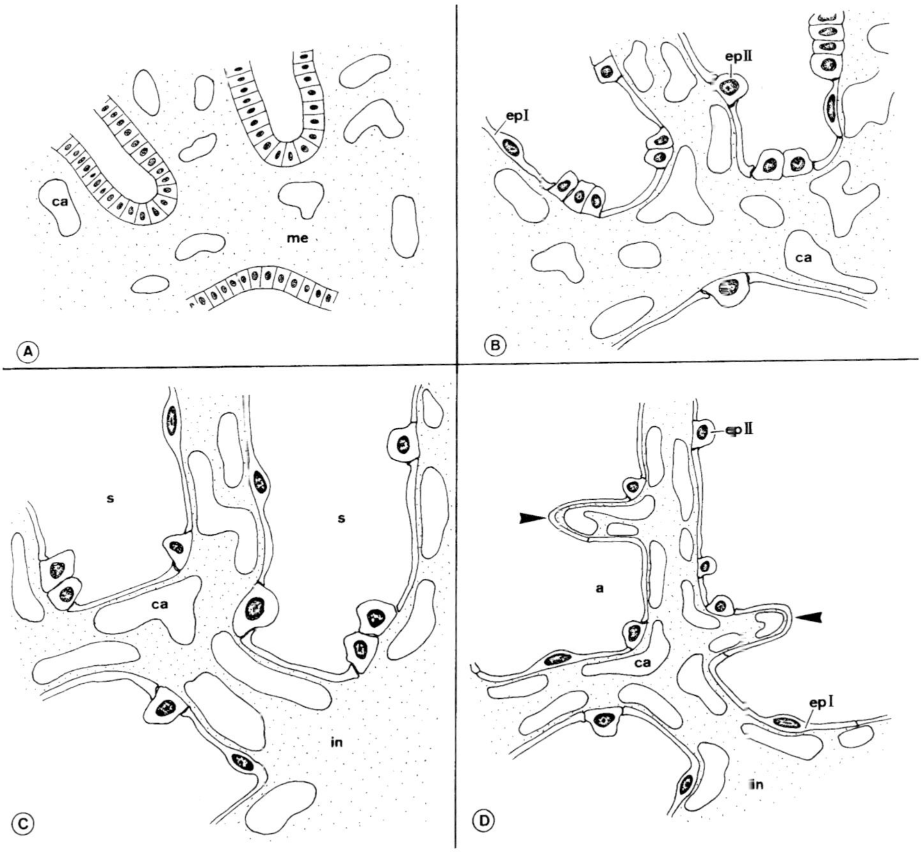

Fig. 5.5 Capillary development. (*A*) During the pseudoglandular stage, the epithelial tubes grow into the loose mesenchyme of zone I: the capillaries form a three-dimensional network. (*B*) During the canalicular stage, capillaries grow markedly and form a dense network. They come to lie closer to the epithelial tubes whose epithelium is differentiating into type I and type II cells. (*C*) In the saccular lung, capillaries form a sleeve around each air space. Intersaccular walls (primary septa) contain a capillary bilayer. (*D*) During alveolization; interalveolar walls (secondary septa) have formed in the saccules by up-folding of one of the two capillary networks (*arrowheads*). All septa are still of the immature (or primitive) type. *a*, alveoli; *ca*, capillary; *epI*, type I epithelial cell; *epII*, type II epithelial cell; *in*, interstitium; *me*, mesenchyme; *s*, saccule.

airway tree. Its most proximal and distal branches are connected to the developing arterial system and through the veins to the left atrium, respectively. During the pseudoglandular stage, the capillaries are arranged in a more or less isotropic, three-dimensional network. With the expansion of the air space system during the canalicular stage, the capillary system is "compressed" or "squeezed" between the air spaces. The meshes of the network rearrange around the air canaliculi (Fig. 5.5 B). During the canalicular stage, the capillaries come to lie at numerous places directly underneath the cuboidal epithelial layer. Wherever this happens, the cuboidal epithelium differentiates and thin type I cells appear to preform the air–blood barrier (Fig. 5-5 B). As a result of this process every air canaliculus becomes ensheathed by a capillary plexus (Fig. 5.5 C). Because each capillary sleeve around the air spaces is also part of a three-dimensional system, it is, and remains, interconnected with the neighboring sleeves. This process of the formation of peri-air-space capillary sleeves concludes toward the end of the saccular stage when all the intersaccular walls contain a double capillary layer (Fig. 5-5 C). As will be discussed later, this structure represents the basis for the alveolization of the lungs (Fig. 5.5 D).

Postnatal Period

Although birth represents a radical environmental change for the lung, it does not have a direct impact on lung development. The alterations induced by birth are much more functional in nature than structural, therefore lung development transits smoothly from the prenatal to the postnatal period.

Most of our knowledge about the postnatal stages of lung development has been obtained from the rat lung. Fortunately, as has been established by comparisons of lung structure during these late stages, human and rat lung development does not really differ in the main features. In both species, lung development completes two postnatal stages before it fades into normal growth: the alveolar stage and the stage of microvascular maturation. The timing of these stages has been much debated and will continue to be disputed because, in addition to technical limitations (such as identification of alveoli in sections), sharp limits can not be determined by statistical approaches in slowly changing processes.

Alveolar Stage (week 36 to postnatal month 18)

Whether the lung contains no alveoli at birth (11) or 20 million (25) or 50 million (43) is almost irrelevant, because most alveoli are formed after birth; the adult complement reaches about 300 million (2, 84).

During the last weeks of fetal life, the alveoli start to appear in the saccular lung; they are delineated by a network of low ridges or crests protruding from the inter-air-space walls. The mechanism of their formation has been extensively studied in the rat lung (16, 19), where the bulk of alveoli are formed within approximately 10 days. Additional alveoli are produced at a slower pace until adulthood (8, 49, 50). The process can be nicely visualized by scanning electron microscopy (Fig. 5.6). The transitory channels and saccules of the saccular lung are incompletely subdivided by

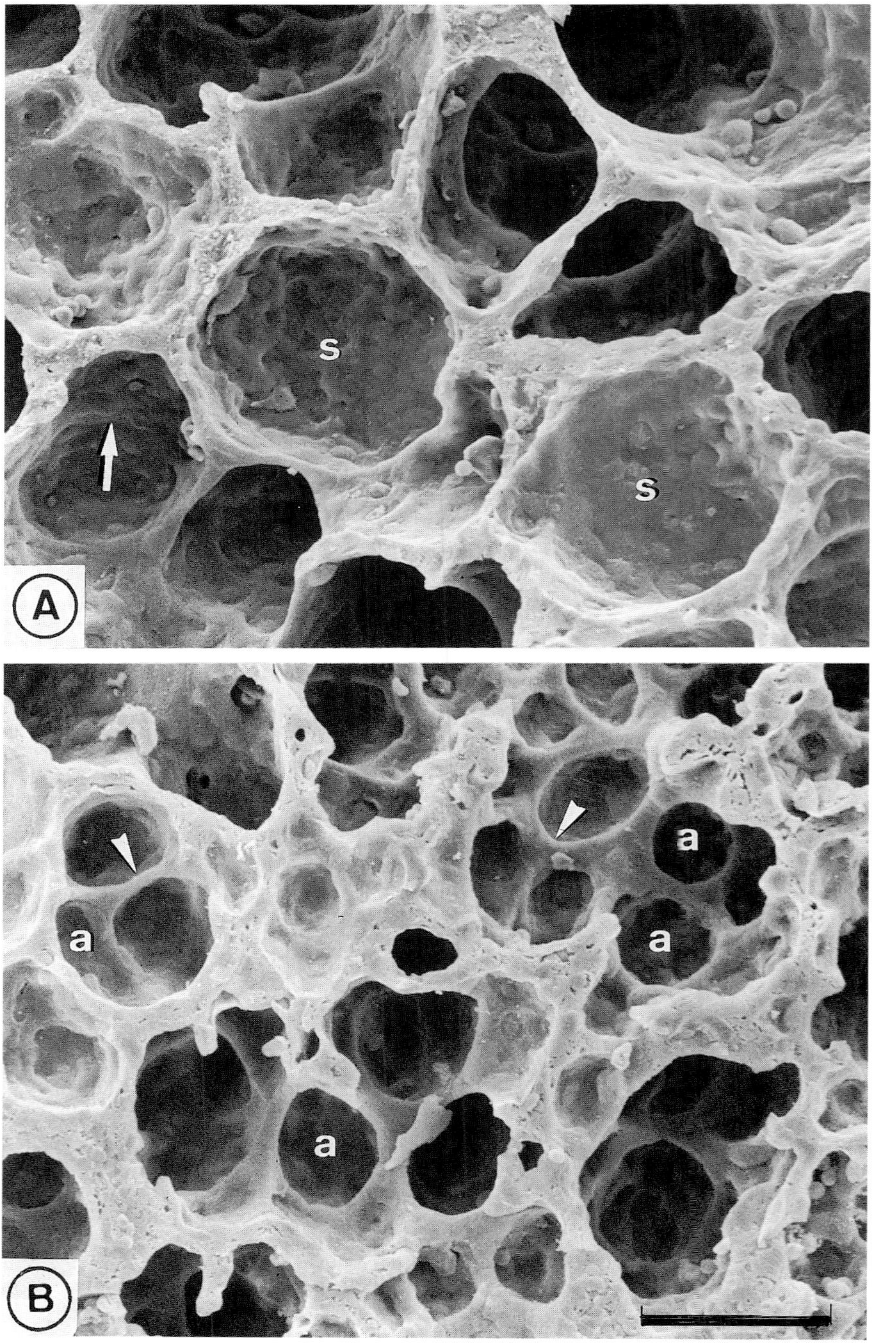

Fig. 5.6 Scanning electron micrographs illustrating the rapid phase of alveolar formation. Comparison of rat lungs aged 4 days and 10 days, respectively, at the same magnification is shown. (*A*) Day 4: The lung parenchyma is made of saccules; very low ridges start to appear, indicating the sites of secondary septa formation (*arrows*). (*B*) Day 10: The saccules have been incompletely subdivided into numerous shallow cups, the alveoli, by newly formed secondary septa, the interalveolar walls (*arrowheads*). *a*, alveoli; *s*, saccules. Bar = 50 μm.

ridges into alveolar ducts or sacs. The resulting interalveolar walls have been termed *secondary septa* because they appear on the primary septa in the saccular lung. Under electron microscopy the secondary septa show a central layer of connective tissue with numerous cells and very little collagen fibrils, flanked on both sides by capillaries, which, depending on the level of sectioning, appear to be interconnected over the edge of the crest (Fig. 5.7). Cross-sectioned fibers of elastin can be detected at the tip of the crest or just below the capillary loop (Fig. 5.7). It has long been known that elastin deposition in the saccular lung marks the site of secondary septa

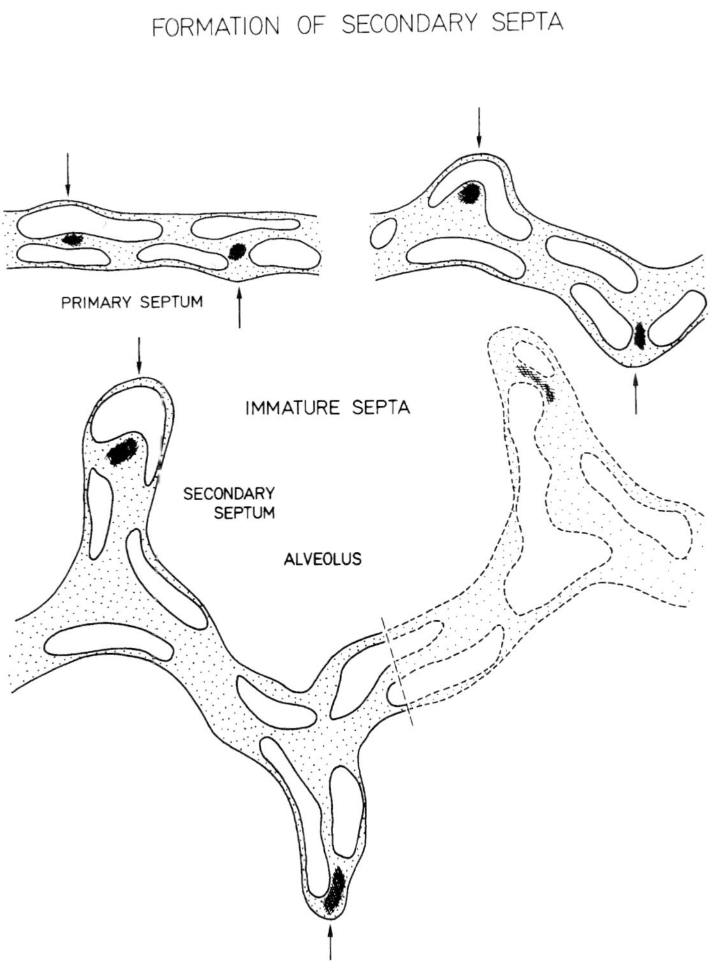

Fig. 5.7 Diagram illustrating the principles of interalveolar wall formation as observed in electron microscopy. Low crests (*arrows*) are formed by alternately lifting up one of the two capillary layers of a primary septum on either side of it. The crests increase in height and become secondary septa. All the septa present are still of the immature type with two capillary layers. Fibers of elastin (*dark spots*) are clearly related to secondary septa formation. [From Burri (18), with permission.]

formation (26). The morphological features suggest that the new interalveolar walls are formed by the alternative up-folding of one of the two capillary layers on either side of a primary septum (Fig. 5.7). As a result of this process, not only the primary but also the secondary septa contain a double capillary layer, (Fig. 5.8 A) i.e., all the parenchymal septa can be described as immature or primitive when compared with the mature septa of the adult lung (Fig. 5.8 B). The latter contain only a single capillary network, and the central capillary abuts the air space on both sides (Fig. 5.1). This means that the alveolar stage *must* be followed by an additional and final stage in lung development, the stage of microvascular maturation.

As was the case for assessing the beginning of the alveolization process, it is equally impossible to determine its end. In the rat, there is a relatively short phase of rapid alveolization (bulk alveolar formation) in the first 2 weeks of life, which is followed by a longer period of alveolar formation at a much slower pace. In the human lung, fast alveolization occurs during the last few weeks of the prenatal period and the first 5 to 6 months of postnatal life. This is apparent because large parts of the human lung look mature at 6 months of age; i.e., many parenchymal septa no longer exhibit the double capillary network needed for the formation of new interalveolar walls. As in the rat, however, this does not mean that alveolar formation is terminated. A slower phase must be assumed to last up to the age of 2 years (43) or even older. Labeling experiments of the growth areas in rats have shown that the lung periphery appears to be the preferred region for the addition of alveoli after bulk alveolization (50). This is in accord with the concept that new interalveolar septa can be formed wherever a capillary layer can be folded up. This is possible at those places where the parenchymal septa have maintained an immature aspect, (which is found even in adult lungs) or, importantly, where a single-layered capillary network abuts connective tissue, as is the case for the pleura and the adventitial layer of bronchi or blood vessels. This is an important observation in view of the fact that the slow formation of further alveoli has been proposed to occur by means other than septation (7, 49, 50, 71) or by the late peripheral addition of new saccules (6, 50). Overlapping the stage of alveolar formation is the next and final stage of development, microvascular maturation.

Stage of Microvascular Maturation (birth to 2–3 years)

This important, final step in lung development has long been ignored in reviews on lung development. As Figure 5.8 illustrates, the mature lung capillary network shows a completely different structural (and maybe functional) design than before and during alveolization. In the saccular and alveolarizing lung, the inter-air–space walls are thick and contain a capillary bilayer, which represents a suboptimal structural layout with respect to gas exchange. It is interesting to note that mammalian species with immature lung capillaries at birth are mostly of the altricial type, whereas the precocial species have interalveolar walls of the adult type (50). The mode by which the lung parenchyma becomes mature is still not completely understood. On the basis of observations made through transmission and scanning electron microscopy we put forward the hypothesis that capillary maturation is the

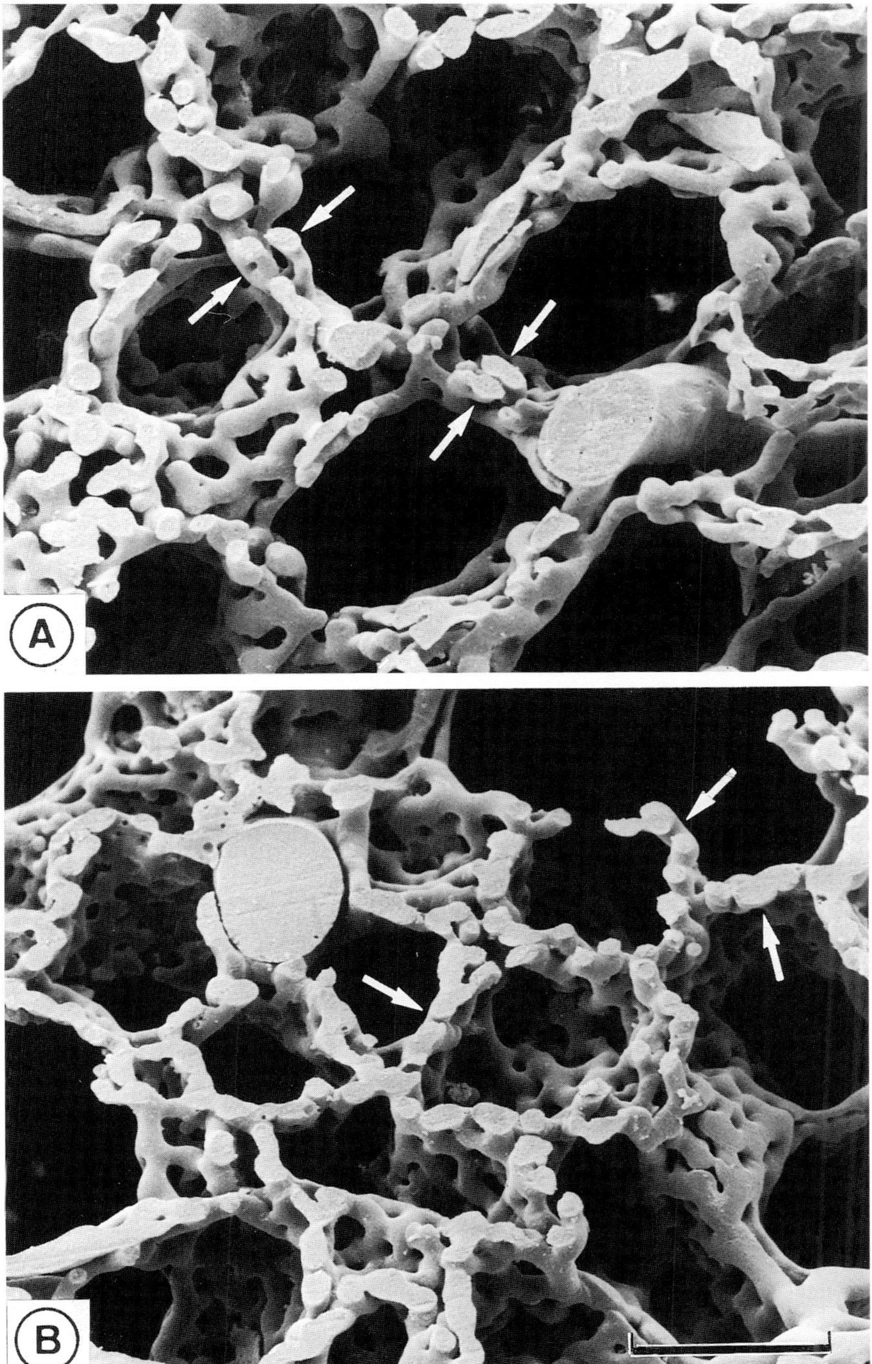

Fig. 5.8 Scanning electron micrograph of Mercox casts of rat aged 4 days (*A*) and 44 days (*B*). Notice the double capillary networks in immature lung septa (*arrows*) and mostly single network in mature interalveolar walls (*arrows in B*). Bar = 50 μm.

result of multiple focal fusions between the adjacent capillary layers, followed by preferential growth of the fused areas (16, 17, 23). These events are induced by a decrease in the mass of interstitial tissue.

Morphometric studies in the rat have shown that interstitial tissue volume of the parenchymal septa decreases in absolute terms from days 14 to 21 despite a volume increase of the lung by about 20% (19). By thinning out the connective tissue layer separating the two capillary networks, the latter come to lie close to each other, touch each other in places, and focally merge their lumina. Capillary wall restructuring allowing capillary merging is a process that has not been studied in detail. It is evident, however, that network alterations and wound repair with sprouting vessels connecting and opening to neighboring ones could not occur without the phenomenon of capillary merging. Furthermore, the following ultrastructural observations and developmental facts support a merging mechanism.

1. During this period a frequent observation is that two capillary lumina are only separated by the cytoplasmic extension of single endothelial cells. We have to keep in mind, however, that such findings must be interpreted with great caution; they could be due to the sectioning of capillary bifurcations.
2. In scanning electron micrographs of vascular casts, the number of interconnections between the two capillary layers seems to increase, but no precise counts are available thus far.
3. The parenchymal capillary networks in the adult lung show two distinct patterns: a dense network in interalveolar walls and a coarse network facing the pleura or abutting the peribronchial or perivascular sheets. This difference could be explained by the fact that a dense network within the alveolar septum is the result of the fusion of two capillary networks. The coarse network is found where there is no merging.
4. The interalveolar pores (pores of Kohn) are practically missing in the immature septa. They develop during the course of septal and capillary restructuration. We have proposed that the decrease in interstitial tissue volume also leads to transseptal epithelial–epithelial cell contacts. Where this happens, there is a reorganization of junctional complexes with a "merging" of the epithelia, an opening in the interalveolar wall, and the formation of Kohn's pores (87). These events require the same processes at the cellular level as capillary merging. The above observations strongly support that merging of capillary lumina represents a major mechanism for capillary maturation. However, capillary merging alone cannot totally transform the lung parenchyma. We suggest therefore that the merged areas expand by preferential growth (23), i.e., they grow more rapidly than the immature areas of the interalveolar wall. Preferential growth of parts or areas of an organ is a well-established phenomenon in organ development (e.g., heart development).

Through the combination of capillary merging and preferential growth of areas of the interalveolar wall containing a single capillary network, the maturation process of the parenchymal septa rapidly spreads throughout the lung.

GROWTH OF THE LUNG CAPILLARY NETWORK

Morphometric studies reveal that the human lung volume increases about 23 times between birth and adulthood (90, 91). The alveolar and capillary surface areas expand about 20 fold and the capillary volume 35 fold during the same period. From these figures we can deduce that the parenchymal capillary network must also multiply the number of its capillary segments to maintain an efficient gas exchange at the lung's inner surface during the growth of the organism.

It is generally assumed that capillary networks grow by sprouting. Some years ago, we proposed an alternative angiogenetic mechanism (21, 23). Investigating microvascular Mercox® casts of rat lungs to study capillary merging, we observed the frequent presence of tiny holes (diameter <1.5 m) in sheet-like areas of the capillary bed (Fig. 5.9). Dismissing the first idea that these were casting artefacts, we found the holes to be highly suggestive of newly formed intercapillary meshes. Evidently, the repeated insertion of new meshes into an existing capillary network would allow for its growth and expansion as well as its increase in complexity (Fig. 5.10). Sprouting would not be needed. This new mode of capillary network growth was termed *intussusceptional* or *intussusceptive microvascular growth* (IMG) by analogy to the

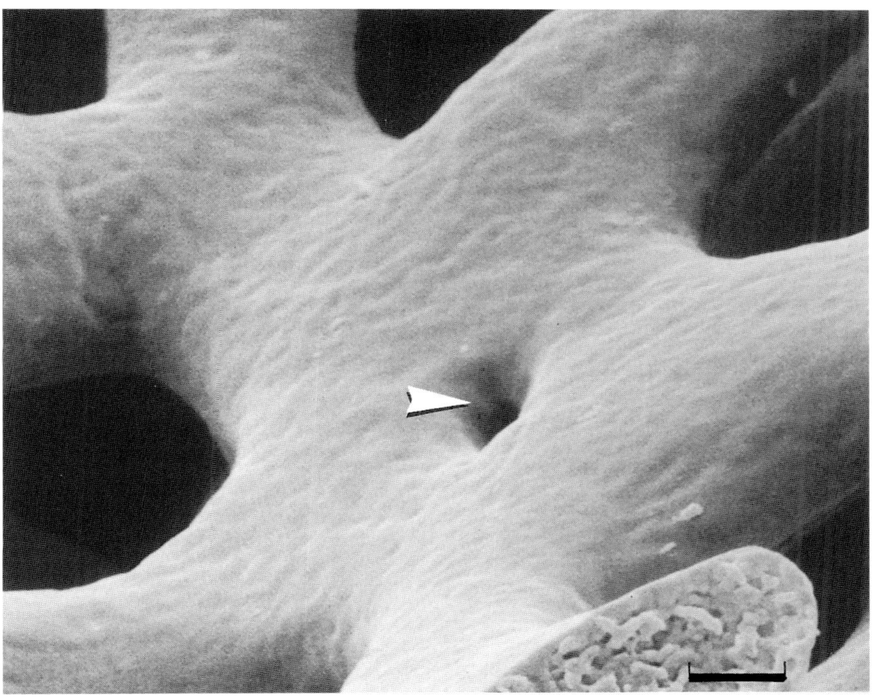

Fig. 5.9 Scanning electron micrograph of a Mercox® cast of rat lung vasculature. In addition to regular intercapillary meshes, there is a tiny transcapillary hole of <2 μm in diameter (*arrowhead*). This hole corresponds to a newly formed transcapillary tissue pillar (see Figs. 5.3 and 5.15). Bar = 2 μm.

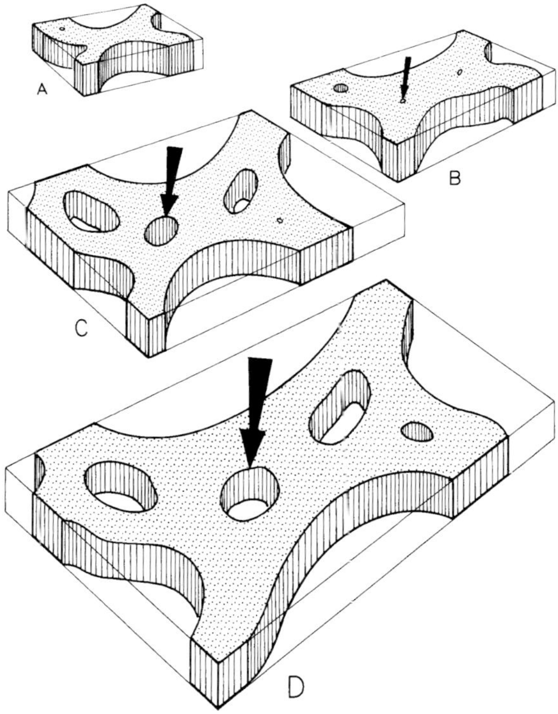

Fig. 5.10 Diagram showing how a capillary network can increase in volume, surface area, and in number of capillary segments or meshes by the insertion of new transluminal tissue pillars (*arrowheads*). [From Caduff et al. (23), with permission.]

growth process in cartilage. Intussusception is the deposition of new particles of formative material among those already present in a tissue or structure. Short (80) had already proposed in 1950 that the capillary network of interalveolar walls could grow by the addition of new meshes. He studied light-microsopic en face views of interaveolar septa in developing rabbit lungs.

By serial-sectioning lung tissue for electron microscopic investigation, the tissue structures correlating to the holes in the casts were found: transcapillary tissue posts or pillars <2.5 μm in diameter-[Fig. 5.3; (21)]. From analysis of the ultrastructure reflecting various stages of their formation, a first mode of pillar production was proposed (Fig. 5.11 A).

Fig. 5.11 (*Facing page*) Intussusceptive microvascular growth. Illustration of various modes of formation of transcapillary tissue pillars. The principle is based on the fusion of endothelial cell leaflets with formation of new intercellular junctions (*arrows*). (*A, B*) A cross-sectioned septum found in the lung; the transcapillary pillar is formed by perforation of a disk-like zone of contact between opposite capillary walls (*arrowheads*). The area is then invaded by connective tissue, in particular by cytoplasmic extensions of myofibroblasts (see Fig. 5.2). In *A*, the zone of contact is symmetrical, in *B*, one side

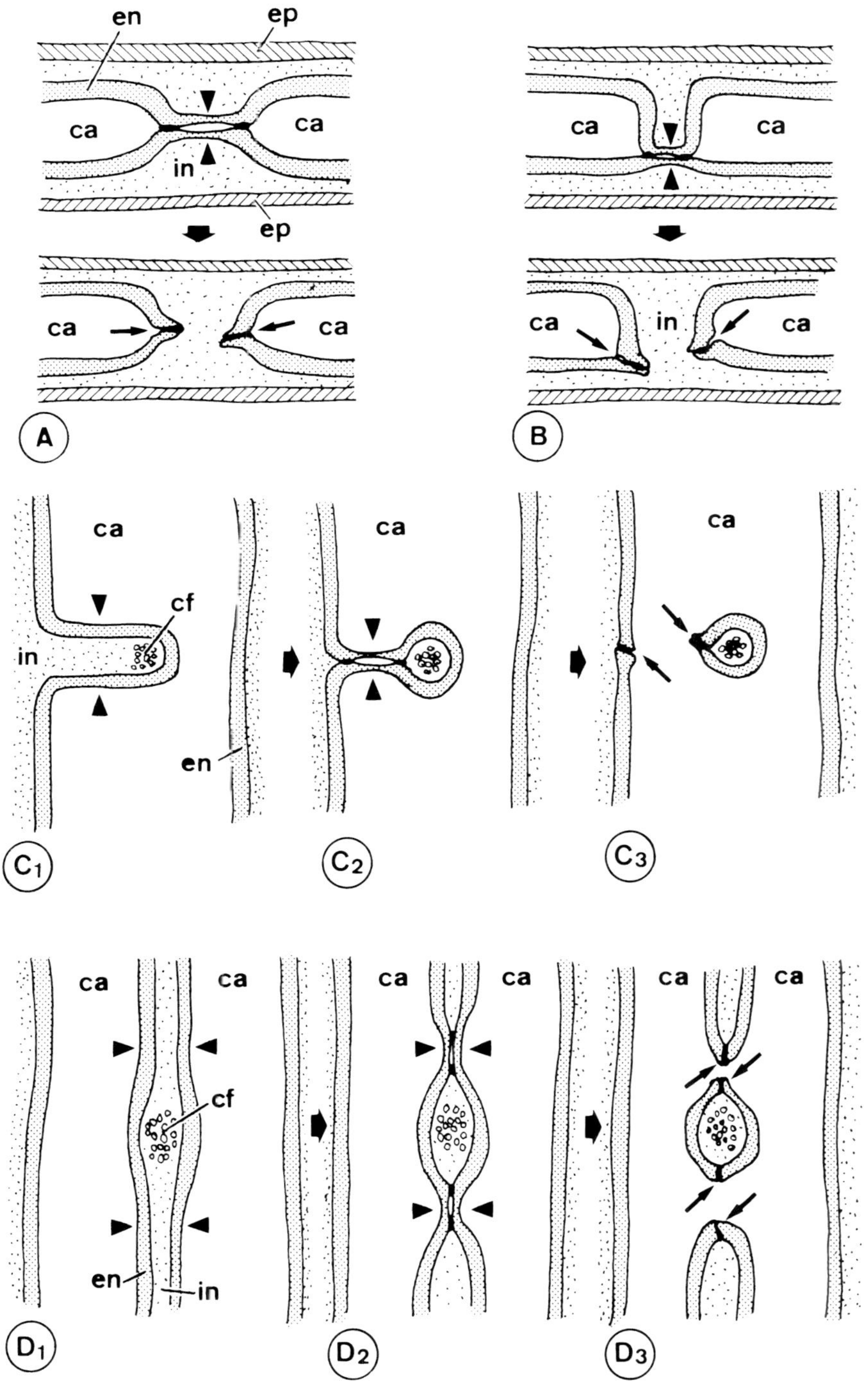

of the capillary wall forms a cone-like protrusion. *(C, D)* Longitudinally sectioned capillaries described in chorioallantoic membrane of chicken. *C1–C3* show intraluminal fold transformed into pillar (cross-sectioned) by perforation of meso-like structure (*arrowheads*). *D1–D3* illustrate intussusceptive microvascular growth by fusions between two adjacent capillaries running in parallel (*arrowheads*). *ca*, capillary lumen; *cf*, collagen fibrils; *en*, endothelium; *ep*, epithelial cover of septum; *in*, interstitium.

In addition, IMG was further documented in various species and organ systems, as well as in tumor growth (64–66, 89). Using the shell-free chicken culture technique (3), which allows observation of capillary flow for several hours, we were able to describe additional and alternative ways of pillar formation, which are summarized in figure 5.11 (67, 68).

The nonsprouting angiogenic mechanism of IMG seems to represent an important principle of capillary growth. It occurs not only in the lung but is widespread and may be a fundamental angiogenic process in vascularized organisms.

INTERFERENCE OF EXOGENOUS RISK FACTORS WITH POSTNATAL LUNG DEVELOPMENT AND GROWTH

The development of the organism is a continuous process with more or less well-defined periods for the development of specific organs and organ structures. Therefore, any exogenous agent with effects on cell division or cell differentiation reaching the organism can induce alterations in those parts of a system most actively involved in developmental steps. With regard to the lung, teratogenic factors (noxious chemicals, physical agents, bacteria and viruses, even untimely hormone applications) will affect mainly the nonparenchymal portions of the lung during the first third of gravidity and more electively, the pulmonary parenchyma during the last two-thirds.

It is beyond the scope of this chapter to review all the teratogenic accidents that can affect the lung during development. We shall concentrate here on the postnatal period in general and deal in particular with recent findings on the phase of alveolization that seems to be extremely susceptible to disturbances induced by environmental, chemical, and hormonal factors. Special attention will be given to the inhibitory effect of glucocorticoids on alveolar formation because it illustrates how the untimely surge of a hormone level in the blood can alter the genetic program.

General Considerations

In postnatal developmental disturbances the lung responds with structural alterations and/or growth retardation.

Food deficiency is a classic and obvious example of growth inhibition: functional and structural alterations of the lung parenchyma have been commonly described as a result of malnutrition (24, 63, 74). The experimental findings are not uniform, however, and therefore often difficult to interpret. Differences in the severity, timing, and duration of malnutrition as well as in diet composition prevent a clear analysis. The most common findings are a loss in tissue recoil and an enlargement of the terminal air spaces. As a consequence, the alveolar surface area is reduced. Wall rupture has been described, and the emphysema-like pattern has been termed "nutritional emphysema" (38, 39). The contradictory and conflicting findings reported in the literature have been carefully disentangled by Gaultier (28). Who distinguished between caloric deprivation and protein deprivation and whether experiments were performed in rats or guinea pigs, the two species most often used and which differ much in timing of alveolization. She concluded that lung growth and alveolar development was most altered when food reduction coincided with or occurred slightly prior to the period of alveolar formation. Kalenga et al., reported that feeding rats a low-protein diet during alveolar formation resulted in decreased lung growth, which was less reduced, however, than body growth, but produced no alterations in alveolar structure (35, 36). The same authors reported a remarkable catch-up growth of the lung upon refeeding.

Exposure of pregnant rats to *cigarette smoke* has negative effects on lung growth and alveolization in offspring. Similar findings have been reported with regard to maternal nicotine injections (45), which significantly reduced elastin synthesis and alveolar formation in neonatal rats.

Perinatal exposure to *hypoxia* in rats, even of very short duration, seems to inhibit lung septation (51, 52). On the other hand, exposure for 3 weeks starting after weaning resulted in higher gas-exchange surface area per 100 g body weight (5, 22).

Hyperoxia has long been known to be toxic for both the lung and nervous system when applied at higher concentrations and for longer periods of time. It is not surprising that it also influences or even damages the developing and growing lung, depending on the exposure concentration. At 40% it caused a significant decrease in lung size and morphometric lung parameters in rats exposed for 3 weeks at the age of 23 days (22). At 60% it led to parenchymal thickening and fibrosis (30) and also provoked an increase in insulin-like growth factor gene expression. At a concentration of 85%, O_2 was reported to induce an up-regulation of various growth factors and a proliferation of fibroblasts (13, 60). When exposure to high oxygen occured at birth, it reduced alveolar formation (71, 79).

Finally *low temperature* was reported to inhibit lung growth (77) in postnatal lambs.

Impaired Alveolization

In the 1980s Massaro and co-workers published findings that low-dose glucocorticoid injections to rats during the first 2 weeks of life inhibited or even abolished alveolization (49). These findings were subsequently confirmed by others (73) and further analyzed by Massaro and co-workers (9, 47). It was demonstrated that other factors, such as changes in the O_2 partial pressure of the inspired air (8, 27, 51, 52, 71, 79), thyroxine (48), and retinoic acid [see review by Massaro and Massaro; (50)] could influence alveolar formation negatively or positively even when applied briefly, but during a critical period. From a clinical point of view, glucocorticoid-induced inhibition of alveolization seems to be the most important observation of all of these findings. The phenomenon has been reported by several authors and it appears to be the best-investigated disturbance of alveolization thus far.

One daily injection of a very low dose of dexamethasone to rats from days 2 or 3 to the age of 2 weeks not only seriously inhibited lung parenchyma septation but induced also a rapid thinning of the intersaccular walls (47). This latter result led us to hypothesize that glucocorticoids did not inhibit lung septation directly, but could do so indirectly by inducing a precocious maturation of the capillary system. To provide evidence for this hypothesis (81), we treated rats with 0.1 μg dexamethasone phosphate (Decadron®) from postnatal days 2 to 15. The morphologic and morphometric analysis of their lungs at various time points revealed that alveolar formation was markedly impaired and that microvascular maturity of interalveolar septa was significantly increased in treated rats on days 10 and 13. Even on day 4, 2 days after treatment began it was possible to distinguish the treated lungs from controls by light microscopy: the inter-air-space walls of the treated lungs clearly appeared thinner. The amount of interstitial tissue in the saccular walls was significantly decreased in treated animals. In control animals this change normally occurs in the third week, when capillary maturation occurs. At day 60, the last time point investigated, Decadron-treated rats had emphysematous-looking lungs. These findings are in accord with the hypothesis that bulk alveolar formation is impaired by glucocorticoids, because they precociously induce capillary maturation. In other words, the larger the areas with mature intersaccular walls, the fewer alveoli can form.

Interestingly, glucocorticoid treatment does not inhibit the slow alveolization that occurs after weaning (7). This is in agreement with the concept that these alveoli form mainly at the lung periphery, at the border between the pleura and the perivascular and peribronchial connective sheaths, where there is no microvascular maturation.

Another observation was made at the age of 21 days, i.e., at about 1 week after Decadron withdrawal. The inter-air-space walls were suddenly thicker and the arithmetic mean thickness (a measure for tissue mass) was higher in experimental animals than in controls. Also, areas with a double capillary network were more prominent and lipid-containing interstitial fibroblasts (which had prematurely disappeared in treated animals) and low secondary septa reappeared. The entire pulmonary parenchyma appeared to have made a step backwards in development. This observed "rebound phenomenon" is in accord with observations made by other authors. Lung fibroblasts, whose activity had been depressed by glucocorticoid treatment, exhibited increased proliferative activity after the treatment ended which resulted in septal thickening (61). An analogous rebound effect was described by Bruce and co-workers (12) in developing rat lungs after exposure to 95% O_2 between days 4 and 14. O_2 exposure induced a marked depression in the level of tropoelastin mRNA as detected by in situ hybridization; these levels, however, peaked postexposure, whereas they were low in controls.

This phenomenon of reactive septal immaturity could account for a compensatory late round of alveolization described by Massaro and co-workers, who found that additional alveoli were formed between 14 and 60 days of age. Therefore, catch-up alveolization after glucocorticoid treatment could be achieved by two mechanisms: first, by increased septation of the lung periphery, and second, by a second round of alveolization as the result of a rebound reaction of the lung parenchyma toward immaturity. With the present state of knowledge, however, the mechanism for the latter phenomenon is hard to explain. Thus to summarize our findings, it is likely that glucocorticoids during the early postnatal period induce precocious maturation of the parenchymal capillary networks and, through this, partly prevent septation. Despite compensatory mechanisms in the lungs of treated animals, the full adult complement of alveoli can no longer be attained.

The author gratefully acknowledges the help of Mrs. B. Itten, L. Jeangros, and B. Krieger and Mr. K. Babl in preparing this manuscript and the figures. Research was supported by grants from the Swiss National Science Foundation (Nr. 31-45831.95) and from the Schweizerische and Bernische Krebsliga.

REFERENCES

1. Alescio, T. and A. Cassini. Induction in vitro of tracheal buds by pulmonary mesenchyme grafted on tracheal epithelium. *J. Exp. Zool.* 150: 83–94, 1962.
2. Angus, G.E. and W.M. Thurlbeck. Number of alveoli in the human lung. *J. Appl. Physiol.* 32: 483–485, 1972.
3. Auerbach, R., L. Kubai, D. Knighton, and J. Folkman. A simple procedure for the long-term cultivation of chicken embryos. *Dev. Biol.* 41: 391–394, 1974.
4. Bartels, H. Freeze-fracture demonstration of communicating junctions between interstitial cells of the pulmonary interalveolar septa. *Am. J. Anat.* 155: 125–129, 1979.
5. Bartlett, D.J. and J.E. Remmers. Effects of high altitude exposure on the lungs of young rats. *Respir. Physiol.* 13: 116–125, 1971.
6. Blanco, L.N. A model of postnatal formation of alveoli in rat lung. *J. Theor. Biol.* 157: 427–446, 1992.
7. Blanco, L. N. and L. Frank. The formation of alveoli in rat lung during the third and fourth postnatal weeks: effect of hyperoxia, dexamethasone, and deferoxamine. *Pediatr. Res.* 34: 334–340, 1993.
8. Blanco, L.N., D. Massaro, and G.D. Massaro. Alveolar size, number, and surface area: developmentally dependent response to 13% O_2. *Am. J. Physiol.* 261: 370–377, 1991.
9. Blanco, L.N., G.D. Massaro, and D. Massaro. Alveolar dimensions and number: developmental and hormonal regulation. *Am. J. Physiol.* 257: L240–L247, 1989.
10. Bluemink, J.G., P. van Maurik, and K.A. Lawson. Intimate cell contacts at the epithelial/mesenchymal interface in embryonic mouse lung. *J. Ultrastruct. Res.* 55: 257–270, 1976.
11. Boyden, E.A. Development and growth of the airways. In: *Lung Biology in Health and Disease. Development of the Lung,* edited by WA. Hodson. New York: Marcel Dekker, 1977, p. 3–35.
12. Bruce, M.C., E.N. Bruce, K. Janiga, and A. Chetty. Hyperoxic exposure of developing rat lung decreases tropoelastin mRNA levels that rebound postexposure. *Am. J. Physiol.* 265: L293–L300, 1993.
13. Buch, S., R.N.N. Han, J. Liu, A. Moore, J.D. Edelson, B.A. Freeman, M. Post, and A.K. Tanswell. Basic fibroblast growth factor and growth factor receptor gene expression in 85% O_2-exposed rat lung. *Am. J. Physiol.* 268: 455–464, 1995.
14. Bucher, U. and L. Reid. Development of the intrasegmental bronchial tree: the pattern of

branching and development of cartilage at various stages of intra-uterine life. *Thorax* 16: 207–218, 1961.

15. Buck, C.A., J.M. Edelman, C.E. Buck, G. Kennedy, and H.S. Baldwin. Expression patterns of adhesion receptors in the developing mouse lung: functional implications. *Cell Adhes. Commun.* 4: 69–87, 1996.
16. Burri, P.H. The postnatal growth of the rat lung. III. Morphology. *Anat. Rec.* 180: 77–98, 1974.
17. Burri, P.H. Development and growth of the human lung. In: *Handbook of physiology, section 3: The respiratory system. Circulation and nonrespiratory functions*, edited by A.P. Fishman and A.B. Fisher. *American Physiology Society* 1985, p. 1–46.
18. Burri, P.H. Development and regeneration of the human lung. In: *Pulmonary diseases and Disorders*, edited by A.P. Fishman. New York: McGraw Hill, 1988, p. 61–78.
19. Burri, P.H., J. Dbaly, and E.R. Weibel. The postnatal growth of the rat lung. I. Morphometry. *Anat. Rec.* 178: 711–730, 1974.
20. Burri, P.H. and M. Moschopulos. Structural analysis of fetal rat lung development. *Anat. Rec.* 234: 399–418, 1992.
21. Burri, P.H. and M.R. Tarek. A novel mechanism of capillary growth in the rat pulmonary microcirculation. *Anat. Rec.* 228: 35–45, 1990.
22. Burri, P.H. and E.R. Weibel. Morphometric estimation of pulmonary diffusion capacity. II. Effect of PO_2 on the growing lung. Adaptation of the growing rat lung to hypoxia and hyperoxia. *Respir. Physiol.* 11: 247–264, 1971.
23. Caduff, J.H., L.C. Fischer, and P.H. Burri. Scanning electron microscopic study of the developing microvasculature in the postnatal rat lung. *Anat. Rec.* 216: 154–164, 1986.
24. Das, R.M. The effects of intermittent starvation on lung development in suckling rats. *Am. J. Pathol.* 117: 326–332, 1984.
25. Davies, G. and L. Reid. Growth of the alveoli and pulmonary arteries in childhood. *Thorax* 25: 669–681, 1970.
26. Dubreuil, G., A. Lacoste, and R. Raymond. Observations sur le développement du poumon humain. *Bull. Histol. Tech. Microsc.* 13: 235–245, 1936.
27. Frank, L., and G.E. McLaughlin. Protection against acute and chronic hyperoxic inhibition of neonatal rat lung development with the 21-aminosteroid drug U74389F. *Pediatr. Res.* 33: 632–638, 1993.
28. Gaultier, C. Malnutrition and lung development. *Pediatr. Pulmonol.* 10: 278–286. 1991.
29. Griffin, M., R. Bhandari, G. Hamilton, Y C. Chan, and J.T. Powell. Alveolar type II cell-fibroblast interactions, synthesis and secretion of surfactant and type I collagen. *J. Cell Sci.* 105: 423–432, 1993.
30. Han, R.N.N., S. Buch, I. Tseu, J. Young, N.A. Christie, H. Fmdova, S.J. Lye, M. Post, and A.K. Tanswell. Changes in structure, mechanics, and insulin-like growth factor-related gene expression in the lungs of newborn rats exposed to air or 60% oxygen. *Pediatr. Res.* 39: 921–929, 1996.
31. Hislop, A. and L. Reid. Intra-pulmonary arterial development during fetal life-branching pattern and structure. *J. Anat.* 113: 35–48, 1972.
32. Hislop, A. and L. Reid. Growth and development of the respiratory system-anatomical development. In: *Scientific Foundations of Paediatrics*, edited by J.A. Davis and J. Dobbing. London: Heinemann, 1981, p. 390–432.
33. Ingbar, D.H., C.B. Weeks, M. Gilmore Hebert, E. Jacobsen, S. Duvick, R. Dowin, S.K. Savik, and J.D. Jamieson. Developmental regulation of Na, K-ATPase in rat lung. *Am. J. Physiol.* 270: L619–L629, 1996.

34. Junod, A.F. Metabolism of vasoactive agents in lung. *Am. Rev. Respir. Dis.* 115: 51S–57S, 1977.
35. Kalenga, M., S A. Tschanz, and P.H. Burri. Protein deficiency and the growing rat lung. I. Nutritional findings and related lung volumes. *Pediatr. Res.* 37: 783–788, 1995.
36. Kalenga, M., S.A. Tschanz, and P H. Burri. Protein deficiency and the growing rat lung. II. Morphometric analysis and morphology. *Pediatr. Res.* 37: 789–795, 1995.
37. Kapanci, Y., A. Assimacopoulos, C. Irle, A. Zwahlen, and G. Gabbiani. 'Contractile interstitial cells' in pulmonary alveolar septa: a possible regulator of ventilation/perfusion ratio? *J. Cell Biol.* 60: 375–392, 1974.
38. Karlinsky, J.B., R.H. Goldstein, B. Ojserkis, and G.L. Snider. Lung mechanics and connective tissue levels in starvation-induced emphysema in hamsters. *Am. J. Physiol.* 251: R282–R288, 1986.
39. Kerr, J.S., D.J. Riley, S. Lanza Jacoby, R.A. Berg, H.C. Spilker, S.Y. Yu, and N.H. Edelman. Nutritional emphysema in the rat. Influence of protein depletion and impaired lung growth. *Am. Rev. Respir. Dis.* 131: 644–650, 1985.
40. Kikkawa, Y., M. Kaibara, E.K. Motoyama, M.M. Orzalesi, and C.D. Cook. Morphologic development of fetal rabbit lung and its acceleration with cortisol. *Am. J. Pathol.* 64: 423–442, 1971.
41. Kitaoka, H., P.H. Burri, and E.R. Weibel. Development of the human fetal airway tree: analysis of the numerical density of airway endtips. *Anat. Rec.* 244: 207–213, 1996.
42. Kotas, R.V., P.M. Farrel, R.E. Ulane, and R.A. Chez. Fetal rhesus monkey lung development: lobar differences and discordances between stability and distensibility. *J. Appl. Physiol.* 43: 92–98, 1977.
43. Langston, C., K. Kida, M. Reed, and W.M. Thurlbeck. Human lung growth in late gestation and in the neonate. *Am. Rev. Respir. Dis.* 129: 607–613, 1984.
44. Luciano, L., E. Reale, and H. Ruska. Buerstenzellen im Alveolarepithel der Rattenlunge. *Z. Zellforsch.* 95: 198–201, 1969.
45. Maritz, G.S., K. M. Woolward, and G. du Toit. Maternal nicotine exposure during pregnancy and development of emphysema-like damage in the offspring. *S. Afr. Med. J.* 83: 195–198, 1993.
46. Mason, R.J., M.C. Williams, H.L. Moses, S. Mohla, and M.A. Berberich. Stem cells in lung development, disease, and therapy. *Am. J. Respir. Cell Mol. Biol.* 16: 355–363, 1997.
47. Massaro, D. and G.D. Massaro. Dexamethasone accelerates postnatal alveolar wall thinning and alters wall composition. *Am. J. Physiol.* 251: R218–R224, 1986.
48. Massaro, D., N. Teich, and G.D. Massaro. Postnatal development of pulmonary alveoli: modulation in rats by thyroid hormones. *Am. J. Physiol.* 250: R51–R55, 1986.
49. Massaro, D., N. Teich, S. Maxwell, G.D. Massaro, and P. Whitney. Postnatal development of alveoli. Regulation and evidence for a critical period in rats. *J. Clin. Invest.* 76: 1297–1305, 1985.
50. Massaro, G.D. and D. Massaro. Formation of pulmonary alveoli and gas-exchange surface area: quantitation and regulation. *Annu. Rev. Physiol.* 58: 73–92, 1996.
51. Massaro, G.D., J. Olivier, C. Dzikowski, and D. Massaro. Postnatal development of lung alveoli: suppression by 13% O_2 and a critical period. *Am. J. Physiol.* 258: L321–L327, 1990.
52. Massaro, G.D., J. Olivier, and D. Massaro. Short-term perinatal 10% O_2 alters postnatal development of lung alveoli. *Am. J. Physiol.* 257: L221–L225, 1989.
53. Matalon, S. Mechanisms and regulation of ion transport in adult mammalian alveolar type 2 pneumocytes. *Am. J. Physiol.* 260 *(Cell Physiol.* 29) : C727–C738, 1991.

54. McCormack, J., D.E. Crawley, and T.W. Evans. New perspectives in the pulmonary circulation and hypoxic pulmonary vasoconstriction. *Pulm. Pharmacol.* 6: 97–108, 1993.
55. McGowan, S.E. and J.S. Torday. The pulmonary lipofibroblast (lipid interstitial cell) and its contributions to alveolar development. *Annu. Rev. Physiol.* 59: 43–62, 1997.
56. Melnick, M., H.A. Choy, and T. Jaskoll. Glucocorticoids, tumor necrosis factor-alpha, and epidermal growth factor regulation of pulmonary morphogenesis: a multivariate in vitro analysis of their related actions. *Dev. Dyn.* 205: 365–378, 1996.
57. Mercurio, A.R. and J.A.G. Rhodin. An electron microscopic study on the type I pneumocyte in the cat: differentiation. *Am. J. Anat.* 146: 255–272, 1976.
58. Mercurio, A.R. and J.A.G. Rhodin. An electron microscopic study on the type I pneumocyte in the cat: pre-natal morphogenesis. *J. Morphol.* 156: 141–156, 1978.
59. Meyrick, B. and L. Reid. Ultrastructure of alveolar lining and its development. In: *Lung Biology in Health and Disease. Development of the Lung*, edited by W.A. Hodson. New York: Marcel Dekker, 1977, p. 135–214.
60. Moore, A.M., S. Buch, R.N.N. Han, B.A. Freeman, M. Post, and A.K. Tanswell. Altered expression of type 1 collagen, TGFb1 and related genes in rat lung exposed to 85% O_2. *Am. J. Physiol.* 268: 178–184, 1995.
61. Morishige, W.K. and N.S. Joun. Influence of glucocorticoids on postnatal lung development in the rat: possible modulation by thyroid hormone. *Endocrinology* 111: 1587–1594, 1982.
62. Moschopulos, M. and P.H. Burri. Morphometric analysis of fetal rat lung development. *Anat. Rec.* 237: 38–48, 1993.
63. Myers, B., M. Dubick, J.A. Last, and R.B. Rucker. Elastin synthesis during perinatal lung development in the rat. *Biochim. Biophys. Acta* 761: 17–22, 1983.
64. Nagy, J.A., E.S. Morgan, K.T. Herzberg, E.J. Manseau, A.M. Dvorak, and H.F. Dvorak. Pathogenesis of ascites tumor growth: angiogenesis, vascular remodeling, and stroma formation in the peritoneal lining. *Cancer Res.* 55: 376–385, 1995.
65. Patan, S., M.J. Alvarez, J.C. Schittny, and P.H. Burri. Intussusceptive microvascular growth: a common alternative to capillary sprouting. *Arch. Histol. Cytol.* 55: 65-75, 1992.
66. Patan, S., B. Haenni, and P.H. Burri. Evidence for intussusceptive capillary growth in the chicken chorio-allantoic membrane (CAM). *Anat. Embryol.* 187: 121–130, 1993.
67. Patan, S., B. Haenni, and P.H. Burri. Implementation of intussusceptive capillary growth in the chicken chorio-allantoic membrane (CAM): 1. Pillar formation by folding of the capillary wall. *Microvasc. Res.* 51: 80–98, 1996.
68. Patan, S., B. Haenni, and P.H. Burri. Implementation of intussusceptive microvascular growth in the chicken chorio-allantoic membrane (CAM): 2. Pillar formation by capillary fusion. *Microvasc. Res.* 53: 33–52, 1997.
69. Post, M. Tissue interactions. In: *The Lung: Scientific Foundations*, edited by R.G. Crystal, J.B. West, E.R. Weibel, and P.J. Barnes. Philadelphia: Lippincott-Raven, 1997, p. 1003–1011.
70. Pump, K.K. Distribution of bronchial arteries in the human lung. *Chest* 62: 447–451, 1972.
71. Randell, S.H., R.R. Mercer, and S.L. Young. Postnatal growth of pulmonary acini and alveoli in normal and oxygen-exposed rats studied by serial section reconstructions. *Am. J. Anat.* 186: 55–68, 1989.
72. Rannels, D.E., and S.R. Rannels. Influence of the extracellular matrix on type 2 cell differentiation. *Chest* 96: 165–173, 1989.

73. Sahebjami, H. and M. Domino. Effects of postnatal dexamethasone treatment on development of alveoli in adult rats. *Exp. Lung Res.* 15: 961–973, 1989.
74. Sahebjami, H., C.L. Vassallo, and J.A. Wirman. Lung mechanics and ultrastructure in prolonged starvation. *Am. Rev. Respir. Dis.* 117: 77–83, 1978.
75. Shannon, J.M. Induction of alveolar type 2 cell differentiation in fetal tracheal epithelium by grafted distal lung mesenchyme. *Dev. Biol.* 166: 600–614, 1994.
76. Spooner, B.S., and N.K. Wessells. Mammalian lung development: Interactions in primordium formation and bronchial morphogenesis. *J. Exp. Zool.* 175: 445–454, 1970.
77. Symonds, M.E., D.C. Andrews, D.S. Buss, L. Clarke, C J. Darby, P. Johnson, and M.A. Lomax. Environmental effects on thermoregulation and breathing patterns during early postnatal development in hand-reared lambs. *Exp. Physiol.* 80: 779–792, 1995.
78. Ten Have Opbroek, A.A.W. Immunological study of lung development in the mouse embryo.II. First appearance of the great alveolar cell, as shown by immunofluorescence microscopy. *Dev. Biol.* 69: 408–423, 1979.
79. Thibeault, D.W., B. Heimes, M. Rezaiekhaligh, and S. Mabry. Chronic modifications of lung and heart development in glucocorticoid-treated newborn rats exposed to hyperoxia or room air. *Pediatr. Pulmonol.* 16: 81–88, 1993.
80. Thurlbeck, W.M. Postnatal growth and development of the lung. *Am. Rev. Respir. Dis.* 111: 803–844, 1975.
81. Tschanz, S.A., B.M. Damke, and P.H. Burri. Influence of postnatally administered glucocorticoids on rat lung growth. *Biol. Neonate* 68: 229–245, 1995.
82. Verbeken, E.K., M. Cauberghs, and K.P. Van de Woestijne. Membranous bronchioles and connective tissue network of normal and emphysematous lungs. *J. Appl. Physiol.* 81: 2468–2480, 1996.
83. Wasowicz, M., S. Yokoyama, K. Kashima, and I. Nakayama. The connective tissue compartment in the terminal region of the developing rat lung. An ultrastructural study. *Acta Anat* 156: 268–282, 1996.
84. Weibel, E R. *Morphometry of the Human Lung*. Heidelberg: Springer-Verlag, 1963.
85. Weibel, E. R., and H. Bachofen. Structural design of alveolar septum and fluid exchange. In: *Pulmonary Edema*, edited by A. P. Fishman, and E.M. Renkin. Bethesda, MD: American Physiology Society, 1979, p. 1–20.
86. Weichselbaum, M., A.W. Everett, and M.P. Sparrow. Mapping the innervation of the bronchial tree in fetal and postnatal pig lung using antibodies to PGP 9.5 and SV 2. *Am. J. Respir. Cell Mol. Biol.* 1-9, 1996.
87. Weiss, M.J. and P.H. Burri. Formation of interalveolar pores in the rat lung. *Anat. Rec.* 244: 481–489, 1996.
88. Whitsett, J. A. and L. Zhou. Use of transgenic mice to study autocrine-paracrine signaling in lung morphogenesis and differentiation. *Clin. Perinatol.* 23: 753–769, 1996.
89. Wilting, J., B. Christ, M. Bokeloh, and H.A. Weich. In vivo effects of vascular endothelial growth factor on the chicken chorioallantoic membrane. *Cell Tissue Res.* 274: 163–172, 1993.
90. Zeltner, T.B., and P.H. Burri. The postnatal development and growth of the human lung. II.Morphology. *Respir. Physiol.* 67: 269–282, 1987.
91. Zeltner, T.B., J.H. Caduff, P. Gehr, J. Pfenninger, and P.H. Burri. The postnatal development and growth of the human lung. I. Morphometry. *Respir. Physiol.* 67: 247–267, 1987.
92. Zhou, L., L. Lim, R.H. Costa, and J.A. Whitsett. Thyroid transcription factor-1, hepatocyte nuclear factor-3β, surfactant protein B, C, and Clara cell secretory protein in developing mouse lung. *J. Histochem. Cytochem.* 44: 1183–1193, 1996.

chapter 6

DEVELOPMENT OF THE PULMONARY VASCULATURE

Nicholas W. Morrell, Mary C. M. Weiser, and Kurt R. Stenmark

The cardiovascular system is the first organ system that forms during embryonic development. The primitive blood vessels must be in place to accommodate the cardiac output of the fetal heart which begins to beat as early as the 14th day of gestation in humans. Since the endothelial cell defines the lumen of the developing vasculature, it can be said to be one of the first cells in the organism to acquire a specialized function. The continued growth of endothelial tubes is necessitated by the nutritional and respiratory demands of the embryonic tissues beyond the reach of simple diffusion. Thus the spatial pattern of the developing vasculature is defined initially by the endothelial tubes and appears to be under strict developmental control. The continued growth of the endothelial tubes during organ morphogenesis is critical for the normal development of that organ. Development of larger blood vessels (i.e. arteries, arterioles, venules, and veins) from these initial vessels involves recruitment of smooth muscle cell (SMC) precursor cells into the region surrounding the endothelial tubes with subsequent morphogenesis of the appropriate blood vessel. This process requires that cells in the developing vessel, committed to becoming SMC, acquire specific functions and properties that distinguish them from other cell types. In addition, these cells must function to control blood flow while also participating in the process forming a complex vascular structure. Thus dramatic changes in cellular (SMC) proliferation, matrix production, and contractile protein expression take place over the course of vascular development. The SMC in the adult vessel wall perform mostly contractile functions but must also retain the capability of re-expressing certain characteristics of earlier development (migration/proliferation and matrix production) in response to injury.

Our knowledge of the events controlling the early formation and differentiation of the pulmonary vasculature remains rudimentary. Therefore, much of the following description of factors involved in early morphogenesis has been extrapolated from what is known regarding the formation of the vasculature in other organs. The specialized nature of the pulmonary endothelium, in particular, and the pulmonary vasculature, in general, requires that further work be directed toward understanding factors specific to the pulmonary circulation.

DEVELOPMENT OF THE PULMONARY ENDOTHELIUM

Early Origins of the Endothelium

During a process called *gastrulation* in the early embryo, mesodermal cells derived from the embryonic epithelium migrate throughout the extraembryonic membranes and the embryo itself (9). Within the embryo, progenitor endothelial cells, or angioblasts, differentiate within the mesoderm (150). Initially, angioblasts do not form a lumen and display none of the characteristic markers of mature endothelium (see below). They then either migrate and fuse with other angioblasts or capillaries, or they form a vessel in situ (36). Vascularization of individual organ rudiments may take place by the ingrowth of capillaries from the pre-existing embryonic network (a process known as *angiogenesis*), or by the differentiation of angioblasts from within the mesoderm of the developing organ (known as *vasculogenesis*). The relative contribution of these two processes to the vascularization of a particular organ varies. Vasculogenesis predominates in organs of endodermal origin, e.g., lung, pancreas, and spleen (151, 163), whereas angiogenesis prevails in organs of ectodermal or mesenchymal origin e.g., kidney and brain (168). During in situ vasculogenesis in the coronary vessels, endothelial precursors proliferate to form clones of endothelial cells which fuse to form capillary channels (134). The consequence of this process, if it is also true of the lung vasculature, is that the endothelium has a polyclonal origin, which may partly explain endothelial heterogeneity in the adult lung.

These primitive capillary plexuses are extensively remodeled by the processes of endothelial migration, proliferation, and apoptosis, leading to vascular growth, fusion, and regression, prior to assuming their adult distribution. Many of the embryonic vessels formed are ultimately redundant and disappear (161). The highly migratory and invasive nature of the embryonic endothelial cell contrasts with its quiescent nature in the adult. It is likely that with the onset of flow in larger vessels, endothelial cells are subjected to mechanical stresses that will play some part in vessel development and remodeling. However, understanding of these processes is at an early stage.

Structural Morphogenesis of the Pulmonary Circulation

The most proximal part of the pulmonary circulation, the pulmonary trunk, is derived from the truncus arteriosus, which becomes divided into the aorta and pulmonary trunk by 8 weeks of gestation in humans by growth of the spiral aorticopulmonary septum (19). The pulmonary trunk connects to the pulmonary arch arteries, which are derived from the sixth branchial arch arteries, the most caudal of the branchial arch arteries (37), by 7 weeks of gestation in humans. There is no consensus as to the mode of development of the sixth branchial arch artery, but recent reappraisal suggests that these pulmonary arch arteries originate from a strand of endothelial precursors that connect the ventral wall of the dorsal aortae to the pulmonary trunk (45, 47). These strands become lumenized, initially at the sites of connection with pulmonary trunk and dorsal aortae, then in between (46). The origin of the intrapulmonary arteries has been variously described by early investigators as endothelial sprouts from either the aortic sac (37) or from the dorsal aortae (95), or as originating from a network of capillaries around the foregut (25, 192). The latter observation comes closest to the results of more recent studies that utilized a monoclonal antibody (aMB1) specific for endothelial cells and their precursors (46). These recent studies suggest that the pulmonary artery and vein develop in situ within the splanchnic mesoderm surrounding the foregut. This splanchnic plexus of vessels then connects up to pre-existing vessels. Thus it is now generally believed that the distal pulmonary arteries and veins, and alveolar capillaries, are derived from the splanchnic plexus, which arises by in situ vasculogenesis within the mesenchyme surrounding the primordial lung bud, rather than by ingrowth of existing vessels (45c, 151, 186). However, angiogenesis may also be involved in the formation of more proximal vessels (186), and it seems likely that blood vessels grow through sprouting of the pre-existing vascular bed during continued lung growth, especially during the process of alveolarization.

The ductus arteriosus is also formed from the left sixth branchial arch (37). The pulmonary veins drain into the systemic venous system until day 28 to 30 of gestation, when they join the proximal pulmonary vein and left atrium (29). The bronchial arteries, which supply systemic arterial blood to the walls of larger bronchi and pulmonary arteries, also form in situ from the expanded splanchnic plexus (46). During two subsequent stages of development, the splanchnic plexus is transiently connected to systemic arteries and veins. During the second of these connections the bronchial arteries and veins are formed (46), by 12 weeks of gestation in humans (20).

Thus, at the end of 16 weeks of gestation in humans, all preacinar bronchi are in place (26) and are accompanied by the pulmonary and bronchial arteries (91). However, although the conducting airways and arteries are formed by the end of this so-called pseudoglandular stage (5–17 weeks) of lung development, the development of the gas-exchanging surface of the lung has just begun. The canalicular stage (17–26 weeks) encompasses the early development of the pulmonary parenchyma during which there is a great increase in the number of lung capillaries (28). The capillaries begin to arrange themselves around the air spaces and come into close apposition with the overlying cuboidal epithelium. At sites of apposition, thinning of the epithelium occurs to form what will be the first air–blood barrier portions. During the saccular stage (24th week to birth) the airways end in clusters of thin-walled saccules, and by term have formed the last generations of airways, the alveolar ducts. Capillaries form a bilayer within the relatively broad and cellular intersaccular septa at this stage. The period of alveolarization is largely a postnatal phenomenon, with more than 90% of all alveoli being formed after birth in humans. During the period of alveolarization the initially thick interalveolar septa are attenuated and the double capillary layer fuses to a single layer to assume the adult form (28). It is possible that the apposition of air spaces to capillaries may play a role in quiescing the extensive capillary remodeling, since alveolar type II epithelial cells secrete a factor that prevents apoptosis in endothelial cells (215).

Endothelial Cell Heterogeneity

It is now well established that different endothelial phenotypes exist in the adult systemic and pulmonary circulations (114, 203, 220). Heterogeneity exists between endothelium of different organs, between endothelial cells from large and small vessels within the same organ (114), and between endothelial cells in the same vascular region (43, 203). However, the embryonic origin of these diverse phenotypes remains unknown. In particular, it is not clear whether these phenotypes originate from separate endothelial precursors or represent phenotypic modulation of cells from the same embryonic origin. These mechanisms are not mutually exclusive and it is likely that both mechanisms play a role in determining the phenotype of an endothelial cell in a particular location in a given organ. Thus, in the coronary circulation the endothelium appears to have a polyclonal origin, and vessels form by the coalescence of discontinuous colonies (134). On the other hand, endothelial cells tend to dedifferentiate in culture and endothelial phenotype can be influenced by extracellular matrix constituents and by co-culture with other cells derived from the vascular wall, for example, pericytes (5).

Mechanisms Controlling Angiogenesis and Vasculogenesis

Primarily because of studies in tumor angiogenesis, the mechanisms contributing to capillary blood vessel growth are becoming increasingly understood. Two areas require special mention: (*1*) cell–extracellular matrix and cell–cell interactions and (*2*) growth factors. Shown in Table 6.1 are some of the molecular factors demonstrated to be of importance in vascular growth, these are discussed below.

Cell–Extracellular Matrix Interactions

The extracellular matrix, composed of collagens, glycoproteins, and proteoglycans, plays a central role in morphogenesis. In the process of angiogenesis, extracellular matrix may regulate vascular growth and orientation, since extracellular matrix

Table 6.1 Molecular Factors Likely to be Involved at Different Stages of Blood Vessel Formation

Molecules	*Localization*
Mesoderm formation	
VEGFR-2	Mesodermal cells
ets-1	Mesodermal cells
Fibronectin	Extracellular matrix
Aggregation of angioblasts	
VEGFR-2	Angioblasts
VEGFR-1	Angioblasts
VE-cadherin	Angioblasts
tie-2 / tek	Angioblasts
ets-1	Angioblasts
PECAM-1	Angioblasts
Fibronectin	Extracellular matrix
VEGF	Endoderm
Endothelial differentiation and formation of primary capillary plexus	
VEGFR-2	Endothelial cells
VEGFR-1	Endothelial cells
VE-cadherin	Endothelial cells
tie-2 / tek	Endothelial cells
tie-1	Endothelial cells
E-selectin	Endothelial cells
ets-1	Endothelial cells
PECAM-1	Endothelial cells
Integrins (e.g., $\alpha5\ \beta_3$)	Endothelial cells
Fibronectin	Extracellular matrix
Laminin	Extracellular matrix
Collagen IV	Extracellular matrix
VEGF	Endoderm
Smooth muscle cell recruitment and differentiation	
tie-2	Endothelial cells
PDGF-BB	Endothelial cells
PDGF-AA	Endothelial cells
HB-EGF	Endothelial cells
bFGF	Endothelial cells
Thromboxane A2	Endothelial cells
Angiotensin II	Endothelial cells
Endothelin	Endothelial cells
Leukotrienes	Endothelial cells
Substance P	Endothelial cells
Serotonin	Endothelial cells
Angiopoietin	Mesenchyme
TGF-β	Mesenchyme
Laminin	Basement membrane
Type IV collagen	Basement membrane
Perlecan	Basement membrane
Heperan sulphates	Basement membrane

components induce and maintain differentiation of endothelial cells, and modulate their response to angiogenic growth factors and inhibitors (79, 129). In the adult and fetus, the ablumenal surface of endothelial cells is in contact with basement membrane. The endothelial basement membrane is morphologically similar to that of other cells and contains several typical basement membrane components, such as laminin, type IV collagen, and basement membrane proteoglycan. It is believed that the basement membrane is produced by endothelial cells, maintains the polarity of these cells, and sustains their well-differentiated state.

Examination of the distribution of extracellular matrix components during differentiation of vessels in the chick chorioallantoic membrane (8) demonstrated a developmentally regulated pattern of expression of fibronectin, laminin, and type IV collagen. Fibronectin (MW 440 kDa), which binds to cells via integrin receptors, appears transiently in the capillary basement membranes at very early stages of vessel formation (8), preceding by 2 days the appearance of an ultrastructurally identifiable basal lamina. It is suggested, therefore, that fibronectin plays a role in the early aggregation of mesenchymal cells to form capillary tubes. Fibronectin is also expressed in the endothelial basement membrane during the angiogenic vascularization of the brain (163), it appears to promote migration and proliferation (96, 207), and it prevents apoptosis (224) of endothelial cells. In support of these roles, mice embryos lacking the fibronectin gene fail to develop a normal vasculature (70) and die in utero.

Laminin, a large noncollagenous glycoprotein (MW 800 kDa) consisting of at least three separate polypeptide chains (A, B1, and B2) held together by disulfide bonds (107), has been shown to promote cell attachment, migration, differentiation, and cell growth (81). During vasculogenesis and angiogenesis in the embryo, expression of laminin in the endothelial basement membrane is delayed compared with fibronectin; laminin probably has a role in early endothelial maturation (8, 163). Furthermore, laminin appears to be essential to the early differentiation on reconstituted basement membrane proteins of endothelial cells into tubular structures (113). Attachment of laminin to endothelial cells is mediated by the binding of an RGD peptide–containing sequence in the A chain of laminin to a cell-surface integrin receptor, while a YIGSR peptide site in the B1 chain induces cell–cell interactions and the resulting tube formation (82). In addition, microvascular endothelial cells have been shown to grow more rapidly on laminin than on fibronectin, or on collagens type I, III, or IV although large vessel endothelial cells may have different requirements (60).

Type IV collagen (MW 540 kDa) is a triple helical molecule arranged in a highly cross-linked network. It is the major structural component of the mature basement membrane and binds the other components. Collagen IV has been shown to promote cell attachment and differentiation primarily through a specific family of cell-surface integrin receptors (167). Type IV collagen appears later than fibronectin and laminin in the basement membrane during angiogenesis (8, 60) and its appearance coincides with a reduction in endothelial cell division. In cell culture, endothelial cells grown on substrata containing the basement membrane collagens, types IV and V, tend more readily to form tube-like structures and to proliferate less rapidly than cells grown on substrata of the interstitial collagens, types I and III (129). Furthermore, poorly differentiated, proliferating endothelial cells express predominantly type I and III collagens and form occasional tube-like structures only after prolonged periods in culture. These tube-like structures are associated with endothelial expression of types IV and V collagen and laminin (128). These findings are consistent with a role for basement membrane collagens type IV and V in stabilizing the structure of newly formed vessel walls, perhaps by binding cells to the extracellular matrix and maintaining endothelial differentiation. Other components of the basement membrane include heparan sulfate proteoglycan (750 kDa) and the glycoprotein entactin (MW 150 kDa). The roles of these molecules in angiogenesis remains to be elucidated.

As would be expected from the demonstration that all cell:matrix interactions are crucial during angiogenesis, integrins have also been critically linked to vascular development. The cell surface receptor for fibronectin, von Willebrand factor, and fibrin is the integrin $\alpha v\beta 3$. This integrin receptor initiates a calcium-dependent signaling pathway leading to endothelial cell migration and is expressed during angiogenesis and in wound granulation tissue but not in normal skin (24). Antibodies to $\alpha v\beta 3$ integrin were found to block angiogenesis in the chick chorioallantoic membrane and blocked angiogenesis induced by tumor neurosa's factor (TNF)α or basic fibroblast growth factor (bFGF) (24). Another integrin, the $\alpha V\beta 5$ receptor, has also recently been implicated in the angiogenic process (64a). Endothelial cells in ocular tissue from patients with proliferative diabetic retinopathy demonstrate increased expression of $\alpha V\beta 5$. Increasingly, VEGF-induced angiogenesis was inhibited by $\alpha V\beta 5$ mAbs but not $\alpha V\beta 3$ mAbs, while bFGF-induced angiogenesis was blocked by anti- $\alpha V\beta 3$ mAbs but not $\alpha V\beta 5$ mAbs (64b).

Cell-Cell Interactions

Angiogenesis may ultimately depend on the ability of endothelial cells to sever their normal cell–cell attachments, to migrate along or through extracellular matrix, and then to reform cell–cell attachments to form new capillaries. In the early stages of vascular development, interactions between endothelial cells and extracellular matrix may be dominant. During later stages, adhesive interactions between endothelial cells appear necessary to promote organization and to stabilize the vascular tubes.

Small cell adhesion molecules have also been implicated in capillary morphogenesis. E-selectin is expressed by bovine capillary endothelial cells (144). Antibodies to E-selectin prevents the formation of capillary tubes in culture. The cell surface ligand involved in binding E-selectin contains sialyl Lewis-X and/or sialyl Lewis A, since antibodies to these carbohydrate epitopes compete with E-selectin and inhibit tube formation (144). Furthermore, during vasculogenesis in the chick lung, alpha 4 integrin and VCAM-1 are expressed by mesenchymal precursors of vascular endothelium and smooth muscle (185).

Platelet endothelial cell adhesion molecule-1 (PECAM/CD31) is a member of the immunoglobulin superfamily that concentrates at intercellular junctions of endothelial cells (138a), but is also found on platelets and leukocytes. An important characteristic of PECAM-1 is its ability to mediate cell adhesion through multiple ligand interactions. It is able to interact with both itself or with a number of non-PECAM-1 molecules including αVβ3, CD38, and an unidentified proteoglycan. Engagement of surface PECAM-1 may transduce intracellular signals that activate the function of integrins (45a). Recent studies demonstrating that anti-PECAM-1 antibodies block cytokine-induced rat corneal neovascularization and vascular ingrowth into implanted gels in mice (45b) strong suggesting an important role for PECAM-1 in angiogenesis.

Growth Factors

The concept that soluble factors can promote angiogenesis was first realized from studies of tumor-induced angiogenesis (83). Since then, a variety of soluble polypeptides have been described that promote angiogenesis. Most mitogens for endothelium have turned out to belong to a large family of molecules called *fibroblast growth factors* (FGFs) or *heparin binding growth factors* (HBGFs) (27, 58).

Factors involved in early endothelial growth and differentiation are now being identified. In amphibians, FGF-like factors are known to be involved in the induction of primitive mesoderm, from which endothelial cells ultimately differentiate (190). In addition, endothelial cell differentiation and formation of vascular structures in avian embryos can be induced in vitro by incubation of pluripotent embryonic cells with basic or acidic FGF (56), but not with other growth factors such as transforming growth factor (TGF)-β, TGF-α, and epidermal growth factor (EGF). In fact TGF-β1 may be involved in the regression of endothelial tubes (117). Moreover, expression of dominant-negative mutants of the FGF receptor in amphibians inhibits vasculogenic mesoderm induction and endothelial cell differentiation (4). Basic (b) and acidic (a) FGFs appear to be expressed transiently in the fetal rat lung in both epithelial and mesenchymal cells (67) and bound to the extracellular matrix (77). Messenger RNA for FGF receptors is expressed during early stages of lung development in the mouse (152, 153) but at much lower levels in the older fetus and neonate. In situ hybridization studies localized the FGF receptor 1 (FGFR1) to the lung mesenchyme, whereas the FGFR2 was expressed mainly in lung epithelium (152, 153). On the basis of these findings it is possible to suggest a role for FGFs mediated by the FGFR1 in continued lung vessel growth or differentiation. This role may be in growth and differentiation of medial and adventitial layers, rather than the endothelium. It has been reported that late-gestation fetal lung small-vessel endothelial cells do synthesize DNA in response to endogenous FGFs, and neutralizing antibodies to bFGF do reduce bFGF-induced DNA synthesis (199). However, there are doubts for such a role in embryonic angiogenesis per se. First, there is no good correlation between the temporal and spatial expression of aFGF or bFGF mRNA and blood vessel growth during brain angiogenesis (172). Second, there is no evidence that FGF receptors are expressed by endothelial cells in vivo. Thus, despite the abundance of literature relating to the angiogenic properties of the FGFs (65), it is not known how this family of growth factors contributes specifically to lung vascular formation and differentiation.

Although the platelet-derived growth factors (PDGF) are recognized as major mitogens for mesenchymal cells, evidence for a role in embryonic angiogenesis has been scant until recently. In situ hybridization studies of human placenta have shown that most capillary endothelial cells co-express the PDGF-B and PDGF β-receptor genes (92). This observation indicates that PDGF-B may participate in placental angiogenesis by forming autostimulatory loops in capillary endothelial cells to promote cell proliferation. More recently, it has been demonstrated that intraembryonic small vessels of the mouse also express the PDGF β-receptor (188).

Vascular endothelial growth factor (VEGF) was first described as a molecule able to promote vascular permeability, hence the alternative name of vascular permeability factor (VPF), and was subsequently shown to be angiogenic (54). This growth factor is expressed early by the embryonic endoderm (23). The underlying mesoderm expresses the VEGF receptor-2 (VEGFR-2), which is one of a family of tyrosine kinase receptors (also known as flk-1 in the mouse or KDR in human) and is the first molecule known to be expressed by the population of mesodermal cells that subsequently give rise to angioblasts (55, 219). As well as being present at sites of vasculogenesis, VEGF and flk-1 are detected in the blood vessels of all highly vascularized tissues during development, including lung (135, 219). The expression of VEGF by the endoderm and flk-1 by the underlying mesoderm suggests a paracrine relationship between the germ layers. VEGFR-1 (also known as flt) is also expressed in the mesoderm at an early stage (23). Clearly, the presence of the flt (152) and flk-1 (135) receptors specifically confined to endothelial cells suggests an important role for their ligand, VEGF, in vasculogenesis and angiogenesis. Indeed, injection of exogenous VEGF into quail embryos profoundly alters vascular development with inappropriate neovascularization and excessive fusion of vessels (48). In addition, mouse embryos homozygous for a targeted mutation in the flt-1 locus assemble endothelial cells into abnormal vascular channels and die in utero (59).

In the developing lung, VEGF expression is confined mainly to the bronchial epithelium (187, 197). However, the receptors for VEGF, flt, and flk-1 are found only on endothelial cells (142,162). It seems possible that this arrangement of receptor and ligand may guide the spatial differentiation of endothelial tubes during lung morphogenesis, perhaps by chemotaxis of endothelial precursors (55).

Another family of receptor tyrosine kinases (RTK) recently shown to be important in vascular development are tek, and tie. Like flt and flk-1, the expression of these RTKs is almost exclusively restricted to the endothelial cell lineage (50, 51, 52, 55, 170, 172). Messenger RNAs for flk-1, tek, and tie are detected sequentially at one- half-day intervals starting at embryonic day 7 in the mouse, suggesting a unique role for each of the RTKs during vascularization of the mouse embryo (49). All three receptors are expressed at low levels in the adult (52, 110, 219) but flk-1 and tie expression are up-regulated with induction of angiogenesis (110, 174). Homozygous tek null embryos (embryonic lethal) are able to initiate a properly patterned vasculature, but they have signs of vascular hemorrhaging and considerably fewer endothelial cells than their normal littermates (51). Thus, these experiments suggest that tek may play a critical role in endothelial proliferation and/or differentiation. Of the RTKs only tie expression has been studied in any detail in the developing lung vasculature (110, 172). In the 12th day mouse lung tie expression is localized to capillary structures and the endothelium of large vessels. Unlike other organs where down-regulation of tie occurs, the lung capillaries continue to express tie abundantly in the adult (110). The first known ligand for tie, angiopoeitin-1, has recently been described and this receptor-ligand loop has been shown to be important in accumulation of SMCs around the developing vessel wall (see below). It is likely that the investigation of signal transduction via this receptor tyrosine kinase family will lead to a better understanding of the molecular mechanisms of blood vessel formation.

Anti-Angiogenic Factors

Current evidence supports the idea that angiogenes is ultimately regulated by a balance between angiogenic stimulators and anti-angiogenic factors (86a). Several anti-angiogenic factors have recently been described. One, angiopoitin 2, is a protein approximately 60% homologous to Ang 1 that also binds with high affinity to Tie 2. However, in contrast to Ang 1, Ang 2 binding does not trigger Tie 2 phosphorylation. In fact, increasing concentrations of Ang 2 substantially blocks Ang 1 activity suggesting that Ang 2 may be an endogenous inhibitor of Ang 1. Consistent with this is the finding that transgenic mice overexpressing Ang 2 have a phenotype similar to mice deficient in Ang 1 (129a).

Some of the most potent inhibitors of angiogenesis are internal fragments of extracellular matrix proteins that themselves are derived from larger proteins. Much attention has focused on angiostatin and endostatin (86b, 171a). Angiostatin is a degradation product of plasminogen A number of metaloproteinases have been reported to release angiostatin from plasminogen including stromelysin-1 (MMP-3, human matrilysin (MMP-7), and human neutrophil gelatinase B (MMP-9) (151a). Endostatin is an internal fragment of collagen XVII, an unusual collagen that localizes to perivascular basement membranes (146a). Both have been shown to inhibit endothelial cell proliferation in vitro and to inhibit tumor growth and angiogenesis (34a, 146a).

Endothelial Cell Differentiation: Expression of Endothelial Antigens

Although in avians a number of antigens have been identified that appear to be specific for endothelial cells and their precursors, the lack of similar antigens in mammals has hampered attempts to track the fate of endothelial precursors during development. Recently, however, it was reported that an antigen designated CD34 is expressed by vascular endothelium in adult mice and on hemopoietic cells and blood vessels during development (222).

The cellular adhesion molecules responsible for leukocyte recruitment, ICAM-1 and VCAM, are expressed and are further inducible by lipopolysaccharide at an early stage of murine embryonic development (90).

DEVELOPMENT OF PULMONARY ARTERIAL SMOOTH MUSCLE

Origins of Smooth Muscle Cells in Pulmonary Vasculature

The blood vessel initially consists of a single layer of endothelial cells embedded in mesoderm and a scaffolding of extracellular matrix. Development of larger blood vessels (i.e., arteries and veins) from these initial vessels involves recruitment of SMC precursor cells into the region with subsequent proliferation and then differentiation into mature SMC. Morphological studies have shown that during vasculogenesis, "putative" smooth muscle precursor cells appear at stage 11 (day 2) in the developing chick embryo as one to two layers of relatively undifferentiated mesenchymal cells that surround the developing endothelial cells of forming vessels (148, 159). By stage 19 (at 72 h), the cells that surround the endothelial cell layer are recognizably different from undifferentiated mesenchyme but are clearly not mature smooth muscle cells in that they lack basement membranes and attachment bodies. However, the cells have abundant thin filaments and may already possess contractile activity (159). After stage 22 (3.5 days) there is continuous accumulation of smooth muscle and veins and arteries become distinguishable.

Until very recently, the mechanisms involved in the recruitment and differentiation of mesenchymal cells to SMC or pericytes, a crucial step in vessel assembly, has been unclear. However, recent observations first describing the TIE2 receptor on endothelial cells (171) and subsequently the discovery of angiopoietin-1, the first described TIE2 receptor ligand produced by mesenchymal cells, suggest a receptor-ligand loop that is crucial to early vessel assembly (42, 196). In a model proposed by Folkman and D'Amore, angiopoietin-1, produced by undifferentiated mesenchymal cells, activates the TIE2 receptor on endothelial cells, which in turn leads to the production and/or release of a recruiting signal for mesenchymal cells [Fig. 6.1A; (57)]. In support of this hypothesis is the observation that the absence of angiopoetin-1 results in vessels that do not properly recruit supporting cells to the vascular wall. Unlike VEGF, angiopoietin-1 is neither a mitogen for endothelium, nor does it induce tube formation. Most data indicate that the recruiting signal produced by endothelial cells in response to angiopoetin-1 activation involves PDGF-BB, at least in the case of the pericyte. At the level of the SMC, this recruitment may also involve PDGF-AA or HB-EGF (heparin-binding epidermal growth factor), another SMC chemotactic factor and mitogen. Evidence supporting the role of PDGF-BB is derived primarily from studies in mice where PDGF-B ligand null mice die perinatally from hemorrhage and have no pericytes in the kidney vasculature (122) or throughout the microvasculature. Once mesenchymal cells arrive and contact endothelium, TGF-β may be activated [Fig. 6.1B; (5)]. The TGF-β may then induce differentiation of the mesenchymal cells into pericytes and SMC inhibit endothelial cell proliferation, and stimulate matrix deposition. Experiments have shown that 50% of TGF-β null mice die from a severe deficit in yolk-sac vasculogenesis, which is thought to result from improper interactions between epithelial and mesenchymal cells (47a). It is also important to note that incorporation of committed SMC around the endothelial

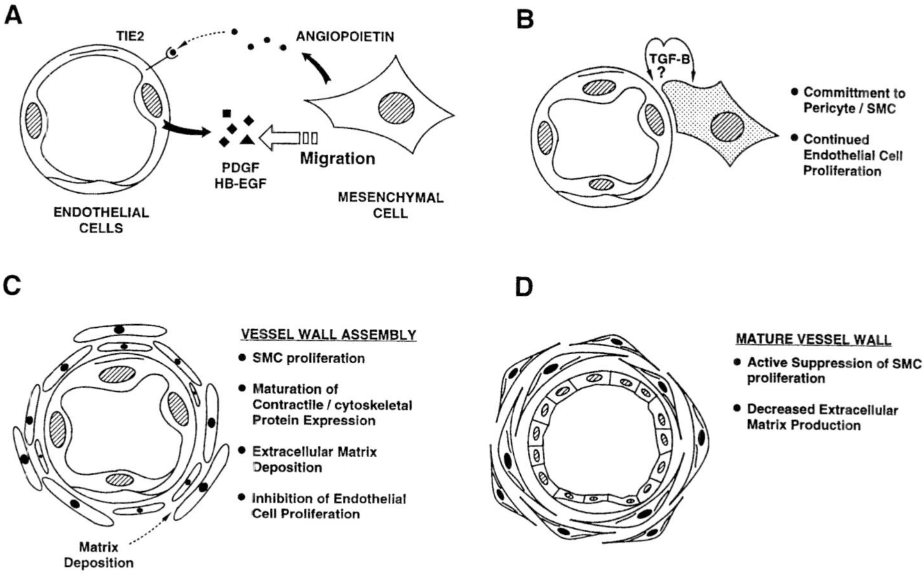

Fig. 6.1 A proposed model for the development of a mature vessel wall. Under this model, angiopoietin, produced by undifferentiated mesenchymal cells, binds to and activates the TIE2 receptor on endothelial cells (*A*), resulting in release of a recruitment/chemotactic signal (e.g., PDGF, HB-EGF) for mesenchymal cells. Migration of mesenchymal cells to the developing endothelial tube and subsequent contact with the endothelium may cause the activation of signals [(*B*), e.g, TGF-β] necessary for the commitment of mesenchymal cells to SMC-specific lineages. The developing vessel then undergoes structural assembly (*C*), which includes the inhibition of endothelial cell proliferation, rapid SMC proliferation, and extracellular matrix deposition. Throughout this period, differentiation to a more mature cell occurs as SMC gradually accumulate contractile and cytoskeletal proteins. By the time the adult blood vessel morphology is reached (*D*), the primary function of SMC becomes contraction and, as such, SMC become extremely quiescent, respond poorly to mitogenic stimulation, and produce minimal matrix proteins.

tube corresponds with establishment of blood flow and an increase in blood pressure within the endothelial tube (109, 148). This observation leads to the speculation that mechanical forces play an important role in recruitment and differentiation of SMC during the early arterialization process.

Consideration of the embryologic origin of SMC in the pulmonary circulation is also important because recent studies suggest different functional capabilities of SMC derived from different sources. As was suggested above, both vasculogenic and angiogenic mechanisms contribute to vessel formation in the lung. Gross mapping of the embryological origins of SMC in the pulmonary circulation, at least in the avian species, has been accomplished using interspecies grafting techniques (chicken:quail, chimeras). Results of these studies demonstrate that the main pulmonary artery is derived from the sixth aortic arch artery and contains cells primarily of neural crest origin. The SMC within lung parenchyma originate from ventrolateral mesoderm, arise uniquely in the lung buds themselves and are not the result of ingrowth from the sixth arch (210a). The different embryologic origins of cells in the proximal and distal pulmonary circulation may therefore contribute to unique phenotypic and functional differences observed later in life.

SMC Replication During Development

Continuous accretion and rapid proliferation of "committed" SMC characterizes later stages of embryonic vascular development (day 12 or 13 through day 18 in the rat). Cook et al. have evaluated the replication rates of aortic SMC throughout development in the rat (38). Smooth muscle cells were found to replicate at extremely high rates (>80% per day) throughout embryonic life (days 13–18). At the embryonic-to-fetal transition (between embryonic days 17 and 19), the SMC replication rate dramatically declines to approximately 40% per day. During postnatal life, SMC gradually acquire a quiescent phenotype, reaching a replication rate of <0.06% per day in the adult. A recent study has shown a nearly identical pattern in large pulmonary vessels during development (13). Vascular SMC therefore undergo a >2000-fold decrease in replication rate from embryonic to adult life (Fig. 6.2).

Currently available data suggest that SMC replication during early development in the rat (up to embryonic day 17) is accomplished by an autonomous (self-driven) fashion and is not related to secretion of mitogens. The early embryonic SMC exhibit poor mitogenic responses to serum and growth factors, providing further support to the idea that growth is intrinsically regulated (38). The dramatic decline in in vivo proliferation observed between embryonic and fetal periods (days 17–19) was shown to correspond with the loss of autonomous growth capacity by SMC cultured from the great vessels of animals at these time points [Fig. 6.2; (38)]. Further data suggest that the switch from autonomous to serum- and growth factor–dependent growth may be associated with the developmental acquisition of a *trans*-acting "adult" factor capable of suppressing autonomous DNA replication (130). Thus, SMC replication during early embryonic vascular development seems to be genetically predetermined and independent of the secretion of mitogens by other cells or tissues.

In the fetal and neonatal period, in contrast to the embryonic period, mechanisms involving growth factors are likely involved in the regulation of vascular cell growth. Recent studies utilizing a neonatal calf model have directly tested this hypothesis (44). Smooth muscle cells cultured from neonatal calves were compared with cells cultured from adult animals and tested for size differences, serum-stimulated proliferation, susceptibility to senescence, resistance to serum withdrawal, autocrine growth capacity and responsiveness to growth factors. Neonatal SMC were significantly smaller in size, grew faster, and reached higher plateau density and were less susceptible to senescence under serum-stimulated conditions than adult cells. They were also more resistant to induction of a quiescent state, had spontaneous autocrine growth capacity, and were more responsive to mitogens including insulin growth factor (IGF)-1, PMA, and the combination. Neonatal cells also had increased activated protein Kinase C (PKC) activity under basal conditions compared with adult cells. Increased activity of this central signaling pathway could contribute to enhanced responsiveness to mitogens observed in neonatal cells. Thus, the increased growth capacity of isolated neonatal pulmonary artery SMC was dependent on cell size, age at time of cell harvest, IGF-1, and autoactivation of PKC (44).

The precise factors that drive SMC proliferation in vivo during fetal and neona-

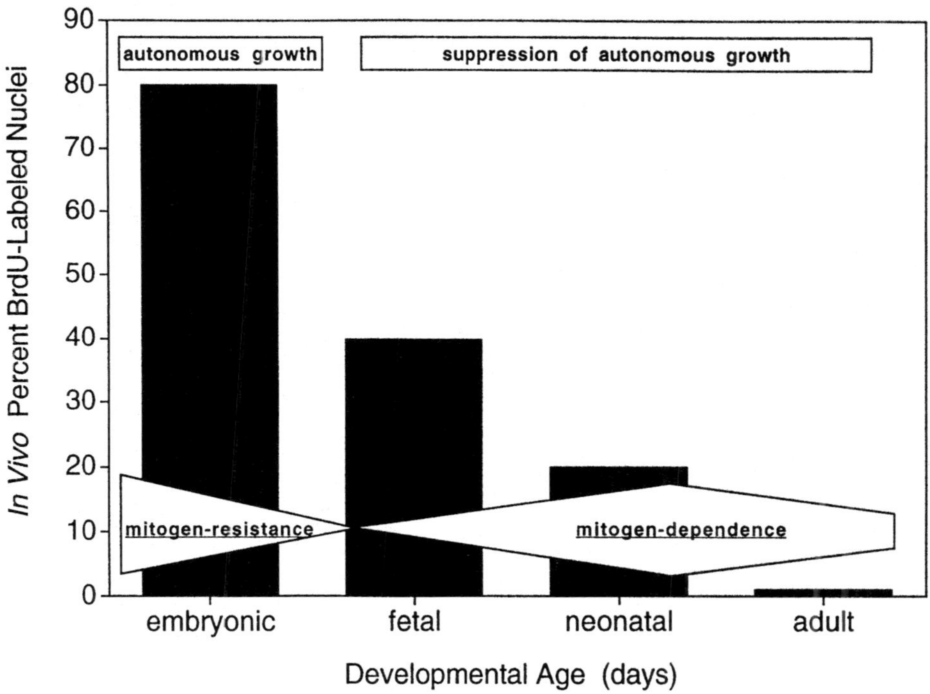

Fig. 6.2 The SMC growth properties during rat aortic development. Embryonic SMC exhibit very high in vivo replication rates which dramatically decline at the embryonic-to-fetal transition (bars). during postnatal life, replication continues to gradually decrease and SMC acquire a quiescent phenotype, showing replication rates of <0.06% per day in the adult. Corresponding to the in vivo changes in SMC replication, cultured embryonic SMC demonstrate a significant capacity for autonomous, mitogen-independent growth that is lost by fetal life, very likely due to the developmental acquisition of intra- and extracellular factors capable of active growth suppression. Cultured embryonic SMC exhibit poor mitogenic responses to serum and growth factors, further suggesting that early embryonic SMC growth is intrinsically regulated. In contrast, although in vivo growth is minimal, cultured postnatal SMC demonstrate significant proliferative responses to exogenous mitogens with early neonatal SMC exhibiting exaggerated responses compared to adult SMC. [Modified from Cook et al., 1993 (38)].

tal development are largely unknown. Many studies have confirmed roles for various growth factors in influencing SMC proliferation in vitro, although the in vivo roles of these factors during this phase of blood vessel development have not been firmly established. It is reasonable to suggest that endothelial cells, through secretion of growth factors, play an important role in the arterialization process. Indeed, cultured endothelial cells have been shown to secrete a variety of SMC growth factors, including PDGF and bFGF (45, 74), as well as growth inhibitors such as heparin and TGF-β (21, 35). Some of these same factors may influence the differentiation state of SMC. For instance, exogenous heparin has been reported to increase SMC α-SM actin content while an as-yet unidentified aortic endothelial-derived mitogen may act as a potent suppressor of SMC differentiation. Table 6.2 lists many of the growth factors, cytokines, and lipids produced by vascular wall cells that are known to influence the in vitro growth, matrix synthetic, and differentiation state of SMC (also recently reviewed in refs. 137, 148).

Several vasoactive mediators produced by the vascular endothelium may also play roles in vascular development. Blood flow to the lung is limited during fetal life, and regulation by locally produced vasoconstrictors has been shown to be important (94, 137). These same vasoconstrictors, including thromboxane A2 (98), angiotensin II

Table 6.2 Factors Regulating SMC Growth and Matrix Protein Synthesis

Factors	*SMC growth*	*Elastin*	*Type I collagen*
IGF-I	↑	↑	↑
IGF-II	↑	↑	↑
TGF-β	↑ / ↓	↑	↑
PDGF	↑	↑	↑ / ↔
Leukotriene C_4(LTC_4)	↑	ND	↑
PAF	↑	↑	ND
IL-1	↑ / ↓	↓	↑ / ↓
EGF	↑	↓	↔
Prostaglandins (PGE_2, PGI_2)	↓	↔ / ↓	↓
Interferons	↓	↓	↓
Protein Kinase C activation (PKC)	↑	↓	↓
bFGF	↑	ND	ND
aFGF	↑	ND	ND
Insulin	↑		
TGF-α	ND	ND	ND
HB-EGF	↑	ND	ND
PD-ECGF	↔	ND	ND
VEGF (VPF)	↔	ND	ND
Serotonin	↑	ND	ND
Histamine	↑	ND	ND
TNF-α	↓	ND	ND
Heparan sulfates	↓	ND	ND

ND, not determined.

(102), endothelin (16), leukotrienes (149), substance P (145), and 5-hydroxytryptamine (167), may exert growth-promoting effects on vascular SMC. Recent studies have suggested potential roles for angiotensin II and endothelin-1 in vascular development (see below).

Extracellular Matrix Protein Changes During Development

Extracellular matrix (ECM) protein production by vascular wall cells also changes significantly during the course of normal development. The ECM not only provides structural integrity to the developing vessel and a lattice work to which cells can anchor themselves but also provides informational clues that effect a variety of cell processes, including proliferation, migration, differentiation, and the synthesis of further types of matrix molecules. It has become clear that "information" encoded in or received by the ECM can be transmitted to the internal domain of the cell (30, 164). The connective tissue elements of the vascular wall are complex and include molecules from virtually every class of extracellular matrix: elastin, collagens, proteoglycans, and structural and adhesive glycoproteins. The relative proportions of each matrix component appear to reflect either the physical and functional properties expected of a particular vascular segment or the forces to which that vascular segment is exposed. Thus, pulmonary vascular protein composition changes significantly with development and with type and location of the vessel studied (136).

For example, elastin is the most abundant protein in major arteries subjected to large pulsatile pressures generated by cardiac contraction (121). Elastogenic progenitor cells, giving rise to at least some of the smooth muscle cells that constitute the aorta and other elastic vessels, arise from mesenchyme adjacent to the myocardium (177). Elastogenic activity in these cells, at least in developing chick aorta, appears in an orderly, sequential, proximal-to-distal deployment, beginning nearest the heart and advancing downstream into all nascent elastic vessels. In the developing rat aorta, peak tropoelastin (TE) mRNA synthesis occurs during late fetal and early postnatal life and remains high through the first postnatal month (133, 140). By two months, TE mRNA expression is virtually undetectable and no significant TE is produced by normal adult vascular smooth muscle cells (133, 155, 193). The developmentally confined period of elastin production suggests that TE mRNA expression is accurately controlled by tissue- and temporal-specific mechanisms, but the precise mechanisms that govern elastogenesis are not known.

Using the neonatal bovine model, we evaluated expression of TE mRNA at various time points in normal fetal and neonatal development as well as in response to hypoxic hypertension (17) to gain a better insight into the factors controlling expression of this gene. Utilizing in situ hybridization and immunohistochemical techniques to simultaneously evaluate TE mRNA expression and cytodifferentiation state of the cell, respectively, we found that TE mRNA exhibited a biphasic pattern of expression during fetal development that seemed to be influenced by two major factors: the differentiation state of the SMC and the arterial pressure. In early fetal development (less than 100 days of gestation), TE mRNA was expressed throughout the entire main pulmonary arterial wall. This is a time when pressure in the pulmonary circulation is low and SMC are poorly differentiated, based on expression of various muscle-specific proteins. In mid-gestation (180 days), TE mRNA expression decreased starting in the outer media, which coincided with the appearance of immunoreactivity to cytodifferentiation-related markers (specifically, desmin, SM-myosin, and calponin) in cells of the outermost media. During late gestation (250–270 days), coincident with the rise in fetal pulmonary arterial pressure, TE mRNA was re-expressed throughout the entire vessel wall in a heterogeneic pattern that correlated with the existence of distinct SMC phenotypes within the arterial media. The TE mRNA was expressed in all SMC populations except those in the outer media, which were expressing metavinculin (L3-"C" cells, see Fig. 6.1, Table 6.3). After birth, TE mRNA expression in the vessel wall rapidly declined such that by 1 month no TE mRNA signal was detected (12). However, if newborn calves were exposed to hypoxia on the first day of life and developed severe pulmonary hypertension, TE mRNA persisted at high levels in all SMC subpopulations except those marked by expression of metavinculin (12, 17). These data demonstrated the existence of specific SMC subpopulations within the vascular media which differed dramatically in their matrix-producing capabilities, suggesting differential roles for unique SMC subpopulations in elastogenesis during normal development and in the pathogenesis of vascular disease.

As distance from the heart increases, a progressive decrease in the amount of vascular elastin and a progressive increase in the amount of collagen is observed (41). Mature cross-linked collagen is much stiffer than elastin and thus confers different structural properties to the vessel wall. Collagens are an important family of

Table 6.3 Expression of Contractile and Cytoskeletol Proteins by SMC During Vascular Development

	α-SM-actin	*SM-2/SM-1 ratio*	*NM-MMC*	*M-VN*	*h-Cd*	*Cp*
Fetal media						
8–10 weeks	+	+	+++	–	–	–
22–25 weeks	++	++	++	–	–	–
Infant media						
2–3 months	ND	++	++	+	+	ND
6 months	+++	+++	+	++	++	++
18 months	ND	ND	ND	+++	+++	+++
Adult media	+++	+++	–	++–	+++	+++
Subendothelial intima (normal, adult)	+++	ND	++	++	++	++
Atherosclerotic plaque	+	ND	+++	+	+	+

α-SM-actin, alpha smooth muscle actin; SM-1 and SM-2, smooth-muscle myosin heavy chain isoforms, 204 kDa and 200 kDa, respectively; NM-MHC, non-muscle myosin heavy chain; M-VN, metavinculin; h-Cd, high-molecular-weight (smooth muscle) caldesmon; Cp, calponin; ND, not determined.

structural proteins localized in the basement membrane and interstitial spaces of the vascular wall. Many excellent studies have evaluated accumulation of collagen in both systemic and pulmonary vessels during normal development (104, 216). The amount of collagen in a vessel wall depends on both age and site of the vessel studied. Furthermore, the amount of this fibrous protein, like elastin, can be correlated with differences in vascular wall tension that normally occur in different arteries during growth.

Immunohistochemical studies have evaluated the appearance and distribution of various collagen types in the developing pulmonary artery. The interstitial collagens are deposited in the order of types V, III, and then I during embryonic development (136). The amount of types I and V collagen in the pulmonary arterial media increases with age. Particularly striking is the paucity of type I collagen in resistance-sized pulmonary arteries of the newborn compared with the adult lung (53, 136). Interesting functional implications can be drawn from these studies. Type I collagen is characterized by a high tensile strength; large quantities of this protein are prominent in tissues that are relatively indistensible. On the other hand, type III collagen is present in distensible connective tissues (e.g., the uterus). The relative lack of type I collagen in developing pulmonary vessels may help explain the plasticity required of the pulmonary arteries in fetal and early neonatal life. Cells composing the vessel wall change rapidly in shape and position during the first hours of life. The vessel walls themselves are continually remodeled with growth. These events may be facilitated by a paucity of type I collagen. However, although present in small amounts, type I collagen appears to be crucial for the maintenance of vascular integrity during normal development because mutant mice, deficient in type I collagen, die at about 15 days of gestation with ruptured major blood vessels (112).

Components of the ECM such as collagen, laminin, fibronectin, and perlecan have been shown to be capable of influencing proliferation, migration, and differentiation of cultured endothelial cells and SMC (60, 87, 88), suggesting that changes in production during development not only will be seen but will directly influence vascular function. The distribution of these proteins and the sequence of their appearance have been studied in various tissues during development in attempts to determine whether ECM components play a role in regulating the growth and patterning of blood vessels in vivo. Information on the timing of basement membrane formation during vascular development is of crucial importance to our understanding of the role that the extracellular matrix may play in the control of SMC replication, migration, gene expression, and growth responsiveness during development and in response to injury.

Fibronectin is one of the earliest components to be deposited in the vascular basal laminae. The appearance of fibronectin in the perivascular ECM precedes by at least 2 days the appearance of ultrastructurally identifiable basal lamina, which are not evident until day 6 (8). The location of fibronection relative to the developing blood vessels is consistent with its playing a role in certain critical stages in the formation of capillaries and larger vessels. The presence of fibronectin in the allantois, where the primitive blood vessels are first formed, suggests that this molecule participates in the early aggregation of mesenchymal cells to form capillary tubes. As in other embryonic tissues, fibronectin could promote the migration of capillary endothelial cells because it is known to stimulate the migration of vascular endothelial cells in vitro (18, 207). As fibronectin levels peak in developing arterioles and venules of the CAM, glycosaminoglycans (7) and type IV collagen are first detected. The ability of fibronectin to bind to cell surfaces as well as matrix components such as collagen and proteoglycans (96, 166) makes it reasonable to suppose that fibronectin plays a role in the progressive accumulation and organization of the basal lamina to the endothelial and SMC it envelops. Fibronectin content then diminishes in the basal laminae with time, and is usually a minor component of adult vascular basal laminae. It is important to also note that the mRNA for fibronectin undergoes extensive alternative splicing that results in at least 10 different fibronectin variants (111). At least two of these alternatively spliced peptides appear to be developmentally regulated in vascular SMC. For example, the aortic media of the 10- to 12-week-old human fetus expresses fibronectin protein that binds to monoclonal antibodies recognizing both extradomain A (ED-A) and extradomain B (ED-B) fibronectin sequences. With continued development to 20–25 weeks, the proportion of ED-A antibody recognizing fibronectin decreases fivefold and that for ED-B decreases twofold. By adulthood, no ED-A- or ED-B-recognizing fibronecting sequences can be found in the vessel media. However, ED-A is seen in SMC in the normal adult arterial intima (74).

Laminin also appears early in vessel walls, although later than fibronectin. Laminin has been shown to promote the morphological differentiation of cultured human capillary and venous endothelial cells into capillary-like structures (113). Laminin has also been shown to promote the maintenance of the contractile phenotype and other differentiated properties of cultured arterial SMC, which in the absence of laminin tend to loose their microfilaments and assume a more undifferentiated and synthetically active phenotype (87).

Type IV collagen is the last basement membrane collagen to appear in the matrix surrounding CAM vessels. It is not present during the earliest stages of vessel development, when endothelial cells are proliferating rapidly, but appears only as endothelial cell division starts to slow (8). Type IV collagen appears in the vascular basal laminae at approximately the same time as sulfated proteoglycans. Similar to laminin, type IV collagen has been shown to enable cultured SMC to maintain a contractile phenotype (87) and thus could be involved in the progressive differentiation that occurs later in vascular development.

Endogenous heparin-like molecules are believed to play critical roles in the control of vascular SMC replication (14, 34, 66, 201), migration (131), and differentiated functions (124, 202). The pattern of expression of perlecan, the predominant basement membrane heparan sulfate proteoglycan (HSPG), during pulmonary and aortic development has recently been described in the rat (13, 213). Expression of perlecan mRNA and protein in the aortic SMC was first observed at embryonal day 19, a time which marks a dramatic decline in SMC replication rate and a change in growth phenotype (213). Expression of perlecan message and protein was high throughout fetal and early neonatal life, and remained readily detectable in the adult aorta. Furthermore, both in vivo and in vitro data suggest that the expression of perlecan by vascular SMC is regulated by apparent developmental age as well as by cellular growth state. The developmental timing of perlecan expression suggests that this HSPG may play a determining role in the cessation of SMC replication during vascular morphogenesis and may participate in maintaining SMC in a quiescent state in the adult blood vessel wall. Alternatively or in addition, perlecan expression by quiescent SMC may reflect the deposition of a "protective" growth-suppressive and differentiation-promoting basement membrane. Removal of such growth-inhibitory influences may be a major determinant of the extent of SMC replication following injury.

Integrins

Integrins, or cell surface receptors for extracellular matrix proteins, are directly involved in signaling mechanisms that regulate SMC migration, anchorage of cells during vasoconstriction, interaction of smooth muscle cells with basement membrane, and integration of extracellular matrix components and the cytoskeletal framework. Integrins are heterodimers consisting of an α subunit linked noncovalently to a nonrelated β subunit. Currently, 16 α and 8 β subunits have been described (96), with the combination of αβ-specifying receptor subtype. Furthermore, the number and type of integrins expressed by different cell types varies significantly—many integrins are cell type specific and their expression pattern appears to be developmentally regulated (76a). Analysis of the integrin repertoire in adult human vascular SMC reveals mainly α1β1 and small amounts of α3β1, α5β1, and αVβ1. In vascular SMC, expression of α1β1 integrin appears early during SMC differentiation and remains detectable throughout life. Similarly, at least in the human, α3β1 integrin expression is low in the fetus and slowly increases after birth. In contrast, α5β1 is present in early vascular development but its expression is greatly diminished in the adult vessel wall. It is believed that the specific expression pattern of integrins by SMC provides them with the ability to recognize collagens, laminin, and fibronectin and, therefore, centers specific biological activity. For instance, it has been suggested that specific interaction between collagen-laminin receptors, α1β1 and α3β1 integrins, and corresponding components of basement membrane (particularly α1β2-g1 laminin) promotes maturation of SMC and maintenance of a differentiated state.

Changes in Contractile and Cytoskeletal Protein Expression During Development

Significant changes also occur in the expression of contractile and cytoskeletal proteins during normal development. However, as yet, complete mapping of the time course of changes in expression of each of the known SMC differentiation marker proteins over the entire developmental time course has not been completed in a single species. Certain clear patterns are emerging suggesting that there is a continuum of phenotypes that exists between the committed but undifferentiated SMC precursor cell at one end of the spectrum and the fully contractile mature SMC at the other end. The SMC of different lineages may progress along unique differentiation pathways and not all cells express all proteins associated with fully differentiated SMC (Table 6.3).

The earliest known marker of SMC is smooth muscle α-actin, which is induced coincident with recruitment of presumptive SMC precursors into the vessel wall. With maturation there is a switch from predominant expression of non-muscle β-actin by neonatal aortic smooth muscle cells to predominant expression of smooth muscle (SM)-specific α-actin isoforms by adult SMC (108). In addition to this shift from non-muscle β-actin to the SM-specific form of a-actin during maturation, the cellular content of tropomyosin, and certain cytoskeletal proteins (vimentin and desmin) in SMC increases with age (139, 148). Recently the SM2 isoform of SM-myosin heavy chain (SM-MHC) was found to be expressed only in adult blood vessels, whereas the SM1 isoform was found to be expressed earlier in development (116, 169). Newborn rat aortic SMC underexpressing α-actin isoforms exhibit a higher replication rate than α-actin-positive cells, suggesting an inverse correlation between acquisition of the adult phenotype and cell replication. However, it must be noted that during development contractile and synthetic function of SMC are clearly not mutually exclusive. The SMC in developing vessels simultaneously express multiple SM contractile proteins, a variety of ECM proteins, and are capable of proliferating (148, 178).

Studies in the developing human aorta have recently evaluated expression of the regulatory contractile proteins h-caldesmon and calponin in conjunction with expression of α-SM-actin and SM-MHC (62, 73, 76). Actin and myosin are expressed far earlier in development than caldesmon and calponin, which suggests that these latter proteins, because they are involved in the regulation of contraction, may serve as markers of more highly differentiated smooth muscle cells. In addition, expression of metavinculin, a marker of microfilament-membrane association sites, also occurs in more differentiated smooth muscle cells later in development (75).

Clearly then, substantial differences exist in the proliferative, secretory, and contractile phenotypes between fetal and adult vascular wall cells. It is reasonable to assume that many more such differences exist at the gene and protein level and that these differences may play pivotal roles in the control of SMC replication and differentiation during vascular development. It is also reasonable to assume that these differences in gene expression could contribute to significant differences in the response to injurious stimuli exhibited by cells at different times during vascular development.

Developmental Changes in Ion Channels and Receptors: Relation to Changes in Vascular Tone

Vascular SMC express numerous ion channels and membrane receptors that are critical in influencing the cells' contractile behavior through effects on its electrical activities and sensitivity to stimulation by hormones, neurotransmitters, and contractile agonists. The specific repertoire of ion channels and receptors that are expressed varies widely between different vascular beds and is a key determinant of the contractile responsiveness of the SMC. Most of these receptors and ion channels also change during the differentiation/maturation of the SMC. For example, expression of angiotensin II receptor subtypes changes during development. In the fetal rat aorta (embryonic day 18) AT2 type receptors predominate, whereas in adult aorta AT1 type receptors are almost exclusively expressed. There is also evidence for developmental regulation of a number of other contractile agonist receptors in vascular SMC, including muscarinic M1, M2, and M3 receptors (38); vasopressin V1 and V2 receptors; α1-adrenergic receptors; and β-adrenergic receptors. However, no studies have as yet demonstrated when these contractile agonist receptors are first expressed by cells in the developing vessel cell.

Recent studies by Cornfield and colleagues have also demonstrated marked changes in ion channel activity and distribution during pulmonary vascular development (39). They have shown that there are significant increases in the ability of the pulmonary circulation to constrict to hypoxia following birth and that these differences are intrinsic to changes in the SMC. Maturational changes in the expression of K^+ channels are related to changes in the vascular reactivity of the pulmonary circulation during development. Specifically, K^+ ATP channel activity increased with maturation and membrane potential and hypoxic constriction in adult SMC are controlled by delayed rectifier K^+ channels.

Factors Actively Contributing to Differentiation and Growth Suppression in Adult Smooth Muscle Cells

In vivo, adult SMC are replicatively quiescent and relatively unresponsive to mitogens that stimulate cultured SMC. Exposure of SMC to exogenous mitogens alone, either in vivo or in cultured tissue explants, does not appear to be sufficient to initiate DNA synthesis, suggesting the presence of potent growth-suppressive mechanisms operative in the adult vessel wall. Both intracellular and extracellular factors probably contribute to SMC quiescence in the adult blood vessel wall. Intracellular factors that have been shown to exist in SMC include tumor suppressor genes, whose loss-of-function mutations or inactivation (e.g., by binding to viral gene products) can lead to a loss of normal growth control (123). Similarly, the existence of an adult factor capable of suppressing the autonomous growth phenotype of embryonic SMC has been inferred from adult:embryonic SMC heterokaryon studies (130). This factor is likely to be functionally related to tissue-specific "extinguishers" such as fibroblast TSE-1 (100), which suppresses liver-specific gene expression in fibroblast:hepatoma fusion cells. Other specific extinguishers also exist and appear to play important roles in regulating the expression of differentiation-specific genes (182). Finally, Blau and colleagues have shown that the 3′ untranslated regions of several skeletal muscle–specific mRNAs exert growth-inhibitory, tumor-suppressive, and differentiation-promoting activity (160). Their data suggest that the expression of differentiation-specific mRNAs may, in turn, contribute to the maintenance of the quiescent, differentiated state. A similar situation may exist for vascular SMC.

Extracellular factors that may contribute to developmental growth suppression in vascular SMC include growth factors, whose disappearance during development might lead to "passive growth arrest," and growth inhibitors such as those of the TGF-β superfamily (105). Components of the extracellular matrix also appear to contribute substantially to the control of SMC growth and differentiation. For example, when actively replicating "synthetic" SMC are cultured on basement membrane components isolated from the Engelbreth-Holm-Swarm (EHS) mouse tumor (commercially available as Matrigel), they become growth inhibited, activate MAP kinases less efficiently in response to mitogens, and exhibit more "differentiated" functions (124, 214). Fibronectin appears to facilitate the expression of a "synthetic" SMC phenotype, while other matrix components (e.g., laminin) may induce the expression of a "contractile" phenotype and inhibit SMC proliferation (201, 202). Components of the basement membrane–extracellular matrix that have been reported to inhibit SMC replication or to promote SMC differentiation include heparan sulfates, laminin, and collagen type IV (202, 227). Other studies have indicated that the developmentally timed expression of perlecan, the predominant basement membrane heparan sulfate proteoglycan, may contribute substantially to the establishment and/or maintenance of SMC quiescence in the mature blood vessel wall, and may regulate the expression of certain growth-essential transcription factors [(213, 214); see Fig. 6.1C]. The mechanism(s) by which perlecan or heparin-like molecules regulate SMC replication and gene expression is not yet clear, but may include a number of parallel growth-inhibitory pathways (6).

Heterogeneity of Smooth Muscle Cell Phenotype in the Vascular Wall

In addition to the developmentally regulated differences in SMC phenotype, there is a growing body of literature based on both in vivo and in vitro studies documenting the existence of phenotypic heterogeneity within the resident SMC population of a given tissue at a specified developmental stage.

In Vivo

The hypothesis that multiple distinct SMC subpopulations comprise the normal mammalian arterial media is supported by previous observations in the systemic circulation. Several laboratories have reported the existence of SMC of different size, shape, and differentiation state in the mature systemic vessel wall (147, 189, 223). Recent studies have demonstrated that the pulmonary artery is also composed of multiple phenotypically distinct (as defined by cytoskeletal and matrix protein expression) SMC subpopulations (61, 156, 193, 195). Further, the data demonstrated that these cells progress along different developmental pathways, thus suggesting the existence of distinct vascular SMC lineages (61). The observation of multiple SMC subpopulations comprising the arterial media raises an important question as to why this cellular diversity exists. Numerous functions are required of vascular

SMC under both normal and pathologic conditions, including contraction, proliferation, and synthesis of matrix proteins. Different SMC functions may require different SMC phenotypes. Accordingly, it is highly likely that, in response to pathologic stimuli, some medial SMC maintain their normal, mainly "contractile," functions whereas others exhibit elevated proliferation and/or matrix protein synthesis. This diversity in cellular responses would lend itself to a better maintenance of vascular homeostasis in the setting of hypoxic injury. Most functions could continue without severe or fatal compromise as would occur if all (or most) cells shifted simultaneously from one phenotype ("contractile") to another ("proliferative" and/or "synthetic").

In Vitro

Recent in vitro studies also support the hypothesis that phenotypically distinct SMC subpopulations exist within the normal arterial media that exhibit unique and selective responses to the same stimulus. Vascular SMC of multiple phenotypes have been isolated and maintained in culture over many passages. Smooth muscle cells distinct in morphology, growth factor requirements, saturation density, and expression of cytoskeletal/contractile proteins, growth factors, and extracellular matrix molecules have been derived from systemic vessels from rats of different ages and injured vessels. For example, subpopulations of PDGF-independent and PDGF-dependent SMC have been isolated from the arterial media of neonatal rats (120, 173) and a subpopulation of SMC less sensitive to the growth-inhibitory effects of heparin have been isolated from the adult rat aortic media (11). Most recently, two morphologically distinct SMC populations, isolated from the mature rat aortic media, were shown to differ dramatically in their ionic responses to vasoactive agonists (143). Similar to data obtained from rat studies, two stable SMC subpopulations were isolated from human systemic arteries that demonstrate markedly different growth properties (68). In vitro data from our laboratory (63, 64) demonstrate that multiple morphologically and phenotypically distinct SMC subpopulations can be selectively isolated from the mature bovine main pulmonary artery. These SMC subpopulations exhibit dramatically different responses to growth-promoting and -inhibiting stimuli. Stable clones of SMC retaining unique characteristics have been obtained from the systemic circulation as well as from pulmonary arteries (165, 173).

FUNCTIONAL CHANGES IN THE PULMONARY CIRCULATION DURING DEVELOPMENT

The normal adult pulmonary circulation is a low-resistance, high-flow, vascular bed with little or no resting tone. In contrast, the fetal pulmonary circulation is characterized by high vascular resistance and low flow with only 8%–10% of the combined cardiac output of the fetus passing through the lungs (89); the remainder passes through the foramen ovale or ductus arteriosus into the descending aorta to the placenta where the blood is oxygenated. With the closure of the ductus at birth, pulmonary blood flow must increase eight to ten fold. To accommodate the increased blood flow, the pulmonary vascular resistance falls rapidly following birth and pulmonary arterial pressure falls to normal adult levels within hours or days. Thus the developing pulmonary circulation must be able to maintain high vascular resistance in utero, while anticipating the abrupt transition that occurs at birth. Although many factors participate in the regulation of vascular tone, the endothelium plays a central role by sensing changes in flow and oxygen tension, and producing vasodilators and vasoconstrictors that act on underlying smooth muscle. Vasoactive factors derived from the endothelium clearly contribute to the elevated fetal pulmonary vascular resistance and to the rapid transition at birth. The following section summarizes our present knowledge regarding the developmental regulation of some important endothelium-derived factors that influence pulmonary vascular tone.

Vasoconstrictors

Endothelin

The endothelium (ET) is the main site of production of the endothelins. Although this group of peptides was originally characterized as powerful vasoconstrictors, it is becoming clear that their effects vary depending on the predominant receptor subtype present and the initial tone of the vascular bed. In addition, endothelins may be mitogenic and chemotactic to pulmonary artery fibroblasts and smooth muscle cells, raising the possibility that these peptides may contribute to growth of the normal pulmonary circulation and to pathological remodeling in pulmonary hypertension (198).

To date, three structurally similar peptides have been designated: endothelin-1, endothelin-2, and endothelin-3 (ET-1, ET-2, and ET-3), each produced by a separate gene (97). Endothelin-1 is the best characterized of the ET family and is formed within the endothelial cell by a two-stage process. Preproendothelin-1, a 212 amino acid precursor, is cleaved by an endopeptidase to form proendothelin-1, or bigET-1, a 38 amino acid peptide. BigET-1 is then converted to ET-1 (21 amino acids) by endothelin-converting enzyme (ECE) and released mainly at the abluminal surface of the endothelial cell (10, 221).

Endothelin receptors exist in at least two separate isoforms, ETA and ETB. The ETA receptor displays high affinity for ET-1 and ET-2, is generally present on smooth muscle cells, and mediates vasoconstriction. The ETB receptor is located mainly on endothelial cells, binds all three endothelins, and mediates vasodilatation via release of nitric oxide or prostacyclin, or via ATP-gated K channels (228).

Infusion of ET-1 into the pulmonary circulation of the late gestation ovine fetus results in complex changes in vascular resistance that are time and tone dependent (217, 228). Generally, vasodilatation is initially observed; vasoconstriction occurs with prolonged infusion. Inhibition of the ETA receptor with BQ123, a cyclic pentapeptide, also results in vasodilatation, a response thought to be mediated by preferential binding of endothelin to the ETB receptor. This hypothesis is supported by the observation that ETB agonists evoke vasodilatation, and combined ETA/ETB antagonists evoke no response in the ovine fetal pulmonary circulation (99). Intrapulmonary infusion of bigET-1 causes an increase in pulmonary arterial pressure, without vasodilatation (101). Possibly, ECE acting on bigET-1 produces ET-1, which then preferentially binds to smooth muscle cell ETA receptors mediating vasoconstriction. However, the experiments seem to suggest a limited role for endogenously produced ET-1 in the maintenance of high fetal pulmonary vascular resistance, and inhibition of ECE by the non-specific metalloproteinase phosphoramidon did not alter fetal pulmonary vascular resistance (101).

The cellular localization and levels of expression of endothelins, receptor subtypes, and ECE during development are less well characterized than the physiologic responses. High levels of ET-1 and ET-3 mRNA are expressed during lung development (127). In rat fetus at 19 of 21 days, in situ hybridization studies for ET mRNA reveal that most of the signal is localized to bronchial epithelial cells, with lower levels over small vessels. Endothelin mRNA and peptide expression has been found in the human fetal lung as early as 12 weeks of gestation (71). In the adult lung, endothelin-binding sites are widely distributed throughout the bronchial and vascular systems and the lung parenchyma (226). The ETA receptors predominate on smooth muscle and ETB predominate in the lung parenchyma (93, 141). The ETB receptor also predominates on endothelial cells, suggesting a role for endothelin in modulation of endothelial cell function (84). Recent studies evaluating homozygous ET-1 null mutation mice (Edn-1) confirm that ET-1 is essential to normal development of the heart and great vessels. Edn-1–/–mice displayed cardiovascular malformations including interrupted aortic arch, tubular hypoplasia of the aortic arch, aberrant right subclavian artery, and ventricular septal defect with abnormalities of the outflow tract (115).

Endothelin-converting enzyme is widely expressed in adult endothelial cells (197) but its expression during fetal lung development remains to be studied.

Angiotensin

Angiotensin II (ANG II) is an octapeptide vasoconstrictor, cleaved from the decapeptide angiotensin I (ANG I), mainly by the action of angiotensin-converting enzyme (ACE). Angiotensin I is produced from angiotensinogen by the action of renin. Angiotensin II is a powerful vasoconstrictor in the pulmonary circulation and can stimulate specific intracellular growth events in vascular SMC (69, 72, 176). It has been shown to stimulate protein and DNA synthesis, to up-regulate c-*fos* and c-*myc* expression, and to stimulate PDGF-A chain gene expression in vascular SMC (15, 175). Moreover, ANG II has been shown to increase selectively the expression of α-SM-actin and myosin heavy chain by rat aortic SMC in culture (206) and to affect the synthesis of extracellular matrix proteins by SMC (176). Recently, evidence has accumulated to support the notion of a local-angiotensin generating system within the vascular wall, with ANG II functioning as a paracrine or autocrine growth factor. In humans, two isoforms of the ANG II receptor have been described and cloned, the

AT_1 and AT_2 receptor subtypes. In rodents, two splice variants of the AT_1 receptor exist, the AT_{1a} and AT_{1b}.

The role of endogenous or exogenous ANG II in fetal pulmonary vascular hemodynamics is unknown, although these studies are now possible with the advent of subtype-specific ANG II receptor antagonists. Toxicology studies indicate that ACE inhibition in human pregnancy is teratogenic, resulting in growth retardation, renal tubular dysplasia, and pulmonary hypoplasia. The results suggest that ANG II may be important in fetal lung growth (157).

Expression of ACE (138) and angiotensin receptors (80, 138, 179–181, 204, 205) are developmentally regulated in the fetal lung. In the rat, lung ACE activity is about 10 times lower at birth than in the mature animal (138, 211, 212). The dramatic increase in postnatal ACE activity is due to a combination of increased number of pulmonary capillaries (154) and an increase in the expression level of ACE in endothelial cells (138). Morrell et al. demonstrated that ACE expression commences in the endothelium of large proximal pulmonary arteries in the pseudoglandular lung and extends distally during gestation. This distal extension is associated with the expression of α smooth muscle actin in the media of developing pulmonary arteries, suggesting a role for ANG II in differentiation of the arterial media (138). This is supported by the observation of transient AT_1 receptor mRNA expression in mesenchymal cells condensing around endothelial channels in the lung, coincident with the distal extension of ACE expression (138). The availability of knockout mice deficient in ACE and ANG II receptors will help to determine whether ANG II contributes to pulmonary vascular growth and differentiation. A role for the AT_2 receptor subtype in developmental growth emerged from observations of high levels of AT_2 receptor expression in the developing aorta (210), however knockout mice deficient in AT_2 receptors exhibited no abnormality of vascular structure (85).

Vasodilators

Nitric oxide

The production of nitric oxide (NO) by the endothelium is dependent on the intracellular conversion of L-arginine to L-citrulline catalyzed by NO synthase (NOS). Endothelial NO causes relaxation of underlying SMC by activation of SMC-soluble guanylate cyclase, resulting in an increased intracellular concentration of cGMP. Cyclic GMP is rapidly hydrolyzed within the SMC by phosphodiesterases, so constitutive release of NO by endothelial cells is necessary to maintain basal tone in many vascular beds. Endothelium-dependent vasodilators, such as acetylcholine and bradykinin, act by increasing basal production of NO.

The normal adult pulmonary circulation has little resting tone and it has been postulated that the low resting tone is maintained by NO production. However, inhibition of NOS by analoges of L-arginine cause a variable degree of vasoconstriction depending on the species studied. In the rat, L-NMMA has little effect on resting pulmonary arterial tone in isolated perfused rat lungs (218). Although, the modulatory role for NO on pulmonary vascular tone in the adult is minimal, evidence suggests that NO has an important role in the transition that occurs at birth and in lowering pulmonary vascular resistance in the neonate. Experiments conducted in organ bath-mounted intrapulmonary arterial rings from newborn pigs (125, 225) and pre- and postnatal lambs (2) indicated that endothelium-dependent vasorelaxation to acetylcholine, ADP or A23187, is present but limited in the late-gestation and newborn animal but increases with postnatal maturation. However, the response to the endothelium-independent vasodilator, sodium nitroprusside, is well developed in fetal pulmonary arterial rings, suggesting that the ability of SMC guanylate cyclase to produce cGMP predates the maturation of endothelial NO production (2). Measurement of cGMP levels as an index of NO production in isolated ovine pulmonary arteries has also provided evidence for the developmental regulation of NO synthesis (184) and has demonstrated the oxygen-dependent regulation of NO synthesis in pulmonary artery rings, as distinct from arteries derived from the systemic circulation.

The developmentally regulated increase in sensitivity to endothelium-dependent vasorelaxants may be due to a number of possible mechanisms. These include increased expression of NOS, enhancement of NOS activity by calcium-calmodulin-related mechanisms, greater bioavailability of co-factors required for NOS activity such as NADPH and tetrahydrobiopterin, or changes in activity of phosphodiesterases responsible for the breakdown of cGMP. Limitation of NOS substrate availability has also been proposed, since pre-incubation of ovine pulmonary arterial rings with L-arginine was found by one group to augment greatly the response of late-gestation fetal vessels to endothelium-dependent vasodilators (2). Such substrate limitation has not been confirmed by other investigators (184).

Studies in chronically instrumented ovine fetuses have provided evidence that endogenous NO modulates fetal pulmonary vascular tone as early as 0.78 term (106), and the response to endothelium-dependent vasodilators increases toward term (1, 31, 106). Furthermore, the fetal pulmonary vasculature responds to inhaled exogenous NO by vasodilatation (106). At birth, the normal increase in pulmonary blood flow and decrease in pulmonary vascular resistance is greatly reduced by intrapulmonary infusion of nitro-L-arginine. The NO-mediated fall in pulmonary vascular resistance at birth may be partly due to induction of NOS by changes in shear stress in small pulmonary arteries, and by oxygen-dependent modulation of NOS activity (184). The importance of NO-mediated pulmonary artery relaxation at birth is also demonstrated in experiments in which the preterm ovine fetus is made hypertensive by ductal ligation: on delivery, these animals demonstrate preferential impairment of endothelium-dependent vasodilation, whereas responsiveness to exogenous NO remains relatively intact (132).

Thus functional studies in isolated pulmonary arterial rings and in intact animals indicate that endothelium-dependent, NO-mediated vasorelaxation of the pulmonary circulation develops to a limited extent in the fetus, contributes to the fall in pulmonary vascular resistance at birth, but reaches maximal responsiveness only in the adult. Clearly, the net response to an endothelium-dependent vasodilator is complex and depends on a number of possible factors involved in the generation and transduction of NO-mediated events, in addition to interactions with other endothelium-derived vasodilators and vasoconstrictors. Studies of the expression of endothelial NOS, and smooth muscle cell guanylyl cyclase and phosphodiesterases are required to clarify the ontogeny of the separate components of endothelium-dependent vasorelaxation. To date, studies have focussed on the ontogeny of NOS expression in the ovine (86) and rodent (103, 146) lung. Two studies in rats have shown endothelial NOS mRNA and protein to increase during the latter part of gestation (103, 146). However, one study showed that eNOS expression fell immediately following birth (146), whereas the other found that eNOS expression increased markedly during the first few hours after birth and declined thereafter to very low levels in the adult (103). In contrast to these findings in the rat, Halbower et al., using immunohistochemistry in the ovine lung, found that eNOS was highly expressed during early fetal life, with the highest levels observed at 50% gestation (86). By birth, much lower levels were seen and immunostaining was lowest in adult sheep. The lack of consistency between these studies awaits further clarification, but taken together they suggest that low pulmonary vascular tone in the adult is not dependent on eNOS expression and that eNOS expression in the early fetus may mediate functions beyond control of vascular tone.

Eicosanoids

Metabolism of arachidonic acid predominantly within the endothelial cell, but also in the SMC (22, 158), leads to local production of vasoactive eicosanoids. Arachidonic acid is metabolized through the lipoxygenase pathway to form leukotrienes, or through the cyclooxygenase pathway to form prostaglandins. The cyclooxygenase pathway appears to predominate in the fetal pulmonary circulation, and of the vasoactive prostaglandins, the vasodilator prostaglandin I2, or prostacyclin, has greatest influence on vascular tone (200), since inhibition of cyclooxygenase induces pulmonary vasoconstriction in the fetus (126) and enhances acute hypoxic pulmonary vasoconstriction in the neonate (78).

Although early studies suggested that lung leukotrienes may contribute to increased pulmonary vascular tone in the fetus (118, 191, 194), subsequent direct measurements of leukotriene levels in fetal and adult lung have shown that leukotriene content of fetal lung fluid is extremely low and much lower than adult levels (3). In addition, there was no change in lung leukotrienes during the transition in ovine fetuses (3).

Prostacyclin, the major prostanoid metabolite in fetal lung, can be shown to be produced in fetal pulmonary vessels in vitro (200) and causes potent vasodilatation when infused into the fetal pulmonary circulation (34). In addition, a number of studies have shown increased prostacyclin production during normal transition (3, 119), and acute cyclooxygenase inhibition modestly attenuates the drop in pulmonary vascular resistance at birth (40) but does not inhibit the normal fall in vascular resistance induced by oxygenation and ventilation of the ovine fetus (209). Prostacyclin synthesis appears to be regulated by oxygen tension and shear stress (158, 183, 208) in cultured cells.

The developmental regulation of prostacyclin synthesis in the pulmonary artery has been studied in an elegant series of experiments by Brannon et al. (22). These studies showed that prostacyclin synthesis increases during late gestation in the pulmonary, but not mesenteric, arteries and is due to an increase in cyclooxygenase-1 expression and activity (22).

Prostaglandins of the D and E series cause vasodilation when infused into the fetal lung (32, 33). Prostglandin E1 is important in maintaining patency of the fetal ductus, and it seems likely that a change in the production of local prostaglandins stimulated by a change in the oxygen environment at birth leads to closure of the ductus arteriosus.

REFERENCES

1. Abman, S.H., B.A. Chatfield, S.L. Hall, and I.F. McMurtry. Role of endothelium-derived relaxing factor during transition of the pulmonary circulation at birth. *Am. J. Physiol.* 259: H1921–H1927, 1990.
2. Abman, S.H., B.A. Chatfield, D.M. Rodman, S.L. Hall, and I.F. McMurtry. Maturational changes in endothelium-derived relaxing factor activity of ovine pulmonary arteries in vitro. *Am. J. Physiol.* 260: L280–L285, 1991.
3. Abman, S.H. and K.R. Stenmark. Changes in lung eicosanoid content during normal and abnormal transition in perinatal lambs. *Am. J. Physiol.* 262: L214–L222, 1992.
4. Amaya, E., T.J. Musci, and M.W. Kirschner. Expression of a dominant negative mutant of the FGF receptor disrupts mesoderm formation in *Xenopus* embryos. *Cell* 66: 257–270, 1991.
5. Antonelli-Orlidge, A., K.B. Saunders, S.R. Smith, and P.A. D'Amore. An activated form of transforming growth factor beta is produced by cocultures of endothelial cells and pericytes. *Proc. Natl. Acad. Sci. USA* 86: 4544–4548, 1989.
6. Au, Y.P., R.D. Kenagy, M.M. Clowes, and A.W. Clowes. Mechanisms of inhibition by heparin of vascular smooth muscle cell proliferation and migration. *Haemostasis* 23: 177–182, 1993.
7. Ausprunk, D.H. Distribution of hyaluronic acid and sulfated glycosaminoglycans during blood vessel development in the chick chorioallantoic membrane. *Am. J. Anat.* 177: 313–331, 1986.
8. Ausprunk, D.H., S.M. Dethlefsen, and E.R. Higgins. Distribution of fibronectin, laminin and type IV collagen during development of blood vessels in the chick chorioallantoic membrane. In: *The Development of the Vascular System, Issues in Biomedicine,* Vol. 14. edited by R.N. Feinberg, G.K. Sherer, and R. Auerbach, Basel: Karger, 1991, p. 93–108.
9. Azar, Y. and H. Eyal-Giladi. Marginal zone cells—the primitive streak-inducing component of the primary hypoblast in the chick. *J. Embryol. Exp. Morphol.* 52: 79–88, 1979.
10. Barnes, K., L.J. Murphy, M. Takahashi, K. Tanzawa, and A.J. Turner. Localization and biochemical characterization of endothelin-converting enzyme. *J. Cardiovasc. Pharmacol.* 26 (Suppl. 3): S37–S39, 1995.
11. Barzu, T., J.-M. Herbert, A. Desmouliere, P. Carayon, and M. Pascal. Characterization of rat aortic smooth muscle cells resistant to the antiproliferative activity of heparin following long-term heparin treatment. *J. Cell. Physiol.* 160: 239–248, 1994.
12. Belknap, J.K., E.C. Orton, B. Ensley, and K.R. Stenmark. Hypoxia increases bromode-

oxyuridine labeling indices in bovine neonatal pulmonary arteries. *Am. J. Respir. Cell. Mol. Biol.* 16: 366–371, 1997.

13. Belknap, J.K., M.C.M. Weiser, S.S. Grieshaber, N.A. Grieshaber, and R.A. Majack, K.R. Stenmark. Relationship between perlecan and tropoelastin gene expression and cell replication in the developing rat pulmonary vasculature. *Am. J. Respir. Cell Mol. Biol.* (In Press).
14. Benitz, W.E., R.T. Kelley, C.M. Anderson, D.E. Lorant, and M. Bernfield. Endothelial heparan sulfate proteoglycan. I. Inhibitory effects on smooth muscle cell proliferation. *Am. J. Resp. Cell. Molec. Biol.* 2: 13–24, 1990.
15. Berk, B.C., V. Verkstein, H.M. Gordon, and T. Tsuda. Angiotension II–stimulated protein synthesis in cultured vascular smooth muscle cells. *Hypertension* 13: 305–314, 1989.
16. Bobik, A., A. Grooms, J.W. Millar, A. Mitchell, and S. Grinpukl. Growth factor activity of endothelin on vascular smooth muscle. *Am. J. Physiol. (Cell. Physiol.)* 258: C408–C415, 1990.
17. Botney, M.D., M.J. Liptay, L.R. Kaiser, J.D. Cooper, W.C. Parks, and R.P. Mecham. Active collagen synthesis by pulmonary vascular cells in human primary pulmonary hypertension. *Am. J. Pathol.* 143: 121–129, 1993.
18. Bowersox, J.C. and N. Sogente. Chemotaxis of aortic endothelial cells in response to fibrin. *Cancer Res.* 42: 2547–2551, 1982.
19. Boyd, J.D. Development of the heart. In: *Handbook of Physiology, Section 2, Circulation, Vol. III,* edited by W.F. Hamilton, Washington, DC: American Physiological Society, 1965, p. 2511–2543.
20. Boyden, E.A. The developing bronchial arteries in a fetus of the twelfth week. *Am. J. Anat.* 129: 357–368, 1970.
21. Brain, S.D., D.C. Crossman, T.L. Buckley, and T.J. Williams. Endothelin-1: demonstration of potent effects on the microcirculation of human and other species. *J. Cardiovasc. Pharmacol.* 13: 147–149, 1989.
22. Brannon, T.S., A.J. North, L.B. Wells, and P.W. Shaul. Prostacyclin synthesis in ovine pulmonary artery is developmentally regulated by changes in cyclooxygenase-1 gene expression. *J. Clin. Invest.* 93: 2230–2235, 1994.
23. Breier, G., M. Clauss, and W. Risau. Coardinate expression of vascular endothelial growth factor receptor-1 (flt-1) and its ligand suggests a paracrine regulation of of murine vascular development. *Dev. Dyn.* 204: 228–239, 1995.
24. Brooks, P.C., R.A.F. Clark, and D.A. Cheresh. Requirement of vascular integrin $\alpha v\beta 3$ for angiogenesis. *Science* 264: 569–571, 1994.
25. Brown, A.J. The development of the pulmonary vein in the domestic cat. *Anat. Rec.* 7: 299–329, 1913.
26. Bucher, U. and L. Reid. Development of the intrasegmental bronchial tree: the pattern of branching and development of cartilage at various stages of intra-uterine life. *Thorax* 16: 207–218, 1961.
27. Burgess, W.H. and T. Maciag. The heparin binding (fibroblast) growth factor family of proteins. *Annu. Rev. Biochem.* 58: 575–601, 1989.
28. Burri, P.H. Fetal and postnatal development of the lung. *Annu. Rev. Physiol.* 46: 617–628, 1984.
29. Butler, H. Some derivatives of the foregut venous plexus of the albino rat, with reference to man. *J. Anat.* 86: 95–109, 1952.
30. Carey, D.J. Control of growth and differentiation of vascular cells by extracellular matrix proteins. *Annu. Rev. Physiol.* 53: 161–177, 1991.

31. Cassin, S., G.S. Dawes, and B.B. Ross. Pulmonary blood flow and vascular resistance in immature fetal lambs. *J. Physiol.* (Lond.) 171: 80–89, 1964.
32. Cassin, S., M.L. Tod, J. Phillips, F. Frisinger, J. Jordan, and C. Gibbs. Effects of prostaglandin D_2 on the perinatal circulation. *Am. J. Physiol.* 240: H755–H760, 1981.
33. Cassin, S., T. Tyler, C. Leffler, and R. Wallis. Pulmonary and systemic vascular responses of perinatal goats to prostaglandin E1 and E2. *Am. J. Physiol.* 236: H828–H832, 1979.
34. Castelott, J.J., M.L. Addonzio, R.D. Rosenberg, and M.J. Karnovsky. Cultured endothelial cells produce a heparin-like inhibitor of smooth muscle cell growth. *J. Cell. Biol.* 90: 372–379, 1981.
34a Claesson-Welsh, L., M. Welsh, N. Ito, B. Anand-Apte, S. Soker, B. Zetter, M. O'Reilly, and J. Folkman. Angiostatin induces endothelial cell apoptosis and activation of focal adhesion kinase independently of the integrin-binding motif RGD. *Proc. Natl. Acad. Sci. USA* 95: 5579–5583, 1998.
35. Clozel, J.-P., C. Saunier, D. Hartemann, and W. Fischli. Effects of cilazapril, a novel angiotensin converting enzyme inhibitor, on the structure of pulmonary arteries of rats exposed to chronic hypoxia. *J. Cardiovasc. Pharmacol.* 17: 36–40, 1991.
36. Coffin, J.D. and T.J. Poole. Embryonic vascular development: immunohistochemical identification of the origin and subsequent morphogenesis of the major vessel primordia in quail embryos. *Development* 102: 735–748, 1988.
37. Congdon, E.D. Transformation of the aortic arch system during the development of the human embryo. *Carnegie Inst. Contrib. Embryol.* 14: 47–110, 1922.
38. Cook, C.L., M.C.M. Weiser, P.E. Schwartz, C.L. Jones, and R.A. Majack. Developmentally timed expression of an embryonic growth phenotype in vascular smooth muscle cells. *Circ. Res.* 74: 189–196, 1993.
39. Cornfield, D.N., H.L. Reeve, S. Tolarova, E.K. Weir, and S. Archer. Oxygen causes fetal pulmonary vasodilation through activation of a calcium-dependent potassium channel. *Proc. Natl. Acad. Sci. USA* 93: 8089–8094, 1996.
40. Davidson, D. Pulmonary hemodynamics at birth: effects of acute cyclooxygenase inhibition in lambs. *J. Appl. Physiol.* 64: 1676–1682, 1988.
41. Davidson, J.M., K.E. Hill, M.L. Mason, and M.G. Giro. Longitudinal gradient of collagen and elastin gene expression in the procine aorta. *J. Biol. Chem.* 260: 1901–1908, 1985.
42. Davis, S., T.H. Aldrich, P.F. Jones, A. Acheson, D.L. Compton, V. Jain, R.E. Ryan, J. Bruno, C. Radziejewski, P.C. Maisonpierre, and G.D. Yancopoulos. Isolation of angiopoietin-1, a ligand for the TIE2 receptor, by secretion-trap expression cloning. *Cell* 87: 1161–1169, 1996.
43. DeFouw, D.O. Structural heterogeneity within the pulmonary microcirculation of the normal rat. *Anat. Rec.* 221: 645–654, 1988.
44. Dempsey, E.C., D.B. Badesch, E. Dobyns, and K.R. Stenmark. Enhanced growth capacity of neonatal pulmonary artery smooth muscle cells in vitro: Dependence on cell size, time of harvest, insulin-like growth factor-1, and auto-activation of protein kinase C. *J. Cell. Physiol.* 160: 469–481, 1994.
45. Dempsey, E.C., S.J. Walchak, J.L Peach, and K.R. Stenmark. Adult bovine PA adventitial fibroblasts, but not matched SMC, have a potential PKC-dependent autocrine growth loop. *Am. Rev. Respir. Dis.* 145: A481, 1992.
45a. DeLisser, H.M. H.S. Baldwin, and S.M. Albelda. Platelet endothelial cell adhesion molecule 1 (PECAM-1/CD31): a multifunctional vascular cell adhesion molecule. *Trends Cardiovasc. Med.* 7: 203–210, 1997.

45b DeLisser, H.M., M. Christofidou-Solomidou, R.M. Strieter, M.D. Burdick, C.S. Robinson, R.S. Wexler, J.S. Kerr, C. Garlanda, J.R. Merwin, J.A. Madri, and S.M. Albelda. Involvement of endothelial PECAM-1/CD31 in angiogensis. *Am J. Pathol.* 151: 671–677, 1997.

45c deMello D.E., D. Sawyer, N. Galvin, and L.M. Reid. Early fetal development of lung vasculature. *Am. J. Respir. Cell. Mol. Biol.* 16: 568–581, 1997.

46. DeRuiter, M.C., A.C. Gittenberger-de-Groot, R.E. Poelmann, L. VanIperen, and M.M. Mentink. Development of the pharyngeal arch system related to the pulmonary and bronchial vessels in the avian embryo. With a concept on systemic-pulmonary collateral artery formation. *Circulation* 87: 1306–1319, 1993.

47. DeRuiter, M.C., A.C. Gittenberger-de Groot, S. Ramos, and R.E. Poelmann. The special status of the pulmonary arch artery in the branchial arch system of the rat. *Anat. Embryol.* 179: 319–325, 1989.

47a. Dickson, M.C., J.S. Martin, F.M. Cousins, A.B. Kulkarni, S. Karlsson, and R.J. Akhurst. Defective hematopoiesis and vasculogenesis in transforming growth factor-beta 1 knock out mice. *Development* 121: 1845–1854, 1995.

48. Drake, C.J. and C.D. Little. Exogenous vascular endothelial growth factor induces malformed and hyperfused vessels during embryonic neovascularization. *Proc. Natl. Acad. Sci. USA* 92: 7657–7661, 1995.

49. Dumont, D.J., G.-H. Fong, M.C. Puri, G. Gradwohl, K. Alitalo, and M.L. Breitman. Vascularization of the mouse embryo: a study of *flk-1, tek,* and *tie,* and vascular endothelial growth factor expression during development. *Dev. Dyn.* 203: 80–92, 1995.

50. Dumont, D.J., G.J. Gradwohl, G.-H. Fong, R. Auerbach, and M.L. Breitman. The endothelial-specific receptor tyrosine kinase, *tek,* is a member of a new subfamily of receptors. *Oncogene* 8: 1293–1301, 1993.

51. Dumont, D.J., G.J. Gradwohl, G.-H. Fong, M.C. Puri, M. Gertsenstein, A. Auerbach, and M.L. Breitman. Dominant-negative and targeted null mutations in the endothelial receptor tyrosine kinase, *tek,* reveal a critical role in vasculogenesis of the embryo. *Genes Dev.* 8: 1897–1909, 1994.

52. Dumont, D.J., T.P. Yamaguchi, R.A. Conlon, J. Rossant, and M.L. Breitman. *tek,* a novel tyrosine kinase gene located on mouse chromosome 4, is expressed in endothelial cells and their presumptive precursors. *Oncogene* 7: 1471–1480, 1992.

53. Durmowicz, A.G., W.C. Parks, D.M. Hyde, R.P. Mecham, and K.R. Stenmark. Persistence, re-expression, and induction of pulmonary arterial fibronectin, tropoelastin, and type I procollagen mRNA expression in neonatal hypoxic pulmonary hypertension. *Am. J. Pathol.* 145: 1411–1420, 1994.

54. Ferrara, N., K.A. Houck, L.B. Jakeman, J. Winer, and D.W. Leung. The vascular endothelial growth factor family of polypeptides. *J. Cell. Biochem.* 47: 211–218, 1991.

55. Flamme, I., G. Breier, and W. Risau. Vascular endothelial growth factor (VEGF) and VEGF receptor 2 (flk-1) are expressed during vasculogenesis and vascular differentiation in the quail embryo. *Dev. Biol.* 169: 699–712, 1995.

56. Flamme, I. and W. Risau. Induction of vasculogenesis and hematopoiesis in vitro. *Development* 116: 435–439, 1992.

57. Folkman, J. and P.A. D'Amore. Blood vessel formation: what is its molecular basis. *Cell* 87: 1153–1155, 1996.

58. Folkman, J. and M. Klagsbrun. Vascular physiology A family of angiogenic peptides. *Nature* 329: 671–672, 1987.

59. Fong, G.H., J. Rossaant, M. Gertsenstein, and M.L. Breitman. Role of the Flt-1 receptor

tyrosine kinase in regulating the assembly of vascular endothelium. *Nature* 376: 66–70, 1995.

60. Form, D.M., B.M. Pratt, and J.A. Madri. Endothelial cell proliferation during angiogenesis. In vitro modulation by basement membrane components. *Lab. Invest.* 55: 521–530, 1986.
61. Frid, M.G., A.A Aldashev, E.C. Dempsey and K.R. Stenmark. Smooth Muscle Cells Isolated From Discrete Compartments of the Mature Vascular Media Exhibit Unique Phenotypes and Distinct Growth Capabilities. *Circ. Res.* 81: 940–952, 1997.
62. Frid, M.G., B.V. Shekhonin, V.E. Koteliansky, and M.A. Glukhova. Phenotypic changes of human smooth muscle cells during development: late expression of heavy caldesmon and calponin. *Dev. Biol.* 153: 185–193, 1992.
63. Frid, M.G., and K.R. Stenmark. An immature smooth muscle cell subpopulation exists in the normal adult bovine pulmonary arterial media. *Am. J. Respir. Crit. Care Med.* 149: A823, 1994.
64. Frid, M.G. and K.R. Stenmark. Distinct adult bovine arterial smooth muscle cell subpopulations exhibit unique growth characteristics in vitro. *Am. J. Respir. Crit. Care Med.* 151: A526, 1995.

64a. Friedlander, M., C.L. Theesfeld, M. Sugita, M. Fruttiger, M.A. Thomas, S. Chang, and D.A. Cheresh. Involvement of integrins αVβ3 and αVβ5 in ocular neovascular diseases. *Proc. Natl. Acad. Sci. USA* 93: 9764–9769, 1996.

64b Friedlander, M., P.C. Brooks, R.W. Shaffer, C.M. Kincaid, J.A. Varner, and D.A. Cheresh. Definition of two angiogenic pathways by distinct αV intigrins. *Science* 270: 1500–1502, 1995.

65. Friesel, R.E. and T. Maciag. Molecular mechanisms of angiogenesis: fibroblast growth factor signal transduction. *FASEB J.* 9: 919–925, 1995.
66. Fritze, L.M., C.F. Reilly, and R.D. Rosenberg. An antiproliferative heparan sulfate species produced by postconfluent smooth muscle cells. *J. Cell. Biol.* 100: 1041–1049, 1985.
67. Fu, Y.-M., P. Spirito, Z.-X. Yu, S. Biro, J. Sasse, J. Lei, V.J. Ferrans, S.E. Epstein, and W. Casscells. Acidic fibroblast growth factor in the developing rat embryo. *J. Cell Biol.* 114: 1261–1273, 1991.
68. Fujita, H., K. Shimokado, C. Yutani, S. Takaichi, J. Masuda, and J. Ogata. Human neonatal and adult vascular smooth muscle cells in culture. *Exp. Mol. Pathol.* 58: 25–39, 1993.
69. Geisterfer, A.A.T., M.J. Peach, and G.K. Owens. Angiotensin II induces hypertrophy, not hyperplasia, of cultured rat aortic smooth muscle cells. *Circ. Res.* 62: 749–756, 1988.
70. George, E.L., E.N. Georges-Labouesse, R.S. Patel-King, H. Rayburn, and R.O. Hynes. Defects in mesoderm, neural tube and vascular development in mouse embryos lacking fibronectin. *Development* 119: 1079–1091, 1993.
71. Giaid, A., J.M. Polak, V. Gaitonde, Q.A. Hamid, G. Moscoso, S. Legon, D. Uwanogho, M. Roncalli, O. Shinmi, T. Sawamura, and D.R. Springall. Distribution of endothelin-like immunoreactivity and mRNA in the developing and adult human lung. *Am. J. Respir. Cell. Mol. Biol.* 4: 50–58, 1991.
72. Gibbons, G.H., R.E. Pratt, and V.J. Dzau. Vascular smooth muscle cell hypertrophy vs. hyperplasia. Autocrine transforming growth factor-β_1 expression determines growth response to angiotensin II. *J. Clin. Invest.* 90: 456–461, 1992.
73. Glukhova, M.A., M.G. Frid, and V.E. Koteliansky. Developmental changes in expression of contractile and cytoskeletal proteins in human aortic smooth muscle. *J. Biol. Chem.* 265: 13042–13046, 1990.

74. Glukhova, M.A., M.G. Frid, B.V. Shekhonin, Y.V. Balabanov, and V.E. Koteliansky. Expression of fibronectin variants in vascular and visceral smooth muscle cells in development. *Dev. Biol.* 141: 193–202, 1990.
75. Glukhova, M.A., A.E. Kabakov, A.M. Belkin, M.G. Frid, O.I. Ornatsky, N.I. Zhidkova, and V.E. Koteliansky. Metavinculin distribution in adult human tissues and cultured cells. *FEBS Lett.* 207: 139–141, 1986.
76. Glukhova, M.A., A.E. Kabakov, M.G. Frid, O.L. Ornatsky, A.M. Belkin, and D.N. Mukhin, et al. Modulation of human aorta smooth muscle cell phenotype: a study of muscle-specific variants of vinculin, caldesmon, and actin expression. *Proc. Natl. Acad. Sci. USA* 85: 9542–9546. 1988.
76a. Glukhova, M.A. and V.E. Koteliansky. Integrins, cytoskeletal and extracellular matrix proteins in developing smooth muscle cells of human aorta. In: *The Vascular Smooth Muscle Cell*, edited by S.M. Schwartz and R.P. Mecham, San Diego: Academic Press, 1995, p. 37–79.
77. Gonzalez, A.-M., M. Buscaglia, M. Ong, and A. Baird. Distribution of basic fibroblast growth factor in the 18 day rat fetus: localization in the basement membranes of diverse tissues. *J. Cell Biol.* 110: 753–765, 1990.
78. Gordon, J.B., M.L. Tod, R.C. Wetzel, M.L. McGeady, N.F. Adkinson, and J.T. Sylvester. Age-dependent effects of indomethacin on hypoxic vasoconstriction in neonatal lamb lungs. *Pediatr. Res.* 23: 580–584, 1988.
79. Gospodarowicz, D. and C. Ill. Extracellular matrix and control of proliferation of vascular endothelial cells. *J. Clin. Invest.* 65: 1351–1364, 1980.
80. Grady, E.F., L.A. Sechi, C.A. Griffin, M. Schambelan, and J.E. Kalinyak. Expression of AT2 receptors in the developing rat fetus. *J. Clin. Invest.* 88: 921–933, 1991.
81. Graf, J., Y. Iwamoto, M. Sasaki, G.R. Martin, H.K. Kleinman, F.A. Robey, and Y. Yamada. Identification of an amino acid sequence in laminin mediating cell attachment, chemotaxis and receptor binding. *Cell* 48: 989–996, 1987.
82. Grant, D.S., K.-I. Tashiro, B. Segui-Real, Y. Yamada, G.R. Martin, and H.K. Kleinman. Two different laminin domains mediate the differentiation of human endothelial cells into capillary-like structures. *Cell* 58: 933–943, 1989.
83. Greenblatt, M. and P. Shubik. Tumor angiogenesis: transfilter diffusion studies in the hamster by the transparent chamber technique. *J. Natl. Cancer Inst.* 41: 111–124, 1968.
84. Hagiwara, H., T. Nagasawa, T. Yamamoto, K.M. Lodhi, T. Ito, N. Takemura, and S. Hirose. Immunochemical characterization and localization of endothelin ETB receptor. *Am. J. Physiol.* 264: R777–R783, 1993.
85. Hain, L., G.S. Barsh, R.E. Pratt, V.J. Dzau, and B.K. Kobilka. Behavioral and cardiovascular effects of disrupting the angiotensin II type 2 receptor in mice. *Nature* 377: 744–747, 1995.
86. Halbower, A.C., R.M. Tuder, W.A. Franklin, J.S. Pollock, U. Förstermann, and S.H. Abman. Maturation-related changes in endothelial nitric oxide synthase immunolocalization in developing ovine lung. *Am. J. Physiol. (Lung Cell. Mol. Physiol.)* 267: L585–L591, 1994.
86a. Hanahan, D. and J. Folkman. Patterns and emerging mechanisms of the angiogenic switch during tumorgenesis. *Cell* 86: 353–364, 1996.
86b. Harris, A. Are angiostatin and endostatin cures for cancer? *Lancet* 351: 1598–1599, 1998.
87. Hedin, U., B.A. Bottger, E. Forsberg, S. Johansson, and J. Thyberg. Diverse effects of fi

bronectin and laminin on phenotypic properties of cultured arterial smooth muscle cells. *J. Cell Biol.* 107: 307–319, 1988.

88. Herbst, T.J., J.B. McCarthy, E.C. Tsilibary, and L.T. Furcht. Differential effects of laminin, intact type IV collagen, and specific domains of type IV collagen on endothelial cell adhesion and migration. *J. Cell Biol.* 106: 1365–1373, 1988.
89. Heymann, M.A., R.K. Creasy, and A.M. Rudolph. Quantitation of blood flow patterns in the foetal lamb in utero. In: *Proceedings of the Sir Joseph Barcroft Symposium: Foetal and Neonatal physiology,* Cambridge: Cambridge University Press, 1973, p. 129–135.
90. Heyward, S.A., N. Dubois-Stringfellow, R. Rapoport, and V.L. Bautch. Expression and inducibility of vascular adhesion receptors in development. *FASEB J.* 9: 956–962, 1995.
91. Hislop, A. and L. Reid. Intrapulmonary arterial development during fetal life—branching pattern and structure. *J. Anat.* 113: 35–48, 1972.
92. Holmgren, L., A. Glaser, S. Pfeifer-Ohlsson, and R. Ohlsson. Angiogenesis during human extraembryonic development involves the spatiotemporal control of PDGF ligand and receptor gene expression. *Development* 113: 749–754, 1991.
93. Hori, S., Y. Komatsu, R. Shigemoto, N. Mizuno, and S. Nakanishi. Distinct tissue distribution and cellular localization of two messenger ribonucleic acids encoding different subtypes of rat endothelin receptors. *Endocrinology* 130: 1885–1895, 1992.
94. Hu, N. and E.B. Clark. Hemodynamics of the stage 12 to stage 29 chick embryo. *Circ. Res.* 65: 1665–1670, 1989.
95. Huntingdon, G.S. The morphology of the pulmonary artery in the mammalia. *Anat. Rec.* 17: 165–189, 1919.
96. Hynes, R.P. Integrins: versatility, modulation and signaling in cell adhesion. *Cell* 69: 11–25, 1992.
97. Inoue, A., M. Yanagisawa, S. Kimura, Y. Kasuya, T. Miyauchi, K. Goto, and T. Masaki. The human endothelin family: three structurally and pharmacologically distinct isopeptides predicted by three separate genes. *Proc. Natl. Acad. Sci. USA* 86: 2863–2867, 1989
98. Ishimitsu, T., Y. Uehara, M. Ishii, T. Ikeda, H. Matsuoka, and T. Sugimoto. Thromboxane and vascular smooth muscle cell growth in genetically hypertensive rats. *Hypertension* 12: 46–51, 1988.
99. Ivy, D.D., J.P. Kinsella, and S.H. Abman. Physiologic characterization of endothelin A and B receptor activity in the ovine fetal pulmonary circulation. *J. Clin. Invest.* 93: 2141–2148, 1994.
100. Jones, K.W., M.H. Shapero, M. Chevrettm, and R.E.K. Fournier. Subtractive hybridization cloning of tissue-specific extinguisher: TSE1 encodes a regulatory subunit of protein kinase A. *Cell* 66: 861–872, 1991.
101. Jones, O.W. and S.H. Abman. Systemic and pulmonary hemodynamic effects of big endothelin-1 and phosphoramidon in the ovine fetus. *Am. J. Physiol.* 266: R929–R955, 1994.
102. Kawahara, Y., M. Sunako, T. Tsuda, H. Fukuzaki, Y. Fukumoto, and Y. Takai Angiotensin II induces expression of the c-f*OS* gene through protein kinase C activation and calcium ion mobilization in cultured vascular smooth muscle cells. *Biochem. Biophys. Res. Commun.* 150: 52–59, 1988.
103. Kawai, N., D.B. Bloch, G. Filippov, D. Rabkina, H.-C. Suen, P.D. Losty, S.P. Janssens, W.M. Zapol, S. de la Monte, and K.D. Bloch. Constitutive endothelial nitric oxide synthase gene expression is regulated during lung development. *Am. J. Physiol.* 268: L589–L595, 1995.

104. Keeley, F.W. and M. Rabinovitch. Vascular matrix metabolism in hypertension. In *Pulmonary Vascular Remodeling*, Vol. 5, edited by J.E. Bishop, J.T. Reeves, and G.J. Laurent. London: Portland Press, 1995, p. 149–169.

105. Kingsley, D.M. The TGF-beta superfamily: new members, new receptors, and new genetic tests of function in different organisms. *Genes Dev.* 8: 133–146, 1994.

106. Kinsella, J.P., D.D. Ivy, and S.H. Abman. Ontogeny of NO activity and response to inhaled NO in the developing ovine pulmonary circulation. *Am. J. Physiol.* 267: H1955–H1961, 1994.

107. Kleinman, H.K., F.B. Cannon, G.W. Laurie, J.R. Hassell, M. Aumailley, V.P. Terranova, G.R. Martin, and M. Dubois-Dalcq. Biological activities of laminin. *J. Cell Biol.* 27: 317–325, 1985.

108. Kocher, O. and G. Gabbiani. Expression of actin mRNA in rat aortic smooth muscle cells during development, experimental intimal thickening, and culture. *Differentiation* 32: 245–251, 1986.

109. Komuro, I., H. Kurihara, T. Sugiyama, M. Yoshizumi, F. Takaku, and Y. Yazaki. Endothelin stimulates c-*fos* and c-*myc* expression and proliferation of vascular smooth muscle cells. *FEBS Lett.* 238: 249–252, 1988.

110. Korhonen, J., A. Polvi, J. Partanen, and K. Alitalo. The mouse *tie* receptor tyrosine kinase gene: expression during embryonic angiogenesis. *Oncogene* 9: 395–403, 1994.

111. Kornblihtt, A.R., K. Umezawa, K. Vige-Pedersen, and F. Baralle. Primary structure os human fibronectin: differential splicing may generate at least 10 polypeptides from a single gene. *EMBO J.* 4: 1755–1759, 1985.

112. Kratochwil, K., M. Dziadek, J. Lohler, K. Harbers, and R. Jaenisch. Normal epithelial branching morphogenesis in the absence of collagen. *Dev. Biol.* 117: 596–606, 1986.

113. Kubota, Y., H.K. Kleinman, G.R. Martin, and T.J. Lawley. Role of laminin and basement membrane in the morphological differentiation of human endothelial cells in capillary-like structures. *J. Cell Biol.* 107: 1589–1598, 1988.

114. Kumar, S., D.C. West, and A. Ager. Heterogeneity in endothelial cells from large vessels and microvessels. *Differentiation* 36: 57–70, 1987.

115. Kurihara, Y., H. Kurihara, H. Oda, K. Maemura, R. Nagai, T. Ishikawa, et al. Aortic arch malformations and ventricular septal defect in mice deficient in endothelin-1. *J. Clin. Invest.* 96: 293–300, 1995.

116. Kuro-O, M., R. Nagai, H. Tsuchimochi, H. Katoh, Y. Yazaki, A. Ohkubo, and F. Takaku. Developmentally regulated expression of vascular smooth muscle myosin heavy chain isoforms. *J. Biol. Chem.* 264: 18272–18275, 1989.

117. Kuzuya, M. and J.L. Kinsella. Reorganization of endothelial cord-like structures on basement membrane complex (Matrigel): involvement of transforming growth factor beta 1. *J. Cell. Physiol.* 161: 267–276, 1994.

118. Lebiodes, J., S.J. Soifer, R.I. Clyman, and M.A. Heymann. Piriprost: a putative leukotriene synthesis inhibitor increases pulmonary blood flow in fetal lambs. *Pediatr. Res.* 22: 350–354, 1987.

119. Leffler, C.W., J.R. Hessler, and R.S. Green. The onset of breathing at birth stimulates pulmonary vascular prostacylin synthesis. *Pediatr. Res.* 18: 938–942, 1984.

120. Lemire, J.M., C.W. Covin, S. White, C.M. Giachelli, and S.M. Schwartz. Characterization of cloned aortic smooth muscle cells from young rats. *Am. J. Pathol.* 144: 1068–1081, 1994.

121. Leung, D.Y.M., S. Glagov, and M.B. Mathews. Elastin and collagen accumulation in rab-

bit ascending aorta and pulmonary trunk during postnatal growth. *Circ. Res.* 41: 316–323, 1977.

122. Leveen, P., M. Pekny, S. Gebre-Medhin, B. Swolin, E. Larsson, and C. Betsholtz. *Genes Dev.* 8: 1875–1887, 1994.
123. Levine, A.J. The tumorsuppressor genes. *Annu. Rev. Biochem.* 62: 623–651, 1993.
124. Li, X., P. Tsai, E.D. Wieder, A. Kribben, V. Van Putten, R.W. Schrier, and R.A. Nemenoff. Vascular smooth muscle cells grown on Matrigel. A model of the contractile phenotype with decreased activation of mitogen-activated protein kinase. *J. Biol. Chem.* 269: 19653–19658, 1994.
125. Liu, S.F., A.A. Hislop, S.G. Haworth, and P.J. Barnes. Developmental changes in endothelium-dependent pulmonary vasodilatation in pigs. *Br. J. Pharmacol.* 106: 324–330, 1992.
126. Lock, J.E., P.M. Olley, S. Soldin, and F. Coceani. Indomethacin-induced pulmonary vasoconstriction in the conscious newborn lamb. *Am. J. Physiol.* 238: H639–H651, 1980.
127. MacCumber, M.W., C.A. Ross, B.M. Glaser, and S.H. Snyder. Endothelin: visualization of mRNAs by in situ hybridization provides evidence for local action. *Proc. Natl. Acad. Sci. USA* 86: 7285–7289, 1989.
128. Madri, J.A. Endothelial cell-matrix interactions. In: *Progress in Thrombosis and Hemostasis*, Vol. 6, edited by T. Spaet, New York: Grune and Stratton, 1982, p. 1–24.
129. Madri, J.A. and S.K. Williams. Capillary endothelial cell cultures: phenotypic modulation by matrix components. *J. Cell Biol.* 97: 153–165, 1983.

129a. Maisonpierre, P.C., C. Suri, P.F. Jones, S. Bartunkova, S.J. Wiegand, C. Radziejewski, D. Compton, J. McClain, T.H. Aldrich, N. Papadopoulos, T.J. Daly, S. Davis, T.N. Sato, and G.D. Yancopoulos. Angiopoitin-2, a natural antagonist for Tie2 that disrupts in vivo angiogenesis. *Science*, 277: 55–60, 1997.

130. Majack, R.A. Extinction of autonomous growth potential in embryonic:adult vascular smooth muscle cell heterokaryons. *J. Clin. Invest.* 95: 464–468, 1995.
131. Majack, R.A. and A.W. Clowes. Inhibition of vascular smooth muscle cell migration by heparin-like glycosaminoglycans. *J. Cell. Physiol.* 118: 253–256, 1984.
132. McQueston, J.A., J.P. Kinsella, D.D. Ivy, I.F. McMurtry, and S.H. Abman. Chronic pulmonary hypertension in utero impairs endothelium-dependent vasodilation. *Am J. Physiol.* 268: H288–H294, 1995.
133. Mecham, R.P., K.R. Stenmark, and W.C. Parks. Connective tissue production by vascular smooth muscle in development and disease. *Chest* 99: 43S–47S, 1991.
134. Mikawa, T. and D.A. Fischman. Retroviral analysis of cardiac morphogenesis: discontinuous formation of coronary vessels. *Proc. Natl. Acad. Sci. USA* 89: 9504–9508, 1992.
135. Millauer B., S. Wizigmann-Voos, H. Schnurch, R. Martinez, N.P. Moller, W. Risau, and A. Ullrich. High-affinity VEGF binding and developmental expression suggest Flk-1 as a major regulator of vasculogenesis and angiogenesis. *Cell* 72: 835–846, 1993.
136. Mills, A.N. and S.G. Haworth. Pattern of connective tissue development in swine pulmonary vasculature by immunolocalization. *J. Pathol.* 153: 171–176, 1987.
137. Morin, F.C. and K.R. Stenmark. Persistent pulmonary hypertension of the newborn. State-of-the-Art. *Am. J. Respir. Crit. Care Med.* 151: 2010–2032, 1995.
138. Morrell, N.W., S.S. Grieshaber, S.M. Danilov, R.A. Majack, and K.R. Stenmark. Developmental regulation of angiotensin converting enzyme and angiotensin type I receptor in the rat pulmonary circulation. *Am. J. Respir. Cell. Mol. Biol.* 14: 526–537, 1996.

138a. Muller, W.A., C.M. Ratti, S.L. McDonnell, and Z.A. Cohn. A human endothelial cell-restricted externally disposed plasmalemmal protein enriched in intercellular junctions. *J. Exp. Med.* 170: 399–414, 1989.

139. Muthuchamy, M., L. Pajak, P. Howles, T. Doetschman, and D.F. Wieczorek Developmental analysis of trypomyosin gene expression in embryonic stem cells and mouse embryos. *Mol. Cell. Biol.* 13: 3311–3323, 1993.
140. Myers, B., M. Dubich, J.A. Last, and R.B. Ruche. Elastin synthesis during perinatal lung development in the rat. *Biochem. Biophys. Acta* 761: 17–22, 1983.
141. Nakamichi, K., M. Ihara, M. Kobayashi, T. Saeki, K. Ishikawa, and M. Yano. Different distribution of endothelin receptor subtypes in pulmonary tissues revealed by the novel selective ligands BQ-123 and [Ala 1,3,11,15]ET-1. *Biochem. Biophys. Res. Commun.* 182: 144–150, 1992.
142. Nemecek, G.M., S.R. Coughlin, D.A. Handley, and M.A. Moskowitz. Stimulation of aortic smooth muscle cell mitogenesis by serotonin. *Proc. Natl. Acad. Sci. USA* 83: 674–678, 1986.
143. Neylon, C.B., P.V. Avdonin, R.J. Dilley, M.A. Larsen, V.A. Tkachuk, and A. Bobik. Different electrical responses to vasoactive agonists in morphologically distinct smooth muscle cell types. *Circ. Res.* 75: 733–741, 1994.
144. Nguyen, M., N.A. Strubel, and J. Bischoff. A role for sialyl Lewis-X/A glycoconjugates in capillary morphogenesis. *Nature* 365: 267–269, 1993.
145. Nilsson, J., A.M. Von Euler, and C.J. Dalsgaard. Stimulation of connective tissue cell growth by substance P and substance K. *Nature* 315: 61–63, 1985.
146. North, A.J.J., R.A. Star, T.S. Brannon, K. Ujiie, L.B. Wells, C.J. Lowenstein, S.H. Snyder, and P.W. Shaul. Nitric oxide synthase type I and type III gene expression are developmentally regulated in rat lung. *Am. J. Physiol.* 266: L635–L641, 1994.
146a. O'Reilly, M.S., T. Boehm, Y. Shing, N. Fukai, G. Vasios, W.S. Lane, E. Flinn, J.R. Birkhead, B.R. Olsen, and J. Folkman. Endostatin: an endogenous inhibitor of angiogenesis and tumor growth. *Cell* 88: 277–285, 1997.
147. Osborn, M., J. Caselitz, and K. Weber. Heterogeneity of intermediate filament expression in vascular smooth muscle: a gradient in desmin positive cells from the rat aortic arch to the level of the arteria iliaca communis. *Differentiation* 20: 196–202, 1981.
148. Owens, G.K. Regulation of differentiation of vascular smooth muscle cells. *Physiol. Rev.* 75: 487–517, 1995.
149. Palmberg, L., H.E. Clawsson, and J. Thyberg. Leukotrienes stimulate initiation of DNA synthesis in cultured arterial smooth muscle cells. *J. Cell Sci.* 88: 151–159, 1987.
150. Pardanaud, L., C. Altman, P. Kitos, F. Dieterlen-Lievre, and C.A. Buck. Vasculogenesis in the early quail blastodisc as studied with a monoclonal antibody recognizing endothelial cells. *Development* 100: 339–349, 1987.
151. Pardanaud, L., F. Yassine, and F. Dieterlen-Li˘8Avre. Relationship between vasculogenesis, angiogenesis and haemopoiesis during avian ontogeny. *Development* 105: 473–485, 1989.
151a. Patterson, B.C. and Q.A. Sang. Angiostatin-converting enzyme activities of human Matrilysin (MMP-7) and Gelatinase B/Type IV collagenase (MMP-9). *J. Biol. Chem.* 272: 28823–28825, 1997.
152. Peters, K.G., C. De Vries, and L.T. Williams. Vascular endothelial growth factor receptor expression during embryogenesis and tissue repair suggests a role in endothelial differentiation and blood vessel growth. *Proc. Natl. Acad. Sci. USA* 90: 8915–8919, 1993.
153. Peters, K.G., S. Werner, G. Chen, and L.T. Williams. Two FGF receptor genes are differ-

entially expressed in epithelial and mesenchymal tissues during limb formation and organogenesis in the mouse. *Development* 114: 233–243, 1992.

154. Pitt, B.R., G. Lister, P. Davies, and L. Reid. Correlation of pulmonary ACE activity and capillary surface area during postnatal development. *J. Appl. Physiol.* 62: 2031–2041, 1987.
155. Powel, J.T. and P.L. Whitney. Postnatal development of rat lung. *Biochem. J.* 188: 1–8, 1980.
156. Prosser, I.W., K.R. Stenmark, M. Suthar, R.P. Mecham, E.C. Crouch, and W.C. Parks. Regional heterogeneity of elastin and collagen gene expression in intralobar arteries in response to hypoxic pulmonary hypertension as demonstrated by in situ hybridization. *Am. J. Pathol.* 135: 1073–1088, 1989.
157. Pryde, P.G., A.B. Sedman, C.E. Nugent, and M. Barr. Angiotensin converting enyme inhibitor fetopathy. *J. Am. Soc. Nephrol.* 3: 1575–1582, 1993.
158. Rabinovitch, M., N. Boudreau, G. Vella, F. Coceani, and P.M. Olley. Oxygen-related prostaglandin sythesis in ductus arteriosus and other vascular cells. *Pediatr. Res.* 26: 330–335, 1989.
159. Rabinovitch, M., W. Gamble, A.S. Nada, O.S. Miettinen, and L. Reid. Rat pulmonary circulation after chronic hypoxia: hemodynamic and structural features. *Am. J. Physiol.* 236: H818–H827, 1979.
160. Rastinejad, F., and H.M. Blau. Genetic complementation reveals a novel regulatory role for 3′ untranslated regions in growth and differentiation. *Cell* 72: 903–917, 1993.
161. Reagan, F.P. Vascularization phenomena in fragments of embryonic bodies completely isolated from yolk-sac entoderm. *Anat. Rec.* 9: 329–341, 1915.
162. Resink, T.J., A.W.A. Hahn, T. Scott-Burden, J. Powell, F. Webber, and F.R. Buhler. Inducible endothelin mRNA expression and peptide secretion in cultured human vascular smooth muscle cells. *Biochem. Biophys. Res. Commun.* 168: 1303–1310, 1990.
163. Risau, W. and V. Lemmon. Changes in the vascular extracellular matrix during embryonic vasculogenesis and angiogenesis. *Dev. Biol.* 125: 441–450, 1988.
164. Roman, J., C.W. Little, and J.A. McDonald. Potential role of RGD-binding integrins in mammalian lung branching morphogenesis. *Development* 112: 551–558, 1991.
165. Rothman, A., T.J. Kulik, M.B. Taubman, B.C, Berk, C.W.J. Smith, and B. Nadal-Ginard. Development and characterization of a cloned rat pulmonary arterial smooth muscle cell line that maintains differentiated properties through multiple subcultures. *Circulation* 86: 1977–1986, 1992.
166. Ruoslahti, E., E. Engvall, and E.G. Hayman. Fibronectin: current concepts of its structure and function. *Collagen Res.* 1: 95–128, 1981.
167. Ruoslahti, E. and M.D. Pierschbacher. New perspectives in cell adhesion. *Science* 238: 491–497, 1987.
168. Sariola, H., P. Ekblom, E. Lehtonen, and L. Saxen. Differentiation and vascularization of the metanephric kidney grafted on the chorioallantoic membrane. *Dev. Biol.* 96: 427–435, 1983.
169. Sartore, S., M. Scatena, A. Chiavegato, E. Faggin, L. Giuriato, and P. Pauletto. Myosin isoform expression in smooth muscle cells during physiological and pathological vascular remodeling. *J Vasc. Res.* 31: 61–81, 1994.
170. Sato, T.N., Y. Qin, C.A. Kozak, and K.L. Audus. *tie–1* and *tie-2* define another class of putative receptor tyrosine kinase genes expressed in early embryonic vascular system. *Proc. Natl. Acad Sci. USA* 90: 9355–9358, 1993.

171. Sato, T.N., Y. Tozawa, U. Deutsch, K. Wolburg-Buchholz, Y, Fujiwara, M. Gendron-Maguire, T. Gridley, H. Wolburg, W. Risau, and Y. Qin. Distinct roles of the receptor tryosine kinases Tie-1 and Tie-2 in blood vessel formation. *Nature* 376: 70–74, 1995.

171a. Sato, T.N. A new approach to fighting cancer? *Proc. Natl. Acad. USA* 95: 5843–5844, 1998.

172. Schnürch, H. and W. Risau. Expression of tie-2, a member of a novel family of receptor tyrosine kinases, in the endothelial cell lineage. *Development* 119: 957–968, 1993.

173. Schwartz, S.M., L. Foy, D.F. Bowen-Pope, and R. Ross. Derivation and properties of platelet-derived growth factor–independent rat smooth muscle cells. *Am. J. Pathol.* 136: 1417–1428, 1990.

174. Schweiki, D., A. Itin, D. Soffer, and E. Keshet. Vascular endothelial growth factor induced by hypoxia may mediate hypoxia-initiated angiogenesis. *Nature* 359: 843–845, 1992.

175. Scott-Burden, T., T.J. Resink, A.W.A. Hahn, and F.R. Buhler. Amiloride sensitive activation of S_6 kinase by angiotensin II in cultured vascular smooth muscle cells. *Biochem. Biophys. Res. Commun.* 151: 583–589, 1988.

176. Scott-Burden, T., T.J. Resink, A.W.A. Hahn, and F.R. Buhler. Angiotensin-induced growth related metabolism is activated in cultured smooth muscle cells from spontaneously hypertensive rats and Wistar-Kyoto rats. *Am. J. Hypertens.* 4: 183–188, 1991.

177. Selmin, O., D. Volpin, and G.M. Bressan. Changes of cellular expression of mRNA for tropoelastin in the intraembryonic arterial vessels o developing chick revealed by in situ hybridization. *Matrix* 11: 347–358, 1991.

178. Shanahan, C.M., P.L. Weissberg, and J.C. Metcalfe. Isolation of gene markers of differentiated and proliferating vascular smooth muscle cells. *Circ. Res.* 73: 193–204, 1993.

179. Shanmugan, S., P. Corvol, and J.-M. Gasc. Ontogeny of the two angiotensin II type I receptor subtypes in rats. *Am. J. Physiol.* 267: E828–E836, 1994.

180. Shanmugan, S., P. Corvol, and J.-M. Gasc. Angiotensin II type II receptor mRNA expression in the developing cardiopulmonary system of the rat. *Hypertension* 28: 91–97, 1996.

181. Shanmugan, S., C. Monnot, P. Corvol, and J.-M. Gasc. Distribution of type 1 angiotensin II receptor subtype messenger RNAs in the rat fetus. *Hypertension* 23: 137–141, 1994.

182. Shapero, M.H., A.A. Langston, and R.E. Fournier. Tissue-specific extinguisher loci in the human genome: a screening study based on random marking and transfer of human chromosomes. *Somat. Cell Mol. Genet.* 20: 215–231, 1994.

183. Shaul, P.W., W.B. Campbell, M.A. Farrar, and R.R. Magness. Oxygen modulates prostacyclin synthesis in ovine fetal pulmonary arteries by an effect on cyclooxygenase. *J. Clin. Invest.* 90: 2147–2155, 1992.

184. Shaul, P.W., M.A. Farrar, and R.R. Magness. Pulmonary endothelial nitric oxide production is developmentally regulated in the fetus and the newborn. *Am. J. Physiol.* 65: H1056–H1063, 1993.

185. Sheppard, A.M., M.D. Onken, G.D. Rosen, P.G. Noakes, and D.C. Dean. Expanding roles for alpha 4 integrin and its ligands in development. *Cell Adhesion Commun.* 2: 27–43, 1994.

186. Sherer, G.K. Vasculogenic mechanisms and epithelio-mesenchymal specificity in endodermal organs. In: *The Development of the Vascular System, Issues in Biomedicine*, Vol. 14, edited by R.N. Feinberg, G.K. Sherer, and R. Auerbach. Basel: Karger, 1991, p. 37–57.

187. Shifren, J.L., N. Doldi, N. Ferrara, S. Mesiano, and R.E. Jaffe. In the human fetus, vascular endothelial growth factor is expressed in epithelial cells and myocytes, but not vascular

endothelium: implications for mode of action. *J. Clin. Endocrinol. Metab.* 79: 316–322, 1994.

188. Shinbrot, E., K.G. Peters, and L.T. Williams. Expression of platelet-derived growth factor beta receptor during organogenesis and tissue differentiation in the mouse embryo. *Dev. Dyn.* 199: 169–175, 1994 .
189. Skalli, O., P. Ropraz, A. Trzeciak, G. Benzonana, D. Gillessen, and G. Gabbiani. A monoclonal antibody against a-smooth muscle actin: a new probe for smooth muscle differentiation. *J. Cell. Biol.* 103: 2787–2796, 1986.
190. Slack, J.M.W., B.G. Darlington, J.K. Heath, and S.F. Godsave. Mesoderm induction in early *Xenopus* embryos by heparin-binding growth factors. *Nature* 326: 197–200, 1987.
191. Soifer, S.J., R.D. Loitz, C. Roman, and M.A. Heyman. Leukotriene end-organ antagonists increase pulmonary blood flow in fetal lambs. *Am. J. Physiol.* 249: H570–H576, 1985.
192. Squier, T.L. On the development of the pulmonary circulation in the chick. *Anat. Rec.* 10: 425–438, 1916.
193. Stenmark, K.R., D.B. Badesch, E.C. Dempsey, M.G. Frid, R.P. Mecham, and W.C. Parks. Regulation of pulmonary vascular wall cell growth: developmental and site-specific heterogeneity. *Eur. Respir. Rev.* 3: 629–637, 1993.
194. Stenmark, K.R., S.L. James, N.F. Voelkel, W.H. Toews, J.T. Reeves, and R.C. Murphy. Leukotriene C4 and D4 in neonates with hypoxaemia and pulmonary hypertension. *N. Engl. J. Med.* 309: 377–380, 1983.
195. Stenmark, K.R., R.P. Mecham, A.G. Durmowicz, and W.C. Parks. Persistence of the fetal pattern of tropoelastin gene expression in severe neonatal pulmonary hypertension *J. Clin. Invest.* 93: 1234–1242, 1994.
196. Suri C., P.F. Jones, S. Patan, S. Bartunkova, P.C. Maisonpierre, S. Davis, T.N. Sato, and G.D. Yancopoulos. Requisite role of angiopoietin-1, and ligand for the TIE2 receptor, during embryonic angiogenesis. *Cell* 87: 1171–1180, 1996.
197. Takahashi, M., K. Fukuda, K. Shimada, K. Barnes, A.J. Turner, M. Ikeda, H. Koike, Y. Yamamoto, and K. Tanzawa. *Biochem. J.* 311: 657–5, 1995.
198. Takuwa, N., Y. Takuwa, M. Yanagisawa, K. Yamashita, and T. Masaki. A novel vasoactive peptide endothelin stimualtes mitogenesis through inositol lipid turnover in swiss 3T3 fibroblasts. *J. Biol. Chem.* 264: 7856–7861, 1989.
199. Tanswell, A.K., R.N. Han, D. Jassal, L.J. Fraher, and M. Post. The response of small vessel endothelial cells from fetal rat lung to growth factors. *J. Dev. Physiol.* 15: 199–209, 1991.
200. Terragno, N.A. and A. Terragno. Prostaglandin metabolism in the fetal and maternal vasculature. *Fed. Proc.* 38: 75–77, 1979.
201. Thyberg, J., U. Hedin, M. Sjolund, L. Palmberg, and B.A. Bottger. Regulation of differentiated properties and proliferation of arterial smooth muscle cells. *Atherosclerosis* 10: 966–990, 1990.
202. Thyberg, J. and A. Hultgardh-Nilsson. Fibronectin and the basement membrane components laminin and collagen type IV influence the phenotypic properties of subcultured rat aortic smooth muscle cells differently. *Cell Tissue Res.* 276: 263–271, 1994.
203. Tomlinson, A., H. Van Vlijmen, A. Loesch, and G. Burnstock. An immunohistochemical study of endothelial cell heterogeneity in the rat: observations in "en face" Hˇ84utchen preparations. *Cell Tissue Res.* 263: 173–181, 1991.
204. Tsutsumi, K., C. Stromberg, M. Viswanathan, and J.M. Saavedra. Angiotensin II receptor subtypes in fetal tissue of the rat: autoradiography, guanine nucleotide sensitivity, and association with phosphoinositide hydrolysis. *Endocrinology* 129: 1075–1082, 1991.

205. Tufro-McReddie, A., J.K. Harrison, A.D. Everett, and R.A. Gomez. Ontogeny of type I angiotensin II receptor gene expression in the rat. *J. Clin. Invest.* 91: 530–537.

206. Turla, M.B., M.M. Thompson, M.H. Corjay, and G.K. Owens. Mechanisms of angiotensin II- and arginine vasopressin-induced increases in protein synthesis and content in cultured rat aortic smooth muscle cells. *Circ. Res.* 68: 288–299, 1991.

207. Ungari, S., R.S. Katari, G. Alessandri, and P.M. Gullino. Cooperation between fibronectin and heparin in the mobilization of capillary endothelium. *Invasion Metast.* 5:193–205, 1985.

208. Van Grondelle, A., G.S. Worthen, D. Ellis, M.M. Mathias, R.C. Murphy, R.J. Strife, J.T. Reeves, and N.F. Voelkel. Altering hemodynamic variables influences PGI_2 production by isolated lungs and endothelial cells. *J. Appl. Physiol.* 57: 388–395,1984.

209. Velvis, H., P. Moore, and M.A. Heymann. Prostaglandin inhibition prevents the fall in pulmonary vascular resistance as a result of rhythmic distension of the lungs in fetal lambs. *Pediatr. Res.* 30: 62–68, 1991.

210. Viswanathan, M., K. Tsutsumi, F.M.A. Correa, and J.M. Saavedra. Changes in expression of angiotensin receptor subtypes in the rat aorta during development. *Biochem. Biophys. Res. Commun.* 179: 1361–1367, 1991.

210a. Waldo, K.L. and M.L. Kirby. Cardiac neural crest contribution to the pulmonary artery and sixth aortic arch artery complex in chick embryos aged 6 to 18 days. *Anat. Rec.* 237: 385–399, 1993.

211. Wallace, K.B., M.D. Bailie, and J.B. Hook. Angiotensin converting enzyme in developing lung and kidney. *Am. J. Physiol.* 234: R141–R145, 1978.

212. Wallace, K.B., M.D. Bailie, and J.B. Hook. Development of angiotensin converting enzyme in fetal rat lungs. *Am. J. Physiol.* 236: R57–R60, 1979.

213. Weiser, M.C.M., J.K. Belknap, S.S. Grieshaber, M.G. Kinsella, and R.A. Majack. Developmental regulation of perlecan gene expression in aortic smooth muscle cells. *Matrix Biol.* 15: 331–340.

214. Weiser, M.C.M., N.A. Grieshaber, P.W. Schwartz, and R.A. Majack. Perlecan regulates Oct-1 gene expression in vascular smooth muscle cells. *Mol. Biol. Cell* 8: 999–1011, 1997.

215. Wendt, C.H., V.A. Polunovsky, M.S. Peterson, P.B. Bitterman, and D.H. Ingbar. Alveolar epithelial cells regulate the induction of endothelial cell apoptosis. *Am. J. Physiol.* 267: C893–C900, 1994.

216. Winlove, C.P., J.E. Bishop, R.C. Chambers, and G.J. Laurent. The structure and function of extracellular matrix in the pulmonary vasculature. In: *Pulmonary Vascular Remodeling,* Vol. 2, edited by J.E. Bishop, J.T. Reeves, and G.J. Laurent. London: Portland, 1995, pp. 21–46.

217. Wong, J., J.R. Fineman, and M.A. Heymann. The role of endothelin and endothelin receptor subtypes in regulation of fetal pulmonary vascular tone. *Pediatr. Res.* 35: 664–670, 1994.

218. Yamaguchi, T., D.M. Rodman, R.F. O'Brien, and I.F. McMurtry. Modulation of pulmonary artery contraction by endotheium-derived relaxing factor. *Eur. J. Pharmacol.* 161: 259–262, 1989.

219. Yamaguchi, T.P., D.J. Dumont, R.A. Conlon, M.L. Breitman, and J. Rossant. Flk-1, an flt-related receptor tyrosine kinase, is an early marker for endothelial cell precursors. *Development* 118: 489–498, 1993.

220. Yamamoto, M., K. Shimokata, and H. Nagura. An immunohistochemical study on phe-

notypic heterogeneity of human pulmonary vascular endothelial cells. *Virchows Arch. A Anat. Histopathol.* 412: 479–486, 1988.

221. Yanagisawa, M., H. Kurihara, S. Kimura, Y. Tomobe, M. Kobayashi, Y. Mitsui, Y. Yasaki, K. Goto, and T. Masaki. A novel potent vasoconstrictor peptide produced by vascular endothelial cells. *Nature* 332: 411–415, 1988.
222. Young, P.E., S. Baumhueter, and L.A. Lasky. The sialomucin CD34 is expressed on hematopoietic cells and blood vessels during murine development. *Blood* 85: 96–105, 1995.
223. Zanellato, A.M., A.C. Borrione, L. Giuriato, M. Tonello, G. Scannapieco, P. Pauletto, and S. Sartore. Myosin isoforms and cell heterogeneity in vascular smooth muscle, I: developing and adult bovine aorta. *Dev. Biol.* 141: 431–446, 1990.
224. Zanetti, R.F.A., M. Sironi, N. Polentarutti, L. Lanfrancone, E. Dejana, and F. Colotta. Inhibition of anchorage-dependent cell spreading triggers apoptosis in cultured human endothelial cells. *J. Cell Biol.* 127: 537–546, 1994.
225. Zellers, T.M. and P.M. Vanhoutte. Endothelium-dependent relaxations of piglet pulmonary arteries augment with maturation. *Pediatr. Res.* 30: 176–180, 1991.
226. Zhao, Y.D., D.R. Springall, Q. Hamid, M.H. Yacoub, M. Levene, and J.M. Polak. Localization and characterization of endothelin-1 binding sites in the transplanted human lung. *J. Cardiovasc. Pharmacol.* 26(Suppl. 3): S336–S340, 1995.
227. Zhou, J., T. Mochizuki, H. Smeets, C. Antignac, P. Laurila, A. dePaepe, K. Tryggvason, and S.T. Reeders. Deletion of the paired alpha 5(IV) and alpha 6(IV) collagen genes in inherited smooth muscle tumors. *Science* 261: 1167–1169, 1993.
228. Ziegler, J.W., D.D. Ivy, J.P. Kinsella, and S.H. Abman. The role of nitric oxide, endothelin, and prostaglandins in the transition of the pulmonary circulation. *Clin. Perinatol.* 22: 387–403, 1995.

chapter 7

NITRIC OXIDE AND ENDOTHELIN IN THE DEVELOPING PULMONARY CIRCULATION: PHYSIOLOGIC AND CLINICAL IMPLICATIONS

Steven H. Abman, John P. Kinsella, and Jean-Christophe Mercier

WITHIN minutes after birth, pulmonary vascular resistance (PVR) rapidly falls from high fetal levels. This allows pulmonary blood flow to increase nearly tenfold and enables the lung to assume its postnatal role in gas exchange. Failure of the pulmonary circulation to successfully achieve and sustain this decrease in PVR causes severe hypoxemia in many neonatal cardiopulmonary disorders, which are referred to as the syndrome persistent pulmonary hypertension of the newborn (PPHN). Mechanisms leading to severe pulmonary hypertension after birth are poorly understood, but they include altered pulmonary vascular reactivity and structure. Persistent pulmonary hypertension of the newborn is a major clinical problem, contributing substantially to morbidity and mortality in both full-term and premature neonates. An understanding of basic mechanisms that underlie normal development of the pulmonary circulation in utero and that contribute to the marked pulmonary vasodilation during the normal transition at birth may provide insight into PPHN and related disorders.

Studies in vascular biology have identified the critical role that the endothelial cell plays in modulating vascular tone, growth, and structure. Although capable of producing multiple products, the vascular endothelium releases two substances that appear to be especially important in vasoregulation of the perinatal lung circulation: nitric oxide (NO) and endothelin-1 (ET-1). Nitric oxide and ET-1 have potent effects on vascular tone and reactivity, and both can modulate endothelial and smooth-muscle cell growth and vessel structure. In many experimental settings, NO and ET-1 have been shown to have opposing effects on vascular tone, growth, and structure. Mechanisms regulating NO and ET-1 production and activities are complex and have been extensively reviewed (43, 71, 72). In this chapter,we review the potential physiologic roles of NO and ET- 1 in the pulmonary circulation during lung development and the transition at birth. We also discuss how changes in the NO-cGMP cascade and the ET-l system may contribute to the pathophysiology of neonatal pulmonary hypertension and briefly discuss implications for the treatment of PPHN.

ROLES OF NO AND ET-1 IN THE DEVELOPING PULMONARY CIRCULATION

Because of the high PVR in the normal fetus, the pulmonary circulation receives less than 10% of combined ventricular output as most of the right ventricular output crosses the ductus arteriosus to the aorta (41, 85, 86). Fetal pulmonary blood flow is low but remains critical for providing the essential substrates, hormones, and oxygen that allow normal lung growth. This is perhaps best illustrated by studies demonstrating that occlusion of the left pulmonary artery during late gestation causes lung hypoplasia and alters maturation in the ovine fetus (96). During fetal life, the pulmonary circulation undergoes striking changes in both structure and function. With advancing fetal age, pulmonary blood flow increases in proportion to lung growth and increased blood vessel number. Along with progressive changes in lung vascular growth, marked changes in lung vascular function also occur during development. Despite an increase in vascular surface area, PVR increases with gestational age when calculated on the basis of fetal lung or body weight. Thus, pulmonary vascular tone appears to actually increase as the fetus nears term. Mechanisms contributing to high fetal PVR include the lack of a gas–liquid interface and low oxygen tension. Low basal production of endogenous vasodilator products (such as prostacyclin and NO), increased production of vasoconstrictors (including ET-l and leukotrienes), and altered smooth muscle cell responsiveness to various stimuli also maintain high PVR in utero.

Over the past four decades, studies from several laboratories have characterized the fetal pulmonary vascular response to diverse physiologic and pharmacologic stimuli, including hypoxia, increased O_2 tension, shear stress, and drugs. Acute pulmonary vasodilation to several stimuli, such as acetylcholine, increased oxygen, and hypoxia, increase with advancing gestation in the ovine fetus (65, 75). The late-gestation fetal lung circulation can be further characterized by its ability to oppose vasodilation; that is, multiple vasodilators (such as increased O_2, acetylcholine, and dilator prostaglandins) increase pulmonary blood flow only transiently, but flow returns toward baseline despite continued treatment (2, 7). This response is also observed during mechanical increases in pulmonary blood flow caused by partial compression of the ductus arteriosus (1). Mechanisms underlying time-dependent increases in PVR despite prolonged exposure to dilator stimuli are uncertain, but suggest that the lung may have autoregulatory properties that maintain high PVR in utero. Maturational changes in pulmonary vascular tone and reactivity may reflect developmentally regulated changes in endothelial or smooth-muscle function. For example, agents that directly stimulate smooth-muscle relaxation independent of endothelial release of vasodilator products, such as cyclic GMP, atrial natriuretic peptide, and K^+ channel agonists, cause more sustained pulmonary vasodilation than endothelium-dependent stimuli (2, 25). In addition, fetal pulmonary arteries have greater myogenic activity than neonatal or adult arteries, which may also serve to oppose vasodilation (13). The roles of the NO-cGMP cascade and the ET-1 system in modulating basal pulmonary vascular tone and reactivity in utero are discussed below.

NO in Fetal Pulmonary Circulation

Maturational changes in endothelial and smooth-muscle function, especially with regard to the NO-cGMP cascade, may account for many changes in pulmonary vasoregulation during fetal life (Fig. 7.1). Nitric oxide is produced by vascular endothelium during conversion of L-arginine to L-citrulline by the enzyme NO synthase [NOS; (43, 72)]. This step requires a unique five-electron oxidation of a terminal guanidinium nitrogen on L-arginine. The NOS activity is also dependent upon availability of other substrates and cofactors, including molecular oxygen, tetrahydrobiopterin, NADPH, FAD, FMN, and calmodulin. Nitric oxide synthase functions as a homodimer, with each component consisting of reductase and oxygenase domains. A binding site for calmodulin spans these domains, and after activation by calcium, permits the transfer of electrons from NADPH via the flavins to the heme catalytic site. The exact mechanisms leading to oxidation of L-arginine are not completely known, but they appear to require at least two steps, including *N*-hydroxylation of the guanidinium *N* to transiently yield the intermediate, *N*-hydroxy-L-arginine.

Three NOS isoforms have been identified: two are considered constitutive (type I, neuronal, and type III, endothelial, or eNOS). Activity of the constitutive NOS isoforms are dependent upon changes in intracellular calcium after stimulation by physiologic, biochemical, and pharmacologic stimuli. The third NOS isoform (type II) is the so-called inducible isoform, which is largely regulated by transcriptional mechanisms. Since calmodulin is tightly bound to type II NOS (iNOS), its activity is largely calcium independent and is capable of generating large amounts of NO. Although originally characterized by cell-specific expression by neuronal cells (type I), endothelium (type III), and macrophages (type II), further work has clearly demonstrated that more diverse cells can express each isoform (see below).

Once produced, NO rapidly diffuses to underlying smooth-muscle cells and causes vasodilation by stimulating soluble guanylate cyclase and increasing cGMP production. Elevated cGMP stimulates cGMP kinase, increases calcium-activated K^+

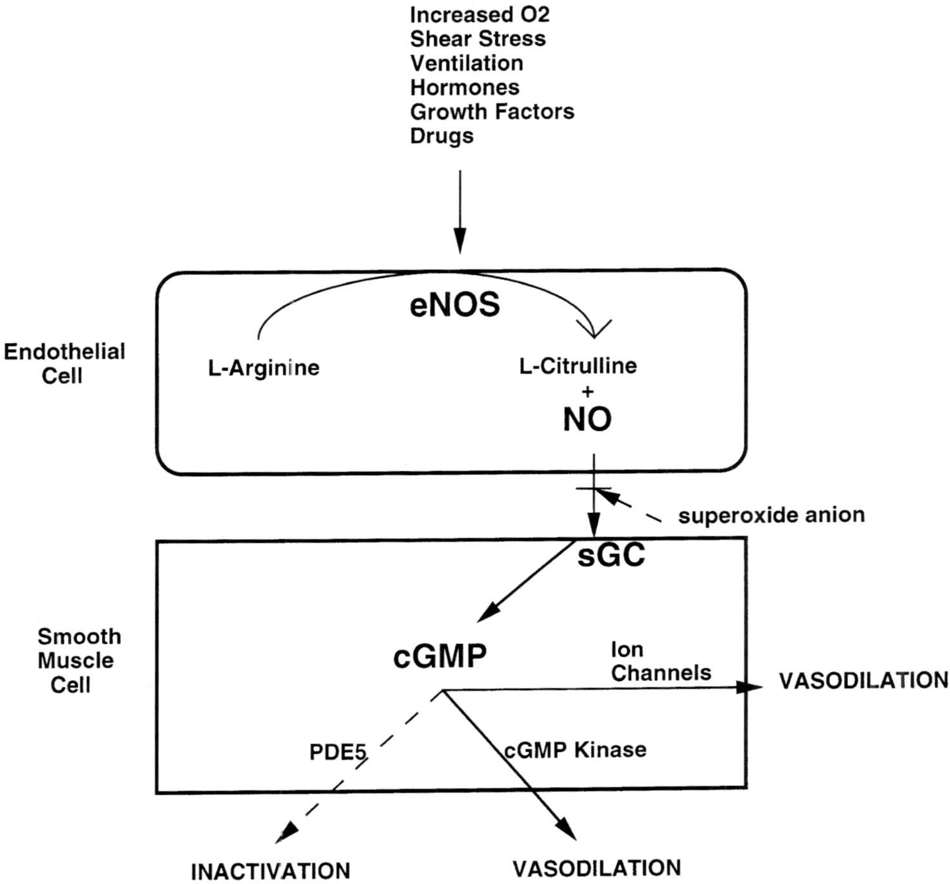

Fig. 7.1 Schematic illustrating the normal NO-cGMP cascade in the perinatal pulmonary circulation. *eNOS*, type III nitric oxide synthase; *sGC*, soluble guanylate cyclase.

channel activity, and causes membrane hyperpolarization (10, 26, 43). This lowers intracellular calcium in the smooth muscle cell by decreasing calcium entry through L-type channels and causes vasodilation. In some experimental systems, NO has been shown to directly stimulate K^+ channels or voltage-gated $Ca2^+$ channels independent of increased cGMP (14, 16). Several investigators have demonstrated that vasodilator responses to multiple hemodynamic (increased flow or shear stress), hormonal, paracrine and pharmacologic stimuli are dependent upon NO release. Nitric oxide activity within the vessel wall is affected by multiple factors, including eNOS content, substrate and co-factor availability, superoxide production (which inactivates NO and forms peroyxynitrite), and superoxide dismutase activity (Table 7.1).

The eNOS activity is also dependent upon its subcellular localization within the endothelial cell (87). Of the three NOS isoforms, type III, or eNOS, is uniquely associated with cell membranes, which is due to the presence of myristoylation and palmitoylation sites on the protein. Acylation of these sites targets eNOS to plasmalemmal microdomains, or caveolae, which may allow for eNOS to be more effectively located for interactions with blood-borne substances, other enzyme or receptor systems contained within caveolae, and the endothelial cytoskeleton (87). Although most studies of the perinatal lung have focused on the role of eNOS in vasoregulation, the other NOS isoforms, including neuronal (type I) NOS and inducible (type II) NOS, have been identified by immunostaining in the rat and human fetal lung (56). Lung nNOS mRNA and protein increases in parallel with eNOS expression during development in the fetal rat (77), but data are limited regarding its site of expression within the fetal lung. Preliminary data from our laboratory has identified type I NOS in bronchial epithelium, vascular endothelium, and mucus glands in the ovine fetus. Inducible (type II) NOS has also been detected by immunostaining in human and rat fetal lung, but quantification of relative changes in lung NOS content and determination of cell type–specific expression during development is lacking. Whether these nonendothelial isoforms contribute to

Table 7.1 Mechanisms that Regulate NO Production from Endothelial Nitric Oxide Synthase (eNOS)

ENOS protein levels
1) *Transcriptional Factors*
Shear stress
O_2 tension
Hypertension
Proliferative state of endothelial cell
Growth factors (e.g., PDGF, VEGF, others)
Hormones (e.g., estradiol)
2) *eNOS mRNA Stability*
3) *Rate of Translation*
4) *Post-translational Modifications*
Phosphorylation
Acylation (palmitoylation, myristovlation)
Disulfide formation (e.g., NO feedback inhibition)
5) *Substrate Availability*
L-arginine, O_2
6) *Co-factor Availability*
NADPH
FAD
FMN
Tetrahydrobioperin
7) *Association with Calcium/Calmodulin*
8) *Intracellular Localization: Cytosol versus Membrane-associated (in caveolae)*
9) *Superoxide Anion/Superoxide Dismutase*

NO-dependent modulation of fetal pulmonary vascular tone is unknown. Treatment of pregnant rats with an iNOS-selective antagonist caused constriction of the great vessels (main pulmonary artery and thoracic aorta) and ductus arteriosus in fetal rats (17). It is unclear, however, whether these changes were due to the direct effects of iNOS blockade in the fetus or secondary to alterations in placental perfusion and fetal oxygenation. Preliminary data in fetal lambs suggest that selective iNOS antagonists (including aminoguanidine, ethylisothiourea, and others) increase fetal PVR at doses that do not inhibit acetylcholine-induced pulmonary vasodilation (78). In contrast, the nonselective NOS antagonist, L-NA, blocks acetylcholine vasodilation and elevates PVR. Although these findings support the speculation that iNOS may also modulate pulmonary vascular tone in utero, further work is needed to clarify the relative roles of the different NOS isoforms in NO production in the fetal lung.

Vascular responsiveness to NO is also dependent upon several smooth-muscle cell enzymes, including soluble guanylate cyclase (sGC), cGMP-specific (types V) phosphodiesterase (PDE5), and cGMP kinase.(Fig. 7.1). Several studies have shown that soluble guanylate cyclase, which produces cGMP in response to NO activation, is active at least as early as 0.75 term in the ovine fetal lung (4, 52). Similarly, PDE5, which limits cGMP-mediated vasodilation by hydrolysis and inactivation of cGMP, is also active in utero (102). Infusions of several selective PDE5 antagonists cause potent and sustained fetal pulmonary vasodilation (102), and fetal lung PDE5 activity is high in comparison with that in postnatal lung (39, 40). Thus, PDE5 activity appears to play a critical role in pulmonary vasoregulation during the perinatal period. Mechanisms regulating sGC and PDE5 mRNA and protein expression or activities are poorly understood.

Several studies have demonstrated the physiologic roles of the NO-cGMP cascade in pulmonary vasoregulation during the perinatal period. Studies of the pulmonary hemodynamic effects of NOS antagonists demonstrated that basal NO release modulates pulmonary vascular tone during late gestation (3). Since NOS blockade increases PVR at least as early as 0.75 gestation (112 days), NOS activity contributes to vasoregulation at least throughout late gestation (52). In addition, NOS inhibition selectively attenuates pulmonary vasodilation to such stimuli as acetylcholine (3), oxygen (68), and increased flow or shear stress (24) in the normal fetus, without altering the vasodilator response to endothelium-independent agonists (including inhaled NO, atrial natriuretic factor, and lemakalim). These findings demonstrate the important role of basal and stimulated NO release in fetal pulmonary vasoregulation. Although present in the early fetus, lung eNOS mRNA and protein increase with advancing gestation in utero and during the early postnatal period in rats (77).

Changes in lung eNOS content appear to parallel functional changes in vasoreactivity as assessed by several in vivo and in vivo studies. Since acetylcholine and oxygen cause pulmonary vasodilation by stimulating NO release (3, 68, 87b, 94), maturational changes in the NO-cGMP cascade are likely to account for past observations of increasing pulmonary vasodilation to these agents with advancing fetal age. In vitro studies suggest that pharmacologic agents that cause vasodilation by stimulating NO release are less potent in fetal than neonatal or adult pulmonary arteries (4). In contrast, pulmonary artery relaxation due to direct stimulation of smooth muscle with sodium nitroprusside (which releases NO) is not different among fetal, newborn and adult vessels (4). Thus, basal eNOS activity influences PVR during late gestation in the ovine fetus, and this maturational change in endothelial cell function may contribute to developmental changes in pulmonary vascular tone and reactivity. Parallel in vivo studies of fetal pulmonary vasoreactivity support these in vitro observations; exogenous NO or agents which directly increase smooth muscle GMP content cause more sustained fetal pulmonary vasodilation than many endothelium-dependent agonists (53).

Although NO production increases cGMP content in vascular smooth muscle, NO-induced vasodilation is limited by the rapid hydrolysis or extrusion of cGMP (12, 18, 43). For example, brief infusions of various PDE5 inhibitors, including dipyridamole. zaprinast, E4021, and DMPPO, cause marked and sustained increases in fetal pulmonary blood flow (102). PDE5 blockers also augment and prolong pulmonary vasodilator responses to acetylcholine and inhaled NO in the normal fetus and in an experimental model of PPHN (39). Maturational studies have also shown that lung PDE5 activity is highest during fetal life, rapidly decreases after birth, and remains low during adult life. Thus, physiologic and biochemical studies demonstrate that high PDE5 activity contributes to high PVR and limits responsiveness to pulmonary vasodilator stimuli in the normal fetus. PDE5 activity also contributes to experimental pulmonary hypertension caused by chronic hypoxia in adult rats (23) and perinatal pulmonary hypertension in fetal lambs (see below).

The role of endogenous NO in the regulation of pulmonary vascular tone during late gestation is well established; however, little is known of its potential role in the pulmonary circulation during earlier stages of lung development. In addition to its effects on vascular tone, cell culture studies have also reported that NO influences vascular endothelial and smooth muscle cell growth in vitro (73, 101). Since eNOS protein is present at a stage of lung development when blood flow is absent or minimal, it has been hypothesized that NO may potentially contribute to angiogenesis during early lung development (38). Whether early eNOS expression implies a role in promoting vascular growth or is merely a marker of growing endothelial cells is unknown. Recent studies report conflicting data regarding the effects of eNOS activity in promoting new vessel formation in different experimental models of angiogenesis. Although NO can inhibit endothelial cell mitogenesis and proliferation, it has also been shown to mediate the angiogenic effects of substance P and vascular endothelial growth factor in vitro (73, 101). Growing bovine aortic endothelial cells in culture express greater eNOS mRNA and protein than confluent cells, but NOS inhibition does not affect their rate of proliferation in vitro (11). Nitric oxide has also been shown to decrease smooth-muscle proliferation in vitro (33), but other studies suggest that NO has biphasic, dose-dependent effects on fetal pulmonary artery smooth-muscle cell growth (99, 92). High doses of NO donors inhibit smooth-muscle cell growth, but low doses cause paradoxical stimulation. Whether NO modulates smooth muscle cell growth in vivo remains controversial. One study purported to show failure of chronic

NOS inhibition to alter pulmonary vascular structure during late gestation in the fetal lamb (29); however, inhibition of basal NO release, as reflected by elevation of PVR, was not achieved, limiting interpretation of this study. Thus, although multiple studies have examined the role of NO in vascular growth and remodeling, its effects vary among experimental settings and remain controversial.

ET-1 in Fetal Pulmonary Circulation

Although several vasoconstrictor products are released by vascular endothelium, none of these products causes the uniquely potent and sustained vasoconstriction of ET-1. As first described by Yanagisawa and co-workers, ET-1 is a 21 amino acid peptide released from endothelial cells during hypoxia (100). Several stimuli, including hemodynamic forces (changes in shear stress, stretch, or pressure) and other factors (including various cytokines, thrombin, and transforming growth factor β), also influence ET-1 release [(91a); Fig. 7.2]. ET-1 is derived from a 212 amino acid precursor (preproendothelin-l) that undergoes proteolysis by a dibasic pair–specific endopeptidase within the endothelial cell. The product of this step is a 39 amino acid protein, bigET-l, which is subsequently cleaved by a metalloprotease enzyme, ET-converting enzyme (ECE), leading to the formation of its vasoactive product, ET-1. The Mechanisms that regulate endopeptidase and ECE gene expression and activities are poorly understood. The ECE gene has been cloned from bovine adrenal cortex cDNA libraries and is characterized by the presence of a zinc-binding motif and multiple sites for glycosylation. Expression of ECE mRNA is highest in vascular endothelium and appears to to be associated with plasma membranes and the Golgi complex. Alternative splicing produces two isoforms of ECE (ECE-1 and ECE-2) that have similar bigET-1 conversion activities. ECE-2 is more sensitive than ECE-1 to inhibition by phosphoramidon, has optimal activity at acidic pH (5.5), and is highly expressed in neuronal tissue. ECE-1 is expressed in vascular endothelium, but not in neuronal tissue, and has optimal activity at neutral pH.

The effects of ET-I on vascular tone and smooth muscle cell growth are mediated through specific ET receptors, designated ETA and ETB. In most vascular beds, ETA and ETB receptors have been localized to smooth-muscle and endothelial cells, respectively, causing either vasoconstriction (via ETA receptor activation) or vasodilation (through ETB receptor activation) (Fig. 7.2). In some experimental settings, the presence of an additional ETB receptor that mediates vasoconstriction has been identified in vascular smooth muscle. The ETB receptor also acts as a clearance mechanism. Regulation of receptor expression contributes to the diverse physiologic effects of ET-1. Cyclic AMP, neuropeptides, and growth factors (epidermal growth factor and basic fibroblast growth factor) increase ET-1 binding sites, whereas dexamethasone and platelet-derived growth factor down-regulate ET receptors (71). Hypoxia or changes in hemodynamics alter the relative densities of ETA and ETB receptors in the pulmonary circulation (see below). Most investigators initially believed that ET-1 is released immediately after production, but it appears that preformed ET-1 can readily be released from storage pools in endothelial cells. Multiple stimuli, such as

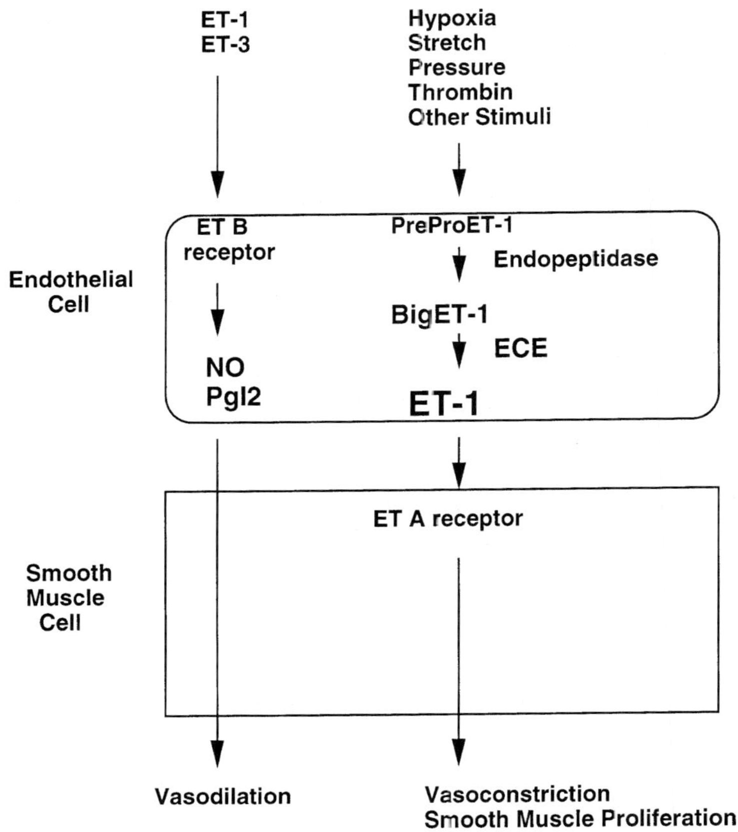

Fig. 7.2 Schematic illustrating the ET-1 system in the normal perinatal pulmonary circulation. *ECE*, endothelin-converting enzyme.

hypoxia, stretch or pressure, thrombin, cytokines, growth factors, and endotoxin increase ET-1 production [(57, 58, 66); Fig. 7.2].

That ET-1 may contribute to fetal pulmonary vasoregulation was first indirectly implied from the detection of preproET-l mRNA in the normal fetal rat lung (67). In addition, clinical studies reported high immunoreactive ET-1 levels from umbilical blood samples from normal neonates at birth (44). Controversy exists, however, regarding the physiologic role of ET-1 in the perinatal lung. To define the physiologic role of ET-1 in the fetal pulmonary circulation, several studies examined the physiologic effects of various agonists and antagonists of the ET system. Early studies reported that rapid bolus infusions of ET-1 cause acute pulmonary vasodilation in normal fetal lambs (21, 22). However, the predominance of evidence supports the hypothesis that endogenous ET-1 acts primarily as a potent vasoconstrictor (95). For example, although infusions of ET-1 cause fetal pulmonary vasodilation, this response is very brief, as hypertension develops during continued treatment (22). In addition, the fetal pulmonary vascular response to ET-1 is tone-dependent; ET-1 causes vasoconstriction when infused into neonatal lambs during mechanical ventilation (21). As discussed above, the net hemodynamic response to ET-1 depends on the relative effects of ETA or ETB receptor stimulation. In the fetal lamb, ET-1 vasodilation is mediated by ETB receptor stimulation. This is supported by findings that intrapulmonary infusions of selective ETB agonists, including ET-3 and sarafotoxin 6c, cause pulmonary vasodilation (99). Since ET-1-mediated vasodilation is attenuated after NOS inhibition, it appears that NO release mediates ETB receptor activity. ETB receptor blockade does not change basal pulmonary vascular tone in the normal lamb lung (40, 45, 98).

In contrast to the transient vasodilator effects of exogenous ET-1, stimulation of endogenous ET-1 release during infusions of its precursor, bigET-I, causes sustained hypertension without pulmonary vasodilation (49). This is likely due to the abluminal release of ET from the endothelium to the underlying smooth muscle, favoring stimulation of the smooth-muscle ETA receptor. The ETA receptor inhibitors block the rise in PVR after bigET1 as effectively as ECE blockade, demonstrating that the ETA receptor mediates vasoconstriction in the fetal lung (49). In addition, ETA blockade causes fetal pulmonary vasodilation (45, 99) and augments the rise in pulmonary blood flow during partial compression of the ductus arteriosus (45). These findings support the hypothesis that the physiologic stimuli that release endogenous ET-1 predominantly causes vasoconstriction through stimulation of ETA receptors. Concomitant ETB receptor activation may serve to attenuate the severity of vasoconstriction through the release of endothelium-derived NO. The ETB receptors may also influence the vascular effects of ET-1 by acting as clearance receptors for circulating ET-1 (71). Thus, along with altered regulation of ET-1 production by endopeptidase or ECE activities, modulation of ET receptor expression serves important regulatory roles in ET-1-mediated vascular responses (see below).

In addition to its vasoconstrictor effects, ET-1 stimulates smooth muscle cell growth and proliferation (28). Chronic ET blockade prevents and reverses hypertensive structural remodeling of small pulmonary arteries in different experimental models of pulmonary hypertension, including chronic hypoxia, genetic (fawn-hooded rats) and perinatal pulmonary hypertension [see below; (15, 46, 71)]. Although released by vascular endothelium, ET-1 is also produced by hypertensive smooth-muscle cells in culture, suggesting an autocrine effect of ET-1 on proliferation that is independent of vascular endothelium. Although ET-1 contributes to high fetal pulmonary vascular tone, it is not clear whether ET-1 also influences vascular growth during early lung development. As a mitogen or comitogen, ET-1 may potentially influence lung vascular growth and structure. Interestingly, recent work reported higher ET-1 mRNA expression in proliferating than confluent endothelial cells in culture (30), but the functional significance in vivo is unclear.

Changes in oxygen tension and hemodynamic forces (blood flow, pressure, stretch, and shear stress) alter ET-1 expression in vitro and in some experimental models of pulmonary hypertension. However, little is known about mechanisms which regulate ET-1 production in the fetal lung. Nitric oxide may directly influence ET-1 production or activity (57, 62). Studies have suggested that NO decreases ET-1 mRNA expression (57) and may decrease ET-1 binding at the receptor level. In general, ET-1 and NO tend to have opposing actions on vasomotor tone and smooth-muscle growth. For example, hypoxia decreases NOS activity but increase ppET-l mRNA and ET-1 peptide release in cultured endothelial cells (57, 58). In vivo, however, chronic hypoxia has mixed effects, depending upon the species and age of the animals. For example, chronic hypoxic pulmonary hypertension increases lung eNOS and iNOS expression in adult rats (59). Nitric oxide can also block ET-1-mediated signaling in smooth muscle through a cGMP-independent mechanism that reduces the affinity of ETA receptors for ET-1. In the fetal lung, NOS inhibition augments ET-1-induced vasoconstriction, and ET blockade augments the rise in pulmonary blood flow during shear stress-induced vasodilation, which is largely due to stimulation of NO release (48). As discussed below, these may have important implications in vasoregulation of the normal fetal lung as well as in the pathophysiology of clinical pulmonary hypertension. For example, decreased NO production or increased NO inactivation may enhance ET-1-mediated pulmonary hypertension through the loss of NO inhibition of ET production, ETA receptor stimulation, or decreased ETB-mediated vasodilation.

Although most studies have focused on the vascular biology of the endothelins, ET-1 and other isoforms (especially ET-3) have been shown to play other important roles during development (71). For example, ET-1-deficient mice have craniofacial abnormalities and die of respiratory failure at birth. ET-3 or ETB receptor–deficient mice have neural crest abnormalities and intestinal disease that mimics aganglionic megacolon (Hirschsprung's disease).

NO AND ET-1 IN THE TRANSITIONAL PULMONARY CIRCULATION

Within minutes after delivery, pulmonary artery pressure falls and blood flow increases nearly tenfold due to the marked vasodilator response to birth-related stimuli. Pioneering work from the laboratories of Drs. Dawes, Strang, Enhorning, and others, first demonstrated the dramatic fall in PVR at birth in the transional lung, and the important role of several birth-related stimuli. Mechanisms contributing to the fall in PVR at birth include establishment of an air–liquid interface, rhythmic lung distension, increased oxygen tension, and altered production of vasoactive substances (41). Physical stimuli, such as increased shear stress, ventilation, and increased oxygen, cause pulmonary vasodilation in part by increasing production of vasodilators, NO, and PgI2 (3, 19, 20, 24, 27, 60). Pretreatment with the arginine analogue, nitro-L-arginine, blocks NOS activity and attenuates the decline in PVR after delivery of near-term fetal lambs (3). These findings suggest that about 50% of the rise in pulmonary blood flow at birth may be directly related to the acute release of NO. Specific mechanisms that cause NO release at birth include the marked rise in shear stress, increased oxygen, and ventilation (3, 24). Recent studies from Cornfield et al. suggest that increased PaO_2 triggers NO release, which augments vasodilation through cGMP kinase-mediated stimulation of K^+ channels (26). The important role of NO activity during the transitional circulation has been confirmed in experiments of chronic treatment of fetal lambs with a NOS antagonist (29). Thus, although NO does not account for the entire fall in PVR at birth, NOS activity appears to be important in achieving postnatal adaptation of the lung circulation. Although these studies were performed in term animals, similar mechanisms also contribute to the rapid decrease in PVR at birth in premature lambs (52). The pulmonary vasodilator responses to ventilation with hypoxic gas mixtures (or, rhythmic distension) of the lung or increased PaO_2 are partly due to stimulation of NO release in premature lambs at least as early as 112–115 days (0.7 term) (52). Other vasodilator products, including PgI2, also modulate changes in pulmonary vascular tone at birth (19, 60, 61, 93). Rhythmic lung distension and shear stress stimulate both PgI2 and NO production in the late-gestation fetus (1, 24); increased O_2 tension triggers NO activity but does not appear to alter PgI2 production in vivo (68, 93).

Along with enhanced release of vasodilators, decreased production or decreased responsiveness to vasoconstrictors, such as leukotrienes (LT) and ET-1, may also contribute to the normal fall in PVR at birth (45, 88, 99). Blockade of ETA receptors augments fetal pulmonary vasodilation caused by increased shear stress during acute compression of the ductus arteriosus (48), leading to the hypothesis that loss of ET constrictor activity may aid the normal fall in PVR at birth. The ET receptor blockade does not alter the rise in pulmonary blood flow at delivery, suggesting that stimulation of ETB (vasodilator) receptors does not directly release NO or PgI2 at birth. It is uncertain whether changes in ET production or receptor activities occur after birth; however, increased ET production and altered receptor density contribute to persistent elevation of PVR in experimental PPHN [(46, 47); see below].

EXPERIMENTAL STUDIES OF NO AND ET-1 IN THE FAILURE OF POSTNATAL ADAPTATION

Some newborns fail to achieve or sustain the normal decline in PVR after birth, and constitute the clinical syndrome known as PPHN (63). As a clinical syndrome, PPHN includes diverse cardiac and pulmonary disorders, such as meconium aspiration syndrome, pneumonia, sepsis, diaphragmatic hernia, respiratory distress syndrome, congenital heart disease, and others. Severe pulmonary hypertension also occurs as an idiopathic disorder, in the absence of significant cardiac or pulmonary disease (in the past, referred to as *persistent fetal circulation*). Although these diverse diseases have features that are distinct from each other, they are generally included within this clinical syndrome because they share a common pathophysiologic feature: high PVR leading to right-to-left shunting of blood across the ductus arteriosus or foramen ovale and marked hypoxemia. Despite multiple therapeutic strategies, morbidity and mortality in neonates with severe PPHN remain high. Although cardiac and lung function contribute significantly to the clinical course of neonates with PPHN, abnormalities of the pulmonary circulation are critical features of

PPHN. This syndrome is characterized by altered pulmonary vascular reactivity, structure, and in some cases, growth. Diseases associated with the syndrome of PPHN are often characterized as fitting into one of three categories: (*1*) maladaptation in which vessels are presumably of normal structural vasoreactivity but have abnormal vasoreactivity; (*2*) excessive muscularization, characterized by increased smooth-muscle cell thickness and increased distal extension of muscle to vessels that are usually nonmuscular; and (*3*) underdevelopment, in which lung hypoplasia is associated with decreased pulmonary artery number (34). Clinically, many conditions combine mixtures of alterations in structure and function; for example, congenital diaphragmatic hernia incorporates elements from each of these categories. It is likely that not all newborns with PPHN have structural lung vascular lesions; altered pulmonary vasoreactivity can be due to an acute or short-term insult (group B streptococcal sepsis, meconium aspiration, and acute asphyxia).

Several experimental models have been studied to explore the pathogenesis and pathophysiology of PPHN (8, 90). Such models have included exposure to acute or chronic hypoxia after birth, chronic hypoxia in utero, placement of meconium into the airways of neonatal animals, sepsis, and others. Although each model demonstrates interesting physiologic changes that may be especially relevant to particular clinical settings, most studies examine only brief changes in the pulmonary circulation, and mechanisms underlying altered lung vascular structure and function of PPHN remain poorly understood. Clinical observations that neonates with severe PPHN who die during the first days after birth already have pathologic signs of chronic pulmonary vascular disease suggest that intrauterine events may play an important role in this syndrome. During late gestation, adverse intrauterine stimuli, such as decreased lung blood flow, changes in substrate or hormonal delivery to the lung, chronic hypoxia, chronic hypertension, or others, may potentially alter lung vascular function and structure, contributing to abnormalities of postnatal adaptation. Mechanisms by which changes in hemodynamic, hormonal, autocrine, and paracrine stimuli affect lung vascular growth and function are complex and uncertain. Several investigators have examined the effects of chronic intrauterine stresses, such as hypoxia or hypertension, and animal models have been developed in order to mimic the clinical problem of PPHN (70). Whether chronic hypoxia alone can cause PPHN is controversial. An early report that maternal hypoxia in rats increases pulmonary vascular smooth muscle thickening in newborns has not been reproduced in maternal rats or guinea pigs with more extensive studies (37). However, animal studies suggest that hypertension, due to either renal artery ligation or partial or complete closure of the ductus arteriosus, can cause structural and physiologic changes that resemble features of clinical PPHN (64).

Pulmonary hypertension induced by early closure of the ductus arteriosus (DA) in fetal lambs alters lung vascular reactivity and structure, causing the failure of postnatal adaptation at delivery and providing an experimental model of PPHN (6, 74). In this model, partial closure of the DA intrauterine pulmonary hypertension acutely increases pulmonary artery pressure and flow, but after 1 h, blood flow returns toward baseline values (1). Over days, pulmonary artery pressure and PVR progressively increase, but flow remains low and PaO_2 is unchanged (6). Thus, this model illustrates the effects of chronic intrauterine hypertension, but not high flow, on intrauterine lung vascular structure and function. Marked right ventricular hypertrophy and structural remodeling of small pulmonary arteries develops after 8 days of hypertension. After delivery, these lambs have persistent elevation of PVR despite mechanical ventilation with high oxygen concentrations (6, 74). Thus, physiologic and structural studies suggest that this experimental model of PPHN mimics many of the abnormalities found in severe idiopathic PPHN in the human newborn.

To test the hypothesis that changes in the NO-cGMP and ET-1 systems can potentially contribute to pulmonary vascular abnormalities in PPHN, our laboratory and others have studied endothelial and smooth muscle cell function in this experimental model (Fig. 7.3). That chronic hypertension can alter NO production or activity was first suggested in physiologic studies of pulmonary vasodilation of hypertensive and control lambs (69). McQueston and co-workers found that pulmonary vasodilator responses to acetylcholine and increased oxygen, which act in part by stimulating NO release, were impaired after chronic hypertension. Responsiveness to atrial natriuretic peptide, which acts independently of NO release by vascular endothelium, remains relatively intact. These findings suggested that intrauterine hypertension impairs endothelial function and that the ability to produce NO may be impaired. Subsequent molecular and biochemical studies have demonstrated that chronic pulmonary hypertension decreases lung eNOS mRNA and protein expression and total NOS activity (94). Thus, these findings support the hypothesis that

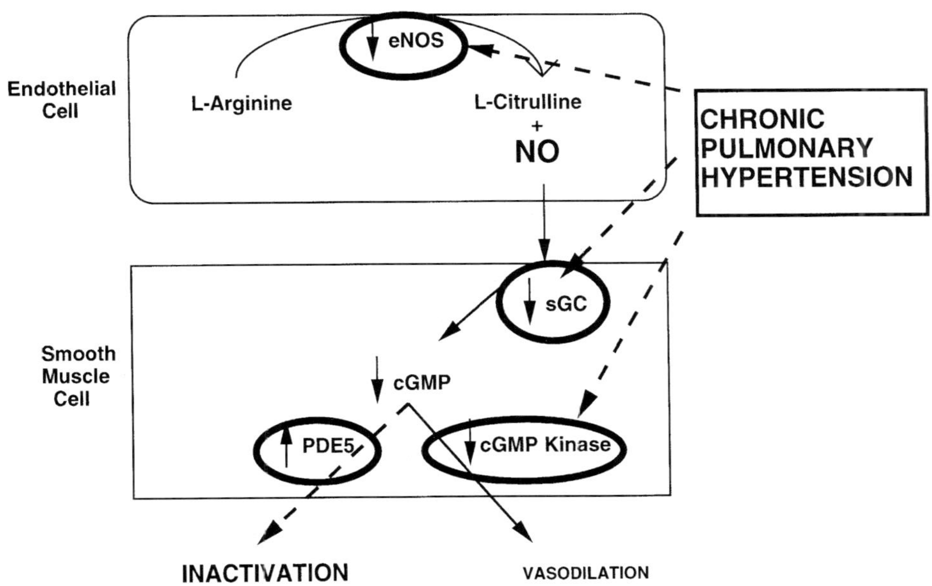

Fig. 7.3 Impaired NO-cGMP cascade in an experimental model of persistent pulmonary hypertension of the newborn. *eNOS*, type III nitric oxide synthase; *sGC*, soluble guanylate cyclase.

vascular injury in utero can decrease vasodilator responsiveness to birth-related stimuli by reducing lung eNOS content and NO production. Whether impaired NOS activity in utero also contributes to hypertensive structural remodeling of pulmonary arteries (including smooth muscle hypertrophy or hyperplasia) is uncertain.

As described above, pulmonary vasodilation to endogenous NO is also dependent upon several other factors, including smooth muscle–soluble guanylate cyclase (sGC) and cGMP-specific phosphodiesterase (type 5; PDE5) activities (43). To determine whether intrauterine hypertension can alter these components of the NO-cGMP cascade, recent studies have examined sGC and PDE5 activities after chronic DA closure in this experimental model. Steinhorn and co-workers reported impaired sGC activity in hypertensive lambs, as reflected by decreased generation of cGMP and reduced vascular relaxation to NO stimulation in vitro (89). In addition, Hanson and co-workers found marked elevation of lung PDE5 activity, suggesting that rapid cGMP hydrolysis may limit cGMP-dependent pulmonary vasodilation after chronic hypertension (39, 40). Thus, decreased lung eNOS protein and activity in the presence of decreased sGC and elevated PDE5 activities limits the ability to sustain smooth-muscle cGMP, favoring vasoconstriction and high PVR in experimental PPHN. These observations may have clinical implications regarding potential strategies for enhancing responsiveness to vasodilator therapy of PPHN (see below).

In addition to abnormalities in the NO-cGMP cascade, alterations in the ET-1 system may also contribute to pulmonary hypertension in PPHN. Although early studies debated whether ET-1 was a marker or mediator of pulmonary hypertension (9, 90, 91a), ET-1 has subsequently been shown to contribute to pulmonary hypertension in several experimental settings, including chronic hypoxia, genetic, inflammatory, and perinatal models. Clinically, circulating ET-1 levels are high in severe PPHN, as well as in other disorders, including acute lung injury (84). Lung ET-1 is increased in adults with severe pulmonary hypertension (35, 36). The consequences of high lung ET-1 production may include marked pulmonary vasoconstriction, pulmonary edema, and augmented lung inflammation. The effects of ET- 1 in pulmonary hypertension could result from excessive production, decreased degradation or altered clearance, or increased sensitivity or augmented responsiveness to ET-1. To examine the potential role of ET-1 in perinatal pulmonary hypertension, we have studied the ET-1 system in our experimental model of PPHN. In comparison with controls, lung-immunoreactive ET- l content was increased threefold after prolonged DA ligation in utero (47). Pharmacologic studies further demonstrated that the pulmonary vasodilator response to ETB receptor stimulation was absent after chronic pulmonary hypertension [(47); Fig. 7.4]. In contrast, the vasodilator response to ETA receptor blockade was enhanced. Similar findings have been found in the surgical diaphragmatic hernia model in the ovine fetus (91b). These findings suggest that multiple changes in the ET-1 system are associated with pulmonary hypertension, including increased lung ET-1 production and altered ET receptor densities. More recent data suggest that hypertension-induced changes in the ET-1 system may occur at the transcriptional level. Ivy and colleagues have reported increased ppET-l mRNA, decreased ETB receptor mRNA, and no change in ETA or ECE mRNA

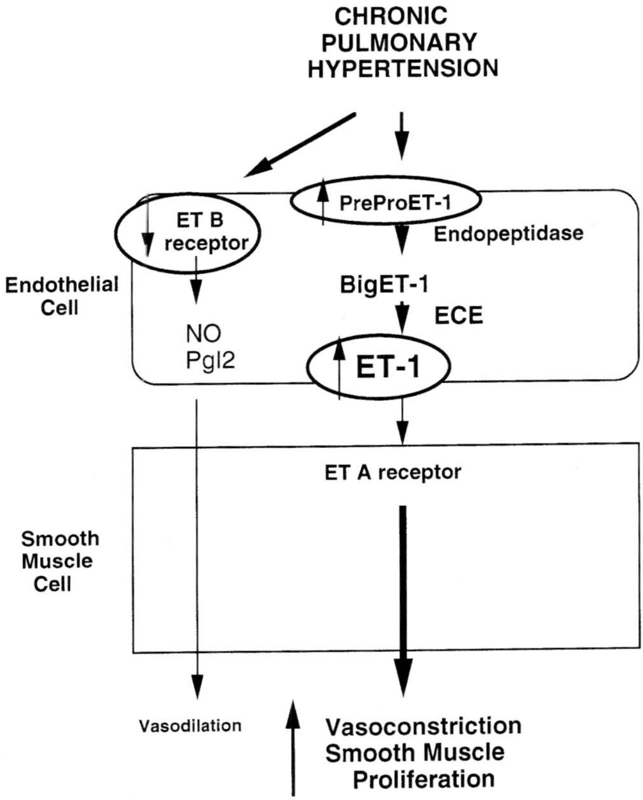

Fig. 7.4 Altered ET-1 system in an experimental model of persistent pulmonary hypertension of the newborn. *ECE,* endothelin-converting enzyme.

(preliminary data). The important contribution of ET-1 in this model of PPHN was recently confirmed by studies in which chronic treatment with a selective ETA receptor blocker (BQ 123) lowered PVR, blocked the development of right ventricular hypertrophy, attenuated lung vascular remodeling, and augmented the vasodilator response at birth (46).

Thus, alterations in the ET-1 and NO-cGMP cascades appear to play essential roles in the pathogenesis and pathophysiology of experimental PPHN. Alterations in these mechanisms and others appear to contribute to altered structure and function of the developing lung circulation, leading to clinical disorders in postnatal cardiorespiratory adaptation. Insights into mechanisms underlying altered vasoreactivity may provide new treatment strategies for clinical PPHN.

CLINICAL IMPLICATIONS

Persistent pulmonary hypertension of the newborn is a clinical syndrome that is associated with diverse neonatal cardiopulmonary disorders, including asphyxia, sepsis, meconium aspiration syndrome, congenital diaphragmatic hernia, respiratory distress syndrome, lung hypoplasia, and others, or it can be "idiopathic." Although originally known as persistent fetal circulation (PFC) from continued postnatal right-to-left shunting of blood across the ductus arteriosus or foramen ovale due to high PVR, the term PPHN syndrome has replaced PFC. Physiologicallv, PPHN is characterized by high PVR and marked pulmonary vasolability, characterized by elevation of pulmonary artery pressure leading to marked right-to-left shunting and hypoxemia. Structural changes, such as smooth-muscle hypertrophy and adventitial thickening with increased extracellular matrix, are present in fatal PPHN (34, 90). Early changes in pulmonary vasoreactivity (due to decreased dilator production, increased vasoconstrictors, or other mechanisms) increase PVR, which over time, may further accelerate pulmonary vascular injury and cause hypertensive structural changes. Variability in clinical courses and outcomes of neonates with PPHN often reflects the variable contributions of myocardial dysfunction, pulmonary parenchymal disease and secondary lung injury from hyperoxia and volutrauma. Morbidity and mortality remain high despite aggressive therapy with hyperoxia, hyperventilation, metabolic alkalosis, and cardiotonic drugs. Attempts to lower PVR with vasodilator drugs, such as tolazoline, sodium nitroprusside, and prostaglandin E1, are often limited because of systemic hypotension, lack of potency, and inability to sustain vasodilation (tachyphylaxis), or other side effects. Thus, although these treatments can be successful, current therapies are often limited by adverse side effects or incomplete responsiveness. Patients who fail conventional therapy often require treatment with extracorporeal membrane oxygenation (ECMO). Although ECMO has improved survival in refractory PPHN, it remains labor intensive, costly, has multiple side effects, requires ligation of the right common carotid artery and internal jugular vein, and is associated with neurodevelopmental sequelae.

Inhaled NO therapy was studied in newborns with severe PPHN after early reports demonstrated its potent and selective pulmonary vasodilator effects in adults with primary pulmonary hypertension and perinatal animals (32, 53, 79). Roberts and co-workers reported acute increases in postductal arterial saturation without systemic hypotension in 6 neonates during brief treatment with inhaled NO at 80 ppm (82). Kinsella and co-workers also reported acute improvement in oxygenation and pulmonary hypertension (as directly assessed by echocardiogram) during brief (up to 4 h) treatment, but used lower doses of inhaled NO (6–20 ppm) (55). In addition to the acute response to inhaled NO, the latter report further demonstrated clinical recovery after continued low-dose NO treatment (55). The efficacy of this low-dose NO strategy was subsequently demonstrated in consecutive patients who met clinical criteria of severe PPHN refractory to conventional therapy, including high-frequency oscillatory ventilation (HFOV), and meeting criteria for ECMO therapy. As reported in the initial report, a low dose (6 ppm) caused sustained improvement in oxygenation without evidence of tachyphylaxis or a need for higher doses. In some cases, clinical responsiveness was sustained with even lower doses of inhaled NO (1–3 ppm). During the initial studies, 13/15 consecutive patients with severe PPHN meeting ECMO criteria were successfully treated without needing ECMO therapy (54, 55). More recently, two multicenter randomized studies have demonstrated the success of inhaled NO therapy in improving oxygenation and decreasing the need for ECMO therapy (76, 79).

Clinical improvement during inhaled NO therapy occurs with many disorders associated with PPHN, such as congenital diaphragmatic hernia (CDH), meconium aspiration syndrome, sepsis, idiopathic disorder, and others (54, 55, 76, 80, 82). Some diseases, especially CDH, appear to be less responsive to treatment than others, and sustained improvement in oxygenation varies among disorders. In addition, not all neonates with acute hypoxemic respiratory failure and pulmonary hypertension respond well to inhaled NO (81). Several mechanisms may explain the clinical variability in responsiveness to inhaled NO therapy. An inability to deliver NO to the pulmonary circulation due to poor lung inflation is the major cause of poor responsiveness. In some settings, administration of NO with HFOV has improved oxygenation more effectively than during conventional ventilation in the same patient. In addition, poor NO responsiveness may be related to myocardial dysfunction or systemic hypotension, severe pulmonary vascular structural disease, and unsuspected or missed anatomic cardiovascular lesions (such as total anomalous pulmonary venous return, coarctation of the aorta, alveolocapillary dysplasia, and others). Another mechanism of poor responsiveness to inhaled NO may be altered smooth-muscle cell responsiveness. As described from animal studies, decreased soluble guanylate cyclase or increased PDE5 activities may limit the vasodilator response to NO. For example, inhibition of PDE5 activity with dipyridamole or zaprinast may augment the vasodilator response to inhaled NO in experimental studies.

Although the primary physiologic abnormality in premature neonates with RDS is surfactant deficiency or dysfunction, severe RDS is associated with pulmonary hypertension. The presence of high PVR is associated with severe lung disease and poor outcome (97). Although pulmonary hypertension in this setting may be due to the mechanical effects of low lung volumes, pulmonary vasoconstriction contributes to high PVR in some patients. As suggested by the marked vasodilator responsiveness to inhaled NO in premature animals (51), low-dose inhaled NO therapy (5 ppm) can improve oxygenation in selected premature neonates with severe RDS (5). In addition to lowering PVR and improving pulmonary blood isiow, low-dose inhaled NO may further improve oxygenation in the absence of severe pulmonary hypertension by reducing intrapulmonary shunt, as demonstrated in ARDS (83). Whether inhaled NO can safely improve oxygenation and mortality without adverse sequelae, such as increased risk of chronic lung disease or intracranial hemorrhage, is under study. Although NO may prove toxic to the premature lung, recent studies suggest that inhaled NO may decrease lung inflammation in experimental RDS in premature lambs (50).

CONCLUSIONS

Experimental studies have clearly shown the important vasoregulatory role of the NO-cGMP cascade in the fetal and transitional pulmonary circulation, and that abnormalities in this system contribute to impaired pulmonary vascular tone and reactivity in an experimental model of PPHN. Although inhaled NO therapy can dramatically improve oxygenation in sick neonates with severe PPHN and premature neonates with RDS, responsiveness is poor in some patients. Further studies of the NO-cGMP cascade may provide helpful insights into novel clinical strategies for more successful treatment of neonatal pulmonary vascular disease. In addition, ET-1 clearly plays a major role in the normal developing lung and in experimental pulmonary hypertension. We speculate that the development and clinical application of ET-1 antagonists may provide an additional therapeutic strategy for severe PPHN.

REFERENCES:

1. Abman, S.H. and F.J. Accurso. Acute effects of partial compression of the ductus arteriosus on the fetal pulmonary circulation. *Am. J. Physiol.* 257: H626–634, 1989.
2. Abman, S.H. and F.J. Accurso. Sustained fetal pulmonary vasodilation during prolonged infusion of atrial natriuretic factor and 8-bromo-guanosine monophosphate. *Am. J. Physiol.* 260: H183–H192, 1991.
3. Abman, S.H., B.A. Chatfield, S.L. Hall, and I.F. McMurtry. Role of endothelium-derived relaxing factor during transition of pulmonary circulation at birth. *Am. J. Physiol.* 259: H1921–H1927, 1990.
4. Abman, S.H., B.A. Chatfield, D.M. Rodman, S.L. Hall, and I.F. McMurtry. Maturation-related changes in endothelium-dependent relaxation of ovine pulmonary arteries. *Am. J. Physiol.* 260: L280–L285, 1991.
5. Abman, S.H., J.P. Kinsella, M.S. Schaffer, and R.B. Wilkening. Inhaled nitric oxide therapy in a premature newborn with severe respiratory distress and pulmonary hypertension. *Pediatrics* 92: 606–609, 1993.
6. Abman, S.H., P.F. Shanley, and F.J. Accurso. Failure of postnatal adaptation of the pulmonary circulation after chronic intrauterine pulmonary hypertension in fetal lambs. *J. Clin. Invest.* 83: 1849–1858, 1989.
7. Accurso, F.J., B. Alpert, R.B. Wilkening, R.G. Petersen, and G. Meschia. Time-dependent response of fetal pulmonary blood flow to an increase in fetal oxygen tension. *Respir. Physiol.* 63: 43–52, 1986.
8. Allen, K. and S.G. Haworth. Impaired adaptation of intrapulmonary arteries to extrauterine life in newborn pigs exposed to hypoxia. An ultrastructural study. *Fed. Proc.* 45: 879, 1986.
9. Allen, S.W., B.A. Chatfield, S.L. Koppenhafer, M.S. Schaffer, R.R. Wolfe, and S.H. Abman. Circulating immunoreactive ET-1 in children with pulmonary hypertension: association with acute hypoxic pulmonary vasoreactivity. *Am. Rev. Respir. Dis.* 148: 519–522, 1993.
10. Archer, S.L., J.M.C. Huang, V. Hampl, D.F. Nelson, P.J. Shultz, and E.K. Weir. NO and cGMP cause vasorelaxation by activation of a charybdotoxin-sensitive K channel by cGMP-dependent protein kinase. *Proc. Natl. Acad. Sci. USA* 91: 7583–7587, 1994.
11. Arnal, J.F., J. Yamin, S. Dockery, and D.G. Harrison. Regulation of endothelial NO synthase mRNA, protein, and activity during cell growth. *Am. J. Physiol.* 267: C1381–C1388, 1994.
12. Beavo, J.A. and D.H. Reifsnyder. Primary sequence of cyclic nucleotide phosphodiesterase isozymes and the design of selective inhibitors. *Trends Pharmacol. Sci.* 11: 150–155, 1990.

13. Belik, J. and N.L. Stephens. Developmental differences in vascular smooth muscle mechanics in pulmonary and systemic circulations. *J. Appl. Physiol.* 74: 682–687, 1993.
14. Bolotina, V.M., S. Najibi, J.J. Palacino, P.H. Pagano, and R.A. Cohen. NO directly activates calcium-dependent potassium channels in vascular smooth muscle. *Nature* 368: 850–853, 1994.
15. Bonvallet, S.T., M.A. Zamora, K. Hasunuma, K. Sato, N. Hanasato, D. Anderson, K. Sato, and T.J. Stelzner. BQ123, an ETA-receptor antagonist, attenuates hypoxic pulmonary hypertension in rats. *Am. J. Physiol.* 266: H1327–H331, 1994.
16. Boulanger, C. and T.F. Luscher. Release of endothelin from the porcine aorta. Inhibition by endothelium-derived nitric oxide. *J. Clin. Invest.* 85: 87–90, 1990.
17. Bustamante, S.A., Y. Pang, S. Romero, M.R. Pierce, C.A. Voelker, J.H. Thompson, M. Sandoval, X. Liu, and M.J. Miller. Inducible NOS and the regulation of central vessel caliber in the fetal rat. *Circulation* 1948–1953, 1996.
18. Braner, D.A., J.R. Fineman, R. Chang, and S.J. Soifer. M&B 22948, a cGMP phosphodiesterase inhibitor, is a pulmonary vasodilator in lambs. *Am. J. Physiol.* 764: H252–H258, 1993.
19. Cassin, S. Role of prostaglandins, thromboxanes and leukotrienes in the control of the pulmonary circulation in the fetus and newborn. *Semin. Perinatol.* 11: 53–63, 1987.
20. Cassin, S., G.S. Dawes, J.C. Mott, B.B. Ross, and L.B. Strang. Vascular resistance of the foetal and newly ventilated lung of the lamb. *J. Physiol. Lond.* 171: 61–79, 1964.
21. Cassin, S., T. Kristova, T. Davis, P. Kadowitz, and G. Gause. Tone-dependent responses to endothelin in the isolated perfused fetal sheep pulmonary circulation in situ. *J. Appl. Physiol.* 70: 1228–1234, 1991.
22. Chatfield, B.A., I.F. McMurtry, S.L. Hall, and S.H. Abman. Hemodynamic effects of endothelin-1 on the ovine fetal pulmonary circulation. *Am. J. Physiol.* 261: R182–R187, 1991.
23. Cohen, A.H., K. Hanson, K. Morris, B. Fouty, I.F. McMurtry, W. Clarke, and D.M. Rodman. Inhibition of cGMP-specific phosphodiesterase selectively vasodilates the pulmonary circulation in chronically hypoxic rats. *J. Clin. Invest.* 97: 172–179, 1996.
24. Cornfield, D.N., B.A. Chatfield, J.A. McQueston, I.F. McMurtry, and S.H. Abman. Effects of birth-related stimuli on L-arginine-dependent pulmonary vasodilation in the ovine fetus. *Am. J. Physiol.* 262: H1474–H1481, 1992.
25. Cornfield, D.N., J.A. McQueston, I.F. McMurtry, D.M. Rodman, and S.H. Abman. Role of ATPsensitive K^+channels in ovine fetal pulmonary vascular tone. *Am. J. Physiol.* 263: H1363–H1368, 1992.
26. Cornfield, D.N., H.L. Reeves, S. Tolarova, E.K. Weir, and S.L. Archer. Oxygen causes fetal pulmonary vasodilation through activation of a calcium-dependent potassium channel. *Proc. Natl. Acad. Sci. USA* 93: 8089–8094, 1996.
27. Davidson, D. and A. Eldemerdash. Endothelium-derived relaxing factor: evidence that it regulates pulmonary vascular resistance in the isolated newborn guinea pig lung. *Pediatr. Res.* 29: 538–542, 1991.
28. Dubin, D., R.E. Pratt, J.P. Cooke, and V.J. Dzau. Endothelin, a potent vasoconstrictor, is a vascular smooth muscle mitogen. *J. Vasc. Med. Biol.* 1: 150–154, 1989.
29. Fineman, J.R., J. Wong, F.C. Morin, L.M. Wild, and S.J. Soifer. Chronic NO inhibition in utero produces persistent pulmonary hypertension in newborn lambs. *J. Clin. Invest.* 93: 9675–9683, 1994.
30. Flowers, M.A., Y. Wang, R.J. Stewart, B. Patel, and P.A. Marsden. Reciprocal regulation of

endothelin-1 and endothelial NOS in proliferating endothelial cells. *Am. J. Physiol.* 269: H1988–H1997, 1995.

32. Fratacci, M.D., C.G. Frostell, T.Y. Chen, and W.M. Zapol. Inhaled NO: a selective pulmonary vasodilator of heparin-protamine vasoconstriction in sheep. Anesthesiology 75: 990–999, 1991.
33. Garg, U.C. and A. Hassid. NO-generating vasodilators and 8-bromo-cGMP inhibit mitogenesis and proliferation of cultured rat vascular smooth muscle ceils. *J. Clin. Invest.* 83: 1774–1777, 1989.
34. Geggel, R.L. and L.M. Reid. The structural basis of persistent pulmonary hypertension of the newborn. *Clin. Perinatol.* 3: 525–549, 1984.
35. Giaid, A. and D. Saleh. Reduced expression of endothelial NO synthase in the lungs of patients with pulmonary hypertension. *N. Engl. J. Med.* 333: 214–221, 1995.
36. Giaid, A., M. Yanagasawa, D. Langleben, R.P. Michel, R. Levy, H. Shennib, S. Kimura, T. Masaki, W.P. Duguid, and D.J. Stewart. Expression of endothelin-l in the lungs of patients with pulmonary hypertension. *N. Engl. J. Med.* 328: 1732–1739, 1993.
37. Goldberg, S.J., R.A. Levy, and B. Siassi. Effects of maternal hypoxia and hyperoxia upon the neonatal pulmonary vasculature. *Pediatrics* 48: 528–533, 1971.
38. Halbower, A.C., R.M. Tuder, W.A. Franklin, J.S. Pollock, U. Forstermann, and S.H. Abman. Maturation-related changes in endothelial NO synthase immunolocalization in the developing ovine lung. *Am. J. Physiol.* 267: L585–L591, 1994.
39. Hanson, K.A., J.A. Beavo, S.H. Abman, and W.R. Clarke. Chronic intrauterine pulmonary hypertension increases lung cGMP hydrolytic activity and decreases cGMP kinase content in the ovine fetus [Abstract]. *Am. J. Respir. Crit. Care Med.* 155: A632, 1997.
40. Hanson, K.A., S. Uezono, J. Beavo, and W.R. Clarke. Developmental regulation of pulmonary cGMP phosphodiesterase activity in fetal and maternal lung [Abstract]. *Am. J. Respir. Crit. Care Med.* 151: A437, 1995.
41. Heymann, M.A. and S.J. Soifer. Control of fetal and neonatal pulmonary circulation. In: *Pulmonary vascular physiology and pathophysiology,* edited by E.K. Weir and J.T. Reeves. New York: Marcel Dekker, 1989, p. 33–50.
42. Hirata, Y., Y.H. Yoshima, S. Eguchi, K. Kanno, T. Imai, K. Ohta, and F. Marumo. ET receptor subtype B mediates synthesis of NO by cultures bovine endothelial cells. *J. Clin. Invest.* 91: 1367–1373, 1993.
43. Hobbs, A.J. and L.J. Ignarro. NO-cGMP signal transduction system. In: *Nitric Oxide and the Lung,* edited by W.M. Zapol and K. Bloch, New York: Marcel Dekker, 1996, p. 1–57.
44. Isozaki-Fukuda, Y., T. Kojima, Y. Hirata, N. Ono, S. Sawaragi, I. Sawaragi, and Y. Kobayashi. Plasma immunoreactive ET-1 concentration in human fetal blood: its relation to asphyxia. *Pediatr. Res.* 30: 244–247, 1991.
45. Ivy, D.D., J.P. Kinsella, and S.H. Abman. Physiologic characterization of endothelin A and B receptor activity in the ovine fetal pulmonary circulation. J. Clin. Invest. 93: 2141–2148, 1994.
46. Ivy, D.D., T.A. Parker, J.W. Ziegler, H.L. Galan, J.P. Kinsella, and S.H. Abman. Prolonged endothelin A receptor blockade attenuates chronic intrauterine pulmonary hypertension. *J. Clin. Invest.* 99: 1179–1186, 1997.
47. Ivy, D.D., J.W. Ziegler, M.F. Dubus, J.J. Fox, J.P. Kinsella, and S.H. Abman. Chronic intrauterine pulmonary hypertension alters endothelin receptor activity in the ovine fetus. *Pediatr. Res.* 39: 335–342, 1995.
48. Ivy, D.D., J.W. Ziegler, J.P. Kinsella, and S.H. Abman. Endothelin blockade augments fetal pulmonary vasodilation. *J. Appl. Physiol.* 81: 2481–2487, 1996.

49. Jones, O.W. and S.H. Abman. Systemic and pulmonary hemodynamic effects of big endothelin-l and phosphoramidon in the ovine fetus. *Am. J. Physiol.* 266: R929–R935, 1994.
50. Kinsella, J.P., A.C. Halbower, J.W. Ziegler, J.F. Fox, D.D. Ivy, and S.H. Abman. Effects of inhaled NO on pulmonary edema and lung neutrophil accumulation in severe experimental hyaline membrane disease. *Pediatr. Res.* 41: 457–463, 1997.
51. Kinsella, J.P., D.D. Ivy, and S.H. Abman. Inhaled nitric oxide improves gas exchange and lowers pulmonary vascular resistance in severe experimental hyaline membrane disease. *Pediatr. Res.* 36: 402–408, 1994.
52. Kinsella, J.P., D.D. Ivy, and S.H. Abman. Ontogeny of NO activity and response to inhaled NO in the developing ovine pulmonary circulation. *Am. J. Physiol.* 267: H1955–H1961, 1994.
53. Kinsella, J.P., J.A. McQueston, A.A. Rosenberg, and S.H. Abman. Hemodynamic effects of exogenous nitric oxide in ovine transitional pulmonary circulation. *Am. J. Physiol.* 263: H875–H880, 1992.
54. Kinsella, J.P., S.R. Neish, D.D. lvy, E. Shaffer, and S.H. Abman. Clinical responses to prolonged treatment of persistent pulmonary hypertension of the newborn. *J. Pediatr.* 123: 103–108, 1993.
55. Kinsella, J.P., S. Neish, E. Shaffer, and S.H. Abman. Low dose inhalational nitric oxide in persistent pulmonary hypertension of the newborn. *Lancet* 340: 819–820, 1992.
56. Kobzik, L., D.S. Bredt, C.J. Lowenstein, J. Drazen, B. Gaston, D. Sugarbaker, and J.S. Stamler. NOS in human and rat lung: immunocytochemical and histochemical localization. *Am. J. Respir. Cell Mol. Biol.* 9: 371–377, 1993.
57. Kourembanas, D., L. McQuillan, G. Leung, and D. Faller. NO regulates the expression of vasoconstrictors and growth factors by vascular endothelium under normoxia and hypoxia. *J. Clin. Invest.* 92: 99–104, 1993.
58. Kourembanas, S., P.A. Marsden, L.P. McQuillan, and D.V. Faller. Hypoxia induces endothelin gene expression and secretion in cultured human endothelium. *J. Clin. Invest.* 88: 1054–1057, 1991.
59. Le Cras, T.D., C. Xue, A. Rengesamy, and R.A. Johns. Chronic hypoxia upregulates endothelial and inducible NO synthase gene and protein expression in rat lung. *Am. J. Physiol.* 270: L164–L170, 1996.
60. Leffler, C.W., J.R. Hessler, and R.S. Green. Mechanism of stimulation of pulmonary prostacyclin synthesis at birth. *Prostaglandins* 28: 877–87, 1984.
61. Leffler, C.W., T.L. Tyler, and S. Cassin. Effect of indomethacin on pulmonary vascular response to ventilation of fetal goats. *Am. J. Physiol.* 234: H346–H351, 1978.
62. Lerman, A., E.K. Sandok, F.L. Hildebrand, and J.C. Burnett. Inhibition of EDRF enhances endothelin-mediated vasoconstriction. *Circulation* 85: 1894–1898, 1992.
63. Levin, D.L., M.A. Heymann, J.A. Kitterman, G.A. Gregory, R.H. Phibbs, and A.M. Rudolph. Persistent pulmonary hypertension of the newborn. *J. Pediatr.* 89: 626–633, 1976.
64. Levin, D.L., A.I. Hyman, M.A. Heymann, and A.M. Rudolph. Fetal hypertension and the development of increased pulmonary vascular smooth muscle: a possible mechanism for persistent pulmonary hypertension of the newborn infant. *J. Pediatr.* 92: 265–269, 1978.
65. Lewis, A.B., M.A. Heymann, and A.M. Rudolph. Gestational changes in pulmonary vascular responses in fetal lambs in utero. *Circ. Res.* 39: 536–541, 1976.
66. Li, H., S. Chen, Y. Chen, Q. Meng, J. Durand, S. Oparil, and T. Elton. Enhanced endothelin-1 and endothelin receptor gene expression in chronic hypoxia. *J. Appl. Physiol.* 77: 1451–1459, 1994.

67. MacCumber, M.W., C.A. Ross, B.M. Glaser, and S.H. Snyder. Endothelin: visualization of mRNAs by in situ hybridization provides evidence for local action. *Proc. Natl. Acad. Sci. USA* 86: 7285–7289, 1989.

68. McQueston, J.A., D.N. Cornfield, I.F. McMurtry, and S.H. Abman. Effects of oxygen and exogenous L-arginine on endothelium-derived relaxing factor activity in the fetal pulmonary circulation. *Am. J. Physiol.* 264: H865–7871, 1993.

69. McQueston, J.A., J.P. Kinsella, D.D. Ivy, I.F. McMurtry, and S.H. Abman. Chronic pulmonary hypertension in utero impairs endothelium-dependent vasodilation. *Am. J. Physiol.* 268: H288–H294, 1995.

70. McQuillan, L.P., G.K. Leung, P.A. Marsden, S.K. Kostyk, and S. Kourembanas. Hypoxia inhibits expression of eNOS via transcriptional and posttranscriptional mechanisms. *Am. J. Physiol.* 267: H1921–H1927, 1994.

71. Michael, J.R. and B.A. Markewitz. Endothelins and the lung. *Am. J. Respir. Crit. Care Med.* 154: 555–581, 1996.

72. Moncada, S., R.M.J. Palmer, and E.A. Higgs. Nitric oxide: physiology, pathophysiology, and pharmacology. *Pharmacol. Rev.* 43: 109–142, 1991.

73. Morbidelli, L., C.H. Chang, J.G. Douglas, H.J. Granger, C.A. Maggi, P. Geppetti, F. Ledda. NO mediates mitogenic effect of VEGF on coronary venular endothelium. *Am. J. Physiol.* 270: H411–H415, 1996.

74. Morin, F.C. Ligating the ductus arteriosus before birth causes persistent pulmonary hypertension in the newborn lamb. *Pediatr. Res.* 25: 245–250, 1989.

75. Morin, F.C., E.A. Egan, W. Ferguson, and C.E.G. Lundgren. Development of pulmonary vascular response to oxygen. *Am. J. Physiol.* 254: H542–H546, 1988.

76. Neonatal Inhaled NO Study Group. Inhaled NO in full-term and nearly full-term infants with hypoxic respiratory failure. *N. Engl. J. Med.* 336: 597–604, 1997.

77. North, A.J., R.A. Star, T.S. Brannon, K. Ujiie, L.B. Wells, C.J. Lowenstien, S.H. Snyder, and P.W. Shaul. NO synthase type I and type III gene expression are developmentally regulated in rat lung. *Am. J. Physiol.* 266: L635–L641, 1994.

78. Rairigh, R., T.D. LeCras, D.D. Ivy, J.P. Kinsella, G. Richter, M. Horan, I. Fan, and S.H. Abman. Role of inducible NOS in regulation of pulmonary vascular tone in the ovine fetus. *J. Clin Invest* 101:15–21, 1998.

79. Roberts, J.D., T. Chen, N. Kawai, J. Wain, P. Dupuy, A. Shimouchi, K. Bloch, D. Polaner, and W.M. Zapol. Inhaled NO reverses pulmonary vasoconstriction in the hypoxic and acidoticnewborn lamb. *Circ. Res.* 72: 246–254, 1993.

80. Roberts, J.D., J.R. Fineman, F.C. Morin, P.W. Shaul, S. Rimar, M.D. Schreiber, R.A. Polin, M.S. Zwass, M.M. Zayek, I. Gross, M.A. Heymann, and W.M. Zapol. Inhaled nitric oxide and persistent pulmonary hypertension of the newborn. *N. Engl. J. Med.* 336: 605–610, 1997.

81. Roberts, J.D., J.P. Kinsella, and S.H. Abman. Inhaled NO in neonatal pulmonary hypertension and severe RDS: experimental and clinical studies. In: *Nitric Oxide and the Lung*, edited by W.M. Zapol and K. Bloch, New York: Marcel Dekker, 1996, p 333–363.

82. Roberts, J.D., D.M. Polaner, P. Lang, and W.M. Zapol. Inhaled nitric oxide in persistent pulmonary hypertension of the newborn. *Lancet* 340: 818–819, 1992.

83. Rossaint, R., K.J. Falcke, F. Lopez, K. Slama, U. Pison, and W.M. Zapol. Inhaled NO for the adult respiratory distress syndrome. *N. Engl. J. Med.* 328: 399–405, 1993.

84. Rosenberg, A.A., J. Kennaugh, S.L. Koppenhafer, M. Loomis, and S.H. Abman. Increased immunoreactive endothelin-1 levels in persistent pulmonary hypertension of the newborn. *J. Pediatr.* 123: 109–114, 1993.

85. Rudolph, A.M. Fetal and neonatal pulmonary circulation. *Annu. Rev. Physiol.* 41: 383–395, 1979.
86. Rudolph A.M., M.A. Heymann, and A.B. Lewis. Physiology and pharmacology of the pulmonary circulation in the fetus and newborn. In: *Development of the lung,* edited by W. Hodson, New York: Marcel Dekker, 1977, p. 497–453.
87. Shaul, P.W., E.J. Smart, L.J. Robinson, Z. German, I.S. Yuhanna, Y. Ying, R.G.W. Anderson, and T. Michel. Acylation targets endothelial NO synthase to plasmalemal calveolae. *J. Biol. Chem.* 271: 6518–6522, 1996.
87b Shaul, P.W., I.S. Yuhanna, Z. German, Z. Chen, R.H. Steinhorn, and F.C. Morin. Pulmonary endothelial nitric oxide synthase gene expression is decreased in fetal lambs with pulmonary hypertension. *Am. J. Physiol.* 272: L1005–L1012, 1997.
88. Soifer, S.J., R.D. Loitz, C. Roman, and M.A. Heymann. Leukotriene end organ antagonists increase pulmonary blood flow infeal lambs. *Am. J. Physiol.* 249: H570–H576, 1985.
89. Steinhorn, R.H., J.A. Russell, and F.C. Morin. Pulmonary arteries from newborn lambs with persistent pulmonary hypertension have decreased sensitivity to NO [Abstract]. *Pediatr. Res.* 35: 354A, 1994.
90. Stenmark, K.R., S.H. Abman, and F.J. Accurso. Etiologic mechanisms of persistent pulmonary hypertension of the newborn. In: *Pulmonary vascular physiology and pathophysiology,* edited by E.K. Weir and J.T. Reeves. New York: Marcel Dekker, 1989, p. 335–402.
91a. Stewart, D.J., R.D. Levy, P. Cernacek, and D. Langleben. Increased plasma endothelin-1 in pulmonary hypertension: marker or mediator of disease? *Ann. Intern. Med.* 114: 464–469, 1991.
91b. Thébaud, B., P. de Lagausie, E. Souil, Y. Aigrain, J.C. Mercier, and A.T. Dinh-Xuan. Pulmonary vasodilation is not impaired in congenital diaphragmatic hernia [Abstract]. *Am. J. Respir. Crit. Care Med.* 155: A948, 1997.
92. Thomae, K.R., D.K. Nakayama, T.R. Billiar, R.L. Simmons, B.R. Pitt, and P. Davies. Effect of NO on fetal pulmonary artery smooth muscle growth. *J. Surg. Res.* 270: H411–H415, 1996.
93. Velvis, H., P. Moore, and M.A. Heymann. Prostaglandin inhibition prevents the fall in pulmonary vascular resistance as the result of rhythmic distension of the lungs in fetal lambs. *Pediatr. Res.* 30: 62–67, 1991.
94. Villamor, E., T.D. Le Cras, M.P. Horan, A.C. Halbower, R.M. Tuder, and S.H. Abman. Chronic intrauterine hypertension impairs endothelial nitric oxide sythase in the ovine fetus. *Am. J. Physiol.* 272: L1013–L1020, 1997.
95. Wang, Y. and F. Coceani. Isolated pulmonary resistance vessels from fetal lambs: contractile behavior and responses to indomethacin and endothelin-1. *Circ. Res.* 71: 320–330, 1992.
96. Wallen, L.D., S.F. Perry, J.T. Alston, and J.E. Maloney. Morphometric study of the role of pulmonary arterial flow in fetal lung growth in sheep. *Pediatr. Res.* 27: 122–127, 1990.
97. Walther, F.J., F.J. Bender, and J.O. Leighton. Persistent pulmonary hypertension in premature neonates with severe RDS. *Pediatrics* 90: 899–904, 1992.
98. Winters, J.W., J. Wong, D. van Dyke, M. Johengen, M.A. Heymann, and J.R. Fineman. Endothelin blockade does not alter the increase in pulmonary blood flow during oxygen ventilation in fetal lambs. *Pediatr. Res.* 40: 152–157, 1996.
99. Wong, J., J.R. Fineman, and M.A. Heymann. The role of endothelin and endothelin re-

ceptor subtypes in regulation of fetal pulmonary vascular tone. *Pediatr. Res.* 35: 664–670, 1994.

100. Yanagisawa, M., H. Kurihara, S. Kirmura, Y. Tomobe, M. Kobayashi, Y. Mitsui, Y. Yazaki, K. Goto, and T. Masaki. A novel potent vasoconstrictor peptide produced by vascular endothelial cells. *Nature* 332: 411–415, 1988.
101. Ziche, M., L. Morbidelli, E. Masini, S. Amerini, H.J. Granger, C.A. Maggi, P. Geppetti, and F. Ledda. NO mediates angiogenesis in vivo and endothelial cell growth and migration in vitro promoted by substance P. *J. Clin. Invest.* 94: 2036–2044, 1994.
102. Ziegler, J.W., D.D. Ivy, J.J. Fox, J.P. Kinsella, W.R. Clarke, and S.H. Abman. Dipyridamole, a cGMP phosphodiesterase inhibitor, causes pulmonary vasodilation in the ovine fetus. *Am. J. Physiol.* 269: H473–H479, 1995.

chapter 8

DEVELOPMENT OF CELLULAR HOST DEFENSE MECHANISMS

Sergei P. Sorokin, Richard F. Hoyt, Jr., and Nancy A.F. McNelly

THE lungs are well guarded against damage from inhaled gases, particulates, and microbes by a variety of local defenses provided by resident cells and hematological defenses provided by leukocytes and their products acting in the lungs. Various mechanisms are used in these defenses, and they come into being at different times during lung development as effector cells differentiate. In general, operation of all such defenses improves as cells become experienced in immunological cross talk or link up with sensory and motor nerves, and the time newly differentiated cells require to reach this state depends on cell type. Physiological processes of more macroscopic scale, represented by pulmonary mechanics and lung reflexes involving the central nervous system, eventually contribute substantially to these host defenses. Discussion of their ontogeny is beyond the scope of this review, which is limited to more intimate cellular interactions.

In the lungs, cellular host defenses that depend primarily on intrinsic lung elements making up the bronchial tree, vessels, connective tissue stroma, and pleura develop as a consequence of general morphogenetic processes. Airway branching appears to be controlled by specific mechanisms. As the developmental plan for the bronchial tree unfolds, additional mechanisms assure that the largest airways soon bear characteristics of bronchi, the intermediate ones of bronchioles, and the terminal ones of thin-walled air–blood barriers ideally suited to respiratory gas exchange. Such regulated events, discussed in detail elsewhere in this book, ensure that cell types appear in a defined order and in their proper places along the airway. In the interim, the lengthening of individual airway branches has come under management by neuroendocrine cells present in the epithelium, and as formation of the bronchial tree nears completion, many of these cells undergo functional metamorphosis into chemoreceptors. Thus many cells essential to respiratory defenses appear as a direct consequence of interaction between the endodermal epithelium of the lung buds and the surrounding pulmonary mesenchyme.

Numerous presumptively immigrant cell populations also contribute to lung defense. These can be classified into two somewhat overlapping groups. The first consists of cells that establish residency early in the rudimentary lungs. They include precursors of intrinsic ganglion cells derived from the neural crest, and quite likely, stem cells for the fetal macrophage lineage. The second group are later arrivals and encompass most of the other leukocytes. Their primarily immunological functions are mainly critical for life after birth when the expanded organ is much more exposed to outside influences. Accordingly, in the epigenetic timetable it is possible for full realization of immunological defense capacity to be delayed until after an otherwise functional lung has been formed.

OVERVIEW OF PULMONARY CELLULAR DEFENSES

Conducting Airways

Throughout the bronchial tree the epithelium has structural provisions and the metabolic capacity to constitute a formidable physical barrier to the outside environment. In the conducting airways, cellular defenses are principally carried out by (*1*) epithelial cells making up the mucociliary clearance apparatus of ciliated and secretory cells and seromucous glands, together with small numbers of cells having monitoring functions, and (2) lymphocytes in bronchus-associated lymphatic tissue (BALT), the pulmonary version of mucosa-associated lymphatic tissue (MALT), providing for immunosurveillance of bronchial and bronchiolar surfaces.

BALT develops variously among different mammals (67) but is never as well organized as the Peyer's patches of gut-associated lymphatic tissue (GALT). It is consistently present in rabbits and rats, less obviously so in mice, guinea pigs, or pigs, and absent from hamsters, dogs, and cats and also from human beings, except when lung infections or smoking-related inflammation intervene. In smokers it develops around lymphatic channels present in the bronchial adventitia rather than in the submucosa (9). BALT possesses a reticular fiber stroma usually formed into solitary follicles, an overlying largely nonciliated "lymphoepithelium," and at the follicular margin, lymphatics and high-endothelial venules (HEV), the hallmark of lymph nodes and Peyer's patches. It is mainly populated by lymphocytes, macrophages, and accessory dendritic cells that function in association with heterophils, eosinophils, mast cells, and globule leukocytes stationed in the periphery. In rats, T cells make up the greater number of lymphocytes and are concentrated in the lower part of the follicle away from the epithelium, flanked by immunoglobulin (Ig)A-expressing B cells. Both IgM and a small number of IgG cells occur in the upper part, and major histocompatibility complex (MHC) class II (Ia antigen)–expressing cells are scattered throughout (65). These include the lymphoepithelium and pulmonary dendritic cells. The latter resemble Langerhans cells of the skin, as distinguished from another epidermal antigen-presenting cell allied to thymocytes, and evidently are related to macrophages. Functionally they are better antigen-presenters but much poorer phagocytes. Dendritic cells occur widely in the conducting airways and respiratory zone of rats but are virtually restricted to extrapulmonary airways of mice. In human GALT, specialized epithelial cells with a characteristically microfolded luminal surface (M cells) are primarily responsible for conveying antigen to underlying lymphocytes; and while such cells have also been described in BALT, the accompanying illustrations have not been convincing. More likely, handling of antigens is relegated to intraepithelial dendritic cells, or else the lymphoepithelium may convey them basalwards by vesicular transport (microendocytosis).

Lymphocytes are found in some number on the airway surface, being immersed in a fluid layer that underlies the mucous sheet. The fluid is provided by secretory mucous and serous cells in the airway epithelium and glands, which synthesize and release various bacterostatic agents (lactoferrin, lysozyme) into it and also produce cytokines and other signaling molecules involved in regulation of inflammatory reactions, recruitment of leukocytes, and other defensive functions. They also add the secretory piece to Ig A prior to its release onto the surface (Table 8.1). In addition, as demonstrated in vitro (55), surface T cells, in part derived from BALT, may be directly activated by the bronchial epithelium in the absence of foreign antigen. This appears to occur if lymphocyte function antigen-3 (LFA-3) molecules on the epithelial surface are up-regulated and binding occurs to its counterstructure LFA-2 (CD2)

Table 8.1 Nocifensive Substances Secreted by Pulmonary Epithelial Cells

Substance	*Secreted by*
Mucins	Conducting airway epithelium
Antibiotic substances	
Surfactant-associated protein A (SP-A)	Respiratory zone epithelium
Secretory immunoglobulin A	Epithelial and IgA B cells
Complement	Epithelial cells
Lactoferrin	Conducting airway epithelium
Lysozyme	Conducting airway epithelium
Antioxidants	
SP-A	Respiratory zone epithelium
Lactoferrin	Conducting airway epithelium
Glutathione	Epithelial cells
Catalase	Epithelial cells
Vitamin E	Respiratory zone epithelium
Vitamin A	Respiratory zone epithelium
Plasmalogens	Respiratory zone epithelium

(*Continued*)

Table 8.1 Nocifensive Substances Secreted by Pulmonary Epithelial Cells (*continued*)

Substance	*Secreted by*
Antiproteases	
Elafin	Respiratory zone epithelium
Secretory leukoprotease inhibitor	Both
CC10	Clara cells
Chemokines (chemoattractant for)	
C-X-C chemokines (neutrophils)	Epithelial cells
C-C chemokines (monocytes, eosinophils, CD4+ lymphocytes)	Epithelial cells
Platelet-activating factor (eosinophils)	Epithelial cells
Leukotriene B_4 (neutrophils, monocytes, eosinophils)	Both
As-yet unidentified lymphocyte attractants	Epithelial cells
Adhesion molecules	
ICAM-1	Both
Type II human histocompatibility antigens	Both, but primarily expressed by great alveolar cells
Cytokines and agents modulating inflammation	
GM-CSF	Conducting or both?
G-CSF	Conducting or both?
NO	Conducting airway epithelium
Prostaglandin E_2 (PGE_2)	Both
TGF-β	Conducting airway epithelium
IL-6	Epithelial cells
Surfactant	Great alveolar cells
Smooth muscle cell modulators	
Neutral endopeptidase (NEP)	Conducting airway epithelium
Endothelins	Mucous, serous, and Clara cells
Vascular permeability modulators	
Angiotensin converting enzyme (ACE)	Conducting airway epithelium
Carboxypeptidase M	Respiratory zone epithelium
Histamine-degrading enzymes	Epithelial cells
Regulators of interaction between epithelial cells	
Fibronectin	Both
EGF	Both
Lipocortin	Both
TGF-α	Both
Regulatory peptides	
CGRP	PNEC
GRP	PNEC
Calcitonin	PNEC

The designation *both* indicates localization to conducting airway and respiratory zone; *conducting or both* indicates the established source and a probability that the entire epithelium is involved; *epithelial cells* is used when the regional source is unspecified. Several of these substances, notably the cytokines, chemokines, and certain growth factors, are also produced by connective tissue cells. [Based on data from ref. 107 and others cited in the text.]

or some other receptor on the T cells. Activation may result from the binding itself or as a direct or indirect sequel to release of factors by the epithelium.

Lymphocytes as well as blood-borne dendritic or veiled accessory cells and monocytes enter BALT through HEV and return to the bloodstream via pulmonary lymphatics, hilar or tracheobronchial lymph nodes, and the thoracic and right lymphatic ducts. By this means, B or T cells sensitized to antigen in the gut reach the lungs and develop further there, or else cells leave to populate other mucosal sites (6, 13). Before leukocytes can cross out from the bloodstream, however, they must first express appropriate surface homing receptors that enable them to bind complementary addressins on the endothelial surface of HEV.

The Respiratory Zone

In the thin-walled respiratory zone, cellular defenses are maintained by resident macrophages as the first line of defense, abetted by monocyte-derived macrophages and other leukocytes and by blood-borne factors as well as secretions provided by alveolar epithelial cells. Included among these are surface tension–modifying substances produced by great alveolar (type II) cells and various antimicrobial agents, in part synthesized by the alveolar epithelium and released to the serous underlayer of alveolar surface fluid, much as epithelial cells in the conducting airways contribute to bronchial fluids (Table 8.1). In this region, macrophages not only serve as scavengers of particles deposited on the alveolar surfaces but also in the frontline for immunological surveillance, interacting directly with lymphocytes or preferentially through accessory cells if these are present (27). Although the alveolar interstitium is less densely populated by lymphocytes and their near kin than in the conducting airways, a functional equivalent to BALT exists there, and given the extent of the respiratory zone probably exceeds it in total cell volume (66). Mast cells occur in the pleura and sometimes in the interstitium; nevertheless, this is decidedly species variable.

Stromal and Intravascular Elements

Cellular defenses are most frequently thought of in terms of the epithelium and the blood cells, but many contributions are also made by fixed components in the connective tissue compartment of the lungs, such as the fibrocytes, chondrocytes, airway and vascular muscle, and endothelium, beginning with the early developmental role of mesenchymal fibroblasts in interaction with pulmonary endoderm during branching morphogenesis and continuing through production of growth or maturation substances that help to maintain the integrity of the lung tissues. Endothelial cells not only are important for regulating access of leukocytes to extravascular compartments of the lungs but also mediate selective uptake of materials like serotonin from the blood and produce a number of secretory products like platelet-derived growth factors (PDGFs) and endothelins, although not uniquely on their own.

Intravascular macrophages are prominent in pulmonary vessels of certain mammalian species but have been studied most in sheep (113), where they appear to become active phagocytes postnatally (53). Megakaryocytes and/or blood platelets may also become sequestered in pulmonary capillaries. In early fetal life, moderate-sized (10–25 μm) megakaryocytes developed in the liver are the most abundant leukocytes encountered in pulmonary vessels, but postnatally it is more typical for giant polyploid forms to remain at the extravascular site of their formation in hematopoietic tissue and release cytoplasmic fragments into the blood stream. These subsequently are modified into discoid platelets either in the blood stream or lungs (70). Occasionally, however, folded naked nuclei of the larger cells occur there as well.

DEVELOPMENT OF CELLULAR PULMONARY DEFENSE MECHANISMS

Complex pulmonary defense mechanisms rarely are fully integrated when they first appear but are pieced together from constituent elements over a period of time. In general, the development of a specific defensive capacity follows a similar sequence of stages within a range of mammalian species, although gauged by the number of days of gestation or as a proportion of the gestational period, the time scale may differ considerably. Full development of some mechanisms may not be reached until late in prenatal life or after birth in some species, even though partial function may be evident much earlier.

Each time a mature cell divides, some part of the "differentiated state" is lost and must be regained by daughter cells. Since most of the cells in the lungs undergo renewal throughout life, this certainly applies to respiratory defense mechanisms operating in these cells, although the compromise to defensive capacity probably is slight when dividing cells are in the minority. Seemingly, it takes less time to recover defenses in a mature population than to develop them in immature cells, and for this reason the process is easier to analyze if studied the first time the defenses appear.

Ontogeny of Respiratory Defenses Intrinsic to the Bronchial Tree

The Epithelial Sheet

It has long been known that undifferentiated epithelial cells in early fetal lungs store large amounts of glycogen in the cytoplasm and that this usually declines sharply near the time they begin to sprout cilia, synthesize mucus, or express some other distinct differentiated characteristic. The decline coincides with increased activity for enzymes of the citric acid cycle, hexose monophosphate shunt, and the cytochrome respiratory chain. It reflects an underlying switch from a predominantly anaerobic to an aerobic oxidative metabolism, a change that also occurs at a comparable developmental age in organ-cultured fetal lung and hence is intrinsically regulated (80). Increased enzymic activity leads to increased oxidative phosphorylation by mitochondria but also expands the opportunities for using oxidative metabolic pathways in defense mechanisms. Little is known precisely about how these changes lead to defenses listed in Table 8.1; and yet it would be safe to predict that mechanisms for the production of nitric oxide [using reduced nicotine adenine diphosphopyridine nucleotide phosphate (NADPH) generated by the hexose monophosphate shunt], hydrogen peroxide or superoxide anion (using flavoprotein oxidases or enzymes acting as NADPH oxidases), for synthesis of mucins or surfactant (NADPH), for detoxification by Clara cells (NADPH, microsomal mixed-function oxidases) or for chemoreception by neuroendocrine cells (NADPH, plasmalemmal cytochrome β as a terminal oxidase) are essentially inoperative in glycogen-laden cells.

As the fetal bronchial tree is laid down, cell-to-cell junctions in the airway lining and vascular endothelium at first are too discontinuous to prevent leakage of serum into the bronchial lumen. As development proceeds, the tight junctions between epithelial cells become structurally elaborated and continuous except where separated by gap junctions, resulting in a degree of impermeability that permits the ionic composition of the lung fluid to be sustained. Although the integrity of junctions between pulmonary endothelial cells may improve during development, fluid remains able to seep into the interstitial space so that the epithelium alone becomes the effective barrier to the airway lumen. This was scrupulously demonstrated in a developmental series of fetal lamb lungs by correlating permeability measurements with the changing morphology of epithelial tight junctions as represented in freeze-fracture replicas (76). These became functionally tight at the midpoint of gestation and from that time resembled those in adult lungs, having changed from an interrupted network formed by 3–6 rows of particles and short segments of junctional strands at the juxtaluminal borders of cells, to a continuous network of some 5–8 strands. Desmosomes occurred near such tight junctions throughout gestation and gap junctions interrupted them between the glandular and canalicular stages of development. The latter were thought to foster communication between differentiating cells and disappeared once much of this had been completed.

Development of bronchial tree–associated pulmonary defenses is summarized for four species in Table 8.2, placed in the timetable of morphogenetic events. It can be seen that defenses are acquired in the same order among the species represented. Comparison also shows that among species having short gestations, organ-related development is crowded closer to birth. Consequently, these animals may provide better guidance as to which pulmonary defenses are the most critical for successful adjustment to birth and early postnatal life.

Ciliated Cells

Ciliated cells are terminally differentiated elements of conducting airways that are renewed by precursors cycling in the secretory cell pool, and while maturing may produce small amounts of mucous or serous secretions themselves (59, 62). Ciliation begins in the trachea and large bronchi and progresses centrifugally. An initial wave leaves a thin but essentially continuous trail of ciliated cells extended along the airway (Fig. 8.1). This wave is best followed by examining successive stages of the

Table 8.2 Ontogeny of Bronchial Tree–Associated Defenses

Human	*Rabbit*	*Rat*	*Mouse*
Bronchial bud *4–7.5 weeks*	*Bronchial bud* *10.5–14 days*	*Bronchial bud* *11.5–14 days*	*Bronchial bud* *9.5–12 days*
Neuroblasts at hillum	Neuroblasts at hilum	Neuroblasts at hilum	
Pseudoglandular *7.5–16 weeks*	*Pseudoglandular* *15–24 days*	*Pseudoglandular* *15–18 days*	*Pseudoglandular* *13–16 days*
First appearance of PNEC Smooth muscle formation PNEC secretory function Ciliation of major bronchi initiated	First appearance of PNEC Smooth muscle formation PNEC secretory function Ciliation of major bronchi initiated Innervation of NEBs begins	First appearance of PNEC Smooth muscle formation Ciliation of major bronchi initiated Innervation of NEBs begins	First appearance of PNEC Smooth muscle formation PNEC secretory function Ciliation of major bronchi initiated
Canalicular *16–24 weeks*	*Canalicular* *25–27 days*	*Canalicular* *19–20 days*	*Canalicular* *17–18 days*
Some innervation of PNEC Mucus secretion begins	NEB innervation elaborate Mucus secretion begins	PNEC secretory function Many NEBs innervated	
Terminal sac *24–38 weeks*	*Terminal sac* *27–32 days*	*Terminal sac* *21–22 days*	*Terminal sac* *18–19 days*
Clara cells Surfactant	Clara cells Surfactant	Mucus secretion begins Clara cells Surfactant	Mucus secretion begins Clara cells Surfactant
Postnatal BALT under some conditions	Postnatal BALT	Postnatal BALT	Postnatal BALT

PNEC, pulmonary neuroendocrine cells; NEB, neuroepithelial body; BALT, bronchus-associated lymphatic tissue.

[Based on data from refs. 15, 33, 112, and others cited in text.]

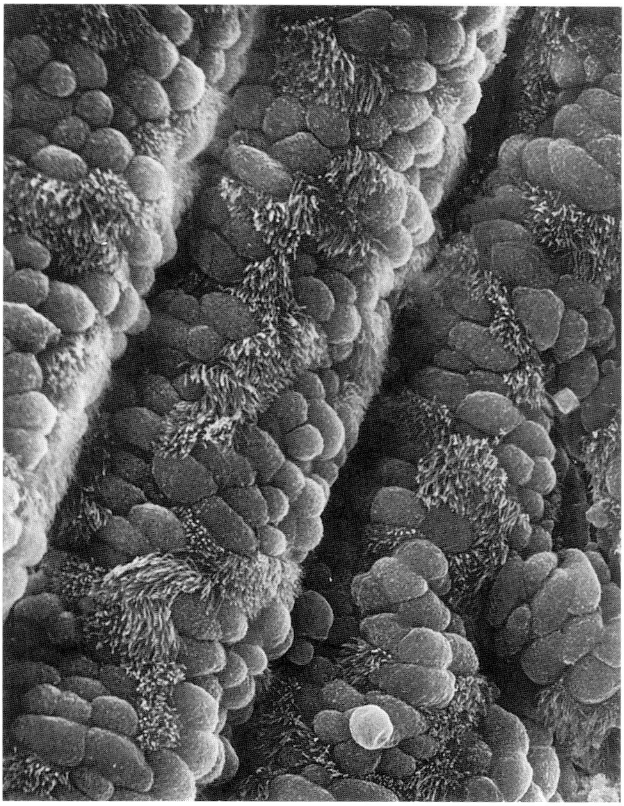

Fig. 8.1 Scanning electron micrograph of bronchial surface in 21-day fetal rat lung. Ciliated cells have not yet come into their majority; those present contact each other, forming thin lines down airway. Magnification, ×900.

developing bronchial trees in a short-gestationed species like the hamster where it passes from the trachea to the bronchioloalveolar portals during the last 3 days of intrauterine life (74). Its progression along the main lobar axis is more rapid than along divergent branches. Contiguity of cells in a trail possibly reflects the need for direct contact in order to pass a signal initiating ciliation as well as to coordinate ciliary beat along the airways. Later additions leave a much larger proportion of the epithelial surface ciliated in large airways than in the bronchioles and respiratory bronchioles where nonciliated Clara cells at first predominate but eventually may be outnumbered (56).

In individual cells, formation of cilia is preceded by assembly of basal bodies, which occurs in close proximity to pre-existing centrioles as well as by "de novo" synthesis. Newly formed basal bodies lengthen and become arrayed under the apical epithelial surface; thereafter they sprout cilia from their outward-facing ends (81). Growth of cilia is by acropetal assembly of components in the elongating ciliary shaft, building on a template of the basal body (Fig. 8-2). Motion begins before the

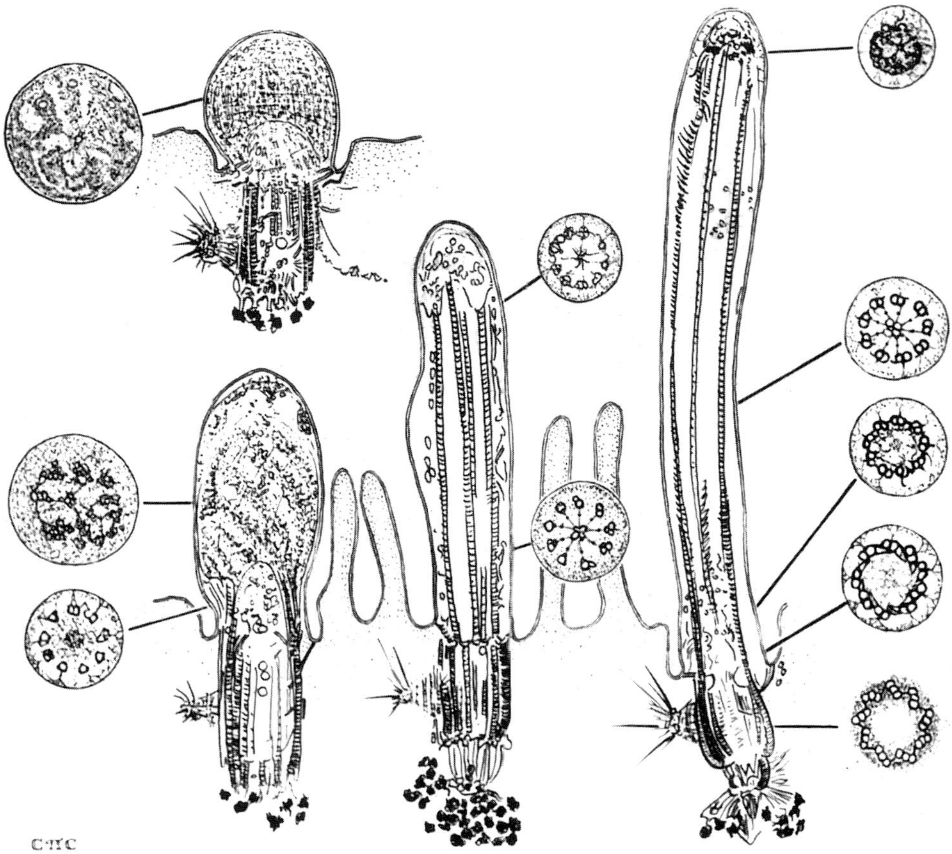

Fig. 8.2 Formation of cilia, progressively from upper left, counterclockwise. Cross sections show internal microtubular organization realized at each stage, correlated with position along elongating ciliary shaft. [Drawing by S.P. Sorokin, based on electron micrographs.]

shaft is fully elongated but not until a "9+2" ultrastructural arrangement of ciliary microtubules has been formed partway along its length. Thus, although rare ciliating cells are first seen in fetal rats at 18 days of gestation, motion is not usually observed until about the 20th day. In living lung cultures, this initially is seen as a "thrill" or flickering at the epithelial surface, which in a day or two becomes conspicuous and coordinated with ciliary action in adjacent cells.

Mucous Cells

Whether in glands or in the bronchial epithelium, mucous cells also follow a centrifugal pattern of differentiation, although extending only to bronchioles. In human lungs, secretions at first appear in glands of the larger airways during the 15th week of gestation and on the surface at 21 weeks. In guinea pigs and rats, they appear just before birth, and in the hamster trachea, at birth (61). Since this population responds to irritation from noxious inhalants or excessively dry air by increased cell division, the proportion of airway surface it occupies postnatally and the collective volume of the glands can vary considerably.

Nonciliated Bronchiolar (Clara) Cells

Like mucous cells in the bronchi, Clara cells provide for renewal of the bronchiolar epithelium, where rapid linear growth continues to occur until fairly late in gestation. Perhaps for this reason differentiation of Clara cell precursors into secretory cells is delayed, the actively replicating elements retaining glycogen until long after virtually all other lining cells of the conducting airways have lost theirs. Indeed, loss of glycogen typically occurs after birth in human beings, rabbits, rats, and mice; in rabbits and rats this is succeeded by an increase in the volume density of secretory granules and mitochondria (56, 72). Secretory granules of Clara cells in human (11) and animal lungs contain a specific protein (CC10) that can bind xenobiotic molecules and may possess anti-inflammatory properties (16). On the day before birth in hamsters, CC10 is at once expressed by all Clara cells in the epithelium instead of in the sequential, proximal-to-distal manner of other differentiating airway components (98). Soon followed by the disappearance of glycogen, it increases postnatally to complete the functional differentiation of these cells. In rats its mRNA becomes localized in the epithelium of conducting airways during the canalicular stage of development (64), but the protein is not expressed in either rats or mice until two days before birth, and it scarcely reaches adult levels before the third postnatal week (78, 106, 116). Consequently, its protective influence becomes available only near term.

Surfactant

As judged by the appearance of multilamellar bodies in glycogen-charged cuboidal cells, surfactant production begins in immature great alveolar cells located in the epithelium of newly formed terminal sacs. This stage of development is reached at about 26 weeks of gestation in human lungs and well before birth in other mammals having long gestations, but in species born immature, and particularly among those with a short period of intrauterine life, terminal sac formation may begin only a day or two before birth. Consequently, in these species, surfactant normally is not secreted until relatively late in gestation. This may retard delivery of associated antimicrobial factors (Table 8.1), although, as observed in great alveolar cells obtained from primary cultures of human fetal lung, release of *surfactant* protein-A (SP-A) is not necessarily tied to secretion of the lamellar bodies (22). Because SP-A stimulates phagocytosis by macrophages (110) and also occurs in Clara cells (45), its primary designation as a *surfactant* protein may not be entirely appropriate.

Pulmonary Neuroendocrine Cells

Pulmonary neuroendocrine cells (PNECs) are the first of the definitive cell types differentiated in mammalian respiratory epithelium. They form multicellular clusters (presumptive neuroepithelial bodies, pNEBs) that appear in a proximal-to-distal wave close behind the zone of terminal budding and ultimately populate the entire conducting airway (60, 74). Mitotic activity soon becomes concentrated in narrow zones of undifferentiated epithelial cells surrounding the clusters (39), and at least one common endocrine cell product, calcitonin gene–related peptide (CGRP), has proved to be an airway mitogen in organ-cultured fetal rat lungs (38). It would seem, therefore, that PNECs assume a mophogenetic role affecting the shape and/or size of the bronchial tree but exerting no selective influence over the differentiation of other cell types.

Ingrowing nerve fibers subsequently convert many endocrine cell clusters into mature neuroepithelial bodies (NEBs). These resemble the carotid bodies both in morphological organization and in sensitivity to pO_2 (115) and extracellular pH (17). Collectively, however, the NEBs far exceed the carotid bodies in total number of chemoreceptive cells, and thanks to their wide distribution along the airway, they provide many more separate inputs (83).

Endocrine secretory products such as CGRP, gastrin-releasing peptide (GRP), and serotonin serve multiple roles as growth factors, neurotransmitters, and regulators of broncho- and vasomotor tone; and hypoxia and low pH of the intraluminal fluid—stimuli to which the cells apparently respond—are not only transient phenomena of mature airways but are characteristic of prenatal lungs. PNECs thus contribute to pulmonary defense in two senses: first by ensuring development of a properly shaped lung inherently less prone to disease than a malformed one, and second by serving throughout later life as local intraepithelial chemoreceptor-effectors linked to the central nervous system.

Brush Cells

These rare, solitary epithelial cells are thinly scattered in the linings of the nasal cavity, the gut, the gall bladder, and the lungs. They are characterized by a thick tuft of microvilli rising from apical and basolateral membranes, from which a robust network of actin filaments is continued into rootlets that reach deep into the cytoplasm. The cells can be identified in tissue sections by their glycogen content or after immunostaining for actin or associated proteins, villin and fimbrin (35). Although they were described years ago as contacted by fine unmyelinated nerve fibers, this has not been verified by desultory reports published since, and they have sometimes been confused with solitary neuroendocrine cells. Brush cells do not contain dense-cored endocrine granules, and they take up few particles (43). Once considered chemoreceptors, they now appear better suited for immunosurveillance, but their function, relationship to other cells, and time of origin remain obscure.

Ontogeny of Nerve-Associated Defenses

Precursors of intrinsic ganglion cells migrating from the vagal neural crest reach the hilus of the lungs at the outset of organogenesis and thereafter extend along the axial structures, laying down nerve tracts and multiplying as they advance. At a later stage of development, sensory nerve processes follow in their wake, and in this way the intrapulmonary groundwork is laid for classic reflexes dependent on airway receptors. Although some of these reflexes may be active at birth, they continue to be refined far into postnatal life, both qualitatively and quantitatively (19).

In a number of well-studied animal species, such as the rat and hamster, intrapulmonary sensory neurons contain CGRP, often colocalized with substance P. They enshroud intrinsic motor ganglion cells in the airway walls and project to the central nervous system. When such CGRP and substance P–containing fibers become associated with NEBs, many of which also contain CGRP, a potentially wide-reaching intrapulmonary peptidergic receptor-effector system is established. This permits action at five different levels: (*1*) local release of peptide from NEBs; (*2*) local release enhanced by axon reflexes within the NEB; (*3*) extension of effector actions by release along the course of sensory nerves; (*4*) involvement of intrapulmonary motor ganglia (true reflex arc); and (*5*) signaling to integrative centers in the brain stem (89).

The elements of such a system exist in human beings but have not been as well defined as in animal models. Lung endocrine cells first appear during the eighth week of gestation and shortly begin producing peptides including GRP, CGRP, and calcitonin. They form clusters, some of which become innervated. These cells persist throughout life in appreciable numbers, apparently being renewed even in old age (8). Nerve fibers containing CGRP or substance P have been described in or beneath the epithelium of the conducting airway as well as among the intrinsic ganglia, and both peptides have been localized in nerve cell bodies of sensory vagal ganglia (21, 34, 108).

As in the enteric nervous system, many CGRP- and substance P–containing sensory nerves in the lung may form "nociceptive systems" on their own, and stimulation by irritating substances such as capsaicin results in neurogenic inflammation (37). This complex process, best studied in the trachea and nasal mucous membrane, involves increased secretion of mucus, vasodilatation, increased blood flow, heightened vascular permeability, adherence of leukocytes to venular endothelium, and their passage into the tissues (4, 58, 71). Presumably the response is mediated directly by local release of peptides from the nerve fibers themselves. In addition to well-documented effects on smooth muscle and glands, substance P and/or CGRP also serve as chemotaxins for a wide variety of leukocytes, up-regulate endothelial cell adhesion molecules, and affect the function of macrophages, eosinophils, and B and T lymphocytes, in some cases at least by binding to specific receptors (1, 4, 5, 37, 68, 71, 79). It thus appears that patterning of the pulmonary nerve network constitutes the local aspect of an important defense mechanism that becomes fully operational only with maturation of the hematopoietic system.

Development of Hematopoietic Defenses

Blood Formation in the Embryo and Fetus

During intrauterine life, the major locus for hematopoiesis shifts from one extrapulmonary site to another (105); differential production of the various kinds of blood cells varies according to site, and leukocytes of different lineages follow separate developmental schedules. Consequently, the composition of leukocyte populations within pulmonary vessels changes considerably during early days of lung development, reflecting initial entry of specific cell types into the circulation.

Figure 8.3 summarizes the origins and development of hematopoietic cells in

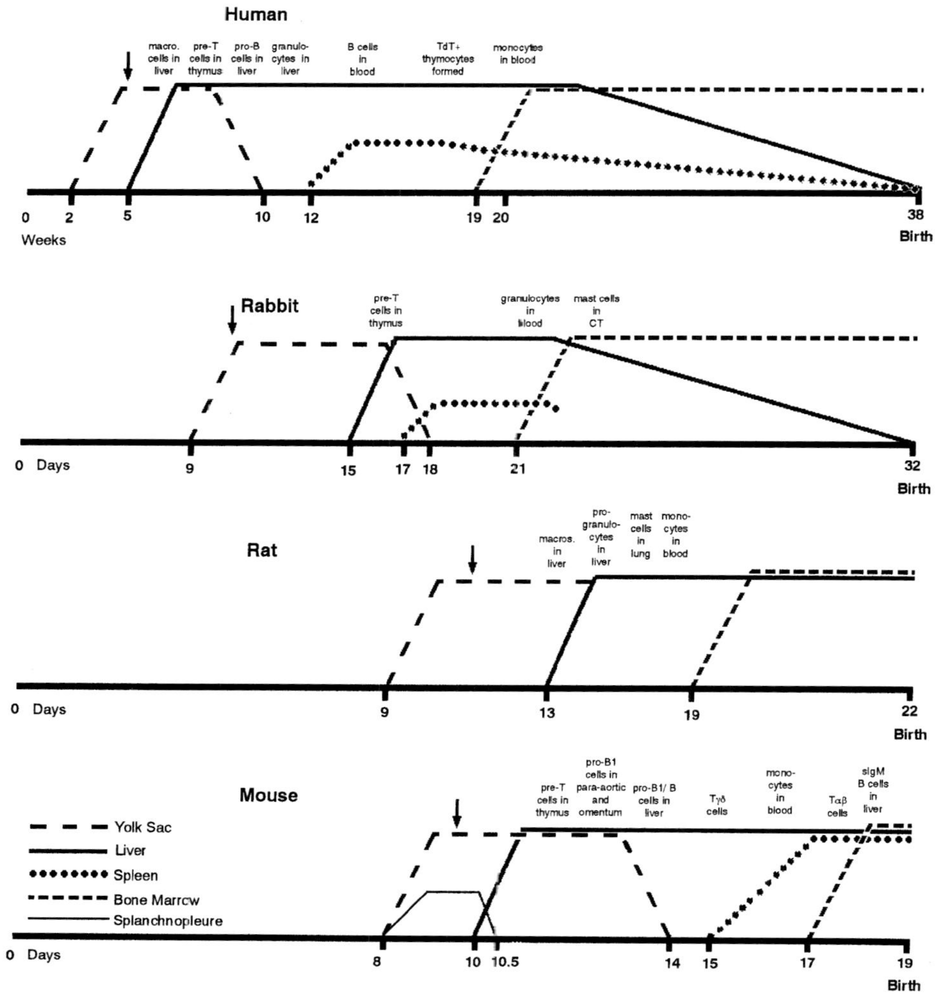

Fig. 8.3 Sites of hematopoiesis during prenatal development. Initial formation occurs in yolk sac and prehepatic sites within the embryo. Thereafter liver, thymus, spleen, and bone marrow progressively become involved. The liver is the main hematopoietic organ before birth; within it cells of the definitive (enucleate) red cell series, megakaryocytes, and the first granulocytes form outside of the sinusoids in association with hepatocytes and macrophages. It also serves as primary lymphatic organ for B lymphocytes. Before lung buds appear (arrows), macrophage precursors are already present in the thorax, and they begin to concentrate in the pulmonary stroma approximately when the liver is first colonized. Differentiated mainstream (TdT^+) thymocytes are released from the thymus midway in human development but near birth in mice and help to establish peripheral lymphatic organs. B1a and 1b cells, fetal subsets of B lymphocytes, arise in the omentum and later in the liver along with conventional B2 cells. These gradually develop the surface receptors (sIgM) needed to respond to foreign antigen. The spleen is a major producer of blood cells only in some species. With ascendance of the marrow, hematopoiesis subsides at the earlier sites but continues in livers of rodents for some 6 weeks after birth and in the spleen throughout life. Postnatally, the body cavities and scattered mucosal sites remain havens for persisting fetal subtypes (TdT^-) of B and T cells. [Based on refs. 7, 46, 95, and others cited in text.]

mammals having long (human), intermediate (rabbit), or short periods of gestation (rats and mice), and the approximate times when certain types of blood cells appear in the circulation or in designated organs. Initial formation occurs in the yolk sac and prehepatic sites within the embryo. In mice the latter occur in the para-aortic splanchnopleure caudal to the anterior intestinal portal where cells develop intra-arterially and within blood islands in the mesentery (23). These sites produce fetal (nucleated) erythroblasts along with primitive macrophages and pluripotent or lineage-restricted stem cells (102), although the yolk sac seems principally dedicated to erythropoiesis.

The liver is the main blood-forming organ before birth; within it cells of the definitive (enucleate) erythrocyte series, megakaryocytes, and the first granulocytes form outside of the sinusoids in association with hepatocytes and macrophages. It is also the main prenatal site for nonantigen-driven proliferation and differentiation *(primary lymphopoiesis)* of B lymphocytes. The thymus begins to function early as primary organ for differentiation of thymic precursors migrating there at first from the yolk sac or liver and later from the bone marrow. These begin to mature only after a prior appearance by macrophage-like cells (40). In mice, thymocytes expressing γ-δ T cell receptors are present during gestational days 15–16, but the predominant, clonotypic α-β T cells of postnatal life do not appear until a day and a half before birth (10). Development of B cells is prolonged, although commitment occurs fairly early. Fetal subsets B1a and 1b arise in the omentum and later in the liver where conventional or B2 cells are also produced; however, B1a cells have also been traced to earlier intraembryonic sites (25). Most B cells are not capable of responding to antigen until fairly late in gestation, after which they may be released into the circulation (Fig. 8.3, sIgM cells). In adults but not in embryos, maturing B and T cells characteristically develop activity for terminal deoxytransferase (TdT), which imbues their receptors with added diversity for recognizing antigens, and in humans such TdT$^+$ thymocytes begin to emerge midway in gestation (111).

The bone marrow takes over as a primary lymphatic organ for B lymphocytes and generates a range of mature red and white cells having the familiar appearance seen in adult life. In certain species, Peyer's patches of gut-associated lymphatic tissue (GALT) may serve as an accessory primary organ for IgA-producing B cells and even a few T cell subsets. Formation of the stroma for *secondary lymphatic organs* (lymph nodules and nodes, white pulp of the spleen, and parts of the marrow) begins insidiously in later prenatal life. Expansion awaits the arrival of sufficient numbers of B- and T cells, further maturation resulting from their interaction, and foreign antigen to drive clonal proliferation of the cells. This normally occurs after birth. The neonatal B cell population remains dominated by fetal phenotypes (B1a and B1b) that are stimulated only by class antigens, respond rather poorly to T cell signals, do not differentiate into plasma cells, and secrete very little antibody, which is of the IgM class (104). Thus, until late in gestation, little antibody circulates in fetal blood vessels, and almost none is of fetal origin (Fig. 8.4). Prenatal IgG is produced by maternal lymphocytes and increasingly crosses the placenta towards birth.

Regarding progenitors of blood cells present during embryonic life, intermedi-

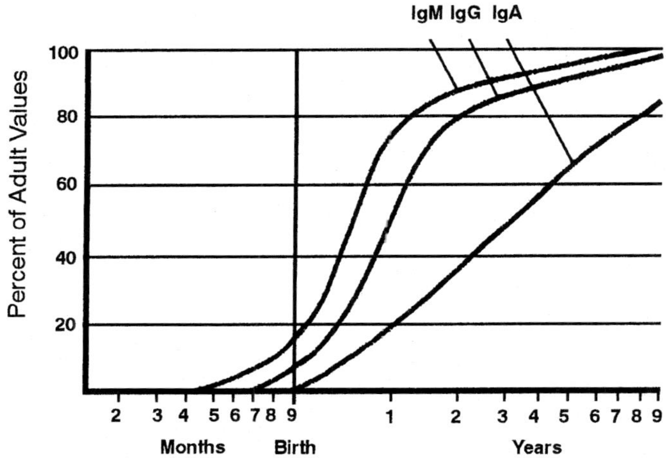

Fig. 8.4 Serum levels of immunoglobulins during prenatal and childhood years of human development. IgM is the main circulating immunoglobulin during intrauterine life and is produced by both B1 and B2 cells. Only IgG is able to cross the placenta and before birth is almost entirely of maternal origin. Infants produce too little on their own to maintain comparable serum levels until past 6 months of age. IgA is associated with mucosal immunity in the alimentary tract and BALT, many of whose B cells are stimulated by antigen presented in the gut before reaching the lungs. Its rise after birth reflects postnatal expansion of these lymphatic tissues. [Modified from Goldman et al. (26)]

ates with the potential to develop into macrophages or B lymphocytes (14), or into macrophages or B or T cells (69), have been shown to exist; and it has been proposed that these derive from a fetal type of hematopoietic stem cell that is superseded by another stem cell predominating during postnatal life. The fetal stem cell may take the form of mesenchyme, endothelium, or hemocytoblast, whereas the stem cell in adults resembles a lymphocyte (Fig. 8.5). The latter gives rise to adult lineages of mainstream (TdT^+) B cells, α-β T cells (49, 77), and probably monocyte-derived macrophages. Fetal B1 and early γ-δ (TdT^-) T lymphocytes together with macrophages descended from the fetal stem cell thus emerge as principal elements of a *paleoimmune system* which may otherwise include natural killer and mast cells. Fetal lineages of B and T cells persist throughout life as a small fraction of the total lymphocyte population, the B1 cells being confined to pleural and peritoneal cavities, and distinct γ δ subsets of T cells (γ5, γ6), respectively providing the skin with specialized epidermal dendritic cells or occupying oral, uterine, and vaginal mucosae (29). These lineages are necessarily self-replicating since the fetal stem cell apparently disappears (41). Fetal macrophages are also self-renewing and seem to generate populations residing in the tissues (101). In contrast, mainstream B cells, T cells, and monocyte-derived macrophages require repeated seeding from the bone marrow or perhaps other sites (spleen, GALT) to maintain population levels.

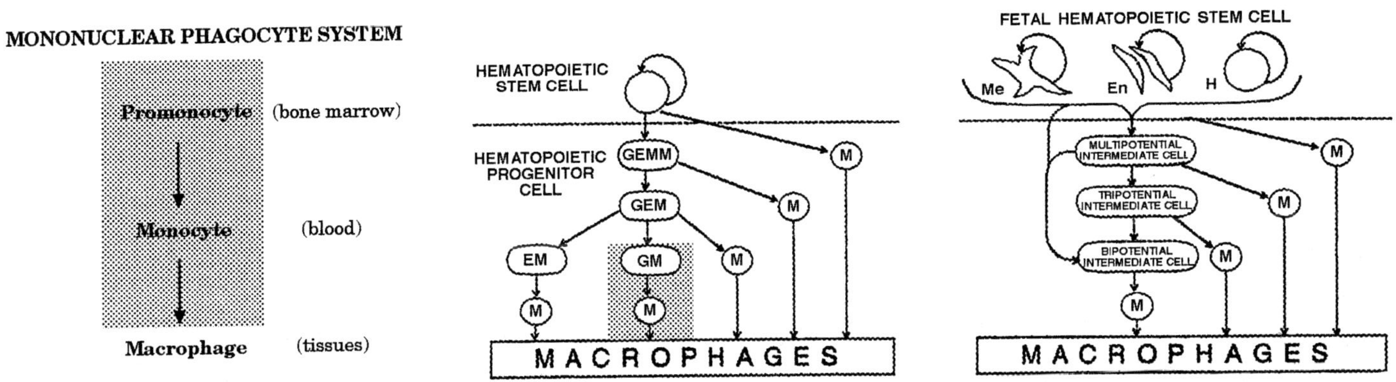

Fig. 8.5 **Left** [after Langevoort et al. (50a)]. Widely held but outdated concept of macrophage (M) origin exclusively from bone marrow monocytes. **Center** [after Wiktor-Jedrzejczak and Gordon (113a)]. In adults macrophages predominately originate from monocytes (shaded area) but also differentiate directly from early progenitors and bipotential cells other than CFU-GM. Greater randomness occurs in the makeup of intermediate progenitors than shown. **GEMM** = granulocyte, erythrocyte, megakaryocyte, macrophage. **Right**. The macrophage population of mammalian embryos and young fetuses is enriched in cells differentiating directly or within a few divisions from stem cells present in hematopoietic tissues. Initially these may be represented by mesenchyme (**Me**), endothelium (**En**), or hemocytoblast (**H**), a primitive blood cell. Angular cells represent this lineage of fetal macrophages.

Early Establishment of Macrophage Precursors in the Lungs
The obvious leukocytic character of macrophages has tended to mask a special relationship that they bear to the respiratory system. In many species, macrophage precursors are present virtually from the onset of lung formation. During subsequent development in vivo, the precursors gradually become converted into recognizable phagocytes with lamellipodia and elevated lysosomal enzyme activity, but relatively few of these have normally appeared by the time of birth (85). The early naturalization of the precursors is as definite as that of pulmonary neuroblasts, and this may signify that the cells are more than bystanders while the lungs are developing. As the first immunologically competent cells to appear in the lungs, they clearly anticipate later development of hemato- and immunological lung defenses.

Identification of the macrophage precursor awaited discovery of a suitable marker for these cells. At this early period, few cell-specific antigens are expressed by macrophages, but a galactose-recognizing lectin marker, *Griffonia simplicifolia* isolectin B_4 (GSA-IB_4), coupled to horseradish peroxidase, binds to cells of this lineage. This enabled the precursor, termed an *angular cell* (Fig. 8.6), to be identified in

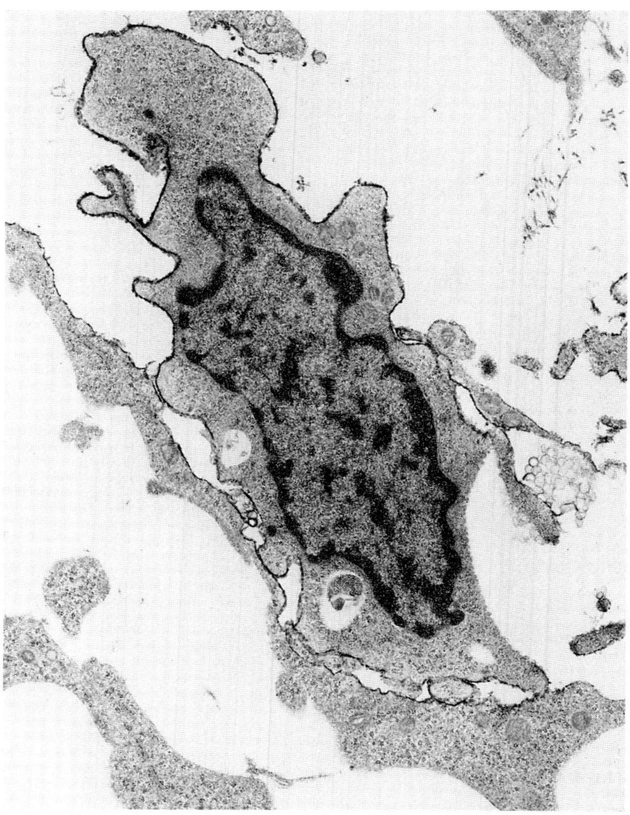

Fig. 8.6 Electron micrograph of angular cell precursor of macrophages in stroma of 14-day fetal rat lung. Peroxidase-coupled GSA-IB_4 coats surface membrane. Magnification, ×8200.

fetal rat lungs and the process and timetable of its conversion to phagocytes to be studied in detail (91). ^{3}H-thymidine autoradiographic studies in 14-day fetal rat lungs revealed that these cells cycle rapidly (labeling index = 34%), keeping pace with other cells in the expanding lung without converting to macrophages, as may be expected of cells establishing residency.

The GSA$^+$ macrophage precursors appear within lung rudiments at the complete embryo stage, near the time the central nervous system, liver, and heart are also being populated by these cells, which in rats occurs 1 to 3 days after similar cells can be seen in rostral connective tissues (84). Since monocyte-derived macrophages are not prevalent at the time, the initial resident population in these organs is "premedullary" and of a distinct fetal lineage. This concept is supported by the recent discovery of "genetic markers" distinguishing embryonic from adult macrophage types: genes for lysozyme (chicken) and heat stable antigen (mouse) are expressed at high levels in macrophages derived from adult bone marrow but at significantly lower levels in those from embryonic yolk sac and fetal liver (20). The extent to which these cells survive past birth is less certain, but indirect evidence lies in the fact that the alveolar macrophage pool of adults is in part self-renewing (75, 103) and the fetal lineage is remarkably long-lived in organ-cultured lungs (92, 93).

Differentiation of Fetal Lung Macrophages

Until very recently, little had been learned about the differentiation pathways followed by fetal macrophages, principally because the cell retains considerable flexibility for much of its life span and appears to stave off terminal differentiation. Furthermore, it doesn't have a unique receptor complex like those on B cells (IgM) or T cells (TCR-CD3), which during their prolonged formation express a variety of intracellular and surface markers that serve to define stages of differentiation (31, 42). Nevertheless, while remaining within the macrophage lineage, an angular cell may proceed for varying distances along a given differentiation pathway, or else select from alternate pathways, to acquire the familiar distinct forms of phagocyte, epithelioid, and multinucleate giant cell, and apparently that of nurse cell (trephocyte) or dendritic cell (branched, antigen-presenting) as well.

Monoclonal antibodies to a number of rat macrophage antigens have been developed, and in fetal lungs several (RM-1, TRPM-2, ED-1, ED-2, Ki-M2R) are expressed in different combinations by subpopulations of these cells (32). Although these markers have not yet been correlated with specific functional states, they verify that the heterogeneity recognized among macrophages inhabiting different niches of adult organisms (73) is also observable at an early age.

Factors Influencing Development of Fetal Lung Macrophages

If embryonic (late bronchial bud stage) lungs of rats or hamsters are organ cultured on a rich serum-containing medium, a very large population of macrophages is soon generated from angular cells in the connective tissue stroma (82). During this process, the labeling index of GSA$^+$ cells remains stable, indicating that population growth of the nascent macrophages is not slowed by differentiation. Under these conditions, the main thrust of differentiation is directed toward development of competent phagocytes, and this progresses by a series of steps. The first is conversion of angular cells to nascent macrophages, and in fetal rat lungs this has a half-time of ~8 h (91). The resulting cells are morphologically recognizable as macrophages but lack the synthetic machinery and surface expression of many antigens characterizing mature macrophages. Thereafter, differentiation proceeds in an orderly sequence of events, best documented in rats (Fig. 8.7). Conversion affects the disposition of the cytoskeleton and is accompanied by gradual expression of Fc receptors, which at first leads merely to binding of particles and only later to ingestion. The cells also develop the ability to bind erythrocytes opsonized by complement factor C3b as well as to ingest particles efficiently using nonimmune mechanisms (86, 90). The resulting improved capacity for endocytosis precedes expansion of the lysosomal digestive system by several days. Over the same period the cells begin to synthesize a series of surface markers and cytokines that may be used during intercellular signaling. Once

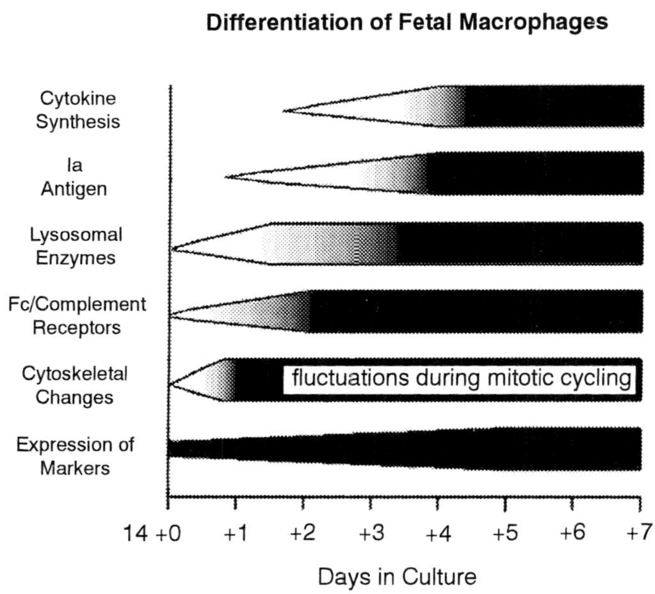

Fig. 8.7 Differentiation of fetal macrophages. As studied in organ-cultured 14-day prenatal rat lungs, the pathway leading from precursor angular cells to mature phagocytic cells is characterized by the sequence of events shown. Macrophage marker RM-1 is expressed by precursors; by day 1 these have converted, and with further differentiation, additional surface antigens become detectable. Cytoskeletal fibers associated with centrioles become very prominent within a few hours of organ culturing but subsequently undergo fluctuations seen in dividing cells. Lysosomal enzymes are represented by activity for nonspecific esterase and acid phosphatase, Ia antigen is reflected by immunostaining with OX-6, and cytokine synthesis includes M-CSF, GM-CSF, and IL-1β.

differentiation is well underway, developing fetal phagocytes become indisinguishable from typical alveolar macrophages.

Studies on the effects of macrophage (M)-, granulocyte/macrophage (GM)-, and granulocyte (G)-colony-stimulating factors (CSFs) and interleukin-3 (IL-3) in organ-cultured 14-day prenatal rat lung show that only M-CSF and GM-CSF stimulate macrophage population growth, compared to unexposed controls (92). Aside from M-CSF, other ligands of the PDGF family differ in their influence over development of fetal macrophages. Whereas the PDGFs are ineffective, stem cell factor (c-*kit* ligand, SCF) stimulates growth of precursors and early differentiating forms, apparently acting in synergy with other cytokines present in the lungs (94). Further studies have shown that M-CSF, GM-CSF, and interleukin 1-beta (IL-1β) are all viable candidates for involvement in conversion, population growth, and differentiation of pulmonary macrophages, because the response to these substances is immediate, and growth can be inhibited by anti-M-CSF, anti-GM-CSF, or the IL-1 receptor antagonist (87). Tumor necrosis factor α also stimulates growth of the population, but its influence on conversion and growth of nascent macrophages is discounted, since effects are delayed. Two transcription blockers, dexamethasone and pyrrolidine dithiocarbamate (PDTC), an inhibitor of nuclear factor NF-κB, both profoundly suppress macrophage growth without preventing conversion from precursors. The severity of PDTC inhibition signifies that NF-κB is important for transmitting proliferative signals in these cells.

Morphologically, cells exposed to exogenous M-CSF resemble phagocytes developed in serum-rich control medium, whereas those exposed to GM-CSF look undifferentiated and include more giant cells in the population (92). This recalls results obtained when alveolar macrophages lavaged from adult rat lungs were cultured in the presence of the same cytokines (52), indicating that GM-CSF alters the appearance of fetal and adult macrophages in the same manner. Thus certain cytokines can influence selection among macrophage differentiation pathways.

Relationship Between Fetal Lung Macrophages and Pulmonary Dendritic Cells

As mentioned earlier, under standard conditions virtually all angular cells in organ-cultured fetal rat lungs proceed along a differentiation pathway leading to phagocytic cells. In contrast, development of rat lungs in vivo is characterized by proportionately greater development of dendritic cells (Fig. 8.8) than of phagocytic macrophages (57, 85). There the dendritic cells have been traced to an Ia antigen-expressing (OX-6$^+$) cell first seen in the pulmonary stroma on fetal day 15. In vivo, nearly all Ia$^+$ cells have a dendritic morphology, whereas in standard organ cultures the only Ia$^+$ cells to develop are bona fide macrophages (88). From this one can surmise that dendritic cells and macrophages stem from the same precursor—the angular cell—which predates both of them in the lung. Thus far, no other candidate-precursor for dendritic cells has been identified so early in pulmonary mesenchyme, nor have precursors for nonmacrophage lineages of antigen-presenting (OX-6$^+$) cells been found there. In adults, dendritic cells have been traced to a post-granulo-

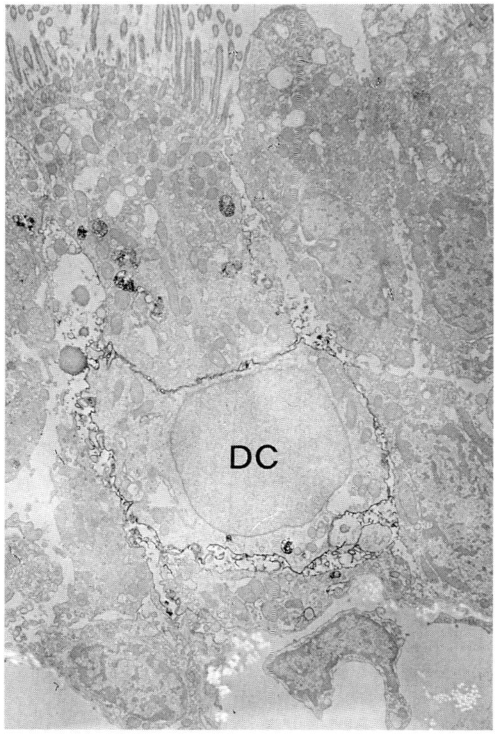

Fig. 8.8 Electron micrograph of dendritic cell (DC) intercalated between tracheal epithelial cells of rat injected with interferon-γ. Characteristically, cell is fringed by branching processes. Immunostaining reveals presence of Ia (OX-6+) antigen on plasmalemma. Magnification, ×3580. [From Kradin et al. (50) courtesy E.E. Schneeberger, with permission of the publisher.]

cyte/macrophage colony–forming unit intermediate (post-CFU-GM) in the bone marrow that can also produce macrophages (100), and like macrophages, pulmonary dendritic cells apparently derive in part from the bone marrow postnatally (36). Nevertheless, in a recent study in which 6- to 7- week postnatal mice (in control, dexamethasone-, or interferon (IFN)-γ-exposed groups) were injected intravenously with carboxyfluorescein-labeled, marrow-derived Ia$^+$ dendritic cells, *none* were found in the pulmonary interstitium or airway epithelium, despite an increase in nonfluorescent Ia$^+$ pulmonary dendritic cells in the IFN-treated group (99). These findings support the alternate possibility of derivation from a resident Ia$^-$ precursor. Our own recent experiments show that in organ-cultured 15-day fetal rat lungs, the direction of angular cell differentiation can be shifted to favor expression of dendritic cell characteristics (branching, expression of Ia antigen and OX-62, an $\alpha_E\beta7$ integrin) if suitable cytokines are added to the standard medium (IL-4/GM-CSF or TNFα/SCF/GM-CSF), and consequently that dendritic cells can also arise from these early residents in rudimentary lungs.

Ontogeny of Respiratory Defenses Provided by Connective Tissues

The Stroma as a Source of Growth Factors

Various growth factors synthesized in developing lungs may be involved with repair as well as formation of lung tissues; these are discussed elsewhere in this book. Other mitogens produced by stromal cells affect leukocytes—the development of macrophages in particular—and consequently, their relevance to lung defense is more immediately apparent.

A Specialized Hematopoietic Environment

Inasmuch as M-CSF, GM-CSF, and IL-1 are all available in the stroma of pseudoglandular rat lungs (88) and some after birth (51), the lungs patently provide factors critical for macrophage survival—M-CSF particularly—from virtually the onset of organogenesis, and in this environment angular cells proliferate actively. During the first 24 h in vitro, explanted fetal lungs undergo a period of "post-explantation shock," reflected as a sharp drop in ^{3}H-thymidine incorporation by stromal cells (91). This mildly proinflammatory environment apparently favors development of phagocytes rather than dendritic cells, since macrophage population growth is lowered if indomethacin is present in the culture medium at explantation (93). Under organ culture conditions, therefore, it is possible that access to the membrane-bound isoform of M-CSF on damaged or dying fibroblasts raises M-CSF levels sufficiently to trigger conversion of angular cells and direct them toward development into macrophages. It has been shown that cells bearing the M-CSF receptor (c-*fms* product) can obtain the cytokine in this manner (96), and this also seems to be the way that macrophages stimulated by soluble M-CSF latch onto tumor cells bearing the membrane-bound isoform before killing them (44). Thus the pulmonary stroma serves as a hematopoietic tissue that supports the macrophage lineage, and alterations to its microenvironment can influence the path selected by differentiating cells.

Endothelial Cells

The endothelial linings of blood vessels in early fetal lungs pose fewer structural obstacles to emigration of blood cells than those present later on. Thus initially it may be easy for amoeboid leukocytes but not stiffer lymphocytes to squeeze through because the intercellular junctions between endothelial cells are less tight than in adults, the underlying basal lamina less robust, and the pulmonary circulation sluggish. In adult lungs, pulmonary capillaries are not much more difficult to cross because intercellular junctions never become continuous; nevertheless, before passing into lung tissues even pliant granulocytes must first be drawn to the endothelium by specific chemotactic agents and become attached to the surface through binding of mutually compatible adhesion molecules on the respective cell surfaces.

Complement fragments are classic taxins involved in leukocyte migration. Besides these, "C-C chemokines" such as monocyte chemoattractant protein-1 (MCP-1), RANTES, and macrophage inflammatory proteins MIP-1α and 3α, mainly attract mononuclear cells. Some draw eosinophils as well (54), but C-C eotaxin is more selective for them. "C-X-C chemokines" like IL-8 and MIP-2 generally attract neutrophils, although C-X-C stromal-derived factor 1 (SDF1) preferentially acts on resting lymphocytes. IL-8 is produced by a variety of cells including epithelial, endothelial, and other stromal cells and MIP-2 by macrophages (30, 54a).

Adhesion of leukocytes to endothelium is mediated by expression of various surface molecules, the most important for regulating traffic apparently being the selectins, proteins expressed either by most blood cells (L-selectin), megakaryocytes and platelets (P-selectin), or endothelial cells (both E- and P-selectins). They bind to mucin-like counterreceptors on the surface of the complementary cell. In a fast-flowing bloodstream, initial tethering (capture) of the leukocyte is most efficiently managed through binding of L-selectin to its ligand on the endothelium because these receptors are most concentrated at the tips of short processes forming a fringe about the cell. Motion is subsequently halted due to progressive involvement by P-selectin (fast rolling) and E-selectin (slow rolling). Thereafter, adhesion is ensured through interaction of β-integrin molecules on the leukocyte membrane with intercellular adhesion molecules (ICAMs) on the endothelial surface; the former normally crowd portions of the leukocyte membrane nearest the cell body rather than the fringe and so are not primarily involved with tethering. The arrested cell then crosses out of the blood vessel between endothelial cells, being guided by chemotaxins. Although the ligand for L-selectin (GlyCAM-1) is constitutively expressed by endothelial cells, expression of E-selectin is always transient. Some leukocytes may express ligands for both endothelial selectins besides their own homing molecule; this enhances their ability to bind to endothelial cells, to platelets, or to a previously bound cell. Additional differences in the exact manner specific cell types use the adhesion molecules can also affect the composition of the recruited population. For instance, during slow rolling monocytes may employ α_4 integrins that neutrophils do not possess (47). Moreover, T cells lacking L-selectin and the ligand for E-selectin may still be brought to adhesion using the interaction between the integrin VLA-4 ($\alpha_4\beta1$) and its ligand VCAM-1 (3).

In bronchial lymphatic tissue, rapid passage of lymphocytes into pulmonary compartments is effected through high endothelial venules which are induced by local microenvironmental factors. Basic endothelial mechanisms for capture and diapedesis of leukocytes are similar to those used in ordinary capillaries or venules, except that the density of ligands for L-selectin is greater and shear forces in the vessels are lower, which favors detention of lymphocytes. In addition, a prominent glycocalyx on the endothelial cells helps to retain fibronectin and laminin that are secreted onto the surface where these proteins normally found in basal laminae tangibly help to secure the blood cells (24).

All of the preceding factors would influence the selection of blood cells leaving the vessels in fetal lungs. During that period, buildup of B cells would hardly be encouraged, since L-selectin is expressed by immature hematopoietic cells but not by B lymphocytes until virgin cells acquire immunocompetence, and then it is only expressed at low levels (48). Furthermore, since a substantial requirement for induction of E-selectin, VCAM-1, and HEVs is the presence of proinflammatory cytokines like TNF-α or IL-1, this means that in the absence of inflammation, comparatively little emigration of leukocytes is likely to take place. Little is yet known about the occurrence of chemokines and vascular adhesive factors in prenatal life. However, in fetal mice, message and product for eotaxin and its receptor are expressed by endocardium and vascular endothelium in yolk sac and liver (72a). SDF1 is involved with the migration of myeloid precursor cells from fetal liver to the bone marrow and with maturation of B cells; mice lacking the SDF1 gene barely survive past birth (64a). In addition, transcripts for MIP-3α have been identified in midterm human fetal lung (72b).

In relation to the secretory functions of fetal endothelium, endothelin-1 is present in the lungs of late-gestation lambs and helps to regulate basal pulmonary vascular tone through interaction with vasodilator and vascoconstrictor receptors located on endothelial cells and vascular smooth muscle. After birth greater activation of the former results in decreased vascular tone for a time, possibly through stimulation of nitric oxide production or activation of ATP-dependent potassium channels (114).

Cellular Interactions and Defense of Prenatal Lungs

One of the important questions raised is why the macrophage lineage is established in the lungs so early. It cannot primarily be in response to apoptosis, since this occurs on a modest scale in fetal lungs, compared to other developing organs like the metanephric kidneys, where a moderate rate of cell death is maintained for an extended period, or the fetal foot pad, where it is intense for a short period. It rather augurs macrophage involvement in setting up immunological respiratory defenses either through engagement with reactive cells or in helping to establish intrapulmonary lymphatic tissues. As yet, little attention has been paid to defensive intercellular interactions that may normally occur in prenatal lungs, but they could be expected to include a variety of cytokine-mediated conversations (IL-1, TNF-α, IL-6, IL-2, IL-4, IFN-γ, etc.) initially among lung cells, macrophages, and mast cells which become established along the bronchial wall precociously (85). On their own, macrophages can produce nitric oxide or interferons, the latter being effective against viruses. When eventually a few T cells appear, the γ-δ-types would predominate at first; and while these "march to a different drummer" from α-β T cells—because they possess Fc receptors and do not require antigen processing to become activated—their effector responses nevertheless are similar to the mainstream cells (29, 12). B1 cells present in the late prenatal period react to carbohydrates and lipids as well as protein antigens but normally produce few antibodies until after birth. The broad specificities of these IgM antibodies pose an advantage because they are effective against many microorganisms having carbohydrate coats, and the bacterial lipopolysaccharide that the cells respond to also activates macrophages. The disadvantage is that many of these antibodies cross-react with autoantigens, but because their affinity for antigens is low, this usually is not troublesome. Nevertheless, the heterophile antibodies and isoagglutinins for blood groups A and B that B1 cells synthesize are clinically significant (2).

A report describing immunocytochemical marker expression in a series of fetal and postnatal human tracheas provides a glimpse into the level of responsiveness to be met in fetal life (97). Before birth, a few IgM-, IgD-, and IgG-producing B cells were sometimes found, and fewer CD3+ T cells were present, whereas IgA or IgE cells were not seen until after birth, when they increased rapidly, and T cells began to infiltrate the epithelium. Unexpectedly, small amounts of secretory component were detectable on the tracheal surface before birth, preceding the IgA cells. Epithelial MHC class II expression was absent until a week after birth, and thereafter became widespread. The limited prenatal responses were considered locally activated.

Development of BALT

The appearance of BALT normally is delayed past birth even in rabbits and rats, in which it is constitutively formed (67); postnatal development is largely attributable to contact with foreign antigen and associated proinflammatory responses (18). Early steps leading to formation of BALT are poorly comprehended. Nevertheless, judging from the tissue's definite histological organization and preferential localization abutting the pulmonary artery near bronchial branch points, a definite program must exist. Infections (chorioamnionitis, intrauterine pneumonia) can lead to precocious development of BALT in mid-term human fetuses (28); consequently, covert preparations quite likely anticipate its normally postnatal manifestation. Various experiments on lymph nodes and chronically inflamed parts of nonlymphatic organs have shown that macrophage-like cells, especially those bearing antigens, and the availability of inflammatory cytokines such as TNF-α, IL-1, IL-6, and interferon-γ are more important than B or T cells for inducing formation of HEVs (24, 63, 109). As discussed earlier, if angular cells in pseudoglandular rat lungs are adequately stimulated, they quickly become able to synthesize all these inflammatory cytokines (Fig. 8.7), and it soon becomes possible for them to interact with mast cells as well. Therefore, mechanisms to up-regulate leukocyte adhesion molecules and form HEVs are potentially available at an early stage, and with the likelihood that pulmonary dendritic cells result from alternate differentiation of angular cells, the tie between the fetal macrophage lineage and formation of BALT becomes stronger. Given the tendency for dendritic cells to home to the bronchial wall, favorable microenvironmental conditions would be created there for establishment of BALT.

Once formation of BALT is underway, fetal macrophages may take on a second role as nurse cells for lymphocytes maturing inside. Postnatally, rounded clusters of developing lymphocytes have been illustrated in electron micrographs of BALT and GALT where the cells are enveloped by thin processes from surrounding macrophages (6). These observations have been confirmed in rats with the discovery of clusters in the T cell area of BALT (65). In fetal rat thymus, such nurse cell/lymphocyte clusters have been frequently observed; and while many undoubtedly represent associations between thymocytes and epithelial-reticular cells, others are formed between thymocytes and macrophages. And because these appear before monocyte-derived macrophages are prevalent, they are of fetal lineage (40).

SYNOPSIS

The first half of this chapter indicates that with a normal fetus developing under favorable conditions, a wide range of defense mechanisms will progressively become established in the lungs. Since many, like mucociliary clearance, production of surfactant, and even the basic patterning of the intrapulmonary nerve network, are the outcome of morphogenetic mechanisms that can be seen unfolding in organ culture, programming for these defenses clearly is included in the genetic instructions contained within pulmonary cells or in the emigrating cells that establish early residence. In a sheltered intrauterine environment blood cells are formed, and associated immunological defense strategies are also quietly set up, many normally to be used only during harsher conditions of postnatal life. Nonetheless, past certain points in development many of the hematological and other defenses are sufficiently in place to function in a coordinated way if called on prematurely, even though this may happen well before term. As yet little experimental work has been performed to find just where these points occur, so that, except as a limited range of players at an early stage may indicate the extent of defense mechanisms then possible, or as observations by a pathologist may illustrate which responses fetal tissues attempt against prenatal infections at different developmental stages, the question is largely unanswered.

The second half of the chapter dwells heavily on cells of the fetal macrophage lineage because their significance for the development of lung defenses has been underappreciated. From this, five main points emerge. (*1*) The macrophage precursors appear very early in developing organs, including the lungs. (*2*) They soon are capable of rapid conversion into active forms. (*3*) They are also the first representatives of the immune system to establish residency in these organs. (*4*) During much of prenatal life, immunological defenses rely mainly on local cell-mediated interactions, rather than on serum-borne antibodies, and many of them must involve macrophages. (*5*) In adult lungs, descendants of fetal macrophages likely contribute to the self-renewing portion of the alveolar macrophage population, supplemented as needed by monocyte-derived cells entering from outside the lungs.

REFERENCES

1. Aguayo, S.M. and Y.E. Miller. Neuropeptides in inflammation and tissue repair. In: *Handbook of Inflammation, Vol. 6: Mediators of the Inflammatory Process,* edited by P.M. Henson and R.C. Murphy. New York: Elsevier, 1989, p. 219–244.
2. Allison, A.C. and Y. Nawata. Cytokines mediating the proliferation and differentiation of B-1 lymphocytes and their role in ontogeny and phylogeny. *Ann. N.Y. Acad. Sci.* 651: 200–219, 1992.

3. Alon, R., P.D. Kassner, M.W. Carr, E.B. Finger, M.E. Hemler, and T.A. Springer. The integrin VLA-4 supports tethering and rolling in flow on VCAM-1. *J. Cell Biol.* 128: 1243–1253, 1995.
4. Baraniuk, J.N., and M. Kaliner. Neuropeptides and nasal secretion. *Am. J. Physiol.* 261: L223–L235, 1991.
5. Barnes, P.J., J.N. Baraniuk, and M.G. Belvisi. Neuropeptides in the respiratory tract. *Am. Rev. Respir. Dis.* 144: 1391–1399, 1991.
6. Bienenstock, J. and D. Befus. Gut- and bronchus-associated lymphoid tissue. *Am. J. Anat.* 170: 437–445, 1984.
7. Bloom, W. Embryogenesis of mammalian blood. In: *Handbook of Hematology*, Vol. II, edited by H. Downey. New York: Paul B. Hoeber. 1938, p. 865–1151.
8. Boers, J.E., J.L.M. den Brok, J. Koudstaal, J.W. Arends, and F.B.J.M. Thunnissen. Number and proliferation of neuroendocrine cells in normal human airway epithelium. *Am. J. Respir. Crit. Care Med.* 154: 758–763, 1996.
9. Bosken, C.H., J. Hards, K. Gatter, and J.G. Hogg. Characterization of the inflammatory reaction in the peripheral airways of cigarette smokers using immunocytochemistry. *Am. Rev. Respir. Dis.* 145: 911–917, 1992.
10. Brenner, M.B., J.L. Strominger, and M.S. Krangel. The gamma delta T cell receptor. *Adv. Immunol.* 43: 133–192, 1988.
11. Broers, J.L.V., S.M. Jensen, W.D. Travis, H. Pass, J.A. Whitsett, G. Singh, S.L. Katyal, A.M. Gazdar, J.D. Minna, and R.I. Linnoila. Expression of surfactant associated protein-A and Clara cell 10 kilodalton mRNA in neoplastic and non-neoplastic human lung tissue as detected by *in situ* hybridization. *Lab. Invest.* 66: 337–346, 1992.
12. Chien, Y., R. Jores, and M.P. Crowley. Recognition by γ/δ T cells. *Annu. Rev. Immunol.* 14: 511–532, 1996.
13. Cripps, A.W., M.L. Dunkley, R.L. Clancy, F. Wallace, A. Buret, and D.C. Taylor. An animal model to study the mechanisms of immunity induced in the respiratory tract by intestinal immunization. *Adv. Exp. Med. Biol.* 371b: 749–753, 1995.
14. Cumano, A., C.J. Paige, N.N. Iscove, and G. Brady. Bipotential precursors of B cells and macrophages in murine fetal liver. *Nature* 356: 612–615, 1992.
15. Cutz, E. Cytomorphology and differentiation of airway epithelium in developing human lung. In: *Lung Carcinomas*, edited by E.M. McDowell. New York: Churchill Livingston, 1987, p. 1–41.
16. Dodge, D.E., R.B. Rucker, G. Singh, and C.G. Plopper. Quantitative comparison of intracellular concentration and volume of Clara cell 10 KD protein in rat bronchi and bronchioles based on laser scanning confocal microscopy. *J. Histochem. Cytochem.* 41: 1171–1184, 1993.
17. Ebina, M., R.F. Hoyt, Jr., N.A.F. McNelly, S P. Sorokin, and R.I. Linnoila. Effects of hydrogen and bicarbonate ions on endocrine cells in fetal rat lung organ cultures. *Am. J. Physiol.* 272: L178–L186, 1997.
18. Emery, J.L. and F. Dinsdale. The postnatal development of lymphoreticular aggregates and lymph nodes in infants' lungs. *J. Clin. Pathol.* 26: 539–545, 1973.
19. Farber, J.P. Development of pulmonary and chest wall reflexes influencing breathing. In: *Developmental Neurobiology of Breathing*, edited by G.G. Haddad and J.P. Farber. New York: Marcel Dekker, 1991, p. 245–269.
20. Faust, N., M.C. Huber, A.E. Sippel, and C. Bonifer. Different macrophage populations develop from embryonic/fetal and adult hematopoietic tissues. *Exp. Hematol.* 25: 432–444, 1997.

21. Fischer, A. and B. Hoffmann. Nitric oxide synthase in neurons and nerve fibers of lower airways and in vagal sensory ganglia of man. Correlation with neuropeptides. *Am. J. Respir. Crit. Care Med.* 154: 209–216, 1996.
22. Froh, D., L.W. Gonzales, and P.L. Ballard. Secretion of surfactant protein A and phosphatidylcholine from type II cells of human fetal lung. *Am. J. Respir. Cell Mol. Biol.* 8: 556–561, 1993.
23. Garcia-Porrero, J.A., I.E. Godin, and F. Dieterlen-Lievre. Potential intraembryonic hemogenic sites at pre-liver stages in the mouse. *Anat. Embryol.* 192: 425–435, 1995.
24. Girard, J-P. and T.A. Springer. High endothelial venules (HEVs): specialized endothelium for lymphocyte migration. *Immunol. Today* 16: 449–457, 1995.
25. Godin, I.E., J.A. Garcia-Porrero, A. Coutinho, F. Dieterlen-Lievre, and M.A.R. Marcos. Para-aortic splanchnopleura from early mouse embryos contains B1a cell progenitors. *Nature* 364: 67–70, 1993.
26. Goldman, A.S., A.J. Ham Pong, and R.M. Goldblum. Host defenses: development and maternal contributions. *Adv. Pediatr.* 32: 71–100, 1985.
27. Gong, J.L., K.M. McCarthy, R.A. Rogers, and E.E. Schneeberger. Interstitial lung macrophages interact with dendritic cells to present antigenic peptides derived from particulate antigens to T cells. *Immunology* 81: 343–351, 1994.
28. Gould, S.J. and P.G. Isaacson. Bronchus-associated lymphoid tissue (BALT) in human fetal and infant lung. *J. Pathol.* 169: 229–234, 1993.
29. Haas, W., P. Pereira, and S. Tonegawa. Gamma/delta cells. *Annu. Rev. Immunol.* 11: 637–685, 1993.
30. Hashimoto, S., J.-F. Pittet, K. Hong, H. Folkesson, G. Bagby, L. Kobzik, C. Frevert, K. Watanabe, S. Tsurufuji, and J. Wiener-Kronish. Depletion of alveolar macrophages decreases neutrophil chemotaxis to Pseudomonas airspace infections. *Am. J. Physiol.* 270: L819–L828, 1996.
31. Havran, W.L. and J.P. Allison. Developmentally ordered appearance of thymocytes expressing different T-cell antigen receptors. *Nature* 335: 443–445, 1988.
32. Higashi, K., M. Naito, M. Takeya, M. Ando, S. Araki, and K. Takahashi. Ontogenetic development, differentiation, and phenotypic expression of macrophages in fetal rat lungs. *J. Leukoc. Biol.* 51: 444–454, 1992.
33. Hilfer, S.R. Development of terminal buds in the fetal mouse lung. *Scan. Electron Microsc.* 3: 1387–1401, 1983.
34. Hislop, A.A., J. Wharton, K.M. Allen, J.M. Polak, and S.G. Haworth. Immunohistochemical localization of peptide-containing nerves in human airways: age-related changes. *Am. J. Respir. Cell Mol. Biol.* 3: 191–198, 1990.
35. Hofer, D. and D. Drenckhahn. Identification of brush cells in the alimentary and respiratory system by antibodies to villin and fimbrin. *Histochemistry* 98: 237–242, 1992.
36. Holt, P.G., S. Haining, D.J. Nelson, and J.D. Sedgwick. Origin and steady-state turnover of class II MHC-bearing dendritic cells in the epithelium of the conducting airways. *J. Immunol.* 153: 256–261, 1994.
37. Holzer, P. Local effector functions of capsaicin-sensitive sensory nerve endings: involvement of tachykinins, calcitonin gene-related peptide, and other neuropeptides. *Neuroscience* 24: 739–768, 1988
38. Hoyt, R.F., Jr., N.A. McNelly, and S.P. Sorokin. Calcitonin gene-related peptide (CGRP) as regional mitogen for tracheobronchial epithelium of organ cultured fetal rat lungs. *Am. Rev. Respir. Dis.* 147: A498, 1993.

39. Hoyt, R.F., Jr., S.P. Sorokin, E.M. McDowell, and N.A. McNelly. Neuroepithelial bodies and growth of the airway epithelium in developing hamster lung. *Anat. Rec.* 236: 15–22, 1993.

40. Hsiao, L., K. Takahashi, M. Takeya, and T. Arao. Differentiation and maturation of macrophages into interdigitating cells and their multicellular complex formation in the fetal and postnatal rat thymus. *Thymus* 17: 219–235, 1991.

41. Ikuta, K., T. Kina, I. MacNeil, N. Uchida, B. Peault, Y.-H. Chien, and I.L. Weissman. A developmental switch in thymic lymphocyte maturation potential occurs at the level of hematopoietic stem cells. *Cell* 62: 863–874, 1990.

42. Ikuta, K., N. Uchida, J. Friedman, and I.L. Weissman. Lymphocyte development from stem cells. *Annu. Rev. Immunol.* 10: 759–783, 1992.

43. Ito, T., H. Kitamura, Y. Inayama, A. Nozawa, and M. Kanasawa. Uptake and intracellular transport of cationic ferritin in the bronchiolar and alveolar epithelia of the rat. *Cell Tissue Res.* 268: 335–340, 1992.

44. Jadus, M.R., M.C.N. Irwin, M.R. Irwin, R.D. Horansky, S. Sekhon, K.A. Pepper, D.B. Kohn, and H.T. Wepsic. Macrophages can recognize and kill tumor cells bearing the membrane isoform of macrophage colony-stimulating factor. *Blood* 87: 5232–5241, 1996.

45. Kalina, M., R.J. Mason, and J.M. Shannon. Surfactant protein C is expressed in alveolar type II cells but not in Clara cells in rat lung. *Am. J. Respir. Cell Mol. Biol.* 6: 594–600, 1992.

46. Kamani N.R. and S.D. Douglas. Structure and development of the immune system. In: *Basic and Clinical Immunology*, edited by D.P. Stites and A.I. Terr. Norwalk, CT: Appleton and Lange, 1991, p. 9–33.

47. Kansas, G.S. Selectins and their ligands: current concepts and controversies. Blood 88: 3259–3287, 1996.

48. Kansas, G.S. and M.O. Dailey. Expression of adhesion structures during B cell development in man. *J. Immunol.* 142: 3058–3062, 1989.

49. Kantor, A.B. and L.A. Herzenberg. Origin of murine B cell lineages. *Annu. Rev. Immunol.* 11: 501–538, 1993.

50. Kradin, R.L., K.M. McCarthy, W. Xia, D. Lazarus, and E.E. Schneeberger. Accessory cells of the lung. I. Interferon-gamma increases Ia+ dendritic cells in the lung without augmenting their accessory activities. *Am. J. Respir. Cell Mol. Biol.* 4: 210–218, 1991.

50a. Langevoort, H.L., Z.A. Cohn, J.G. Hirsch, J.H. Humphrey, W.G. Spector, and R. van Furth. The nomenclature of mononuclear phagocytic cells. In: *Mononuclear Phagocytes*, edited by R. van Furth. Philadelphia, PA: F.A. Davis, 1970, p. 1–6.

51. Lehnert, B.E., Y.E. Valdez, N.M. Lehnert, M.S. Park, and M.D. Englen. Stimulation of rat and murine alveolar macrophage proliferation by lung fibroblasts. *Am. J. Respir. Cell Mol. Biol.* 11: 375–385, 1994.

52. Lemaire, I., H. Yang, W. Lauzon, and N. Gendron. M-CSF and GM-CSF promote alveolar macrophage differentiation into multinucleated giant cells with distinct phenotypes. *J. Leukoc. Biol.* 60: 509–518, 1996.

53. Longworth, K.E., K.H. Albertine, and N.C. Staub. Ultrastructural quantification of pulmonary intravascular macrophages in newborn and 2-week-old lambs. *Anat. Rec.* 246: 238–244, 1996.

54. Lukacs, N.W., T.J. Standiford, S.W. Chensue, R.G. Kunkel, R.M. Strieter, and S.L. Kunkel. C-C chemokine-induced eosinophil chemotaxis during allergic airway inflammation. *J. Leukoc. Biol.* 60: 573–578, 1996.

54a. Luster, A.D. Chemokines—chemotactic cytokines that mediate inflammation. *New England J. Med.* 338: 436–445, 1998.

55. Lutter, R., B. Bruinier, B.E.A. Hol, F.H. Krouwels, T.A. Out, and H.M. Jansen. Physical interaction between lung epithelial cells and T lymphocytes. *Adv. Exp. Med. Biol.* 371a: 257–263, 1995.

56. Massaro, G. Nonciliated bronchiolar epithelial (Clara) cells. In: *Lung Cell Biology*, edited by D. Massaro. New York: Marcel Dekker, 1989, p. 81–114.

57. McCarthy, K.M., J.L. Gong, J.R. Telford, and E.E. Schneeberger. Ontogeny of Ia+ accessory cells in fetal and newborn rat lung. *Am. J. Respir. Cell Mol. Biol.* 6: 349–356, 1992.

58. McDonald, D.M. Neurogenic inflammation in the respiratory tract: actions of sensory nerve mediators on blood vessels and epithelium of the airway mucosa. *Am. Rev. Respir. Dis.* 136: S65–S72, 1987.

59. McDowell, E.M., P.J. Becci, W. Schurch, and B.F. Trump. The respiratory epithelium. VII. Epidermoid metaplasia of hamster tracheal epithelium during regeneration following mechanical injury. *J. Natl. Cancer Inst.* 62: 995–1008, 1979.

60. McDowell, E.M., R.F. Hoyt, Jr., and S.P. Sorokin. Ontogeny of endocrine cells in the respiratory system of Syrian golden hamsters. II. Intrapulmonary airways and alveoli. *Cell Tissue Res.* 275: 157–167, 1994.

61. McDowell, E.M., C. Newkirk, and B. Coleman. Development of hamster tracheal epithelium: I. A quantitative morphological study in the fetus. *Anat. Rec.* 213: 429–447, 1985.

62. McDowell, E.M., C. Newkirk, and B. Coleman. Development of hamster tracheal epithelium: II. Cell proliferation in the fetus. *Anat. Rec.* 213: 448–456, 1985.

63. Mebius, R.E., J. Bauer, A.J.T. Twisk, J. Breve, and G. Kraal. The functional activity of high endothelial venules: a role for the subcapsular sinus macrophages in the lymph node. *Immunobiology* 182: 277–291, 1991.

64. Meneghetti, A., W.V. Cardoso, J.S. Brody, and M.C. Williams. Epithelial marker genes are expressed in cultured embryonic rat lung and in vivo with similar spatial and temporal patterns. *J. Histochem. Cytochem.* 44: 1173–1182, 1996.

64a. Nagasawa, T., S. Hirota, K. Tachibana, N. Takakura, S. Nishikawa, Y. Kitamura, N. Yoshida, H. Kikutani, and T. Kishimoto. Defects of B-cell lymphopoiesis and bone-marrow myelopoiesis in mice lacking the CXC chemokine PBSF/SDF-1. *Nature* 382: 635–638, 1996.

65. Otsuki, Y., Y. Ito, and S. Magari. Lymphocyte subpopulations in high endothelial venules and lymphatic capillaries of bronchus-associated lymphoid tissue (BALT) in the rat. *Am. J. Anat.* 184: 139–146, 1989.

66. Pabst, R. Ia BALT a major component of the human lung immune system? *Immunol. Today* 13: 119–122, 1992.

67. Pabst, R. and I. Gehrke. Is the bronchus-associated lymphoid tissue (BALT) an integral structure of the lung in normal mammals, including humans? *Am. J. Respir. Cell Mol. Biol.* 3: 131–135, 1990.

68. Payan, D.G. and E.J. Goetzl. Substance P receptor-dependent responses of leukocytes in pulmonary inflammation. *Am. Rev. Respir. Dis.* 136: S39–S43, 1987.

69. Peault, B., I. Khazaal, and I.L. Weissman. In vitro development of B cells and macrophages from early mouse fetal thymocytes. *Eur. J. Immunol.* 24: 781–784, 1994.

70. Pennington, D.G. The cellular biology of megakaryocytes. *Blood Cells* 5: 5–10, 1979.

71. Philip, G., A.M. Sanico, and A. Togias. Inflammatory cellular influx follows capsaicin nasal challenge. *Am. J. Respir. Crit. Care Med.* 153: 1222–1229, 1996.

72. Plopper, C.G., J.L. Alley, C.J. Serabjit-Singh, and R.M. Philpott. Cytodifferentiation of the nonciliated bronchiolar epithelial (Clara) cell during rabbit lung maturation: an ultrastructural and morphometric study. *Am. J. Anat.* 167: 329–357, 1983.

72a. Quackenbush, E.J., V. Aguirre, B.K. Wershil, and J.C. Gutierrez-Ramos. Eotaxin influences the development of embyronic hematopoietic progenitors in the mouse. *J. Leukoc. Biol.* 62: 661–666, 1997.

72b. Rossi, D.L., A.P. Vicari, K. Franz-Bacon, T.K. McClanahan, and A. Zlotnik. Identification through bioinformatics of two new macrophage proinflammatory human chemokines MIP 3α and MIP 3β. *J. Immunol.* 158: 1033–1036, 1997.

73. Rutherford, M.S., A. Witsell, and L.B. Schook. Mechanisms generating functionally heterogeneous macrophages: chaos revisited. *J. Leukoc. Biol.* 53: 602–618, 1993.

74. Sarikas, S.N., R.F. Hoyt, Jr., and S.P. Sorokin. Small-granule APUD cells in relation to airway branching and growth: a quantitative, cartographic study in Syrian golden hamster. *Anat. Rec.* 213: 410–420, 1985.

75. Sawyer, R.T. The ontogeny of pulmonary alveolar macrophages in parabiotic mice. *J. Leukoc. Biol.* 40: 347–354, 1986.

76. Schneeberger, E.E., D.V. Walters, and R.E. Olver. Development of intercellular junctions in the pulmonary epithelium of the foetal lamb. *J. Cell Sci.* 32: 307–324, 1978.

77. Shortman, K. and L. Wu. Early T lymphocyte progenitors. *Annu. Rev. Immunol.* 14: 29–47, 1996.

78. Singh, G. and S.L. Katyal. An immunologic study of the secretory products of rat Clara cells. *J. Histochem. Cytochem.* 32: 49–54, 1984

79. Smith, C.J., J.N. Barker, R.W. Morris, C.M. MacDonald, and T.H. Lee. Neuropeptides induce rapid expression of endothelial cell adhesion molecules and elicit granulocytic infiltration in human skin. *J. Immunol.* 151: 3274–3282, 1993.

80. Sorokin, S.P. A study of development in organ cultures of mammalian lungs. *Dev. Biol.* 3: 60–83, 1961.

81. Sorokin, S.P. Reconstructions of centriole formation and ciliogenesis in mammalian lungs. *J. Cell Sci.* 3: 207–230, 1968.

82. Sorokin, S.P. and R.F. Hoyt, Jr. Pure population of non-monocyte-derived macrophages arising in organ cultures of embryonic rat lungs. *Anat. Rec.* 217: 35–52, 1987.

83. Sorokin, S.P. and R.F. Hoyt, Jr. On the supposed function of neuroepithelial bodies in adult mammalian lungs. *News Physiol. Sci.* 5: 89–95, 1990.

84. Sorokin, S.P., R.F. Hoyt, Jr., D.G. Blunt, and N.A. McNelly. Macrophage development. II. Early ontogeny of macrophage populations in brain, liver, and lungs of rat embryos as revealed by a lectin marker. *Anat. Rec.* 232: 527–550, 1992.

85. Sorokin, S.P., R.F. Hoyt, Jr., and M.M. Grant. Development of macrophages in the lungs of fetal rabbits, rats, and hamsters. *Anat. Rec.* 208: 103–121, 1984.

86. Sorokin, S.P., R.F. Hoyt, Jr., and N.A. McNelly. Non-immune phagocytosis by "premedullary" lung macrophages: effects of concanavalin A, tuftsin, and macrophage-inhibitory peptide. *Anat. Rec.* 223: 55–61, 1989.

87. Sorokin, S.P., R.F. Hoyt, Jr., and N.A.F. McNelly. Factors influencing fetal macrophage development: I. Reactions of the tumor necrosis factor-α cascade and their inhibitors. *Anat. Rec.* 246: 481–497, 1996.

88. Sorokin, S.P., R.F. Hoyt, Jr., W.R. Reenstra, and N.A.F. McNelly. Factors influencing fetal macrophage development: III. Immunocytochemical localization of cytokines and time-resolved expression of differentiation markers in organ-cultured rat lungs. *Anat. Rec.* 248: 93–103, 1997.

89. Sorokin, S.P., R.F. Hoyt, Jr., and M.J. Shaffer. Ontogeny of neuroepithelial bodies: correlations with mitogenesis and innervation. *Microsc. Res. Tech.* 37: 43–61, 1997.
90. Sorokin. S.P., L. Kobzik, R.F. Hoyt, Jr., and J.J. Godleski. Development of surface membrane characteristics of "premedullary" macrophages in organ cultures of embryonic rat and hamster lungs. *J. Histochem. Cytochem.* 37: 365–376, 1989.
91. Sorokin, S.P., N.A. McNelly, D.G. Blunt, and R.F. Hoyt, Jr. Macrophage development. III. Transformation of pulmonary macrophages from precursors in fetal lungs and their later maturation in organ culture. *Anat. Rec.* 232: 551–571, 1992.
92. Sorokin, S.P., N.A. McNelly, and R.F. Hoyt. Jr. Macrophage development. IV. Effects of blood factors on macrophages from prenatal rat lung cultures. *Anat. Rec.* 233: 415–428, 1992.
93. Sorokin, S.P., N.A. McNelly, and R.F. Hoyt, Jr. Exogenous cytokines enhance survival of macrophages from organ cultured embryonic rat tissues. *Anat. Rec.* 240: 398–406. 1994.
94. Sorokin, S.P., N.A.F. McNelly, and R.F. Hoyt, Jr. Factors influencing fetal macrophage development. II. Effects of the PDGF subfamily of protein-tyrosine kinase receptor ligands as studied in organ-cultured rat lungs. *Anat. Rec.* 246: 498–506, 1996.
95. Stall, A.M., S. Adams, L.A. Herzenberg, and A.B. Kantor. Characteristics and development of the murine B-1b (Ly-1 B Sister) cell population. *Ann. N.Y. Acad. Sci.* 651: 33–43, 1992.
96. Stein, J., G.V. Borzillo, and C.W. Rettenmier. Direct stimulation of cells expressing receptors for macrophage colony-stimulating factor (CSF-1) by a plasma membrane-bound precursor of human CSF-1. *Blood* 76: 1308–1314, 1990.
97. Stoltenberg, L., P.S. Thrane, and T.O. Rognum. Development of immune response markers in the trachea in the fetal period and the first year of life. *Pediatr. Allergy Immunol.* 4: 13–19, 1993.
98. Strum, J.M., G. Singh, S.L. Katyal, and E.M. McDowell. Immunocytochemical localization of Clara cell protein by light and electron microscopy in conducting airways of fetal and neonatal hamster lung. *Anat Rec.* 227: 77–86, 1990.
99. Suda, T., R.J. Callahan, R.A. Wilkenson, N. van Rooijen, and E.E. Schneeberger. Interferon-gamma reduces Ia+ dendritic cell traffic to the lung. *J. Leukoc. Biol.* 60: 519–527, 1996.
100. Szabolcs, P., D. Avigan, S. Gezelter, D.H. Ciocon, M.A. Moore, R.M. Steinman, and J.W. Young. Dendritic cells and macrophages can mature independently from a human bone marrow-derived, post-colony-forming unit intermediate. *Blood* 87: 4520–4530, 1996.
101. Takahashi, K. Heterogeneity of macrophage development, differentiation, and maturation. In: *Lymphoreticular Cells, Fundamentals and Pathology*, edited by K. Takahashi and S.-H. Kim. Kumamoto: Lymphoreticular Cell Foundation, 1992, p. 1–21.
102. Takahashi, K. and M. Naito. Development, differentiation, and proliferation of macrophages in the rat yolk sac. *Tissue Cell* 25: 351–362, 1993.
103. Tarling, J.D., H. Lin, and S. Hsu. Self-renewal of pulmonary alveolar macrophages: evidence from radiation chimera studies. *J. Leukoc. Biol.* 45: 87–96, 1987.
104. Tarlinton, D. B-cell differentiation in the bone marrow and the periphery. *Immunol. Rev.* 137: 203–229, 1994.
105. Tavassoli, M. Embryonic and fetal hemopoiesis: an overview. *Blood Cells* 17: 269–281, 1991.
106. Ten Have-Opbroek, A.A.W. and E.C.P. de Vries. Clara cell differentiation in the mouse: ultrastructural morphology and cytochemistry for surfactant protein A and Clara cell 10 kD protein. *Microsc. Res. Tech.* 26: 400–411, 1993.

107. Thompson, A.B., R.A. Robbins, D.J. Romberger, J.H. Sisson, J.R. Spurzem, H. Teschler, and S.I. Rennard. Immunological functions of the pulmonary epithelium. *Eur. Respir. J.* 8: 127–149, 1995.

108. Uddman, R., A. Lutz, and F. Sundler. Occurrence and distribution of calcitonin gene-related peptide in the mammalian respiratory tract and middle ear. *Cell Tissue Res.* 241: 551–555, 1985.

109. van Deurs, B. and C. Ropke. The postnatal development of high-endothelial venules in lymph nodes of mice. *Anat. Rec.* 181: 659–678, 1975.

110. van Iwaarden, F., B. Welmers, J. Verhoef, H.P. Haagsman, and L.M.G. van Golde. Pulmonary surfactant protein A enhances the host-defense mechanism of rat alveolar macrophages. *Am. J. Respir. Cell Mol. Biol.* 2: 91–98, 1990.

111. von Gaudecker, B. The development of the human thymus microenvironment. In: *The Human Thymus,* edited by H.K. Hermelink. Berlin: Springer-Verlag, 1986, p. 1–14.

112. Wang, A., L. Patrone, J.M. McDonald, and D. Sheppard. Expression of the integrin subunit α9 in the murine embryo. *Dev. Dyn.* 204: 421–431, 1995.

113. Warner, A.E., R.M. Molina, and J.D. Brain. Uptake of blood-borne bacteria by pulmonary intravascular macrophages and consequent inflammatory responses in sheep. *Am. Rev. Respir. Dis.* 136: 683–690, 1987.

113a. Wiktor-Jedrzejczak, W., and S. Gordon. Cytokine regulation of the macrophage (MØ) system studied using the colony stimulating factor-l-deficient *op/op* mouse. *Physiol. Rev.* 76: 927–947, 1996

114. Wong, J., J.R. Fineman, and M.A. Heymann. The role of endothelin and endothelin receptor subtypes in regulation of fetal pulmonary vascular tone. *Pediatr. Res.* 35: 664–670, 1994.

115. Youngson, C., C. Nurse, H. Yeger, and E. Cutz. Oxygen sensing in airway chemoreceptors. *Nature* 365: 153–155, 1993.

116. Zhou, L., L. Lim, R.H. Costa, and J.A. Whitsett. Thyroid transcription factor-1, hepatocyte nuclear factor 3β, surfactant protein B, C, and Clara cell secretory protein in developing mouse lung. *J. Histochem. Cytochem.* 44: 1183–1193, 1996.

chapter 9

DEVELOPMENT OF LUNG EPITHELIAL ION TRANSPORT: IMPLICATIONS FOR NEONATAL LUNG DISEASE

Olli Pitkänen and Hugh O'Brodovich

AT birth, the lungs must immediately assume the essential job of gas exchange. There are many associated environmental changes taking place at birth, including an approximate fivefold increase in partial pressure of oxygen (PO_2) as air-breathing commences, and tenfold increase in the pulmonary blood flow. For a successful transition to postnatal life, the lungs must also have developed a structural interface between the capillary microcirculation and the epithelium, have a robust antioxidant enzyme defence, and have mature synthetic pathways for surfactant synthesis.

Experiments have now demonstrated that active ion transport regulates lung liquid movement across the fetal and perinatal lung epithelium. During fetal life, lung liquid secretion, which is essential for normal lung development, is driven by active secretion of chloride into the luminal space. Near the end of gestation, the lungs develop the necessary capacity to absorb fluid to enable an essentially dry air-filled alveolus during postnatal life. This capacity results from the maturation of cellular processes that permit commencement of active transport of Na^+ from the luminal (apical) to interstitial (basolateral) side of the epithelial monolayer. The transition from Cl^- secretion to Na^+ absorption, and the pathophysiologic implications when these processes fail, will be the focus of this chapter.

FLUID SECRETION IN EARLY FETAL LUNG DEVELOPMENT

Early Lung Development

The lungs start their development as a diverticulum arising from the foregut. Consequently, the epithelium of the lung originates from the endoderm, and the surrounding connective tissue from the mesoderm. This initial embryonic stage of lung development takes place at 10 to 11 days postconception in mice (term = 19–20 days), 12–13 days postconception in rats (term = 22 days), and 26 days postconception in humans (6, 25). The diverticulum is then separated from the foregut by two parallel grooves that grow deeper and join together. This first recognizable part of the lung primordium will form the larynx and the trachea, and from this stage on, the airway primordium elongates and grows distally in a dichotomous manner (27).

The cells of the primitive epithelium covering the emerging airways are columnar, arranged in a stratified fashion, and remain uncommitted during this stage of lung development. For the airways to grow distally, the leading edge of the epithelium must advance through the mesenchyme which, in its own right, may and frequently does influence the function of the epithelium. During lung development, the mesenchyme itself is continuously undergoing modification that may alter its impact upon the epithelium as the mesenchyme is replete with growth factors and hormones. There is unequivocal evidence that epithelial–mesenchymal interactions are important in maintaining the branching pattern of the developing airways and experiments suggest that the mesenchyme affects the phenotype of the developing epithelium. It is also known that the regulation of airway branching and development is dependent upon direct contact between the mesenchymal fibroblasts and the adjacent epithelium (5, 63).

During the embryonic stage of lung development the airways lack luminal fluid (6). However, as the airway branching continues, the lung acquires the appearance of an exocrine gland (pseudoglandular stage of lung development). The distal airways become lined with a cuboidal epithelium and fluid fills the developing lung's lumen. This fetal lung liquid is produced by the airway epithelium with the epithelium retaining the ability to secrete fluid throughout gestation (10, 34, 113). At this stage (approximately 50% of term), the epithelium has developed tight junctions, as evidenced by morphologic criteria, and the ability to actively secrete fluid (93, 94).

Mechanisms of Fluid Secretion

Fetal lung fluid has been studied in numerous mammalian species, including primates. The findings that are consistent between species are that the lung liquid concentrations (relative to plasma) of Cl^- are higher, K^+ is slightly higher, and Na^+ is similar (Table 9.1). In the developing lamb and guinea pig, the pH value and bicarbonate concentrations are lower, whereas they are similar to plasma values in primate and canine lung liquid (7, 43, 88, 94, 109). The protein concentration in the

Table 9.1 Mean Values for Concentrations of Ions in Fetal Lung Liquid and Plasma of Laboratory Animals

Species (Ref.)	*Na / mEq/L*	*K / mEq/L*	*Cl^- / mEq/L*	*HCO_3^-/ mEq/L*
Dog (43)	137/140	9/6	129/111	22/25
Guinea pig (88)	135/130	11.8/8.9	145/95	1.9/24
Lamb (7)	150/150	6.3/3.3	157/107	2.8/24
Rhesus monkey (88)	161/144	5.5/3.5	138/109	29/22

lung liquid is approximately 1% of plasma concentrations throughout the gestation, thus corroborating the presence of tight junctions necessary for fluid transport (3, 23, 94). These biochemical measurements together with other experiments (3, 93), including the observation that there is lung liquid accumulation after proximal airway ligation (60), have lead to the conclusion that the developing lung epithelium secretes fluid by actively transporting Cl^- against its electrochemical gradient. Additional evidence suggesting active Cl^- transport as the mechanism for fetal lung fluid secretion arises from the observations that loop diuretics, capable of blocking the basolateral co-transport of Cl^-, will decrease lung liquid secretion in animals and cell culture systems (10, 30, 34, 71, 113).

The present model for Cl^- secretion emphasizes the central role of the basolateral Na^+/K^+ ATPase in maintaining high intracellular K^+ and low Na^+ concentrations (upper part in Fig. 9.1). Na^+ re-enters the cell down its electrochemical gradient via the $Na^+/K^+/2Cl^-$ co-transporter located on the basolateral membrane. K^+ may leave the cell through basolateral K^+ channels; however, the negative intracellular membrane potential results in Cl^- being above its electrochemical equilibrium so that it can exit the cell against an unfavorable chemical gradient [in epithelial cells the intracellular vs. extracellular Cl^- concentration is approximately 40:110 mM; (114)]. When there is an apical membrane pathway for Cl^- it can flow out of the cell into the lung's lumen. Na^+ will follow Cl^-, presumably by a paracellular route, with water likely passing between the cells since the water permeable pores, referred to as *aquaporins*, do not appear to be expressed in the lung epithelium during early fetal life (104).

Although in vivo measurements have unraveled the overall mechanism of lung liquid secretion, the specific properties and identification of the cells that harbor the Cl^- channels and the nature of these Cl^- channels are incompletely understood. Similarly, the relative importance to lung liquid secretion of the different Cl^- channels that have been identified in developing lung epithelia is unknown. Large conductance (375 pS) Cl^- channels have been detected in developing airway cells and type II pneumocytes (61). These channels are located in the apical membrane, appear to be active at physiological resting membrane potentials, and are inhibited by guanine nucleotide analogues. A smaller (25 pS) Cl^- channel was demonstrated in the same type II pneumocyte preparation (61). The ClC-2 channel, which is present in epithelial and nonepithelial tissues, is expressed during mid- and late gestation in the surface of developing lung airway epithelium with a subsequent down-regulation of expression

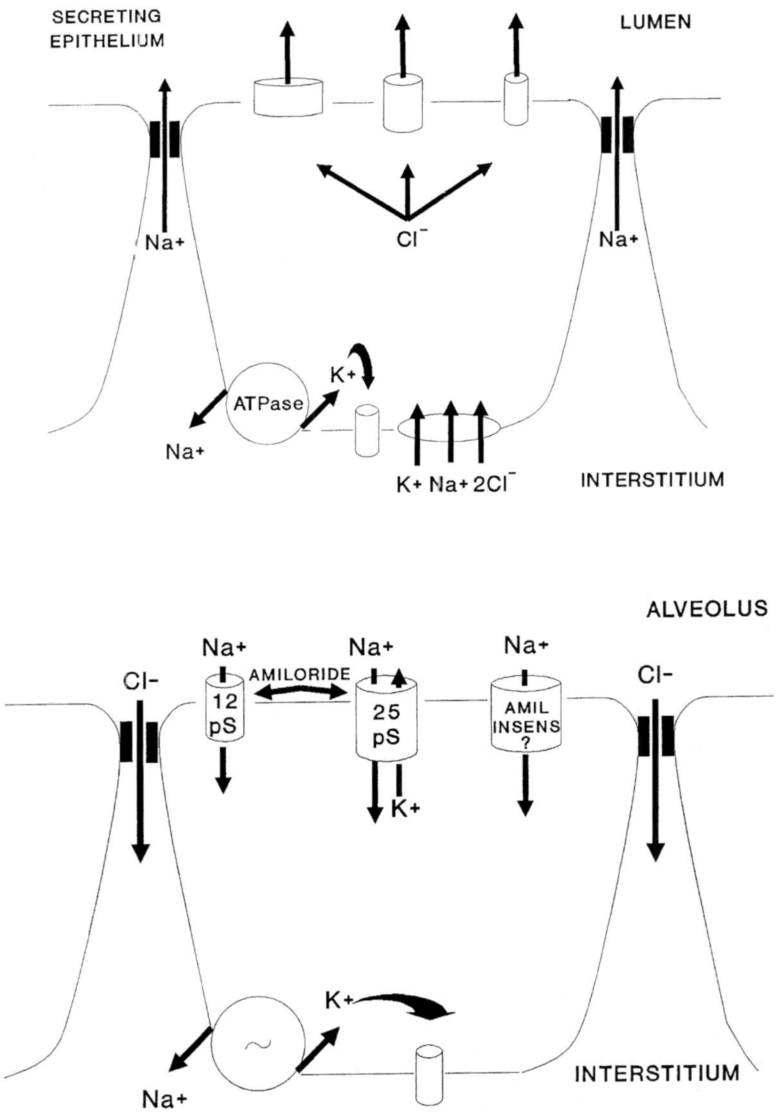

Fig. 9.1 Models of epithelial ion transport during fetal lung liquid secretion (*top*) and perinatal adsorption (*bottom*) for a detailed description see text. [By permission from H. O'Brodovich. *Proc. Assoc. Am. Physicians* 108: 345–355, 1996 (82).]

during postnatal life (79). This pattern of expression is consistent with the pattern of liquid secretion in the intact lung. The discovery and cloning of the cystic fibrosis transmembrane conductance regulator (CFTR), a Cl^- channel defective in cystic fibrosis, made it possible to study both the role and ontogeny of this channel in the secretion of lung fluid. The CFTR mRNA is present in cultured human fetal lung explants from the first trimester onward, and its expression is predominantly confined to the epithelium of the proximal lung (72). The CFTR protein has been detected in lung epithelial cells from second-trimester lungs, with its expression paralleling intraluminal fluid secretion and the demonstration of cAMP-mediated increase in transepithelial ion transport (73, 74). However, the importance of CFTR in the developing lung's Cl^- secretion is unclear since patients with CF are born with intact lungs (77). Furthermore, recent findings have indicated that the fluid secretion of CFTR-deficient fetal murine tracheas in culture continued undisturbed (12). There also is evidence of a Ca^{2+} activated Cl^- channel in developing lung (65). These observations, combined with the demonstration that knockout CFTR transgenic mice do not experience lower airway disease during postnatal life, support the hypothesis that, at least in the murine lung, there are Cl^- channels, other than CFTR, that are involved in fetal lung epithelial Cl^- ion and liquid secretion (12).

Effect of Abnormal Fluid Secretion on Early Lung Development

The lung epithelium secretes liquid during the pseudoglandular stage of lung development which ranges from 2 to 4 months gestation in human, 3 to 8 weeks gestation in the lamb, 18 to 24 days gestation in the rabbit, and 13 to 18 days gestation in the rat (6, 27). This secretion continues throughout the pregnancy, with the amount of lung liquid normalized to total lung weight remaining relatively constant (23, 97, 113, 122).

Much of the Cl^- rich liquid secreted by the pulmonary epithelium enters the amniotic space where it accounts for up to 50% of the amniotic fluid; the remainder results from fetal urine (109). The continuous secretion of liquid by the lungs against the amniotic fluid pressure, combined with the impediment to flow resulting from intermittently closed vocal cords, results in a positive intraluminal pressure. This positive pressure provides support around which lung growth can occur and the positive pressure also appears to be important for the structural and biochemical maturation of the developing lung (26). Laboratory experiments and observations made in fetuses with airway abnormalities have led to the conclusion that lung growth is accelerated when the amount of liquid is increased within the lungs' lumen (8, 9, 78, 107). Interestingly, in experimental animals with hypoplastic lungs, the lung growth can be considerably improved if the outflow of liquid from the hypoplastic lungs is obstructed at the tracheal level (80, 107). Animal experiments and certain pathological conditions in humans such as congenital renal agenesis (Potter's syndrome) have shown that a decrease in lung lumenal and amniotic liquid severely impedes lung growth (78, 80, 107). Also, pharmacologic inhibition of liquid secretion in embryonic lung organ explants may produce adverse effects on lung growth (108).

THE POTENTIAL FOR FLUID ABSORPTION IN THE MATURE FETAL LUNG

The Fetal Lung and its Epithelium during Late Gestation

At a macroscopic level, the lung grows into the embryonic mesenchyme through a separation of the diverticulum from the foregut. As the growth continues with further airway development, the distal regions of lungs' lumen begin to widen and ultimately make contact with the developing pulmonary vasculature. By these later stages of fetal lung development, the mass of the lung and its lumenal surface area has dramatically increased (27, 76). At the microscopic level, the proximal lining of the future airway epithelium consists of glycogen-rich columnar cells. Then, as lung development proceeds, there is a thinning of the epithelium in the distal regions of the lung, with the epithelium acquiring a cuboidal appearance. During the transition from the canalicular to saccular stage of lung development, the primitive air space known as *saccules* appear at the end of the airways. There is a co-existent morphological change in the cuboidal epithelial cells lining the saccules; they lose glycogen and lamellar bodies appear within their cytoplasm. These lamellar body-containing cells are type II pneumocytes and they are capable of elaborating surfactant into to the distal lung lumen. In regions where blood vessels form an intimate contact with the epithelium, the cuboidal cells flatten to cover an extremely large surface area to become type I pneumocytes that do not have lamellar bodies and have very few organelles. Type I pneumocytes are crucial components of the mature air–blood barrier (6, 27).

Factors Inducing Fluid Absorption in the Intrauterine Fetal Lung

As the birth draws near, the fetal lung must develop mechanism(s) that permit efficient removal of the liquid from its lumen. There are data indicating that during later gestation, the amount of CFTR mRNA (112) and CFTR functional activity [(65); Fig. 9.2] decrease in the lung epithelium, suggesting a preparation for diminution of lung liquid secretion.

The process of fluid absorption has been extensively studied in sheep and rabbits. Fluid secretion continues throughout fetal life; however, with the onset of labor there is a reduction of lung liquid volume, as inferred from increased ratios of wet-to-dry lung weight of term animals delivered through cesarean section (4, 22, 24). The factors regulating the labor-induced lung liquid reabsorption and at what stage of fetal development the lungs can first respond to these stimuli have been the focus of much interest. During the final 20% of gestation, the ovine fetal lungs respond to catecholamine stimulation by rapidly switching from net liquid secretion to fluid absorption (26, 122). Adrenaline increases the potential difference between the airway lumen and plasma from –3.6 to –5.4 mV (lumen negative) and induces an amiloride-sensitive absorption of Na^+ and fluid (92).

The ability of the fetal lung to respond to sympathomimetic agents is influenced by thyroid and glucocorticosteroid hormones. Both hormones are needed to enable an adrenaline-induced lung liquid reabsorption in fetal lambs that had undergone thyroidectomy (18), but, a more prolonged glucocorticosteroid stimulus can mature this response in euthyroid fetal lambs (120). In the latter case, however, it is unknown if the glucocorticosteroid infusion also increased thyroid hormone levels. Although thyroid and glucocorticosteroid hormones may enhance the formation of β- adrenergic receptors, the maturation of the downstream signal transduction path-

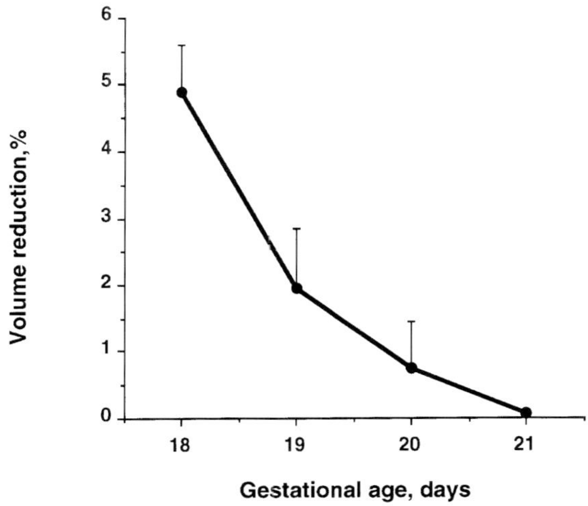

Fig 9.2 Activity of CFTR C1⁻ channel in rat fetal distal lung epithelial cells (*FDLE*) decreases toward end gestation. The FDLE in culture were stimulated by 8–Br–cAMP to induce flow of C1⁻ through CFTR which was demonstrated as simultaneous reduction in cell volume. [Adapted from MacLeod et al. (65), with permission.]

way is also very important. It has been shown that mature, but not immature, fetal lambs respond to membrane-permeant analogues of cAMP or methylxanthine-induced increases in endogenous cAMP levels (38, 119, 122–124). It is also known that arginine vasopressin can curtail fetal lung liquid secretion (33, 35) and that fetal lung liquid absorption can be triggered by intrauterine decreases in umbilical blood flow via amiloride insensitive pathways (52).

Mechanisms of Fluid Absorption by Mature Lung Epithelium

Fetal lung liquid absorption is coupled with Na^+ transport from the lumen to the interstitium and vasculature. This vectorial Na^+ transport is now known to be an inherent characteristic of the mature peri- and postnatal distal lung epithelium in vivo and in vitro. In vivo, it was shown that fetal lambs undergoing intravenous infusions of adrenergic agents would have their fluid-absorptive response blocked when amiloride (a Na^+ channel blocker that has been used in the treatment of systemic hypertension) was placed into the air space liquid (92). Similarly, the effects of arginine vasopressin (52) and aminophylline (38) on fetal lamb lung liquid production are reversed by amiloride. The physiologic importance of this amiloride-blockable process at birth was demonstrated when newborn guinea pigs developed respiratory distress, hypoxemia, and persistently elevated lung water contents when amiloride or its more potent Na^+ channel-blocking analogues were placed into their air space liquid immediately prior to birth (85, 86). The amiloride-sensitive lung liquid absorption has been interpreted as the parallel movement of water prompted by the osmotic gradient produced by vectorial active transport of Na^+ by the lung's epithelium.

The presently favored model to explain this vectorial Na^+ transport utilizes a basolateral Na^+/K^+ ATPase to generate a gradient for Na^+ entry into the epithelial cell (lower part in Fig. 9.1). When Na^+ channels located on the apical side of the epithelium become active, there is an apical-to-basal pathway for transporting the osmotically active Na^+ ion. It is known that type II pneumocytes, which are typically found within the corners of alveoli in the mature lung, possess both Na^+/K^+ ATPase and Na^+ channels (55, 83, 89, 90, 106). The net movement of Na^+ to the basolateral direction induces a parallel movement of Cl^- and fluid through the paracellular route, or the transcellular pathway utilizing specific water channels, i.e., aquaporins (81, 82, 104, 122). An active role of aquaporins could explain the observed fluid-absorbing effects of arginine vasopressin on the perinatal epithelium (35, 52, 119).

There is biochemical and electrophysiologic evidence for more than one type of Na^+-permeant ion channel within the lung epithelium. Patch clamp studies have identified 25 pS nonselective cation (47, 96), along with 12 pS (115) and 4 pS (116) highly Na^+-selective Na^+ channels in the apical membrane of alveolar epithelium. These Na^+-permeant pathways are amiloride sensitive. Membrane vesicle (66, 69), Ussing chamber, and whole-cell patch clamp studies (125) also indicate that there are both H-type (high amiloride affinity) and L-type [low amiloride affinity or ethylisopropyl amiloride (EIPA) sensitive] Na^+ channels on these perinatal distal lung epithelial cells' plasma membranes. Only the L-type Na^+ channel has been described in adult lung (67, 69). Whether these different alveolar epithelial Na^+ channels are in different epithelial cell subtypes, and whether they arise from the same or different genes is unknown.

At present, there has only been one amiloride-sensitive epithelial Na^+ channel (ENaC) cloned. The highly homologous α, β, and γ subunits of ENaC were identified using functional expression cloning techniques (28, 29, 62). The importance of these genes and their related family is reflected by their high degree of conservation across species with homologues subsequently cloned from the amphibian *Xenopus laevis*, nonprimate mammals such as the cow, and the human (in this chapter, rENaC, mENaC, hENaC refer to the *r*at, *m*ouse, or *h*uman analogues of ENaC). The encoded protein even shares sequence homology with proteins involved in neurodegeneration in a mutation occurring in the worm *C. elegans*, and a subunit of rENaC can correct the genetic defect in *C. elegans* genetic "knock-in" experiments (53).

The stoichiometry of the three ENaC subunits is unknown, but oocyte expression studies suggest that the α subunit is essential for formation of an amiloride-sensitive Na^+-conducting ion channel, whereas both the β and γ subunits are required for normal levels of activity (29). This channel is expressed in the appropriate Na^+-transporting tissues, including the distal colon, kidney (28), and lung (29, 75, 83). As described below, the expression of ENaC, at least at the mRNA level, in the lung is regulated by both the degree of lung maturity and by hormones.

MECHANISMS REGULATING THE ONTOGENY OF Na^+ TRANSPORT IN THE DEVELOPING LUNG

Fetal Immaturity

The ability of the lung's epithelium to commence Na^+ transport in response to vasoactive mediators, such as catecholamines, is markedly dependent upon the maturation of the fetus. As described above, adrenaline can induce absorption of lung fluid and Na^+ in fetal sheep after 130 days of gestation (term 147 days). However, between 120 and 130 days, only a reduction of fluid secretion or continuing lung secretion is seen in response to catecholamines (26) or membrane-permeant analogues of cAMP (124). Consistent with these observations is that arginine vasopressin's effect on lung liquid secretion is absent in an immature lamb fetus, with progressively greater effect occurring in more mature animals (33, 99, 119). These in vivo observations have triggered experiments seeking to elucidate the ontogeny of components of the epithelial Na^+ transport.

There is some information with regard to the cellular mechanism responsible for the inability of the immature lung to commence Na^+ absorption. The levels of mRNA (55, 90, 95), protein, and activity (21, 55) of the Na^+/K^+ ATPase in distal lung epithelium only increase with advancing fetal maturity. Similarly, α-rENaC mRNA is not detected during the early stages of fetal rat lung development (83) and α-hENaC mRNA was not detected in early-gestation human fetal lungs (75, 116). Although the mRNA coding for the α-rENaC does increases prior to birth (83), the β-and γ- rENaC subunits are differentially regulated with maximal expression shortly after birth (111). On a functional basis, bioelectric (103) and lung explant (14) studies similarly indicate that the mature, relative to the immature, fetal distal rat lung epithelium has significant capacity for Na^+ transport. Recently, it has also been shown the mature fetal distal lung epithelium from human possesses bioelectric properties similar to those described for rats (11).

Fetal Mesenchyme's Effect on Lung Epithelial Ion Transport

As mentioned above, the extracellular matrix (mesenchyme) undergoes continuous dynamic change in the developing lungs. The effect of the matrix is growth inductive at the leading edge of the developing fetal distal lung epithelium (6). Factors must exist in the mesenchyme that command the epithelium to form ciliated and mucus-secreting cells in the tracheal area, ciliated and Clara cells in the domain of future smaller airways, and type I and II pneumocytes in the distal lung. Several characteristics of the basement membranes lying between the two types of the alveolar epithelial cells postnatally have been identified (6, 64). The basement membrane underlying type II alveolar epithelial cell is rich in types I and IV collagen, whereas fibronectin is abundant under the type I epithelial cell (6, 64). The composition of the matrix per se may direct differentiation, but the various soluble growth factors and hormones that are bound to the mesenchyme may influence the surrounding cells (6, 64, 118).

Apart from the morphological development of the lung, the extracellular matrix may govern ion transport of the epithelium. This is highlighted by studies with primary cultures of polarized distal lung epithelial cell monolayers that were mounted in Ussing chambers for measurements of ion transport activity. Cott studied the bioelectric response of the monolayers to the substratum upon which they were cultured. Substratum consisting of laminin, which is found in basement membranes, favored high transepithelial resistance with slightly reduced net transport of ions across the monolayer compared with monolayers that had been grown on collagen substratum. In addition, the cells that were grown on laminin were flattened and had a morphologic appearance more consistent with type I pneumocytes (40). This contrasts with laminin's ability to preserve lamellar bodies and lipid biosynthesis in cultured distal lung epithelial cells, a characteristic more like that of type II pneumocytes (42). Recently, Pitkänen et al. compared the effect of fetal lung cell–derived matrix substratum and individual matrix components on the ion-transporting characteristics of overlying fetal distal lung epithelia (101). In these experiments, none of the single-matrix components of a developing mesenchyme induced differences in bioelectric baseline properties of distal lung epithelia isolated at the canalicular stage on lung development. In contrast, a matrix produced from canalicular-staged mixed lung cells induced a more immature ion-transporting phenotype epithelia (lower amiloride sensitivity and evidence of Cl^- secretion; Fig. 9.3) in overlying distal lung.

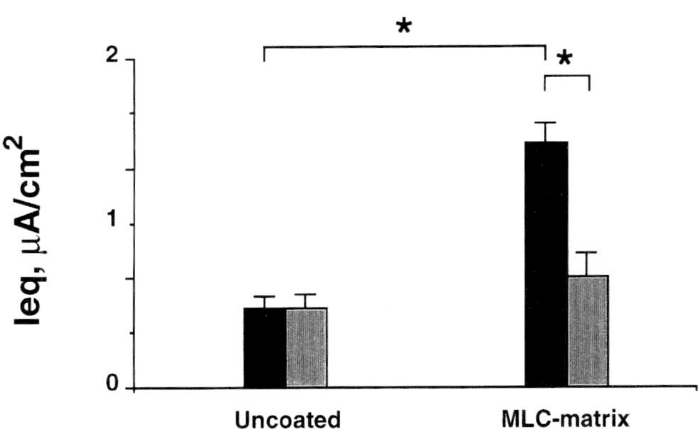

Fig. 9.3 Extracellular matrix produced by fetal mixed lung cells (*MLC-matrix*) maintains fetal ion transporting phenotype in fetal distal lung epithelial cells (FDLE) cultured at perinatal atmosphere. *Black columns*: The FDLE cultured on MLC–matrix and mounted in Ussing chambers in physiologic Hanks cell culture buffer had high amiloride–insensitive equivalent short-circuit currents (*Ieq*) when compared with cells cultured on uncoated tissue culture support. *Hatched columns*: The high amiloride–insensitive Ieq disappeared in a low-$C1^-$ buffer solution, suggesting that FDLE were secreting $C1^-$ on MLC–matrix (*P<0.05). [Adapted from Pitkänen et al. (101), with permission.]

A cellular mechanism for these bioelectric changes may be provided by the subsequent observations that the same immature mixed lung cell matrix decreased the mRNA levels of α, β, and γ-rENaC in the distal lung epithelia (104). These observations suggest a fundamental role for the extracellular matrix in the maturation of the developing distal lung epithelial phenotype.

Hormonal Influences on Lung Epithelial Na^+ Transport

As discussed above, the mature, but not immature, fetal lung commences Na^+ absorption in response to appropriate circulating vasoactive mediators. This deficiency in the fetal lung is likely due to immaturity in the expression of Na^+/K^+ ATPase and ENaC. Consistent with a developmental regulation of lung epithelial Na^+ transport is the observation that the capacity for adrenaline-induced lung liquid reabsorption which increases during later gestation can be abolished by adrenalectomy (121). Also, thyroidectomized, and hence developmentally immature, lambs who reach full term gestation cannot convert from fluid secretion to fluid absorption in response to catecholamines (13). However, if these thyroidectomized lambs receive thyroid hormone, the lungs become capable of a normal Na^+-absorptive response to epinephrine-stimulated cAMP signal transduction pathway (17). Interestingly, in later experiments it was found that the lung liquid absorption commences precociously at 116–120 days of gestation in fetuses treated with T3 and cortisol in concentrations encountered during labor at full term gestation [0.5 ng/ml and 59 ng/ml, respectively; (16, 17, 18)].

Glucocorticosteroid treatment of otherwise normal immature fetal lambs (120) can, by itself, mature the Na^+-absorptive response; although it is uncertain whether the steroid treatment induces an increase in endogenous thyroid hormone levels. It is known, however, that glucocorticosteroids similarly increase Na^+ transport by cultured monolayers of rat distal lung epithelium (41).

The cloning of ENaC has now provided us with information regarding the hormonal regulation of the expression of the lung epithelial Na^+ channels. Glucocorticosteroids increase α-ENaC mRNA (36) in primary cultures of fetal rat distal lung epithelium and in vivo experiments have demonstrated a differential regulation of ENaC subunits by glucocorticosteroids; α, but neither β nor γ-ENaC mRNA levels increase within 8 h of treatment (83, 111). This similarly occurs in the kidney, and it is of interest that aldosterone mediates this effect via mineralocorticoid receptors in the kidney (117), but increases α-ENaC in lung epithelia by stimulating glucocorticosteroid receptors (36).

LUNG ION TRANSPORT AND FLUID MOVEMENT AT BIRTH

Lung Liquid Is Cleared After Birth in a Biphasic Pattern

Labor decreases the amount of lung fluid; however, a significant amount of lung liquid still remains in the lung to be cleared after delivery (4, 22–24). Recent observations suggest that two different mechanisms are important in removal of lung fluid from the alveoli immediately after birth.

The first of these processes is short lived and related to the barrier functions of the epithelium (Fig. 9.4). This mechanism may be important in providing sufficient time for full activation of Na^+ transport–dependent fluid absorption. Egan et al. (46) first demonstrated that the alveolar epithelial membrane "pores" transiently enlarged following spontaneous ventilation of near-term and newborn lambs. The authors hypothesized that the increased pore size could facilitate lung liquid (protein-

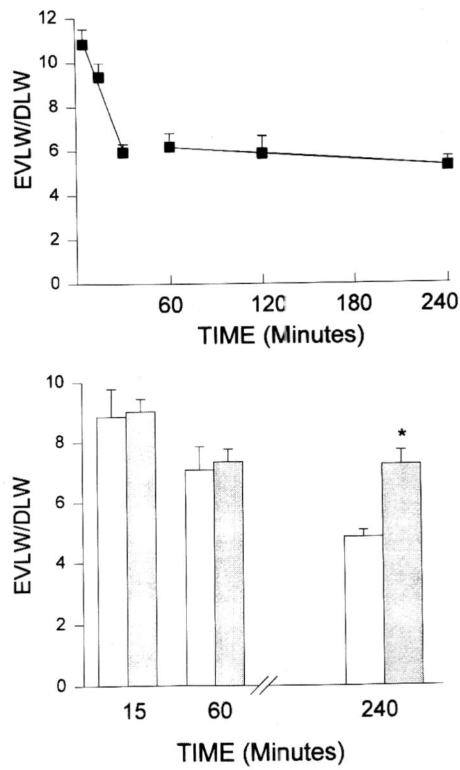

Fig. 9.4 Perinatal liquid is cleared from lungs in two distinct phases. Initially, fluid absorption is independent of Na^+ transport and utilizes passive forces. The second phase, however, is Na^+ dependent and can be impeded by prior administration of amiloride intratracheally. (Upper panel) Newborn guinea pigs were killed at fixed perinatal time points followed by weighing of the lungs corrected for the weight of blood. To illustrate fluid clearance, the wet–lung weights (*EVLW*) were normalized against the respective dried ones (*DLW*). The EVLW/DLW ratio decreased rapidly during the first minutes after birth, which was followed by a slower pace of fluid clearance. (Lower panel) Only the second phase of pulmonary fluid clearance was inhibited by intratracheal administration of 10^{-4}M amiloride prior to birth (*open bars,* saline control; *solid bars,* amiloride). [By permission from H. O'Brodovich. *Proc. Asso. Am. Physicians* 108: 345–355, 1996 (32).]

poor salt and water) removal from the lumen without allowing any or significant movement of the plasma proteins to the opposite direction (46). This concept was later extended by the demonstration that the clearance of lung liquid after birth was associated with the appearance of peribronchovascular cuffs of liquid (22, 24) and that shortly after birth, there is a return to normal epithelial resistance to the movement of a small-sized solute placed in the air space (58). It was conjectured that the lung tissue–protein concentration elicited an oncotic force for the absorption of the luminal protein-poor lung liquid (24). The transient increase in "pore size" is likely required since the normal alveolar epithelial membrane restricts the movement of ions, and ions are theoretically capable of generating a large amount of osmotic pressure (recall that the usual plasma protein concentration is only equivalent to approximately 1.5 mOsm versus the approximate 280 mOsm from extracellular Na^+ and Cl^- concentrations).

A prolonged or greater increase in alveolar epithelial "pore size" would not be desirable as protein would start to move across into the remaining airspace liquid. Thus, it seems logical that this initial process is short lived and that there is another mechanism for salt and water transport after the first minutes of life. As described above, there were much correlative and pharmacologic data from in vivo and in vivo experiments to suggest that the second mechanism participating in the postnatal clearance of lung liquid after birth is active transport of Na^+ by the lung epithelium. Recent genetic experiments have validated the importance of this Na^+ transport. Knockout mice lacking the α subunit of the mENaC had defective tracheal Na^+ transport, and died shortly after birth from their inability to clear lung liquid after birth (54). Microscopic examination suggested no morphological derangement during the lung development of the homozygous knockout mice (54).

As discussed in Mechanisms of Fluid Secretion, there are much data suggesting that there are likely different Cl^- channels participating in fetal lung liquid secretion, and above we provide biochemical and electrophysiologic data suggesting that there may be different lung epithelial Na^+ channels participating in lung fluid absorption. Additional supportive evidence for at least two Na^+ channels within lung epithelial cells comes from "nature's own human genetic experiments." Recently, it was observed that humans suffering from a renal disorder known as pseudohypoaldosteronism type I can have frameshift, premature stop or missense mutations in their α- and β-hENaC subunits (37). This disorder is characterized by severe dehydration in term neonates, due to sodium losses in the urine, and it is of interest that their renal condition tends to improve with age. Surprisingly, in view of the above genetic experiments in mice with absent α-mENaC function, these humans with pseudohypoaldosteronism type I did not have a history of respiratory distress at birth (37). One explanation for this apparent discrepancy is that the human lung has additional amiloride-sensitive or -insensitive epithelial Na^+ channels that can compensate for the lack of α-hENaC; an alternative explanation is that in the human, the β and γ subunits of hENaC can form a functional channel in vivo. There is precedent for the former suggestion, as humans who are a "knockout" for CFTR are born with fit lungs compatible with postnatal life, but later develop cystic fibrosis lower-airway disease, which ultimately leads to their death. In addition, all genetic experiments performed to date in mice show that knockout CFTR mice do not develop lower-airway disease. The explanation for this discrepancy may reside in the data suggesting the presence of alternative calcium-activated Cl^- channels in the lower airways of the mouse lung that could allow compensation for the lack of CFTR Cl^- channel function (12, 65, 79).

Oxygen as a "Switch" for Conversion of the Perinatal Lung from Fluid Secretion to Permanent Fluid Absorption

As discussed above, vasoactive mediators, such as catecholamines and arginine vasopressin, can acutely convert the fetal lung from fluid secretion to fluid absorption. However, these mediators are unlikely candidates for the messengers that would permanently switch the fetal lung to fluid absorbing organ. Many fetuses undergo periods of stress with concomitant release of these vasoactive mediators, yet they return to secreting fluid if the stress is relieved. What then are the potential signals for this important physiologic process?

Several recent observations suggest that at birth, the rapid physiologic increase in the alveolar partial pressure of oxygen (PO_2) from the fetal level of <25–30 torr up to >100 torr may serve as an important stimulus to trigger the conversion of the lung from a "fetal to postnatal mode of fluid transport." For example, Berry et al. studied the effect of ventilation on epithelial permeability of the perinatal lung (19). Prior to the delivery of the premature ovine fetus, the authors obstructed a major bronchus by balloon to separate a portion of the lung from air-breathing and left the pulmonary circulation undisturbed. Subsequent artificial ventilation resulted in a bidirectional flux of macromolecules between plasma and the alveolar space, not only in the ventilated lung but also in those parts of the lung that were separated from ventilation. This finding may suggest that the higher oxygen concentrations in the ventilated lung may have released circulating messengers or that a small rise in blood flow or its O_2 content altered the permeability of the epithelium of the unventilated lung. This would agree with the experiments by Egan et al. (46) described above.

Our laboratory has recently directly assessed whether an elevated PO_2 could induce changes in the epithelial morphology and barrier function. Indeed, we found (102) that when fetal rat distal lung epithelial monolayers were transferred from an ambient PO_2 of 25 torr (fetal levels) to room air, or even higher oxygen levels (approximately 160 and 350 torr, respectively), the monolayer's tight junctions and bioelectric resistance were significantly reduced in a dose-dependent and transient fashion. This suggests that the increase in PO_2 at birth is an important signal to induce a transient "passive osmotically driven" initial stage of lung liquid absorption after birth. Recall that the air space fluid is essentially protein-free and the interstitial protein concentration is approximately half of the level in plasma.

There are also data indicating that altering the ambient PO_2 from the fetal to higher level can markedly alter lung cell function and gene expression. When pseudoglandular-stage human lung explants were transferred from fetal (1% O_2) to postnatal (21% O_2) there was an augmentation of cAMP-mediated increase in gene expression of surfactant protein A and a subsequent release of the protein from the cell (2). This change in biochemical phenotype of the explants was associated with thinning of the interluminal connective tissue and enlargement of ductal structures (2). Subsequent studies demonstrated PO_2-induced increases in mRNA of surfactant apoproteins A, B, and C together with stimulation of surfactant-associated lipid synthesis (1). An effect of ambient PO_2 on fetal lung fluid production was recently suggested by Barker and Gatzy. Fetal PO_2 promoted the formation of cysts within late-gestation fetal rat lung explants, whereas an increased PO_2 in similar preparations prevented fluid-filled cyst formation (14). In agreement with these studies, we have recently demonstrated that an increase in ambient PO_2 from fetal to postnatal levels both increases the mRNA levels of α-, β-, and γ-rENaC in fetal rat distal lung epithelium and augments the amount of amiloride-sensitive Na^+ transport [Fig. 9.5; 102)]. These responses of the developing fetal lung epithelium to ambient PO_2 seem appropriate for a lung that is preparing for the lifetime of gas exchange via a fluid-free alveolar space. Thus oxygen is exploited by the mammalian lung, not only for cellular energy metabolism but also as a signal to launch the crucial switch that is required for extrauterine life.

Inadequate Epithelial Na^+ Transport in Initiation of Human Neonatal Lung Disease

At birth, the newborn infant is challenged with the need to clear a considerable amount of extracellular water. During the first day of life, the newborn will loose approximately 6% of their initial body weight. The rate of removal of fluid from the lungs is even higher. Various studies have indicated that the lung wet-weight reduces by 30% to 60% during the first 24 h after birth [Fig. 9.4; (4, 24, 54, 86)]. Failure to rapidly clear lung air space from fluid not surprisingly results in an inability to properly exchange gases and difficulty in inflating lungs; the situation is equivalent to alveolar pulmonary edema. The following is a brief summary of the two perinatal lung diseases that are initiated, at least in part, by immature and ineffective epithelial Na^+ transport. A more detailed description is available in a recent review (82).

Occasionally in a full-term human infant there is a self-limited period of respiratory distress lasting 1 to 3 days that may require supplemental oxygen and occasionally assisted ventilation but almost invariably is associated with full recovery. In this condition, the lungs have normal amounts of surfactant and normal morphologic appearance. This form of respiratory distress (transient tachypnea of the newborn or TTN) is more frequently seen in babies delivered by cesarean section, probably because of the larger amount of residual fetal lung liquid that these infants have to clear (22). This condition may result from defective Na^+ transport since observations on human infants with TTN have demonstrated a defective bioelectric response of the respiratory epithelium to amiloride, and that this property improves as the infant recovers (49). Further support comes from the animal studies described

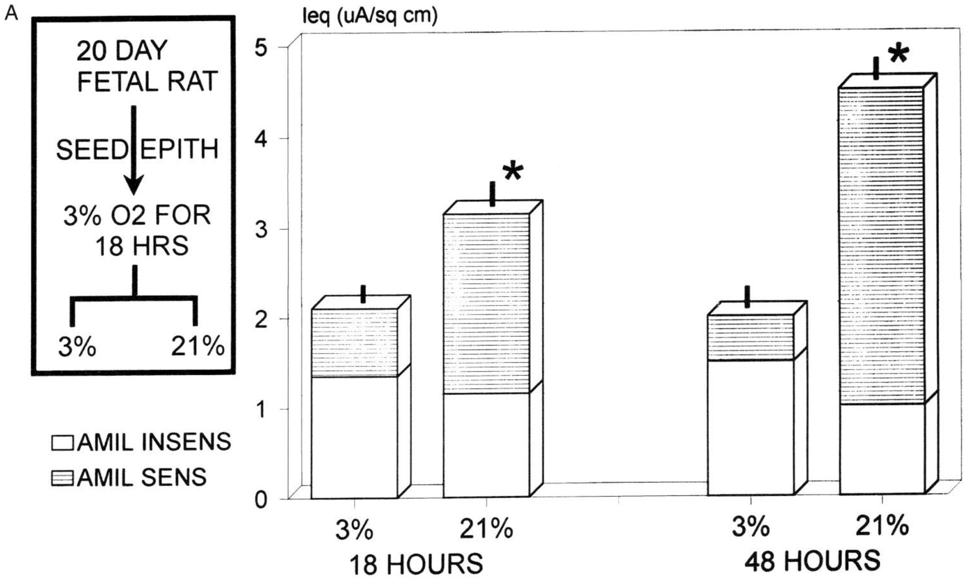

Fig. 9.5 The PO_2 of environment regulates Na^+ transport by fetal distal lung epithelial cells (FDLE) isolated at end gestation. (*A*) Transfer of FDLE from a normal fetal PO_2 of 3% to 21% O_2 increased both the total equivalent short-circuit current (*Ieq, whole column*) and amiloride-sensitive fraction of the total Ieq (*stripes*) at 18 h by 2.2-fold. A further increase of amiloride-sensitive Ieq up to 3.9-fold occurred by 48 h after transfer. $^*P < 0.05$ relative to cells remaining at 3% O_2. *(continued)*

above where pharmacologic and genetic experiments have demonstrated the importance of Na^+ transport in the clearance of fetal lung liquid (54, 85, 86).

A more severe form of noninfective respiratory distress frequently develops in premature infants. It has been referred to by several names, including *hyaline membrane disease* (HMD), the *idiopathic respiratory distress syndrome* (IRDS), *respiratory distress syndrome type I,* or just the *respiratory distress syndrome* (RDS). The variety of names largely result from an ever-improving understanding of the pathogenesis of this disorder over the years. Regardless of the nomenclature, it is a much more severe illness from which the infants may recover within a few days or may go on to severe chronic lung disease or death. There are several pathophysiologic processes that contribute to this disorder and, as described elsewhere in this book, a relative deficiency in surfactant in these preterm infants is a critical initiating factor. Other aspects of lung structure and function may also be incompletely developed, including the structural framework (collagen and elastin content and deposition) and antioxidant systems. These most likely contribute to subsequent and ongoing lung damage as supplemental oxygen is administered and assisted ventilation is carried out to maintain life. There are also data indicating that immaturity of the surfactant system and air space fluid movement may interact with each other, as administration of exogenous surfactant diminishes the prematurely born lung's abnormal epithelial permeability to macromolecules (45) and markedly improves the gas-exchanging ability of a fluid-filled postnatal lung with normal amounts of surfactant (84).

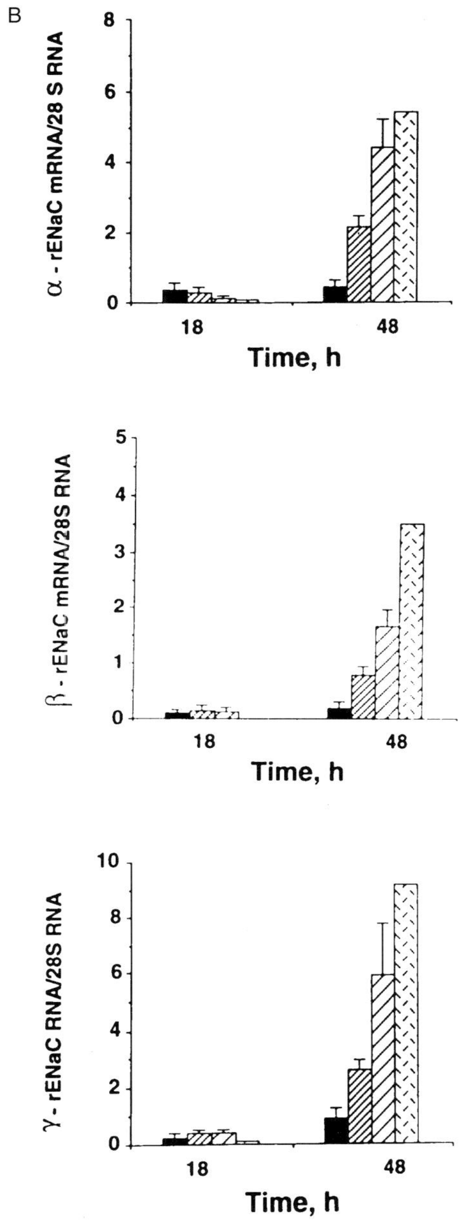

Fig. 9.5 (*continued*)
(*B*) α-, β-, and γ-rENaC mRNA content in three FDLE cultures after transfer from 3% O_2 (*black bars*) to 21% (*narrow stripes*) or 50% 0_2 (*wide stripes*). The average expression of the rENaC subunits of two cultures maintained at 21% O_2 from the beginning of the primary cell isolation is also shown (*stippled columns*). α-, β-, and γ-rENac mRNA content in FDLE cultures was determined by quantitative scanning of Northern blots probed with the respective ^{32}P-cDNA probes as described in Pitkänen et al. (102). [By permission from H. O'Brodovich. *Proc. Assoc. Am. Physicians* 108: 345–355, 1996 (82).]

As discussed in preceding sections of this chapter, there are now much data from observational, pharmacologic, and genetic experiments that indicate in animals that there is an inability of the lung to stop secreting fluid into its air spaces and start absorbing fluid from its air spaces at comparable stages of gestation when human infants develop HMD. Indeed, air space fluid, and not microatelectasis, is the predominate reason for the reduction in total lung capacity in primate models of HMD (56). There are also data from human studies to support these speculations. In the 1960s, deSa demonstrated that human infants had higher lung water content if they were born prematurely and that the lung water burden was greater with increasing immaturity. Of equal importance, these studies demonstrated that in RDS, the infants experienced an increase, rather than a decline, in lung water content (44). These human studies were understandably limited in their experimental design, however, the conclusions are likely valid since comparable data have been obtained in primates (56). Excess air space fluid thus clearly plays a role in the pathogenesis of this disease.

Is there evidence to suggest that the preterm human lung also has inadequate Na^+ transport and can the explain this excess fluid in the premature infant with HMD? It is now known that the human lung actively transports Na^+ (70, 105), human fetal distal lung epithelial monolayers (11) have bioelectric properties similar to rat distal lung epithelia (85, 89), and the mRNA for hENaC is not detected in the immature human lung (75, 116). Thus, extrapolation from other mammalian and primate studies to the human infant seems reasonable. Finally, and most importantly, Barker et al. recently demonstrated that preterm infants with RDS have abnormal amiloride-sensitive Na^+ transport in their nasal epithelium and that this corrects towards normal as the respiratory distress improves (15). Therefore, in vitro and in vivo experiments strongly suggests that defective Na^+ transport is a mechanism that, in addition to surfactant deficiency, leads to the development of HMD in the prematurely born infant.

Mature term infants have approximately tenfold greater amounts of surfactant relative to preterm infants or adults (59), and this likely enables the infant to survive the "salt water drowning" that occurs from the presence of fetal lung liquid within the newborn infant air spaces (Fig. 9.6). A normal fluid-reabsorptive capacity then clears the lung liquid while the "excess" amount of surfactant is capable of maintaining a normal surface tension at the air–liquid interface. In HMD there is both inadequate fluid and Na^+ reabsorption and a relative surfactant deficiency, so the premature infant develops a severe respiratory distress syndrome that is typically characterized by severe lung injury.

Abnormal Na^+ Transport in the Progression of Neonatal Lung Disease

Bronchopulmonary dysplasia (BPD) is a chronic lung disease that occurs in premature infants who do not rapidly recover from HMD. The pathogenesis of BPD is considered multifactorial and a partial list would include persistent lung edema resulting from defective lung water clearance and abnormal epithelial permeability (57),

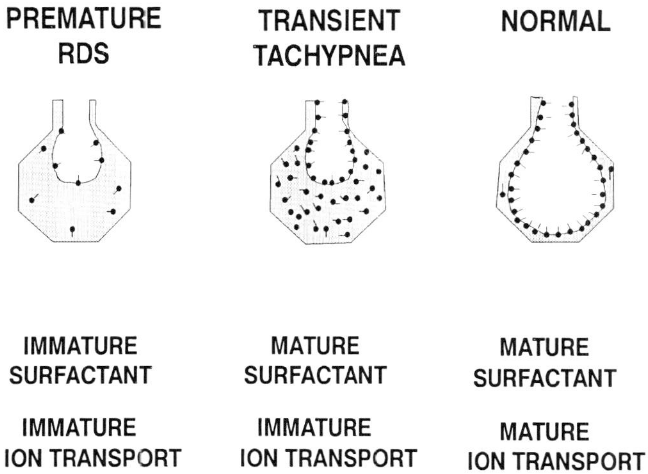

Fig. 9.6 Models for newborn noninfective lung disease. In the mature term infants, "normal" amount of surfactant is approximately tenfold greater than the amount in preterm fetuses or adults (59). This enables the infant to survive the "salt water drowning" that results from the fetal lung liquid that normally fills the air spaces at birth. A normal fluid (Na^+) reabsorptive capacity then clears the lung liquid. In the transient tachypnea syndrome there is an abnormally slow clearance of lung liquid; however, the large amount of surfactant still results in normal surface tension at the air-breathing interface. This results in mild to moderate respiratory distress which resolves within 24–48 h as Na^+ transport rapidly matures (49). In contrast, when there is both inadequate fluid (Na^+) reabsorption and a relative surfactant deficiency, the premature infant develops a severe respiratory distress syndrome (hyaline membrane disease) that is typically characterized by severe lung injury. [By permission from H. O'Brodovich. *Proc. Assoc. Am. Physicians* 108: 345–355, 1996 (82).]

lung damage from reactive oxygen intermediates as a result of supplemental oxygen, ventilatory-induced lung injury, the presence of an inflammatory response, perinatal infection, and worsening pulmonary edema from the high pulmonary blood flow from a patent ductus arteriosus (48, 87, 100).

The net effect of the therapeutic administration of supplemental oxygen on epithelial Na^+ transport is not known. High inspired oxygen concentrations will damage the lung in a variety of ways, and may lead to death (50, 68, 91, 98, 102). However, prolonged but nonlethal exposure to higher oxygen concentrations has been demonstrated to have some beneficial aspects, including increased expression of the membrane proteins involved in Na^+ transport. Nonlethal oxygen exposures have been shown to increase Na^+/K^+ ATPase, Na^+ channel protein, and activity in isolated type II pneumocytes (32, 51, 91, 110, 126).

It has been known for some time that there is a noninfective inflammatory response in the lungs of infants who do not recover from HMD and progress to BPD (for review see ref. 87). Our laboratory has investigated the effect of cellular inflammation on the ability of the lung epithelium to transport Na^+ in vitro. Compeau et al. observed that activated macrophages could decrease amiloride-sensitive transport and diminish Na^+ channel activity via *l*-arginine (presumably nitric oxide)–dependent mechanisms (39). The impairment of amiloride-sensitive Na^+ transport was independent of direct cell–cell contact, as it was mediated by a soluble factor, and was associated with a decrease in the expression of rENaC (J.W. Ding, J. Dickie, O. Rotstein, and H. O'Brodovich , unpublished observations). Finally, the longitudinal changes that take place during the repair and fibrosis following oxidant-induced lung damage involve regression to earlier developmental events including dedifferentiation, transformation, and increased division of the progenitor epithelial and mesenchymal cells (5, 76). The resulting aberrant extracellular matrix may precipitate distorted ion transport of the pulmonary epithelium after the initial insult has subsided (101).

REFERENCES:

1. Acarregui, M.J., J.J.Brown, and R.K. Mallampalli. Oxygen modulates surfactant protein mRNA expression and phospholipid production in human fetal lung in vitro. *Am. J. Physiol.* 268: L818–L825, 1995.
2. Acarregui, M.J., J.M.Snyder, and C.R. Mendelson. Oxygen modulates the differentiation of human fetal lung in vitro and its responsiveness to cAMP. *Am. J. Physiol.* 264: L465–L474, 1993.
3. Adams, F.H., T. Fujiwara, and G. Rowshan. The nature and origin of the fluid in fetal lamb lung. *J. Pediatr.* 63: 881–888, 1963.
4. Adams, F.H., M. Yanagisawa, D. Kuzela, and H. Martinek. The disappearance of fetal lung fluid following birth. *J. Pediatr.* 78: 837–843, 1971.
5. Adamson, I.Y.R. Alveolar injury and repair. In: *Electron microscopy of the lung,* edited by D.E. Schraufnagel. New York: Marcel Dekker, 1990, p. 149–176.
6. Adamson, I.Y.R. Development of lung structure. In: *The Lung: Scientific Foundations,* edited by R.G. Crystal, J.B. West, et al. New York: Raven Press, 1991, p. 663–670.
7. Adamson, T.M., R.D.H. Boyd, H.S. Platt, and L.B. Strang. Composition of alveolar liquid in the fetal lamb. *J. Physiol. Lond.* 204: 159–169, 1969.
8. Adzick, N.S., M.R. Harrison, P.L. Glick, R.L. Villa, and W. Finkbeiner. Experimental pulmonary hypoplasia and oligohydramnios: relative contributions of lung fluid and fetal breathing movements. *J. Pediatr. Surg.* 19: 658–665, 1984
9. Alcorn, D., T.M. Adamson, T.F. Lambert, J.E. Maloney, B.C. Ritchie, and P.M. Robinson. Morphological effects of chronic tracheal ligation and drainage in the fetal lamb lung. *J. Anat.* 123: 649–660, 1977.
10. Ballard, S.T., R.C. Boucher, J.T Gatzy, E.M. Krochmal, and J.R. Yankaskas. Volume and ion transport by fetal rat alveolar and tracheal epithelia in submersion culture. *Am. J. Physiol.* 256: F397–F407, 1989.
11. Barker, P.M., R.C. Boucher, and J.R. Yankaskas. Bioelectric properties of cultured monolayers from epithelium of distal human fetal lung. *Am. J. Physiol.* 268: L270–L277, 1995.
12. Barker, P.M., K.K. Brigman, A.M. Paradiso, R.C. Boucher, and J.T. Gatzy. Cl^- secretion by

trachea of CFTR (+/–) and (–/–) fetal mouse. *Am. J. Respir. Cell Mol. Biol.* 13: 307–313, 1995.

13. Barker, P.M., M.J. Brown, C.A. Ramsden, L.B. Strang, and D.V Walters. The effect of thyreoidectomy in the fetal sheep on lung liquid reabsorption induced by adrenaline or cyclic AMP. *J. Physiol. Lond.* 407: 373–383, 1988.
14. Barker, P.M. and J.T. Gatzy. Effect of gas composition on liquid secretion by explants of distal lung fetal rat in submersion culture. *Am. J. Physiol. (Lung Cell. Mol. Physiol.)* 265: L512–L517, 1993.
15. Barker, P.M., C.W. Gowen, E.E. Lawson, and M.R. Knowles. Decreased sodium ion absorption across nasal epithelium of very preterm infants with respiratory distress syndrome. *J. Pediatr.* 130: 373–377, 1997.
16. Barker, P.M., M. Markiewicz, K.A. Parker, D.V. Walters, and L.B. Strang. Synergistic action of triiodothyronine and hydrocortisone on epinephrine-induced reabsorption of fetal lung liquid. *Pediatr. Res.* 27: 588–591, 1990.
17. Barker, P.M., L.B. Strang, and D.V. Walters. The role of thyroid hormones in maturation of the adrenaline-sensitive lung liquid reabsorptive mechanism in fetal sheep. *J. Physiol. Lond.* 424: 473–485, 1990.
18. Barker, P.M., D.V. Walters, M. Markiewicz, and L.B. Strang. Development of the lung liquid reabsorptive mechanism in fetal sheep: synergism of triiodothyronine and hydrocortisone. *J. Physiol. Lond.* 433: 435–449, 1991.
19. Berry, D., A. Jobe, and M. Ikegami. Leakage of macromolecules in ventilated segments of preterm lamb lungs. *J. Appl. Physiol.* 70: 423–429, 1991.
20. Bland, R.D. Lung epithelial ion transport and fluid movement during the perinatal period. *Am. J. Physiol.* 259: L30–L37, 1990.
21. Bland, R.D. and C.A.R. Boyd. Cation transport in lung epithelial cells derived from fetal, newborn, and adult rabbits. *J. Appl. Physiol.* 61: 507–515, 1986.
22. Bland, R.D., M.A. Bressack, and D.D. McMillan. Labor decreases the lung water content of newborn rabbits. *Am. J. Obstet. Gynecol.* 135: 364–367, 1979.
23. Bland, R.D. and D.W. Nielson. Developmental changes in lung liquid epithelial ion transport and liquid movement. *Annu. Rev. Physiol.* 54: 373–394, 1992.
24. Bland, R.D., D.D. McMillan, M.A. Bressack, and L. Dong. Clearance of liquid from lungs of newborn rabbits. *J. Appl. Physiol.* 49: 171–177, 1980.
25. Brody, J.S. and M.C. Williams. Pulmonary alveolar epithelial cell differentiation. *Annu. Rev. Physiol.* 54: 351–371, 1992.
26. Brown, M.J., R.E. Olver, C.A. Ramsden, L.B. Strang, and D.V. Walters. Effects of adrenaline and of spontaneous labour on the secretion and absorption of lung liquid in the fetal lamb. *J. Physiol. Lond.* 344: 137–152, 1983.
27. Burri, P.H. Fetal and postnatal development of the lung. *Annu. Rev. Physiol.* 46: 617–628, 1984.
28. Canessa, C.M., J.-D. Horisberger, and B.C. Rossier. Epithelial sodium channel related to proteins involved in neurodegeneration. *Nature* 361: 467–470, 1993.
29. Canessa, C.M., L. Schild, G. Buell, B. Thorens, I. Gautschi, J.-D. Horisberger, and B.C. Rossier. Amiloride-sensitive epithelial Na^+ channel is made of three homologous subunits. *Nature* 367: 463–467, 1994.
30. Carlton, D.P., J.J. Cummings, D.L. Chapman, F.R. Poulain, and R.D. Bland. Ion transport regulation of lung liquid secretion in foetal lambs. *J. Dev. Physiol.* 17: 99–107, 1992.
31. Carlton, D.P., J.J. Cummings, R.G. Scheerer, F.R. Poulain, and R.D. Bland. Lung overex-

pansion increases pulmonary microvascular protein permeability in young lambs. *J. Appl. Physiol.* 69: 577–583, 1990.

32. Carter, E.P., S.E. Duvick, C.H. Wendt, J. Dunitz, L. Nici, O.D. Wangensteen, and D.H. Ingbar. Hyperoxia increases active alveolar Na^+ resorption in vivo and type II cell Na,K-ATPase in vitro. *Chest* 105: 75S–78S, 1994.
33. Cassin, S., V. DeMarco, A.M. Perks, H. Kuck, and T.M. Ellis. Regulation of lung liquid secretion in immature fetal sheep: hormonal interaction. *J. Appl. Physiol.* 77: 1445–1450, 1994.
34. Cassin, S., G. Gausse, and A.M. Perks. The effects of bumetanide and furosemide on lung liquid secretion in fetal sheep. Proc. Exp. Biol. Med. 181: 427–431, 1986.
35. Cassin, S. and A.M. Perks. Amiloride inhibits arginine-vasopressin induced decrease in fetal lung liquid secretion. *J. Appl. Physiol.* 75: 1925–1929, 1993.
36. Champigny, G., N .Voilley, E. Lingueglia, V. Friend, P. Barbry, and M. Lazdunski. Regulation of expression of the lung amiloride-sensitive Na^+ channel by steroid hormones. *EMBO J* 13: 2177–2181, 1994.
37. Chang, S.S., S. Grunder, A. Hanukoglu, A. Röler, P.M. Mathew, I. Hanukoglu, L. Schild, Y Lu, R.A. Shimkets, C. Nelson-Williams, B.C. Rossier, and R.O. Lifton. Mutations in the subunits of the epithelial sodium channel cause salt wasting with hyperkalemic acidosis, pseudohypoaldosterinism type 1. *Nat. Genet.* 12: 248–253, 1996.
38. Chapman, D.L., D.P. Carlton, J.J. Cummings, F.R. Poulain, and R.D. Bland. Intrapulmonary terbutaline and aminophylline decrease lung liquid in fetal lambs. *Pediatr. Res.* 29: 357–361, 1991.
39. Compeau, C.G., O.D. Rotstein, H. Tohda, Y. Marunaka, B. Rafii, A.S. Slutsky, and H. O'Brodovich. Endotoxin-stimulated alveolar macrophages impair lung epithelial Na^+ transport by an L-Arg-dependent mechanism. *Am. J. Physiol.* 266: C1330–C1341, 1994.
40. Cott, G.R. Modulation of bioelectric properties across alveolar type II cells by substratum. *Am. J. Physiol.* 257: C678–C688, 1989.
41. Cott, G.R. and A.K. Rao. Hydrocortisone promotes the maturation of Na^+-dependent ion transport across the fetal pulmonary epithelium. *Am. J. Respir. Cell Mol. Biol.* 9: 166–171, 1993.
42. Cott, G.R., S.R. Walker, and R.J. Mason. The effect of substratum and serum on the lipid synthesis and morphology of alveolar Type II cells in vitro. *Exp. Lung Res.* 13: 427–447, 1987.
43. Cotton, C.U., R.C. Boucher, and J.T. Gatzy. Bioelectric properties and ion transport across excised canine fetal and neonatal airways. *J. Appl. Physiol.* 65: 2367–2375, 1988.
44. deSa, D.J. Pulmonary fluid content in infants with respiratory distress. *J. Pathol.* 97: 469–479, 1969.
45. Egan, E.A., W.P. Dillon, and S. Zorn. Fetal lung liquid absorption and alveolar epithelial solute permeability in surfactant deficient, breathing fetal lambs. *Pediatr. Res.* 6: 566–570, 1984.
46. Egan, E.A., R.E. Olver, and L.B. Strang. Changes in non-electrolyte permeability of alveoli and the absorption of lung liquid at the start of breathing in the lamb. *J. Physiol. Lond.* 244: 161–179, 1975.
47. Feng, Z., R.B. Clark, and Y. Berthiaume. Identification of nonselective cation channels in cultured adult rat alveolar type II cells. *Am. J. Respir. Cell Mol. Biol.* 9: 248–254, 1993.
48. Gonzalez, A., I.R.S. Sosenko, J. Chandar, H. Hummler, N. Claure, and E. Bancalari. Influence of infection on patent ductus arteriosus and chronic lung disease in premature infants weighing 1000 grams or less. *J. Pediatr.* 128: 470–478, 1996.

49. Gowen, C.V., E.E. Lawson, J. Gingras, R. Boucher, J.T. Gatzy, and M. Knowles. Electrical potential difference and ion transport across nasal epithelium of term neonates: correlation with mode of delivery, transient tachypnea of the newborn, and respiratory rate. *J. Pediatr.* 113: 121–127, 1988.
50. Haddad, I.Y., G. Pataki, P. Hu, C. Galliani, J.S. Beckman, and S. Matalon. Quantitation of nitrotyrosine levels in lung sections of patients and animals with acute lung injury. *J. Clin. Invest.* 94: 2407–2413, 1994.
51. Haskell, J.F., G. Yue, D.J. Benos, and S. Matalon. Upregulation of sodium conductive pathways in alveolar type II cells in sublethal hyperoxia. *Am. J. Physiol.* 266: L30–L37, 1994.
52. Hooper, S.B., M.J. Wallace, and R. Harding. Amiloride blocks the inhibition of fetal lung liquid secretion caused by AVP but not asphyxia. *J. Appl. Physiol.* 74: 111–115, 1993.
53. Huang, M. and M. Chalfie. Gene interactions affecting mechanosensory transduction in *Caenorhabditis elegans. Nature* 367: 467–470, 1994.
54. Hummler, E., P. Barker, J. Gatzy, F. Beermann, C. Verdumo, A. Schmidt, R. Boucher, and B.C. Rossier. Early death due to defective neonatal lung liquid clearance in α-ENaC-deficient mice. *Nat. Genet.* 12: 325–328, 1996.
55. Ingbar, D.H., C.B. Weeks, M. Gilmore-Hebert, E. Jacobsen, S. Duvick, R. Dowin, S.K. Savik, and J.D. Jamieson. Developmental regulation of Na,K-ATPase in rat lung. *Am. J. Physiol.* 270: L619–L629, 1996.
56. Jackson, C., A. Mackenzie, E. Chi, T. Standaert, W. Truog, and W. Hodson. Mechanisms for reduced total lung capacity at birth and during hyaline membrane disease in premature newborn monkeys. *Am. Rev. Respir. Dis.* 142: 413–419, 1990.
57. Jefferies, A.L., G. Coates, and H.M. O'Brodovich. Pulmonary epithelial permeability in hyaline-membrane disease. *N. Engl. J. Med.* 311: 1075–1080, 1984.
58. Jefferies, A.L. and K.F.Y. Tai. Sequential changes in pulmonary epithelial permeability after birth in term and preterm rabbits. *Biol. Neonate* 66: 86–92, 1994.
59. Jobe, A. and M. Ikegami. State of the art: surfactant for the treatment of respiratory distress syndrome. *Am. Rev. Respir. Dis.* 136: 1256–1275, 1987.
60. Jost, A. and A. Policard. Contribution expérimentale a l'étude du development prénatal du poumon chez la lapin. *Arch. Anat. Microsc. Morphol. Exp.* 37: 323–332, 1948.
61. Kemp, P.J., G.G. MacGregor, and R.E. Olver. G protein-regulated large-conductance chloride channels in freshly isolated fetal type II alveolar epithelial cells. *Am. J. Physiol.* 265: L323–329, 1993.
62. Lingueglia, E., N. Voilley, R. Waldmann, M. Lazdunski, and P. Barbry. Expression cloning of an epithelial amiloride-sensitive Na^+ channel: a new channel type with homologies to *Caenorhabditis elegans* degenerins. *FEBS Lett.* 318: 95–99, 1993.
63. Leung, C.K.H., I.Y.R. Adamson, , and D.H. Bowden. Uptake of ^3H prednisolone by fetal lung explants: role of intercellular contacts in epithelial maturation. *Exp. Lung Res.* 1: 111–120, 1980.
64. Lwebuga-Mukasa, J. Matrix-driven pneumocyte differentiation. *Am. Rev. Respir. Dis.* 144: 452–457, 1991.
65. MacLeod, R.J., J.R. Hamilton, H. Kopelman, and N.B. Sweezey. Developmental differences of cystic fibrosis transmembrane conductance regulator functional expression in rat fetal distal airway epithelial cells. *Pediatr. Res.* 35: 45–49, 1994.
66. Matalon, S., M.L. Bauer, D.J. Benos, T.R. Kleyman, C. Lin, E.R Cragoe, Jr., and H. O'Brodovich. Fetal lung epithelial cells contain two populations of amiloride-sensitive Na^+ channels. *Am. J. Physiol.* 264: L357–364, 1993.

67. Matalon, S., R.J. Bridges, and D.J. Benos. Amiloride inhibitable Na conductive pathways in alveolar type II pneumonocytes. *Am. J. Physiol.* 264: L90–L96, 1991.
68. Matalon, S. and E.A. Egan. Effects of 100% O_2 breathing on permeability of alveolar epithelium to solute. *J. Appl. Physiol.* 50: 859863, 1981.
69. Matalon, S., K.L. Kirk, J.K. Bubien, Y. Oh, P. Hu, G. Yue, R. Shoemaker, E.J.J. Cragoe, and D.J. Benos. Immunocytochemical and functional characterization of Na^+ conductance in adult alveolar pneumonocytes. *Am. J. Physiol.* 262: C1228–C1238, 1992.
70. Matthay, M.A. and J.P. Wiener-Kronish, Intact epithelial barrier function is critical for the resolution of alveolar edema in man. *Am. Rev. Respir. Dis.* 142: 1250–1257, 1990.
71. McCray, P.B. and M.K. Welsh. Developing fetal alveolar epithelial cells secrete fluid in primary culture. *Am. J. Physiol.* 260: L494–L500, 1991.
72. McCray, P.B., Jr., C.L. Wohlford-Lenane, and J.M. Snyder. Localization of cystic fibrosis transmembrane conductance regulator mRNA in human fetal lung tissue by in situ hybridization. *J. Clin. Invest.* 90: 619–625, 1992.
73. McCray, P.B., Jr., W.W. Reenstra, E. Louie, J. Johnson, J.D. Bettencourt, and J. Bastacky. Expression of CFTR and presence of cAMP-mediated fluid secretion in human fetal lung. *Am. J. Physiol.* 262: L472–L481, 1992.
74. McCray, P.B. Jr., J.D. Bettencourt, J. Bastacky, G.M. Denning, and M.J. Welsh. Expression of CFTR and cAMP-stimulated chloride secretory current in cultured human fetal alveolar epithelial cells. *Am. J. Respir. Cell Mol. Biol.* 9: 578–585, 1993.
75. McDonald, F.J., P.M. Snyder, P.B. McCray, and M.J. Welsh. Cloning, expression, and tissue distribution of the human epithelial sodium channel. *Am. J. Physiol.* 268: L728–734, 1995.
76. McGowan, S.E. Extracellular matrix and the regulation of lung development and repair. *FASEB J.* 6: 2895–2904, 1992.
77. McPherson, M.A. and R.L. Dormer. Abnormalities in the intracellular regulation in cystic fibrosis. In: Cystic Fibrosis, edited by J.O. Warner. New York: Churchill Livingstone, 1992, p. 766–784.
78. Moessinger, A.C., R.D. Harding, T.M. Adamson, M. Singh, and G.T. Kiu. Role of lung liquid volume in growth and maturation of the fetal sheep lung. *J. Clin. Invest.* 86: 1270–1277, 1990.
79. Murray, C.B., M.M. Morales, T.R. Flotte, S.A. McGrath-Morrow, W.B. Guggino, W.B. and P.L. Zeitlin. ClC–2: a developmentally dependent chloride channel expressed in the fetal lung and downregulated after birth. *Am. J. Respir. Cell Mol. Biol.* 12: 597–604, 1995.
80. Nardo, L., S.B. Hooper, and R. Harding. Lung hypoplasia can be reversed by short-term obstruction of the trachea in fetal sheep. *Pediatr. Res.* 38: 690–696, 1995.
81. O'Brodovich, H.M. The role of active Na^+ transport by lung epithelium in the clearance of airspace fluid. *New Horizons* 3: 240–247, 1995.
82. O'Brodovich, H.M. Immature epithelial Na^+ channel expression is one of the pathogenetic mechanisms leading to human neonatal respiratory distress syndrome. *Proc. Assoc. Am. Phys.* 108: 345–355, 1996.
83. O'Brodovich, H., C. Canessa, J. Ueda, B. Rafii, B.C. Rossier, and J. Edelson. Expression of the epithelial Na^+ channel in the developing rat lung. *Am. J. Physiol.* 265: C491–C496, 1993.
84. O'Brodovich, H.M. and V. Hannam. Exogenous surfactant rapidly increases PaO_2 in mature rabbits with lungs that contain large amounts of saline. *Am. Rev. Respir. Dis.* 147: 1087–1090, 1993.
85. O'Brodovich, H., V. Hannam, and B. Rafii. Sodium channel but neither Na^+-H^+ nor Na-

glucose symport inhibitors slow neonatal lung water clearance. *Am. J. Respir. Cell Mol. Biol.* 5: 377–384, 1991.

86. O'Brodovich, H., V. Hannam, M. Seear, and J.B.M. Mullen. Amiloride impairs lung water clearance in newborn guinea pigs. *J. Appl. Physiol.* 68: 1758–1762, 1990.
87. O'Brodovich, H.M. and R.B. Mellins. Bronchopulmonary dysplasia. Unresolved neonatal lung injury. *Am. Rev. Respir. Dis.* 132: 694–709, 1985.
88. O'Brodovich, H. and T.A. Merritt. Bicarbonate concentration in rhesus monkey and guinea pig fetal lung liquid. *Am. Rev. Respir. Dis.* 146: 1613–1618, 1992.
89. O'Brodovich, H., B. Rafii, and M. Post. Bioelectric properties of fetal alveolar epithelial monolayers. *Am. J. Physiol.* 258: L201–206, 1990.
90. O'Brodovich, H., O. Staub, B.C. Rossier, K. Geering, , and J.-P. Kraehenbuhl. Ontogeny of α1- and β1-isoforms of Na^+-K^+-ATPase in fetal distal rat lung epithelium. *Am. J. Physiol.* 264: C1137–C1143, 1993.
91. Olivera, W., K. Ridge, L.D.H. Wood, and J.I. Sznajder. Active sodium transport and alveolar epithelial Na-K-ATPase increase during subacute hyperoxia in rats. Am. J. Physiol. 266: L577–L584, 1994.
92. Olver, R.E., C.A. Ramsden, L.B. Strang, and D.V. Walters. The role of amiloride-blockable sodium transport in adrenaline-induced lung liquid reabsorption in the fetal lung. *J. Physiol.* 376: 321–340, 1986.
93. Olver, R.E. and L.B. Strang. Ion fluxes across pulmonary epithelium and the secretion of lung liquid in the foetal lamb. *J. Physiol. Lond.* 241: 327–257, 1974.
94. Olver, R.E., E.E. Schneeberger, and D.V. Walters. Epithelial solute permeability, ion transport and tight junction morphology in the developing lung of the fetal lamb. *J. Physiol. Lond.* 315: 395–412, 1981.
95. Orlowski, J. and J.B. Lingrel. Tissue-specific and developmental regulation of rat Na,K-ATPase catalytic α isoform and β subunit mRNAs. *J. Biol. Chem.* 263: 10436–10442, 1988.
96. Orser, B.A., M. Bertlik, L. Fedorko, and H.M. O'Brodovich. Non-selective cation channel in fetal alveolar type II epithelium. *Biochim. Biophys. Acta (Mol. Cell Struct.)* 1094: 19–26, 1991.
97. Orzalesi, M., M. Motoyama, H.N. Jacobson, Y. Kikkawa, E.O.R. Reynolds, and C.D. Cook. The development of lung liquid in fetal goats. *Pediatrics* 35: 373–381, 1965.
98. Palazzo, R.M., O.D. Wangensteen, and D.E. Niewoehner. Time course of functional repair of the alveolar epithelium after hyperoxic injury. *J. Appl. Physiol.* 73: 1881–1887, 1992.
99. Perks, A.M. and S. Cassin. The effects of arginine vasopressin and other factors on the production of lung liquid in fetal goats. *Chest* 81: 63S–65S, 1982.
100. Pierce, M.R. and E. Bancalari. The role of inflammation in the pathogenesis of bronchopulmonary dysplasia. *Pediatr. Pulmonol.* 19: 371–378, 1995.
101. Pitkänen, O.M., A.K. Tanswell, and H.M. O'Brodovich. Fetal lung cell–derived matrix alters distal lung epithelial ion transport. *Am. J. Physiol.* 268: L762–L771, 1995.
102. Pitkänen, O., A.K. Tanswell, G. Downey, and H. O'Brodovich. Increased PO_2 alters bioelectric properties of fetal lung epithelium. *Am. J. Physiol.* 270: L1060–L1066, 1996.
103. Rao, A.K. and G.R. Cott. Ontogeny of ion transport across fetal pulmonary epithelial cells in monolayer culture. *Am. J. Physiol.* 261: L178–L187, 1991.
104. Ruddy, M.K., J.M. Drazen, O.M. Pitkänen, B. Rafii, H.M. O'Brodovich, and H.W. Harris. Modulation of aquaporin 4 and the amiloride-inhibitable sodium channel in perinatal rat lung epithelial cells. *Am. J. Physiol.* 274: L1066–L1072, 1998.

105. Sakuma, T., G. Okaniwa, T. Nakada, T. Nishimura, S. Fujimura, and M.A. Matthay. Alveolar fluid clearance in the resected human lung. *Am. J. Respir. Crit. Care Med.* 150: 305–310, 1994.
106. Schneeberger, E.E. and K.M. McCarthy. Cytochemical localization of Na^+-K^+-ATPase in rat type II pneumocytes. *J. Appl. Physiol.* 60: 1584–1589, 1986.
107. Scurry, J.P., T.M. Adamson, and L.J. Cussen. Fetal lung growth in laryngeal atresia and tracheal agenesis. *Austr. Pediatr.* J. 25: 47–51, 1989.
108. Souza, P., H. O'Brodovich, and M. Post. Lung fluid restriction affects growth, but not airway branching of embryonic rat lung. *Int. J. Dev Biol.* 39: 629–637, 1995.
109. Strang, L.B. Fetal lung liquid: secretion and reabsorption. *Physiol. Rev.* 71: 991–1016, 1991.
110. Sznajder, J.I., W.G. Olivera, K.M. Ridge, and D.H. Rutschman. Mechanisms of lung liquid clearance during hyperoxia in isolated rat lungs. *Am. J. Respir. Crit. Care Med.* 151: 1519–1525, 1995.
111. Tchepichev, S., J. Ueda, C. Canessa, B.C. Rossier, and H. O'Brodovich. Lung epithelial Na channel subunits are differentially regulated during development and by steroids. *Am. J. Physiol.* 269: C805–C812, 1995.
112. Tizzano, E.F., H. O'Brodovich, D. Chitayat, J.-C. Bènichou, and M. Buchwald. Regional expression of CFTR in developing human respiratory tissues. *Am. J. Respir. Cell. Mol. Biol.* 10: 355–362, 1994.
113. Thom, J. and A.M. Perks. The effects of furosemide and bumetanide on lung liquid production in vitro lungs from fetal guinea pigs. *Can. J. Physiol. Pharmacol.* 68: 1131–1135, 1990.
114. Tohda, H., J.K. Foskett, H. O'Brodovich, and Y. Marunaka. Cl^- regulaton of a Ca^{2+} activated nonselective cation channel in β-agonist-treated fetal distal lung epithelium. *Am. J. Physiol.* 266: C104–C109, 1994.
115. Tohda, H. and Y. Marunaka. Insulin-activated amiloride-blockable nonselective cation and Na^+ channels in the fetal distal lung epithelium. *Gen. Pharmacol.* 26: 755–763, 1995.
116. Voilley, N., E. Lingueglia, G. Champigny, M.-G. Mattéi, R. Waldmann, M. Lazdunski, and P. Barbry. The lung amiloride-sensitive Na^+ channel: biophysical properties, pharmacology, ontogenesis, and molecular cloning. *Proc. Natl. Acad. Sci. USA* 91: 247–251, 1994.
117. Volk, K.A., R.D .Sigmund, P.M. Snyder, J. McDonald, M.J. Welsh, and J.B. Stokes. rENaC is the predominant Na^+ channel in the apical membrane of the rat renal inner medullary collecting duct. *J. Clin. Invest.* 96: 2748–2757, 1995.
118. Vukicevic, S., H. Kleinman, F. Luyten, A. Roberts, N. Roche, , and A.H. Reddi. Identification of multiple active growth factors in basement membrane matrigel suggests caution in interpretation of cellular activity related to extracellular matrix components. *Exp. Cell. Res.* 202: 1–8, 1992.
119. Wallace, M.J., S.B. Hooper, and R. Harding. Regulation of lung liquid secretion by arginine vasopressin in fetal sheep. *Am. J. Physiol.* 258: R104–R111, 1990.
120. Wallace, M.J., S.B. Hooper, and R. Harding. Effects of elevated cortisol concentrations on the volume, secretion, and reabsorption of lung liquid. *Am. J. Physiol.* 269: R881–R887, 1995.
121. Wallace M.J., S.B. Hooper, and R. Harding. Role of the adrenal glands in the maturation of lung liquid secretory mechanisms in fetal sheep *Am. J. Physiol.* 270: R33–R40, 1996.
122. Walters, D.V. Fetal lung liquid: secretion and absorption. In: *Fetus and Neonate: Physiol-*

ogy and Clinical Application. Vol. 2: Breathing, edited by M.A. Hanson, J.A.D. Spencer, and C.H. Rodeck. Cambridge: Cambridge University Press, 1994, p. 42–62.

123. Walters, D.V. and R.E. Olver. The role of catecholamines in lung liquid absorption at birth. *Pediatr. Res.* 12: 239–242, 1978.
124. Walters, D.V., C.A. Ramsden, and R.E. Olver. Dibutyryl cAMP induces a gestation-dependent absorption of fetal lung liquid. *J. Appl. Physiol.* 68: 2054–2059, 1990.
125. Wang, X., T. Kleyman, H. Tohda, Y. Marunaka, and H.M. O'Brodovich. EIPA sensitive Na^+ currents in intact fetal distal lung epithelial cells. *Can. J. Physiol. Pharmacol.* 71: 58–62, 1993.
126. Yue, G., W.J. Russell, D.J. Benos, R.M. Jackson, M.A. Olman, and S. Matalon, Increased expression and activity of sodium channels in alveolar type II cells of hyperoxic rats. *Proc. Natl. Acad. Sci. USA* 92: 8418–8422, 1995.

chapter 10

MECHANISMS OF CELL GROWTH AND TISSUE REPAIR

Annick Clement and Jerome S. Brody

LUNG development and lung repair following injury require a complex series of controlled interactions involving genetic influences, hormonal stimulation, and cell-cell communication. These components regulate the process of cell replication resulting in appropriate lung growth as well as in the re-establishment of the normal architecture of the lung.

CELL CYCLE CONTROL

Proliferation is defined as the increase in cell number resulting from completion of the cell cycle. The intrinsic cell cycle machinery is controlled by external signals such as growth factors and anti-mitogens to integrate cell division with environmental and developmental stimuli. As cells progress through the cell cycle, they undergo several transitions that can be defined as a unidirectional change of state in which a cell that was performing one set of processes shifts its activity to perform a different set of processes (47, 85, 107).

Cell cycle checkpoints are regulatory pathways that control the order and timing of cell cycle transitions and ensure that critical events such as DNA replication and chromosome segregation are completed with fidelity (34, 108). In the past few years, much has been learned about the cell cycle checkpoint that controls G1-S transition and onset of DNA replication. The processes involved exert their greatest effects by targeting particular regulators of G1-phase progression. The present review highlights recent advances in the understanding of the mechanisms controlling

DNA replication and which play a central role in lung growth and lung repair. Progression of eukaryotic cells through G1 phase and G1-S transition is mediated by sequential assembly and activation of key regulators of the cell cycle machinery, the *cyclin-dependent kinases* (CDKs).

Various G1 Cyclin-dependent Kinases and Their Activation

The first CDK that was identified was the product of the *CDC2* gene (34 kDa) in fission yeast; its homolog in mammalian cells is referred to as CDK1. A number of other protein kinases were then identified and designated CDKs on the basis of their ability to bind to a cyclin molecule in human cells. The CDK family shares a high degree of structural homology encoding the domains conserved in all serine/threonine kinases. As the present time, six different proteins have been characterized and have been designated CDK1 to CDK6. The defining property of the CDKs is that they are inactive as monomers and only become active after binding to a cyclin partner (40, 90).

The *cyclins* are another growing family of proteins (65). They were first defined as proteins whose levels vary in a cell cycle manner, but are now identified on the basis of sequence homology. They share a 150 amino acid region of structural homology called the cyclin box, which is responsible for binding to the CDK subunit. It is now well demonstrated that different cyclins can bind to the same CDKs. This flexibility allows CDKs to perform distinct functions during progression through the cell cycle as well as in processes not related to proliferation. Therefore, the specificity of the cyclin–CDK complex is dependent on both the CDK and the cyclin that make up the complex.

In mammals, the G1 CDKs include CDK2, CDK3, CDK4, CDK5, and CDK6. These enzymes form complexes with the G1 cyclins, mostly cyclins D, E, and at the end of G1 cyclin A. Activity of the complexes appears to be regulated by several mechanisms (65, 92). The levels of cyclins are controlled by synthesis and ubipuitin-mediated proteolysis. Cell cycle kinases and phosphatases can either activate or inhibit the complex by modulating phosphorylation of the CDKs. The activatory site of phosphorylation is at threonine 160. Phosphorylating this residue by a kinase termed *Cak* increases the affinity of cyclin binding and converts the CDK into an active enzyme. The catalytic subunit can also be inhibited through dephosphorylation by a phosphatase (Kap1) at the activating threonine residue or phosphorylation of a tyrosine residue (tyrosine 14) (32).

In addition, activity of the cyclin–CDK complex can be negatively regulated by a group pf proteins termed *CDK inhibitory proteins* (CKIs) that might modify their specificity and accessibility to regulators (34, 106–108). The CKIs have been reported to associate with either the cyclin, the catalytic subunit, or the CDK complex, without covalently modifying either the cyclin or catalytic subunit. Several CKIs have been identified on the basis of homology and are currently classified into two groups that were extrapolated further from the first members discovered: p16 and p21. The p16 family consists of $p15^{Ink4B}$, $p16^{Ink4}$, $p18^{Ink4C}$, and $p19^{Ink4D}$. The p21 family includes $p21^{CIP1}$ (also known as WAF1), $p27^{KIP1}$, and $p57^{KIP2}$. The proteins of the p16 family display a certain degree of specificity for CDK4 and CDK6, preventing the association of the CDKs with cyclin D. The p21 family proteins act on a wide range of cyclin–CDK complexes. In addition, $p21^{CIP1}$ has been reported to bind proliferating cell nuclear antigen (PCNA) and to inhibit PCNA-dependent replication in vitro.

Recently, much has been learned about the role and regulation of the various CKIs (40, 90, 92). $p16^{INK4}$ appears to function as a tumor suppressor that is inactivated in a large number of tumors. A recent hypothesis suggests that $p16^{INK4}$ selectively functions in a signaling pathway that detects certain oncogenic perturbations and brakes the cell cycle progression. Expression of the *p21* gene is induced by a wide range of cell growth-regulatory signals including the antiproliferative transforming growth factor β (TGF-β), p53, as well as cellular senescence and DNA damage. Relative levels of $p21^{CIP1}$ seem to be critical in determining the threshold kinase activity of several cyclin–CDK complexes (122). Interestingly, mice homozygous for a null mutation in the p21 gene do not demonstrate a predisposition toward tumorigenesis (118). In addition, in a number of cell types, a correlation was observed between $p21^{CIP1}$ expression and the withdrawal of cells from the cell cycle during differentiation, strongly suggesting a potential role for $p21^{CIP1}$ in normal differentiation. Taken together, these data suggest that appropriate levels of $p21^{CIP1}$ may be critical in normal cell division and animal development (67, 69). $p27^{KIP1}$ is mostly complexed with cyclin D–CDK complexes in proliferating cells. Its level is high in quiescent cells, falls in response to mitogenic stimulation, remains at lower threshold levels in proliferating cells, and increases again when mitogens are withdrawn. Antisense inhibition of $p27^{KIP1}$ synthesis in cycling cells can prevent them from becoming quiescent (25). Interestingly, mice that were nullizygous for the *p27* gene grew faster than control mice with organs containing increased numbers of smaller cells, emphasizing the importance of $p27^{KIP1}$ in regulating both cell size and cell number (83).

Restriction Point Control

The G1 phase is a determinant phase of the cell cycle. During this phase, cells respond to extracellular signals and decide either to progress in the cell cycle and advance toward another division or to withdraw from the cell cycle into a quiescent state called *G0*. G1 events appear to occur sequentially leading to separate the G1 phase into subphases depending on the requirements and effects of specific growth factors, nutrients, and inhibitors. A critical time point late in G1 has been ascertained and termed the *restriction point*. It is now believed that the decision for a cell to divide occurs at this level. Before the restriction point, cells are dependent on signals provided by their environment. Once they pass the restriction point, they become refractory to these signals and follow an autonomous program that leads to mitosis (108, 123).

Passage through the restriction point and progression toward the S phase appears to be controlled by the G1 cyclins and their CDKs. Recent findings propose a sequence in the involvement of these factors (68, 86, 87, 98, 99). The D-type cyclins (D1, D2, and D3) are induced before cyclins E and A. When cells transit from G0 to G1 in response to growth-factor stimulation, synthesis of the D-type cyclins and assembly of these proteins with their CDKs (mostly CDK4 and CDK6) occur. Consequently, activity of cyclin D–CDK complex increases during mid-G1 and reaches a maximum near the G1-S transition. Mitogenic stimulation plays a central role in the activation of the D-type cyclins–CDK complex, as expression of D-type cyclins persists as long as growth factors are present in the cell environment (68, 104, 105). Unlike the D-type cyclins, expression of cyclin E is normally periodic and maximal at the G1-S transition. This induction is associated with the formation of active cyclin E–CDK2 complexes. Once cells enter the S phase, cyclin E is degraded and CDK2 forms complexes with cyclin A. The onset of cyclin A synthesis is observed late in G1 and seems to be essential for the beginning of DNA synthesis, as a defect in formation of cyclin A–CDK2 complexes has been reported to inhibit S-phase entry (107, 108).

Critical substrates of the G1 cylins–CDKs complexes are the retinoblastoma protein Rb and related proteins p107 and p130 (112, 117). Unlike cyclin E, the D-type cyclins can directly bind to Rb and target CDK4 to this protein. In its unphosphorylated form, Rb binds to a family of heterodimeric transcription factors called *E2Fs*. Phosphorylation of Rb releases E2Fs, enabling them to activate genes required for DNA replication, including thymidine kinase, thymidylate synthetase, DNA-polymerase-a, CDC2, as well as cyclin E and E2F. The process of Rb phosphorylation appears to be first triggered by the D-type cyclins–CDK complexes and then by the cyclin E–CDK2 complexes. The onset of Rb phosphorylation leads to upregulation of E2F and cyclin E synthesis, resulting in an increase in cyclin E–CDK2 complexes. Therefore, progression through the restriction point late in G1 is characterized by a process of Rb phosphorylation that shifts from being mitogen-dependent and controlled by D-type cyclins to mitogen-independent through the control of cyclin E–CDK2 complexes (Fig. 10.1)

The finding that most p27 is complexed with cyclin D–CDK suggests that this protein may play a role in restriction point control. $p21^{CIP1}$ seems to be more involved in the late part of G1 progression. Recent studies have begun to provide some insights into the mechanisms by which these CKIs inhibit the cyclin–CDKs. $p21^{CIP1}$ has two cyclin-binding sites termed *Cy1* and *Cy2*, and one site for CDK named the *K site*. $p21^{CIP1}$ utilizes the Cy1 or Cy2 for association with cyclin E and the K site, for association with CDK2. Chen et al. showed that the Cy sites stabilize the interaction of the K site and inhibit kinase activity directly. This simultaneous interaction with cyclin and CDK seems to be essential for optimal kinase inhibition (23). By contrast, isolated cyclin D or CDK4 does not associate with $p21^{CIP1}$, and the cyclin–CDK4 complex exclusively utilizes the Cy1 site for interaction with $p21^{CIP1}$. In this situation only one site is used, which will result in partially inhibited kinase being complexed with $p21^{CIP1}$.

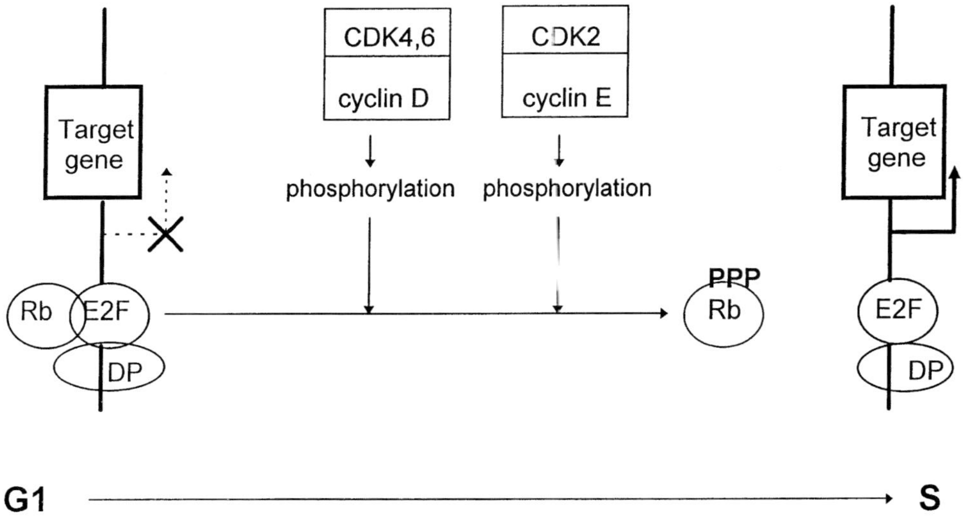

Fig. 10.1 Involvement of retinoblastoma protein (Rb) and its phosphorylation during G1 progression. In its unphosphorylated form, Rb binds to a family of heterodimeric transcription factors called E2Fs, and expression of the target gene is suppressed. Phosphorylation of Rb, which is triggered first by the D-type cyclins–CDK complexes and then cyclin E–CDK2 complexes, releases E2Fs, enabling expression of the target gene.

FETAL LUNG DEVELOPMENT

Surprisingly little is known about the regulation of cell proliferation in the vertebrate embryo. Studies in lower species, particularly *Drosophila,* have detailed the stages in control of embryonic cell proliferation. Initially, maternally derived gene products regulate the early stages of cell division without associated cell growth (thus early embryonic cells become smaller with each division) (33). Embryonic synchronization of cell growth and proliferation is instituted and local control of cell proliferation takes over so that cell division is linked to local morphogenic events and is later coordinated with cell differentiation. Since there is great similarity of cell cycle regulatory molecules between invertebrates and vertebrates, it is likely that the control of cell proliferation and its link to morphogenesis and cell differentiation are similar in flies and mammals.

Patterning Genes

The so-called patterning genes, such as the homeodomain-containing, *Hox* genes, that are homologous to *Drosophila* patterning genes, are transcription factors that establish a series of overlapping domains of expression regulating dorsal–ventral and anterior–posterior patterns in the embryo (62). The distribution of *Hox* genes in time and in place has been charted in the lungs of several species (8, 9, 17, 57). While targets for these transcription factors, are just now being defined, they include cell adhesion molecules, other transcription factors, and growth factors such as the TGF-β and *Wnt* family of genes (see below). Recent studies have shown that the distribution of the *Hox* genes and the pattern of lung development can be altered by morphogenic regulators such as retinoic acid (8, 19, 20). The molecular mechanism of this interaction has been defined, but whether changes on *Hox* genes directly effect lung morphogenesis has not been established. It is of interest that epithelial cell proliferation at the tips of distal lung buds is greater than in central airways during development and retinoic acid abolishes this difference (20).

A number of transcription factors are expressed at high levels in the developing lung and have been shown to regulate lung cell–specific genes (17). The TTF and HNF family of transcriptional activators have been implicated in the expression of a number of epithelial genes (see Chaps. 4 and 14), but they have not been shown to directly influence cell proliferation (60, 120). HFH-11, which is related to the *HNF* genes is expressed in epithelium and mesenchyme of the fetal lung (121). HFH-11 is not expressed in the normal adult lung, but increases dramatically in epithelial cells when epithelial cell proliferation is increased in response to lung injury or to tracheal instillation of FGF-7, which induces lung epithelial cell proliferation. The function of HFH-11 in proliferating cells is not yet clear, but it may induce factors that initiate the proliferation process.

Secreted signaling molecules such as the *hedgehog* and *Wnt* family of genes have been shown to directly increase cell proliferation and are expressed in the developing lung (5, 6, 19). Both of these families of genes were first studied in invertebrates; they induce cell proliferation and act as morphogens (54). Sonic hedgehog (Shh) is expressed at high levels in the epithelial cells of the early embryonic lung, rapidly becoming restricted to epithelial cells of the distal lung tips, and falling to low levels in mid- to late gestation. The Shh receptor, patched (ptc) is expressed in mesenchymal cells at the tips of epithelial buds in the embryonic lung, suggesting that it may be involved in epithelial–mesenchymal interaction. Shh has been shown to regulate members of the BMP family of growth factors, which are related to the TGF family and Wnt family (7); both groups of proteins are expressed in the embryonic lung. Studies in the developing lung bud have also suggested an interaction between Shh and fibroblast growth factors (FGFs), which play an important role in regulating embryonic lung cell proliferation and differentiation (see below). Even less is known about the large family of Wnt proteins (77, 88). The Wnt family of cell growth promoters can function as true oncogenes. The family is increasing in size as new members are continually be discovered, and a large family of Wnt receptors called frizzeled have been cloned (78). Wnt-2 is expressed in the mesenchyme surrounding distal lung buds while Wnt-7b is expressed in lung epithelial cells. It is likely that studies of the role of Wnt and its receptors in lung development will yield important new information.

The role that these molecules play in regulating lung morphogenesis and cell proliferation is just beginning to be defined. A complete description of their distribution is not yet available. Null mutations (gene knockouts) of genes have provided some information, but the elimination of a number of these genes results in embryonic death before the lung is formed, or produces no obvious phenotype, presumably because of the presence of family members that serve similar functions (for example, see ref. 75). Misexpression of these genes or dominant negative mutations that are targeted to specific cells (usually with the SP-C promoter) should begin to provide information about the importance of these molecules in lung development (use of transgenics article). A recent study of transgenic mice with Shh driven by the SP-C promoter has shown that when Shh continues to be expressed at high levels in distal lung epithelial cells, increased mesenchymal and epithelial cell proliferation occur and the interstitium becomes thick with large numbers of fibroblasts, resulting in death in the early postnatal period (5). This study establishes an important role for epithelial Shh in regulating mesenchymal cell proliferation in the lung.

Role of Fibroblast Growth Factors

There is an increasing body of evidence that the FGF family of growth factors plays an important role in regulating cell proliferation and differentiation in the developing lung. A number of FGF receptors and growth factors are expressed in the embryonic lung (see Table 10.1). The importance of the FGF system is suggested by the unique distribution of several of the FGFs and their receptors at the tips of branching epithelial tubes, in positions to control epithelial–mesenchymal interactions. Transgenic animals expressing a dominant negative mutant of the FGFR-2IIIb (that binds FGF-7 as well as other FGFs) develop an embryonic lung bud that continues to grow but no further branching occurs, despite continued cell proliferation; epithelial cell differentiation is also impaired in this model (91). Overexpression of FGF-7 driven by the SP-C promoter results in formation of large peripheral epithelial cysts instead of branching lung buds in the developing lung, suggesting an abnormal pattern of epithelial cell proliferation (109). Recent studies of mesenchyme-free epi thelial lung buds have shown that both FGF-1 and FGF-7 induce epithelial cell

Table 10.1 Fibroblast Growth Factors in the Lung

	Lung Location			Lung Location	
FGF	Epithelial	Mesenchymal	FGFR	Epithelial	Mesenchymal
FGF-1 (aFGF)	+	—	FGFR-1	—	+
FGF-2 (bFGF)	+/-	—			
FGF-3 (int-2)	No report		FGFR-2	+	?
FGF-4	—	—			
FGF-5	—	—	FGFR-3	+	+
FGF-6	No report				
FGF-7 (KGF)	—	+	FGFR-4	+	+
FGF-8	No report				
FGF-9	No report				
FGF-10	—	+			

proliferation, but FGF-1 produces multiple new buds whereas FGF-7 produces large epithelial cysts (18). This difference may be due to the distribution of FGF receptors in the epithelium. The FGFR-2IIIb, to which FGF-7 and FGF-1 bind, is diffusely distributed throughout the epithelial bud and thus FGF-7 would produce uniform proliferation-generating cysts. The FGFR-4, to which FGF-1 also binds, is located at the tips of epithelial tubes and thus, because of the concentration of FGF-binding sites, FGF-1 produces branching epithelial tips. These results likely explain the above-noted dominant negative FGF receptor phenotype. Despite the dramatic effects of FGF-1 and FGF-7 on growth of the mesenchyme-free embryonic lung bud, neither of these growth factors appears to be expressed in the early embryonic lung. However, FGF-10 has recently been cloned and is expressed in the mesenchyme at the tips of epithelial buds (120). FGF-10 appears to act in a fashion that is similar to FGF-1 and may be the FGF that induces early branching in the embryonic lung. The FGFs have also been shown to affect embryonic lung epithelial cell differentiation in vitro (see below); FGF-1 induces SP-B expression while FGF-7 induces SP-A and SP-B expression and the appearance of typical type 2 cell morphology (18).

Role of Retinoblastoma Family Genes and Related Transcription Factors

It had originally been assumed that the cell cycle regulatory genes such as Rb, p107, and p130, the E2F family of protein to which they bound, and the cyclin-CDK proteins were ubiquitously expressed at all times of development and in all cells and tissues. Recent evidence suggests that this is not the case (for a review see ref. 3). A number of studies have now shown that the Rb gene and hypophosphorylated protein are expressed in tissues in association with cell growth arrest and cell differen tiation. In contrast, p107 tends to be expressed in cells that are proliferating and p130, in growth-arrested cells (53).

Despite the apparent importance of the Rb family of genes in regulating cell proliferation and differentiation, disruption of these genes has lead to surprisingly few informative developmental defects. Null mutations of Rb results in death by day 13–14 of gestation in the mouse (49). Pituitary tumors and impaired fetal hepatic hematopoiesis appear to be the only dramatic developmental abnormalities All other tissues, including the lung, appear to be normal, with no evidence of excess cell proliferation. Null mutations of p107 and p130 have produced no evident phenotype. Combined Rb/p107 knockouts die before the lung forms and p107/p130 mutants display some defects in cartilage formation, but die immediately after birth (26, 64). Their lungs, however, appear to be histologically normal. It is presumed that functional overlap between the Rb family accounts for the lack of a more dramatic phenotype in knockout mice and for the minimal apparent effects on cell proliferation.

Tissue-specific inactivation of Rb has been produced by creating transgenic mice with promoter-directed expression of SV40T adenoviral early regions (22). SV40T inactivates both the Rb family proteins and p53, although mutant *SV40T* genes have been engineered to target only the Rb genes. The SP-C promoter has been used to target SV40T to distal lung epithelial cells and the CCSP promoter has been used to target SV40T to Clara cells (70, 116). In both instances, SV40T expression in lung epithelium ultimately leads to excess cell proliferation and formation of tumors in adult mice. However, no abnormalities of fetal lung development or in fetal epithelial lung cell proliferation have been reported in these mice. The lack of uncontrolled epithelial proliferation seems to suggest that these regulation systems are not important in the developing lung. Alternatively, overlapping cell cycle control systems are activated in these mice. Another possibility is that those cells in which Rb has been inactivated undergo apoptosis. This possibility is supported by the finding that Rb functions to coordinate cell cycle withdrawal with programmed cell death in differentiating myocytes (2). In this system, myocytes from Rb null mutants undergo an increased rate of apoptosis as they enter the differentiation pathway; replacing Rb eliminates apoptosis (114). In addition, expression of SV40T driven by a small intestine–specific promoter results in increased apoptosis of intestinal epithelial cells that is p53 independent (22). This suggests that increased numbers of cells resulting from loss of Rb is somehow sensed and dealt with by induction of a cell death program (see below).

The role of Rb in terminal differentiation, irreversible cell growth arrest, has been best studied in developing myoblasts in vitro. Here, Rb is required for terminal differentiation to occur; growth arrest and cell differentiation can occur in the absence of Rb, but the differentiated muscle cells can be induced to re-enter the cell cycle when Rb is not present (103). Expression of the cyclin–CDK inhibitor p21 has also been shown to be correlated with cell differentiation in muscle and other cells [see above; (43)].

As noted above, the E2F family of transcription factors is important in inducing cell proliferation and one of the main functions of the pocket proteins is to bind and inactivate these proteins (1, 115). Relatively little is known about the role of these factors in development. E2F-5, which preferentially binds p130, is expressed early in lung development and its levels tend to fall as the lung matures (45, 48). It has been generally assumed that the various E2Fs target similar genes, although it remains likely that E2F-1, -2, -3 and E2F-4, -5 have different transactivating functions. Null mutations of the E2Fs are just being reported. It came as a surprise that knocking out E2F-1, a putative oncogene, actually lead to formation of tumors in the adult, suggesting that it might also act in some circumstances as a growth suppression gene, presumably by its ability to induce apoptosis (36, 119).

Each member of the D cyclin family of genes is differentially expressed in mouse tissues, thus having the potential of conveying tissue or cell-specific regulation of proliferation (96). Null mutations of specific D cyclins result in decreased cell proliferation in the tissues where the cyclin is specifically expressed.

Role of Apoptosis

Apoptosis, or programmed cell death, has not been critically evaluated in lung development. Programmed cell death occurs during development in all animals that have been studied and likely in all tissues (51). Recently, the molecular mechanisms for this orderly process have begun to be defined (4, 111). Apoptosis has been implicated in various process during development, including restructuring of tissues, adjusting numbers of cells in tissues, and eliminating injured cells or cells with replication defects in DNA. Apoptosis is tightly controlled by a number of genes that can induce or suppress the process. It can be initiated through a number of pathways, including normal developmental programs, conflicting growth signals (as might be the case with absent Rb), DNA damage, and immune modulators (38). The combination of Fas and Fas ligand (FasL) has been associated with immune-modulated cell death and may be involved in postnatal lung growth and in lung repair following injury. Fas is a type I membrane receptor that is a member of the tumor necrosis factor (TNF), nerve growth factor receptor family. FasL belongs to the TNF superfamily. Binding of FasL to Fas initiates programmed cell death. Fas mRNA has been found in the adult lung, and recently Fas has been demonstrated in a subset of alveolar type 2 cells (37). Intratracheal administration of a Fas-binding antibody initiates apoptosis in that subset of type 2 cells. It appears that apoptosis in alveolar epithelial cells may occur during normal postnatal lung growth and that this apoptosis may be Fas mediated. Whether this mechanism is associated with regulation of epithelial cell numbers during fetal lung development and whether it explains the lack of cell accumulation in Rb knockout mice remains to be determined.

POSTNATAL LUNG DEVELOPMENT

The timing and cell type of proliferation during postnatal lung development was charted over 20 years ago (75), but little new information exists about the initiators or regulators of this process. A number of factors, such as oxygen, glucocorticoids, and nutrition, have been shown to influence postnatal lung development (for reviews see refs. 11, 59, 84, 113). Dexamethosone has been shown to impair postnatal alveolar development with associated decreases in fibroblast and alveolar type 1 cell numbers, presumably because of impaired cell proliferation (73). However, there are no mechanistic studies of how these factors impact on cell proliferation and whether they are cell-specific. Furthermore, there is little information about how various growth factors that have been studied in fetal lung development influence early postnatal cell proliferation. Dexamethosone has also been shown to impair type 2 cell proliferation and transition into type 1 cells following lung injury (110), suggesting that glucocorticoid-induced alterations in cell proliferation and/or cell differentiation may be common to both growth and repair. Recently, retinoic acid has been shown to both increase the number of alveoli normally formed in the postnatal period and to counter the effects of glucocorticoids on alveolar formation, although the mechanism of this effect is unclear (74).

One of the most definitive studies of postnatal cell proliferation has shown that PDGF-A is responsible for the selective proliferation of myofibroblasts present in the septal buds of immature alveoli. These septal buds subdivide existing large al veoli during the postnatal period, producing multiple small alveoli with a resultant increase in lung surface area (12–15). They also are a major site of elastin synthesis, which is responsible for the developing elastic recoil that characterizes early postnatal lung development (85). In PDGF-A-chain null mutant mice, septal myofibro blasts do not proliferate, septal buds do not form, alveoli remain large saccules, and little alveolar elastin is deposited (10). This effect is specific to PDGF-A and does not occur in PDGF-B null mutants, and it is specific for alveolar septal myofibroblasts, as elastogenesis proceeds in a normal fashion in lung vessels and airways. The reasons for alveolarization ending and for the adult lung's inability to form new alveoli remain unknown, although some link to the myofibroblast is likely.

LUNG REPAIR: CELLULAR RESPONSE TO DNA DAMAGE

The major threat posed by tissue injury is, at the cellular level, the damage of genetic material. Repair of DNA damage is therefore critical to prevent accumulation of mutations that can disrupt normal cell growth control and lead to gross chromosomal aberrations in daughter cells (28, 101). To counter these threats to genomic integrity, cells can induce mechanisms that arrest the cell cycle, allowing DNA repair to take place in order to prevent replication of damaged genetic templates. In addition to cell cycle arrest, DNA damage may also induce apoptosis to eliminate cells in which damage is beyond repair.

Molecular Basis of the Repair Process

From a number of studies, it is now well established that p53 plays a central role in response to DNA damage by its involvement in cell cycle arrest as well as in apoptosis (66).

p53 Protein

The *p53* gene encodes a nuclear phosphoprotein involved in the control of cell growth. It is one of the most commonly mutated genes found in human tumors. It can function as a sequence-specific DNA-binding protein that positively regulates gene expression (66). The human p53 protein contains 393 amino acids and has been divided structurally and functionally into several domains. The sequence-specific DNA-binding domain of p53 is localized between amino acids 102–292, which is a protease-resistant and independently folded domain containing a Zn^{2+} ion required for its sequence-specific DNA-binding activity. More than 90% of the missense mutations in p53 reside in this sequence-specific DNA-binding domain (46). Products of genes transcriptionally activated by p53 include the following: $p21^{CIP1}$; GADD45, which is induced upon DNA damage and is involved directly in DNA nucleotide excision repair; MDM2, which inactivates p53-mediated transcription and therefore forms an autoregulatory loop with p53 activity; cyclin G, which is a novel cyclin of unknown function with no cell cycle fluctuation levels; and Bax, which is a member of the BCL2 family that promotes apoptosis (79, 100, 124, 125). The first 42 amino acids at the N terminus constitute a transcriptional activation domain that interacts with the basal transcriptional machinery; amino acids 13–23 are identical in a number of species. Proteins that have functional interactions with p53 include the transcriptional TATA-associated factors TAF70 and TAF31, WT1, the oncogene products MDM2 and c-Abl, and the viral proteins such as SV40 T antigen, the adenovirus E1B-55 Kd protein, and the human papilloma virus E6.

p53 and Cell Cycle Arrest

In situations of DNA damage, there is a rapid increase in the level of p53. As mentioned above, one target gene for p53 is the *p21* gene. Indeed, in response to various forms of DNA damage, the activated p53 turns on the *p21* gene (66, 100). Activation of $p21^{CIP1}$ inhibits the activities of cyclin–CDK4 and –CDK2 complexes, preventing phosphorylation and inactivation of Rb and consequently inhibiting the release of transcription factors E2Fs. In addition, $p21^{CIP1}$ binds to PCNA and the formation of p21CIP1–PCNA complexes blocks the role of PCNA as a DNA polymerase processing factor in DNA replication but not its role in DNA repair. $p21^{CIP1}$ is not the sole protein involved in the downstream events in response to p53. Fibroblasts derived from mice deficient in the *p21* gene (null phenotype) display some ability to arrest in G1 in response to DNA damage, which suggests that additional p21-independent pathways may be involved. One potential candidate for p53-induced G1 arrest is GADD45. Recent evidence suggests that GADD45 can interact directly with PCNA and thus block DNA replication and possibly coordinately enhance nucleotide excision repair of damaged DNA.

Study of the mechanisms leading to p53 accumulation in response to DNA damage indicates that de novo transcription is not required. Experiments using cycloheximide have shown that this factor is able to prevent accumulation of p53 protein and partially abrogate the G1 arrest of cells exposed to DNA-damaging agents. This indicates that the increase in p53 protein may be due in part to enhanced translation of pre-existing p53 transcripts (58). The other mechanism includes stabilization of p53. Normally, the p53 protein is kept at a low concentration by its relatively short half-life, which is approximately 15 min. This half-life has been reported to increase by as much as sevenfold in cells after exposure to irradiation. At the present time, the basis for this stabilization remains unclear; the mechanisms discussed include phosphorylation and/or dephosphorylation, homo-oligomerization, and binding to stabilizing proteins (44).

In addition to changes in its levels, involvement of p53 may be modulated by functional modifications. As an example, p53-binding activity has been shown to be subject to redox regulation, the reduced form of p53 displaying increased binding capacity.

p53 and Apoptosis

The processes by which p53 can induce apoptosis are not yet fully understood. The proposed mechanisms include regulation by the Bax protein and activation of proteases of the ICE/Ced-3 class (39, 82). Under certain circumstances, the increase in p53 is associated with changes in the levels of two homologous proteins, Bax and Bcl-2, which have opposing effects on apoptosis. The Bax gene promoter contains consensus p53-binding sites and up-regulation of Bax together with the down-regulation of Bcl-2 has been reported in the presence of enhanced levels of p53. This results in an increased concentration of the Bax-bax homodimers and Bax-bcl-2 heterodimers, thereby potentiating apoptosis.

Mammalian interleukin-1b converting enzyme (ICE) is a cysteine protease that converts interleukin-1b precursor into its mature form. It has been reported that when members of the ICE family are overexpressed, they cause apoptosis. One suggested mechanism involves the Fas ligand. Binding of Fas ligand to Fas induces trimerization of the Fas receptor, which ultimately triggers the ICE protease cascade and leads to degradation of chromosomal DNA. This model of apoptosis signaling by Fas requires further investigation. One central question is how Fas engagement is recruited and regulates the process (82). A link between Bcl-2 and Fas is suggested by results of experiments showing that Bcl-2 could inhibit Fas-mediated apoptosis in vitro as well as in vivo.

The Choice between Cell Cycle Arrest and Apoptosis

In response to DNA damage, signals are generated that ultimately lead to cell cycle arrest or to apoptosis. Recent data suggest a role of the ATM (ataxia telangectasia mutated) gene product in the choice between these two pathways. Ataxia telangectasia (A-T) is an autosomal recessive disease that is characterized by a variety of clinical and cellular defects that appear to be associated with an altered response to DNA damage. Recent cloning of the ATM gene suggests that ATM plays a role in signal transduction (35). Analysis of its sequence has indicated homology with a family of proteins that include phosphoinositide 3-kinase, strongly suggesting a protein kinase activity for ATM. On the basis of recent reports, the following model has emerged. Low levels of DNA damage are sensed by a pathway that involves the ATM protein which may itself be the damage sensor. ATM would be required for the rapid induction of an active form of p53, most likely through phosphorylation, which leads to cell cycle arrest. By contrast, response to high levels of damage can occur in the absence of ATM through a less specific mechanism that is associated with a continuous induction of p53 and this triggers apoptosis. This model may explain that, in A-T cells, X-irradiation cannot induce cell cycle arrest but can trigger p53-dependent apoptosis (35, 56).

Application to Lung Injury

Among the factors involved in the initiation and development of lung diseases, oxidant injury represents a major pathogenic mechanism. This is well explained by the location and anatomy of the lung, which represents an extensive surface area to react with all sources of free radicals. Oxidants include not only the free radicals produced by normal biochemical processes, inflammatory cells, and chemicals or pharmacological agents, but also the free-radical generation as a result of direct exposure of the airway epithelium surface to gas, dust particles, and cigarette smoke (16, 50).

Oxidant injury plays a critical role in respiratory diseases, including pediatric diseases associated with viral infections that represent major causes of pulmonary illnesses in infants and children. It is also a dominant factor in the development of neonatal respiratory distress. The consequences are cytotoxic effects on various pulmonary cell types, which require a rapid induction of repair mechanisms. Any alteration in repair processes will lead to fibrosis with collagen and elastin deposition, and abnormalities in lung development with decreased alveolarization and respiratory surface area expansion (24).

Following oxidant-induced lung injury, repair processes need to be considered not only at a cellular level through mechanisms discussed above but also at the tissue level. Proper tissue healing is based on coordinated cell proliferation and differentiation together with the production and turnover of the extracellular matrix. This coordination is under the control of autocrine and paracrine activity of the cells making up the tissue by means of cytokines that have been shown to regulate all aspects of tissue remodeling (89). Among these factors are TGF-β and the insulin-like growth factors (IGFs).

Role of Transforming Growth Factor β

Transforming growth factor β has three isoforms—TGF-β1, 2, and 3—whose biological properties are nearly identical, and a balance among these isoforms may be critical (72). It is secreted in an inactive (latent) form that requires activation before it can exert a biological effect. Transforming growth factor β binds to three types of receptors (types I, II, and III). Types I and II are transmembrane serine-threonine kinases that interact with one another; this collaboration is required for the initiation and propagation of TGF-β signals. Recent findings support the concept that type I receptors act downstream of the type II receptors. Generation of TGF-β signals is likely to involve phosphorylation of type I receptors by type II receptor kinases. The type III receptor is a membrane-anchored proteoglycan that has no signaling structure but acts to present TGF-β to the other receptors. The in vivo role of TGF-β in wound healing has been shown through acceleration of healing by local application of this factor. In tissue injury, the presence of platelets containing high concentrations of TGF-β and the induction of TGF-β expression in the local cells account for accumulation of TGF-β at the site of injury. When this accumulation becomes excessive, altered healing is observed with development of fibrotic lesions. Fibrosis represents a pathologic excess of the normal process of tissue repair, with sustained production of TGF-β being considered the key molecular mediator. In humans with idiopathic pulmonary fibrosis, TGF-β1 is increased in alveolar walls at the sites at which extracellular matrix has accumulated. It is likely that various cell types may participate in the enhanced production of TGF-β, including fibroblats, alveolar epithelial cells, and alveolar macrophages (27, 41, 44). TGF-β3 has been shown to be the major TGF-β peptide secreted by alveolar type II cells and to exert a paracrine effect on their proliferation, which is inversely proportional to the production of the factor (11a).

By using several types of cell lines, including lung epithelial cells, much has been discovered about the way in which TGF-β may lead to cell cycle arrest in response to oxidative stress (29, 30, 61, 102, 104). The TGF-β-induced G1 cell-cycle arrest has been attributed to the regulatory effects of TGF -β on both the levels and activities of the G1 cyclins and their CDKs, including stimulatory effects on several CKIs such as p21, p27, and p15. Recently, a member of the mitogen-activated protein kinase kinase kinase family has been identified as a mediator in the signaling pathway of the TGF-β family. These findings fit in with reports of regulation of p21 expression through mitogen-activated kinase signaling pathway.

Role of Insulin-like Growth Factors

The IGF system is composed of growth factors IGF-I and IGF-II, receptors (type 1 and type 2), and binding proteins [IGFBPs; (31, 55, 93, 97)]. The growth factors share structural homology with each other and with proinsulin. The type-1 IGF receptor, a transmembrane heterotetramer tyrosine kinase, has a high degree of homology with the insulin receptor and is the only IGF receptor to have IGF-mediated signaling functions. The type-2 IGF receptor is identical to the cation-independent mannose 6-phosphate receptor, which functions in the trafficking of lysosomal enzymes but has no known IGF signaling function. The group of IGFBPs includes six well-characterized proteins (IGFBP1 to 6) that are essential for coordinating and regulating the biological activities of the IGFs. In addition, recent evidence has emerged that the IGFBPs can have direct effects on cellular functions independent of the IGFs.

The findings that IGFs are expressed in lung cells argues for the participation of these factors in regulation of lung development and in repair following injury (71, 76, 116, 117). Indeed, an increase in IGF-I expression has been reported in idiopathic lung fibrosis. Recently, much attention has been paid to IGFBPs. It has been shown that blockage of alveolar type 2 cell proliferation was associated with increased production of IGFBP-2 (80, 118–120). In several systems it has been reported that IGFBP-3 was able to inhibit growth without binding IGF-I and blocking its binding to type-1 IGF receptor and to induce apoptosis (97). A link with TGF-β is supported by the observations that IGFBP-2 and IGFBP-3 can be induced by TGF-β and seem to mediate the potent growth inhibitory action of this factor (21, 42, 63, 81). Moreover, recent findings suggest a nuclear mode of IGFBP action. Whether these proteins are connected to the key regulators of the cell cycle machinery involved in G1 progression remains to be determined (52, 94, 95, 102).

CONCLUSION

Over the past few years, much has been learned about the factors associated with the processes of growth and tissue repair. Each factor is likely involved at a critical time and place following a coordinated cascade of events. It is now crucial to increase our understanding of this cascade so that effective strategies to accelerate normal lung growth or enhance repair after injury can be developed.

REFERENCES

1. Adams, P.D. and W.G.J. Kaelin. Transcriptional control by E2F. *Semin. Cancer Biol.* 6: 83–90, 1995.
2. Almasan, A., Y. Yin, R.E. Kelly, E.Y.H.P. Lee, A. Bradley, W. Li, J.R. Bertino, and G.M. Wahl. Deficiency of retinoblastoma protein leads to inappropriate S-phase entry, acivation of E2F-responsive genes and apoptosis. *Proc. Natl. Acad. Sci. USA* 92: 5436–5440, 1995.
3. Beijersbergen, R.L. and R. Bernards. Cell cycle regulation by the retinoblastoma family of growth inhibitory proteins. *Biochim. Biophys. Acta* 1287: 103–120, 1996.
4. Bellamy, C.O.C., R.C.G. Malcomson, D.J. Harrison, and A.H. Wylie. Cell death in health and disease: the biology and regulation of apoptosis. *Semin. Cancer Biol.* 6: 3–18, 1995.
5. Bellusci, S., Y. Furuta, M.G. Rush, R. Henderson, G. Winnier, and B.L.M. Hogan. Involvement of sonic hedgehog (Shh) in mouse embryonic lung growth and morphogenesis. *Development* 124: 53–63, 1997.
6. Bellusci, S., R. Henderson, G. Winnier, T. Oikawa, and B.L.M. Hogan. Evidence from normal expression and targeted misexpression that bone morphogeneic protein-4 (Bmp-4) plays a role in mouse embryonic lung morphogenesis. *Development* 122: 1963–1702, 1996.
7. Bitgood, M.J. and A.P. McMahon. *Hedgehog* and *Bmp* genes are coexpressed at many diverse sites of cell-cell interaction in the mouse embryo. *Dev. Biol.* 172: 126–138, 1995.
8. Bogue, C.W., I. Gross, H. Vasavada, D.W. Dynia, C.M. Wilson, and H.C. Jacobs. Identification of *Hox* genes in newborn lungs and effects of gestational age and retinoic acid on their expression. *Am. J. Phsiol.* (*Lung Cell. Mol. Physiol.*) 266: L448–454, 1994.
9. Bogue, C.W., L.J. Lou, H. Vasavada, C.M. Wilson, and H.C. Jacobs. Expression of *Hoxb* genes in the developing mouse foregut and lung. *Am. J. Respir. Cell Mol. Biol.* 15: 163–171, 1996.
10. Boström, K. Willets, M. Pekny, P. Levéen, P. Lindhal, H. Hedstrand, M. Pekna, M. Hellström, S. Gebre-Medhin, M. Schalling, M. Nilsson, S. Kurland, J. Törnell, J.K. Heath, and C. Betscholtz. PDGF-A signaling is a critical event in lung alveolar myofibroblast development and alveogenesis. *Cell* 85: 863–873 1996.
11. Brody, J.S. and W.M. Thurlbeck. Development, growth and aging of the lung. In: *Handbook of Physiology: Section 3: The Respiratory System*, edited by A.P. Fishman, P.T. Macklem, and J. Mead. Bethesda, MD: American Physiological Society, 1986, p. 355–386.

11a. Buckley, S., K.C. Bui, M. Hussaini, and D. Warburton. Dynamics of TGF-β3 peptide activity during rat alveolar epithelial cell proliferative recovery from acute hyperoxia. *Am. J. Physiol.* (*Lung Cell. Mol. Physiol.*) 271: L54–L60, 1996.

12. Burri, P.H. The postnatal growth of the rat lung. I. Morphometry. *Anat. Rec.* 178: 711–730, 1974.
13. Burri, P.H. Postnatal growth of the rat lung. III. Morphology. *Anat. Rec.* 180: 77–98, 1974.
14. Burri, P.H. Development and growth of the human lung. In: *Handbook of Physiology. Section 3: The Respiratory System*, edited by A.P. Fishman and A.B. Fisher. Bethesda, MD: American Physiology Society, 1985, p. 1–47.
15. Burri, P. Structural aspects of pre- and postnatal development and growth of the lung. In: *Growth and Development of the Lung*, edited by J. McDonald. New York: Marcel Dekker, 1995.

16. Buttke, T. and P. Sandstrom. Oxidative stress as a mediator of apoptosis. *Viewpoint* 15: 7–10, 1994.
17. Cardoso, W.V. Transcription factors and pattern formation in the developing lung. *Am. J. Physiol.* (*Lung Cell. Mol. Physiol.*) 269 : L429–L442, 1995.
18. Cardoso, W.V., A. Itoh, H. Nogawa, I. Mason, and J.S. Brody. FGF-1 and FGF-7 induce distinct patterns of growth and differentiation in embryonic lung epithelium. *Dev. Dyn.* 208: 398–405, 1997.
19. Cardoso, W.V., S.A. Mitsialis, J.S. Brody and M.C. Williams. Retinoic acid alters the expression of pattern-related genes in the developing rat lung. *Dev. Dyn.* 207: 47–59, 1996.
20. Cardoso, W.V., M.C. Williams, S.A. Mitsialis, M. Joyce-Brady, A.K. Rishi, and J.S. Brody. Retinoic acid changes the pattern of airway branching and alters epithelial cell differentiation in the developing lung in vitro. *Am. J. Respir. Cell Mol. Biol.* 12: 464–476, 1995.
21. Cazals, V., B. Mouhieddine, B. Maitre, K. Chadelat, Y. Le Bouc, J.S Brody, and A. Clement. Insulin-like growth factors, their binding proteins and transforming growth factor-beta 1 in oxidant arrested lung alveolar epithelial cells. *J. Biol. Chem.* 269: 14111–14117, 1994.
22. Chandrasekaran, C., C.M. Coopersmith, and J.I. Gordon. Use of normal and transgenic mice to examine the relationship between terminal differentiation of intestinal epithelial cells and accumulation of their cell cycle regulators. *J. Biol. Chem.* 271: 28414–28421, 1996.
23. Chen, J., P. Saha, S. Kornbluth, B. Dynlacht, and A. Dutta. Cyclin-binding motifs are essential for the function of p21CIP1. *Mol. Cell. Biol.* 16: 4673–4682, 1996.
24. Clement, A. and B. Housset Free radicals and airways injury. In: *Lung Biology in Health and Disease*, edited by J. Chretien and D. Dusser. New York: 1996, p. 355–379.
25. Coats, S., M. Flanagan, J. Nourse, and J. Roberts. Requirement of p27/KIP1 for restriction point control of the fibroblast cell cycle. *Science* 272: 877–880, 1996.
26. Cobrinik, D., M. Lee, G. Hannon, G. Mulligan, N. Bronson, N. Dyson, E. Harlow, D. Beach, R. Weinberg, and T. Jacks. Shared role of the pRb-related p130 and p107 proteins in limb development. *Genes Dev.* 10: 1633–1644, 1996.
27. Corroyer, S., B. Maitre, V. Cazals, and A. Clement. Altered regulation of G1 cyclins in oxidant-inducet growth arrest of lung alveolar epithelial cells. *J. Biol. Chem.* 271: 25117–25125, 1996.
28. Cox, L. and D. Lane. Tumour suppressors, kinases and clamps: how p53 regulates the cell cycle in response to DNA damage. *BioEssays* 17: 501–508, 1995.
29. Datto, M., Y. Li, J. Panus, D. Howe, Y. Xiong, and X. Wang. Transforming growth factor β induces the cyclin-dependent kinase inhibitor p21 through p53-independent mechanism. *Proc. Natl. Acad. Sci. USA* 92: 5545–5549, 1995.
30. Datto, M., Y. Yu, and X. Wang. Functional analysis of the transforming growth factor B responsive elements in the WAF1/Cip1/p21 promoter. *J. Biol. Chem.* 270: 28623–28628, 1995.
31. D'Ercole, A.J. Insulin-like growth factors and their receptors in growth. *Endocrinol. Metab. Clin. North Am.* 25: 573–590, 1996.
32. Desal, D., H. Wessling, R. Fisher, and D. Morgan. Effects of phosphorylation by CAK on cycling binding by CDC2 and CDK2. *Mol. Cell. Biol.* 15 345–350, 1995.
33. Edgar, B.A. and C.F. Lehner. Developmental control of cell cycle regulators: a fly's perspective. *Science* 274: 1646–1652, 1996.
34. Elledge, S. Cell cycle checkpoints: preventing an identity crisis. *Science* 274: 1664–1672, 1996.

35. Enoch, T. and C. Norbury. Cellular responses to DNA damage: cell-cycle checkpoints, apoptosis and the roles of p53 and ATM. *Trends Biochem. Sci.* 20: 426–430, 1995.
36. Field, S. J., F.Y. Tsai, F. Kuo, A.M. Zubiaga, J.W.G. Kaelin, S.H. Orkin, and M.E. Greenberg. E2F-1 functions in mice to promote apoptosis and suppress proliferation. *Cell* 85: 549–561, 1996.
37. Fine, A., N.L. Anderson, T.L. Rothstein, M.C. Williams and B.R. Gochuico. Fas expression in pulmonary alveolar type II cells. *Am. J. Physiol.* 273 (*Lung Cell. Mol. Physiol.* 17): L64–L71, 1997.
38. French, L.E., M. Hahne, I. Viard, G. Radlgruber, K. Zanone, K. Becker, C. Miller, and J. Tschopp. Fas and Fas ligand in embryos and adult mice ligand expression in several immune-priviledged tissues and co-expression in adult tissues characterized by apoptotic cell turnover. *J. Cell Biol.* 133: 355–343, 1996.
39. Friedlander, P., Y. Haupt, C. Prives, and M. Oren. A mutant p53 that discriminates between p53-responsive genes cannot induce apoptosis. *Mol. Cell. Biol.* 16: 4961–4971, 1996.
40. Gao, C. and P. Zelenka. Cyclins, cyclin-dependent kinases and differentiation. *BioEssays* 19: 307–314, 1997.
41. Geng, Y. and R.A. Weinberg. Transforming growth factor-β effects on expression of G1 cyclins and cyclin-dependent protein kinases. *Proc. Natl. Acad. Sci. USA* 90: 10315–10319, 1993.
42. Gucev, Z., Y. Oh, K. Kelley, and R. Rosenfeld. Insulin-like growth factor binding protein 3 mediates retinoic acid-and transforming growth factor β2-induced growth inhibition in human breast cancer cells. *Cancer Res.* 56: 1545–1550, 1996.
43. Halevy, O., B.G. Novitch, D.B. Spicer, S.X. Skapek, J. Rhee, et al. Correlation of terminal cell cycle arrest of skeletal muscle with induction of p21 by myoD. *Science* 267: 1018–1021, 1995.
44. Haupt, Y., R. Maya, A. Kazaz, and M. Oren. MDM2 promotes the rapid degradation of p53. *Nature* 387: 296–303, 1997.
45. Hijmans, E.M., P.M. Voorhoeve, R.L. Beijersbergen, L.J. van Veer, and R. Bernards. E2F-5, a new E2F family member that interacts with p130 in vivo. *Mol. Cell. Biol.* 15: 3082–3089, 1995.
46. Hsu, Y., F. Tang, W. Liu, J. Chuang, M. Lai, and Y. Lin. Transcriptional regulation by p53. *J. Biol. Chem.* 270: 6966–6974, 1995.
47. Hunter, T. Braking the cycle. *Cell* 75: 839–841, 1993.
48. Itoh, A., S. Levinson, T. Morita, S. Kourembanas, J.S. Brody, and S.A. Mitsialis. Structural characterization and specificity of expression of E2F-5; a new member of the E2F family of transcription factors. *Cell. Mol. Biol. Res.* 41: 147–154, 1995.
49. Jacks, T., A. Fazeli, E.M. Schmidt, R.T. Bronson, M.A. Goodell, and R. Weinberg. Effects of an Rb mutation in the mouse. *Nature* 359: 295–300,1992.
50. Jacobson, M. Reactive oxygen species and programmed cell death. *Trends Biochem. Sci.* 21: 83–86, 1996.
51. Jacobson, M.D., M. Weil, and M.C. Raff. Programmed cell death in animal development. *Cell* 88: 347–354, 1997.
52. Jaques, G., K. Noll, B. Wegmann, S. Witten, E. Kogen, R. Radulescu, and K. Havemann. Nuclear localization of insulin-like growth factor binding protein 3 in a lung cancer cell line. *Endocrinology* 138: 1767–1770, 1997.
53. Jiang, Z., E. Zacksenhaus, B.L. Gallie, and R.A. Phillips. The retinoblastoma gene family is differentially expressed during embryogenesis. *Oncogene* 14: 1789–1797, 1997.

54. Johnson, R.L. and C. Tabin. The long and short of hedgehog signalling. *Cell* 81: 313–316, 1995.
55. Jones, J.I. and D.R. Clemmons. Insuline-like growth factors and their binding proteins: biological actions. *Endocr. Rev.* 16: 3–34, 1995.
56. Jung, M., A. Kondratyev, S. Lee, A. Dimtchev, and A. Dristschilo. ATM gene product phosphorylates IkB-a. *Cancer Res.* 57: 24–27, 1997.
57. Kappen, C. *Hox* genes in the lung. *Am. J. Respir. Cell Mol. Biol.* 15:156–162, 1996.
58. Kastan, M. Signalling to P53: where does it all start? *BioEssays* 18: 617–619, 1996.
59. Kauffman, S.L., P.H. Burri, and E.R. Weibel. The postnatal growth of the rat lung II. Autoradiography. *Anat. Rec.* 180: 63–76, 1974.
60. Kelly, S.E., C.J. Bachurski, M.S. Burhans, and S.W. Glasser. Transcription of the lung-specific surfactant protein C gene is mediated by thyroid transcription factor 1. *J. Biol. Chem.* 271: 6881–6888, 1996.
61. Koff, A., M. Ohtsuki, K. Polyak, J.M. Roberts, and J. Massague. Negative regulation of G1 in mammalian cells: inhibition of cyclin-E dependent kinase by TGF-β. *Science* 260: 536–539, 1993.
62. Krumlauf, R. Hox genes in vertebrate development. Cell 78: 191–201, 1994.
63. Lalou, C., C. Cassarre, and M. Binoux. A proteolysis fragment of insulin-like growth factor (IGF) binding protein-3 that fails to bind IGFs inhibits the mitogenic effects of IGF-I and insulin. *Endocrinology* 137: 3206–3212, 1996.
64. Lee, M., B. Williams, G. Mulligan, S. Mukai, R. Bronson, N. Dyson, E. Harlow, and T. Jacks. Targeted disruption of p107; functional overlap between p107 and Rb. *Genes Dev.* 10: 1621–1632, 1996.
65. Lees, E. Cyclin dependent kinase regulation. *Curr. Opin. Cell Biol.* 7: 773–780, 1995.
66. Levine, A. P53, the cellular gatekeeper for growth and division. *Cell* 88: 323–331, 1997.
67. Liu, Y., J. Martindale, M. Gorospe, and N. Holbrook. Regulation of p21 WAF1/CIP1 expression through mitogen-activated protein kinase signaling pathway. *Cancer Res.* 56: 31–35, 1996.
68. Lukas, J., J. Bartkova, M. Rohde, M. Strauss, and J. Bartek. Cyclin D1 is dispensable for G1 control in retinoblastoma gene-deficient cells independently of cdk4 activity. *Mol. Cell. Biol.* 15: 2600–2611, 1995.
69. Macleod, K., N. Sherry, G. Hannon, D. Beach, T. Tokino, K. Kinzler, B. Vogelstein, and T. Jacks. p53-dependent and -independent expression of p21 during cell growth, differentiation, and DNA damage. *Genes Dev.* 9: 935–944, 1995.
70. Magdaleno, S.M., G. Wang, V.L. Mireles, M.K. Ray, M.J. Finegold, and F.J. DeMayo. Cyclin-dependent kinase inhibitor expression in pulmonary Clara cells transformed with SV40 large T antigen in transgenic mice. *Cell Growth Differ.* 8: 145–155, 1997.
71. Maitre, B., A. Clement, M. Williams, and J. Brody. Expression of insulin-like growth factor receptors 1 and 2 in the developing lung and their relation to epithelial cell differentiation. *Am. J. Respir. Cell Mol. Biol.* 13: 262–270, 1995.
72. Massagué, J. TGF-β signaling: receptors, transducers, and mad proteins. *Cell* 85: 947–950, 1996.
73. Massaro, D., N. Teich, S. Maxwell, G.D. Massaro, and P. Whitney. Postnatal development of alveoli. Regulation and evidence for a critical period in rats. *J. Clin. Invest.* 76: 1297–1305, 1985.
74. Massaro, G.D. and D. Massaro. Postnatal treatment with retinoic acid increases the number of pulmonary alveoli in rats. *Am. J. Physiol.* 270 (*Lung Cell. Mol. Physiol.* 14): L305–L310, 1996.

75. Mendelsohn, C., D. Lohnes, D. Decimo, T. Lufkin, M. LeMeur, P. Chambon, and M. Mazrk. Function of retinoic acid receptors (RARs) during lung development. (II) Multiple abnormalities at various stages of organogenesis in RAR double mutants. *Development* 120: 2749–2771, 1994.
76. Moats-Staats, B.M., W.A. Price, L. Xu, W. Jarvis, and A.D. Stiles. Regulation of the insulin-like growth factor system during normal rat lung development. *Am. J. Respir. Cell Mol. Biol.* 12: 56–64, 1995.
77. Moon, R.T., J.D. Brown, and M. Torres. WNTs modulate cell fate and behavior during vertebrate development. *Trends Genet.* 13: 157–162,1997.
78. Moon, R.T., J.D. Brown, J.A. Yang-Snyder, and J.R. Miller. Structurally related receptors and antagonists compete for secreted Wnt signals. *Cell* 88: 725–728, 1997.
79. Morris, G., J. Bischoff, and M. Mathews. Transcriptional activation of the human proliferating-cell nuclear antigen promoter by p53. *Proc. Natl. Acad. Sci. USA* 93: 895–899, 1996.
80. Mouhieddine, O.B., V. Cazals, E. Kuto, Y. Le Bouc, and A. Clement. Glucocorticoid-induced growth arrest of lung alveolarepithelial cells is associated with increased production of insulin like growth factor binding protein-2. *Endocrinology* 137: 287–295, 1996.
81. Mouhieddine, O.B., V. Cazals, B. Maitre, K. Chadelat, Y. Le Bouc, and A.Clement. Insulin-like growth factor II (IGF-II), type 2 IGF receptor and IGF-binding protein-2 gene expression in lung alveolar epithelial cells: relation to proliferation. *Endocrinology* 135: 83–91, 1994.
82. Nagata, S. Apoptosis by death factor. *Cell* 88: 355–365, 1997.
83. Nakayama, K., N. Ishida, M. Shirane, A. Inomata, T. Inoue, N. ShishidoI. Horii, D. Loth, and K. Nakayama. Mice lacking p27/KIP1 display increased body size, multiple organs hyperplasia, retinal dysplasia, and pituitary tumors. *Cell* 85: 707–720, 1996.
84. Nardell, E.A. and J.S. Brody. Determinants of mechanical properties of rat lung during postnatal development. *J. Appl. Physiol.* 53: 140–148,1982.
85. Nasmyth, K. Viewpoint: putting the cell cycle in order. *Science* 274: 1643–1645, 1996.
86. Ohtsubo, M., A. Theodoras, J. Schumacher, J. Roberts, and M. Pagano. Human cyclin E, a nuclear protein essential for the G1-to-S phase transition. *Mol. Cell. Biol.* 15: 2612–2624, 1995.
87. Okamoto, A., W. Jiang, S. Kim, E. Spillare, G. Stoner, I. Weinstein, and C. Harris. Overexpression of human cyclin D1 reduces the transforming growth factor β (TGF-β) type II receptor and growth inhibition by TGF-β1 in immortalized human esophageal epithelial cell line. *Proc. Natl. Acad. Sci. USA* 91: 11576–11580, 1994.
88. Orsulic, S. and M. Peifer. Cell-cell signalling: wingless lands at last. *Curr. Opin. Biol.* 6: 1363–1667, 1996.
89. Perkett, E. Role of growth factors in lung repair and diseases. *Curr. Opin. Pediatr.* 7: 242–249, 1995.
90. Peter, M. and I. Herskowitz. Joining the complex: cyclin-dependent kinase inhibitory proteins and the cell cycle. *Cell* 79: 181–184, 1994.
91. Peters, K.G., S. Werner, X. Liao, S. Wert, J. Whitsett, and L. Williams. Targeted expression of a dominant negative FGF receptor blockes branching morphogenesis and epithelial differentiation in the mouse lung. *EMBO J.* 13: 3296–3301, 1994.
92. Pines, J. The cell cycle kinases. *Cancer Biol.* 5: 305–313, 1994.
93. Price, W. and A. Stiles. New insights into lung growth and development. *Curr. Opin. Pediatr.* 8: 202–208, 1996.
94. Radulescu, R. Nuclear localization signal in insulin-like growth factor-binding protein type 3. *Trends Biochem. Sci.* 19: 278, 1994.

95. Rajah, R., B. Valentinis, and P. Cohen. Insulin-like growth factor (IGF)–binding protein-3 induces apoptosis and mediates the effects of transforming growth factor-B1 on programmed cell death through a p53- and IGF-independent mechanism. *J. Biol. Chem.* 272: 12181–12188,1997.
96. Ravnik, S.E., K. Rhee, and D.J. Wolgemuth. Distinct patterns of expression of the D-type cyclins during testicular development in the mouse. *Dev. Genet.* 16: 171–178, 1995.
97. Rechler, M. Editorial: growth inhibition by insulin-like growth factor (IGF) binding protein3—what's IGF got to do with it? *Endocrinology* 138: 2645–2647, 1997.
98. Resnitzky, D., M. Gossen, H. Bujard, and S. Reed. Acceleration of the G1/S phase transition by expression of the cyclins D1 and E with an inducible system. *Mol. Cell. Biol.* 14: 1669–1679, 1994.
99. Resnitzky, D. and S. Reed. Different roles for cyclins D1 and E in regulation of the G1-to-S transition. *Mol. Cell. Biol.* 15: 3463–3469,1995.
100. Russo, T., N. Zambrano, F. Esposito, R. Ammendola, F. Ciminot, M. Fiscella, J. Jackman, P. O'Connor, C. Anderson, and E. Appella. A p53-independent pathway for activation of WAF/CIP1 expression following oxidative stress. *J. Biol. Chem.* 270: 29386–29391, 1995.
101. Sanchez, Y. and S. Elledge. Stopped for repairs. *BioEssays* 17: 545–548,1995.
102. Sandhu, C., J. Garbe, N. Bhattacharya, J. Daksis, C. Pan, P. Yaswen, J. Koh, J. Slingerland, and M. Stampfer. Transforming growth factor β stabilizes p15 INB4K protein, increases p15 INK4B complexes, and inhibits cyclin D1-cdk4 association in human mammary epithelial cells. *Mol. Cell. Biol.* 17: 2458–2467, 1997.
103. Schneider, J.W., W. Gu, L. Zhu, V. Mahdavi, and B. Nadal-Ginard. Reversal of terminal differentiation mediated by p107 in Rb – muscle cells. *Science* 264: 1467–1470, 1994.
104. Sgambato, A., Y. Doki, I. Schieren, and I. Weinstein. Effects of cyclin E overexpression on cell growth and response to transforming growth factor B depend on cell context and p27Kip1 expression. *Cell Growth Differ.* 8: 393–405, 1997.
105. Sgambato, A., E. Han, P. Zhou, I. Schieren, and I. Weinstein. Overexpression of cyclin E in the HC11 mouse mammary epithelial cell line is associated with growth inhibition and increased expression of p27 Kip1. *Cancer Res.* 56: 1389–1399, 1996.
106. Sherr, C. Mammalian G1 cyclins. *Cell* 73: 1059–1065, 1993.
107. Sherr, C. G1 phase progression: cycling on cue. *Cell* 79: 551–555, 1994.
108. Sherr, C. Cancer cell cycles. *Science* 274: 1672–1677, 1996.
109. Simonet, W.S., M. DeRose, N. Bucay, H.Q. Nguyen, S. Wert, L. Zhou, T.R. Ulrich, D.M. Danienko, and J.A. Whitsett. Pulmonary malformation in transgenic mice expressing human keratinocyte growth factor in the lung. *Proc. Natl. Acad. Sci. USA* 92: 12461–12465, 1995.
110. Smith, L.J. and J.S. Brody. Influence of methylprednisolone on mouse alveolar type 2 cell response to acute lung injury. *Am. Rev. Respir. Dis.* 123: 459–464, 1981.
111. Steller, H. Mechanisms and genes of cellular suicide. *Science* 267: 1445–1448, 1995.
112. Taya, Y., RB kinases and RB-binding proteins: new points of view. *Trends Biochem. Sci.* 22: 14–17, 1997.
113. Thurlbeck, W.M. Postnatal growth and development of the lung. *Am. Rev. Respir. Dis.* 111: 803–844, 1975.
114. Wang, J., K. Guo, K.N. Wills, and K. Walsh. Rb functions to inhibit apoptosis during myocyte differentiation. *Cancer Res.* 57: 351–354,1997.
115. Weinberg, R.A. The retinoblastoma protein and cell cycle control. *Cell* 81: 323–330, 1995.

116. Wikenheiser, K.A., J.C. Clark, R.I. Linnoila, M.T. Stahlman, and J.A. Whitsett. Simian virus 40 large T antigen directed by transcriptional elements of the human surfactant protein C gene produces pulmonary adenocarcinomas in transgenic mice. *Cancer Res.* 52: 5342–5352, 1992.
117. Woo, M., I. Sanchez, and B. Dynlacht. P130 and p107 use a conserved domain to inhibit cellular cyclin-dependent kinase activity. *Mol. Cell. Biol.* 17: 3566–3579, 1997.
118. Wu, H., M. Wade, L. Krall, J. Grisham, Y. Xiong, and T. Dyke. Targeted in vivo expression of the cyclin-dependent kinase inhibitor p21 halts hepatocyte cell-cycle progression, postnatal liver development and regeneration. *Genes Dev.* 10: 245–260, 1995.
119. Yamasaki, L., T. Jacks, R. Bronson, E. Goillot, E. Harlow, and N.J. Dyson. Tumor induction and tissue atrophy in mice lacking E2F-1. *Cell* 85: 537–548, 1996.
120. Yamasaki, M., A. Miyake, S. Tagashira, and N. Itoh. Structure and expression of the rat mRNA encoding a novel member of the fibroblast growth factor family. *J. Biol. Chem.* 271: 15918–15921, 1996.
121. Ye, H. T.F. Kelly, U. Samandi, L. Lim, S. Rubio, D.G. Overdier, K.A. Roebuck, and R.H. Costa. Hepatocyte nuclear factor 3/forkhead homolog 11 is expressed in proliferating epithelial and mesenchymal cells of embryonic and adult tissues. *Mol. Cell. Biol.* 17: 1626–1641, 1997.
122. Zeng, Y. and W. El-Deiry. Regulation of p21WAF1/CIP1 expression by p53-independent pathways. *Oncogene* 12: 1557–1564, 1996.
123. Zetterberg, A., O. Larsson, and K. Wiman. What is the restriction point? *Curr. Opin. Cell Biol.* 7: 835–842, 1995.
124. Zhan, Q., F. Carrier, and A. Fornace. Induction of cellular p53 activity by DNA-damaging agents and growth arrest. *Mol. Cell. Biol.* 13: 4242–4250, 1993.
125. Zhang, L., F. Kashanchi, Q. Zhan, S. Zhan, J. Brady, A. Fornace, P. Seth, and L. Helman. Regulation of insulin-like growth factor II P3 promoter by p53: a potential mechanism for tumorigenesis. *Cancer Res.* 56: 1367–1373, 1996.

chapter 11

BIOACTIVE PEPTIDES AND LUNG DEVELOPMENT

Mary E. Sunday

RECENTLY there has been a surge in interest in the role of specific growth factors or bioactive peptides (Table 11.1) in maturation of type II pneumocytes and other epithelial cells in developing lung. Lung development is a complex process involving multiple interactions between different cell types and secreted factors; among these, epithelial–mesenchymal interactions have been most extensively studied. Cellular processes occurring during this process include cell migration, cell proliferation, apoptosis, and cell differentiation.

In the mid-1980s, the concept of the lung as an endocrine organ was based on studies of pulmonary neuroendocrine (NE) cells and their presumed malignant counterpart, small-cell carcinomas of the lung (SCLCs). It is now clear that non-NE pulmonary cells and tumors can also elaborate bioactive peptides, indicating that paracrine and autocrine mechanisms of cellular signaling occur among a variety of different cell types in the lung as in the immune system. It has been recognized for many decades that lung tumors can produce hormones including catecholamines and bioactive peptides, often referred to as *ectopic hormones*. However, these substances only infrequently give rise to secondary paraneoplastic syndromes such as Cushing's syndrome through production of corticotropin (ACTH) by SCLCs. Many of these substances are not truly ectopic because they have been identified in normal or nonneoplastic lung, with the highest levels often being observed during fetal gestation.

In this review, I will first discuss growth factors derived from non-NE epithelium and/or mesenchymal cells in fetal lung. This overview will be followed by a more in-depth discussion of bioactive neuropeptides in developing lung. Finally, I will present a working hypothesis in an attempt to unify and validate the observations related to multiple bioactive peptides implicated in mammalian fetal lung development.

Table 11.1 Bioactive Peptides Derived from Pulmonary Mesenchymal Cells and/or Nonneuroendocrine (NE) Epithelial Cells

Mesenchymal Peptides
Fibroblast-pneumonocyte factor(s) (FPF)
Keratinocyte growth factor (KGF)
Insulin-like growth factors (IGFs)
Non-NE epithelial peptides
Parathyroid hormone related-protein (PTHrp)
Epidermal growth factor (EGF)
Basic fibroblast growth factor (bFGF)
Platelet-derived growth factor (PDGF)
Bioactive Neuropeptides
Pulmonary neuroendocrine cell peptides
Bombesin-like peptide (BLP)/gastrin-releasing peptide (GRP)
Calcitonin gene-related peptide (CGRP)
Calcitonin
Enkephalin
Corticotrophin (ACTH)
? Corticotrophin releasing hormone (CRH)
Cholecystokinin (CCK)
Substance (SP)
hCG
Pulmonary nerve fiber peptides
Sympathetic, adrenergic
Neuropeptide (NPY)
Parasympathetic, cholinergic
VIP
PHI(M)
Galanin
NPY
Sensory, Non-adrenergic non-cholinergic:
CGRP
Tachykinins: neurokinin A, neurokinin B, eledoisin, neuropeptide K, Substance P

BIOACTIVE PEPTIDES DERIVED FROM NON-NEUROENDOCRINE EPITHELIAL CELLS AND/OR MESENCHYMAL CELLS

Mesenchymal Peptides: Fibroblast-Pneumonocyte Factor(s), Keratinocyte Growth Factor, and Insulin-like Growth Factors

During the canalicular phase of rat lung development, fibroblasts produce fibrolast-pneumonocyte factor (FPF), a soluble factor that stimulates type II cell cholinephosphate cytidylyltransferase enzyme activity, the rate-limiting step in the choline incorporation pathway of phosphatidylcholine synthesis (67). Glucocorticoids enhance pulmonary surfactant production via stimulating FPF activity from fetal lung fibroblasts (55, 67). The use of antenatal glucocorticoids together with exogenous surfactant reduces morbidity and mortality due to surfactant deficiency in respiratory distress syndrome (RDS) (68). Experimentally, antenatal glucocorticoids can augment pre-existing interstitial fibroblast biological activities, such as triglyceride uptake (84), but these processes cannot be stimulated by glucocorticoids prior to the point in gestation when they would increase spontaneously. The stimulation of FPF production by fetal lung fibroblasts can be enhanced by thyroid hormone (68) or inhibited by androgens (14, 51). The inhibitory effect of androgens on FPF production is likely a major factor influencing the slower rate of lung maturation in males, which might be mediated via stimulation of transforming growth factor β (TGF-β) production (85). The TGF-β isoforms, either exogenous or synthesized by non-neuroendocrine epithelium and mesenchymal cells, function to inhibit FPF (86) and EGF-induced type II cell proliferation and maturation (94).

However, FPF has never been isolated, and recent data suggest that its activity may be due to combinations of factors acting together (84). Candidate cytokines with FPF activity include interleukin (IL)-6 and IL-11, which are known to be up-regulated by parathyroid hormone–related protein (PTHrp) in lung fibroblasts exposed to PTHrp (58). However, IL-6 and IL-11 mRNAs are down-regulated by glucocorticoids (26), and hence neither could be the definitive glucocorticoid-inducible gene. One candidate glucocorticoid-inducible cytokine identified in rat fetal lung fibroblasts using subtractive cloning methods was TGF-β3 (90), but this peptide does not have FPF-like activity.

Keratinocyte growth factor (KGF) (53) and insulin-like growth factors (IGFs) (47, 77) are produced by mesenchymal cells in developing lung and have also been implicated in lung growth during development. Treatment of fetal lung with exogenous KGF in organ culture or KGF overexpression driven by the surfactant protein C (SP-C) promoter in transgenic mice (66) led to cystic alveolar hyperplasia of developing fetal lung, a lesion that resembles cystic adenomatoid malformation (66); this suggests that KGF can act as a potent growth factor in developing lung, but that excessive KGF can disrupt normal development and lead to arrested alveolarization (see also Chap. 1 and 4). Targeted mutagenesis of the genes encoding IGF-1, IGF-2, and/or the type-I IGF receptor (40) resulted in homozygous knockout mice with severe growth deficiency that died shortly after birth of respiratory failure; the lungs of mutant neonates are atelectatic but otherwise do not differ histologically from the ventilated and expanded lungs of the normal littermates (40). Increased levels of mRNAs encoding IGF-binding proteins occur during fetal gestation and in adult lung, suggesting that IGF-binding proteins might be the mechanism for modulating actions of the IGF peptides during normal development (47).

Non-NE Epithelial Peptides: Parathyroid Hormone-Related Protein, Epidermal Growth Factor, Basic Fibroblast Growth Factor, and Platelet-Derived Growth Factor

In contrast to glucocorticoids, parathyroid hormone–related protein (PTHrp) can stimulate fibroblast FPF activity in rat fetal lung at least 2-3 days prior to the time when normal differentiation would be initiated (16 versus 19 days post-conceptual age) or prior to the time when mesenchymal maturation can be stimulated in response to exogenous glucocorticoid exposure (52). The PTHrp is an oncofetal hormone that was initially identified as the product of human tumors, including squamous-cell carcinoma of the lung associated with humoral hypercalcemia of malignancy (35). It is known to be produced by a wide range of fetal (37) and adult (35) tissues. In normal lung, PTHrp is produced in developing respiratory epithelium (37), including type II cells. The PTHrp-specific receptor is also expressed in a wide variety of tissues (37), predominantly the adepithelial mesenchyme in the developing lung; in situ hybridization demonstrates receptor mRNAs in mesenchyme at the onset of branching morphogenesis, with the mRNA signal intensity diminishing with increasing distance from the epithelium (37). The timing of PTHrp gene expression in development suggests a possible role in lung branching morphogenesis. Although the biological functions of PTHrp are not yet well understood, in vivo studies in mice homozygous for a disrupted PTHrp allelle (30) point to a role for PTHrp in modulating growth and differentiation. Newborn PTHrp knockout mice die shortly after birth from respiratory insufficiency (30), which appears to be due to surfactant deficiency resulting from arrested lung growth and differentiation (58). The PTHrp stimulates surfactant phospholipid production in rat fetal type II cells, apparently via stimulating mesenchymal–epithelial interactions (58).

Epidermal growth factor (EGF), transforming growth factor α (TGF-α) and amphiregulin (64, 78), basic fibroblast growth factor (bFGF) (24, 54), and platelet-derived growth factor (PD;GF) (25) are produced predominantly by non-neuroendocrine epithelial cells in fetal lung (22, 28, 76). The pattern of mesenchymal expression of EGF receptor mRNAs (91) is similar to that for PTHrp receptors (37). All of these peptides stimulate branching morphogenesis, cell proliferation and type II cell differentiation (94), possibly acting via FPF-like activity. Epidermal growth factor has the ability to stimulate FPF production from fetal lung fibroblasts in culture (61). Fetal mice treated with anti-mouse EGF antiserum in utero were found to have fewer lamellar bodies, which are one of the morphological manifestations of surfactant (96), consistent with diminished type II epithelial cell differentiation, but without an effect on body weight and lung weight. The interpretation of these studies is complicated by the fact that TGF-α and amphiregulin might compensate for decreased tissue levels of EGF because all of these peptides act via the same EGF receptor. The definitive experiment was carried out by three independent laboratories (46, 65, 83): targeted disruption of the mouse EGF receptor led to mice with immature lungs (46, 65), whose survival was contingent on the genetic background of the mice (46, 65, 83). The most striking finding in the lungs of newborn EGF receptor knockout mice was atelectasis (46, 65), but it was not clear whether this was simply due to the general growth retardation of the animals (83). Cumulatively, these results suggest that EGF receptor signaling is not indispensible for lung development and this could reflect redundancy with other bioactive peptides such as FGF and PDGF.

Basic FGF and its receptor have also been localized to the epithelium and mesenchyme of fetal lung by Post and co-workers (24) with a temporal and spatial distribution suggestive of a key role in lung developmental processes. The importance of FGF receptor signaling in lung development has been highlighted by another transgenic mouse model, that of a dominant-negative FGF receptor transgenic mouse in which FGF receptor signaling was blocked specifically in the lung via the SP-C promoter (54). Newborn mice expressing the transgene were completely normal except that instead of having normally developed lungs they had two undifferentiated epithelial tubes extending from the trachea to the diaphragm, a defect that resulted in perinatal death. Thus, the dominant-negative FGF receptor completely blocked airway branching and epithelial differentiation, without prohibiting outgrowth, establishing a key role for FGF signaling in branching morphogenesis of the mammalian lung.

Post et al. have carried out investigations underscoring the importance of PDGF and PDGF receptors in fetal lung development (12, 25, 41, 69, 70). Using immunolocalization and Western blotting, they demonstrated the expression of both PDGF-AA and PDGF-BB homodimer proteins in fetal lung during gestation (25). Using Northern blot and protein analysis of whole fetal lung, they also demonstrated both PDGF α-receptor and PDGF β-receptor (12). Using phosphorothioate antisense PDGF-AA oligodeoxynucleotides, they showed significant inhibition of DNA synthesis, early lung branching, and lung size (69), which could be attenuated by reconstitution with specific peptide. Because the PDGF α-receptor was expressed in the mesenchyme, while PDGF-A mRNA was expressed in the fetal lung epithelium, these data provide further support for epithelial–mesenchymal interactions in early lung branching morphogenesis. Conversely, in similar experiments using antisense oligodeoxynucleotides targeting PDGF-B mRNA, there was inhibition of DNA synthesis, leading to reduced lung size in fetal lung organ cultures, but without any effect on the degree of branching of embryonic rat lung (70). Antisense oligonucleotides for PDGF-B and its receptor were also capable of inhibiting mechanical strain-induced fetal lung cell growth (41), suggesting that PDGF could be a major regulator of fetal growth in response to lung stretch due to breathing movements in utero.

BIOACTIVE NEUROPEPTIDES IN THE LUNG

Most of the current knowledge about effects of neuropeptides in the lung is focussed on molecules derived from intrapulmonary nerve fibers in postnatal lung. Sensory nerve fibers in the lung are believed to play a physiological role as irritant receptors linked to the cough reflex regulating respiratory skeletal muscle and bronchial smooth muscle contractility. These sensory nerves contain a variety of neuropeptides, especially tachykinins, that have been most extensively studied with regard to their contribution to the pathogenesis of neurogenic inflammation or asthma (7). Intrinsic parasympathetic and extrinsic sympathetic nerve fibers originating from the extrapulmonary ganglia are believed to regulate bronchoconstriction and vascular resistance through feedback mechanisms in a similar fashion (73). Increased mucous glandular secretion, ciliary beat frequency, contraction of bronchial musculature, and vasodilation are stimulated by vagal (parasympathetic, cholinergic) fibers; the opposite effects are triggered by sympathetic (adrenergic) fibers as well as by humoral catecholamines (endogenous or exogenous epinephrine or other β-2 adrenergic agonists). Vasoactive intestinal peptide (VIP) has been shown to have the same effects as acetylcholine except for its action as a bronchial smooth-muscle relaxant (7). Neuroendocrine cells could also be implicated in cough reflexes, bronchial and vascular smooth muscle tone, or glandular secretion. In 1990 Lundgren et al. demonstrated that bombesin-like peptide (BLP) [gastrin-releasing protein (GRP) and bombesin], can stimulate glandular secretion of respiratory glycoconjugate in the feline trachea, which is similar to BLP-induced stimulation of glandular secretion in the gastrointestinal tract (82). In a follow-up study, Baraniuk et al. (6) administered BLP topically to human nasal mucosa in vivo and observed dose-dependent stimulation of both serous (lactoferrin) and mucous (glycoconjugate) secretion; these results are similar to those from prior experiments with nasal mucosal explants in vitro. These data suggest that GRP released from trigeminal sensory nerves may bind to BLP receptors on respiratory epithelial cells and submucosal glands to promote neurogenic inflammation.

Pulmonary Neuroendocrine Cell Peptides

Bombesin-like Peptide and Gastrin-Releasing Peptide

Bombesin is a 14 amino acid peptide that was identified by Erspamer in 1971 in skin of the frog *Bombina bombina* (reviewed in 82). A 27 amino acid homolog of bombesin was identified by McDonald et al. in porcine stomach and called *gastrin-releasing peptide* (GRP) because an in vivo bioassay of gastrin release was used to monitor peptide fractions during the purification. Bombesin and GRP are collectively referred to as bombesin-like peptide (BLP) because they share a highly conserved 7 amino acid C terminus that is implicated in both immunogenicity and high-affinity binding to bombesin/GRP-preferring receptors (Fig. 11.1). Consequently, the multiple physiological effects of GRP and bombesin are essentially identical (82). These have been studied most extensively in the brain, gut, pancreas, and thyroid and include both neuroregulatory and growth-modulating effects (15, 45, 82). Some observations on effects of BLP in extrapulmonary systems are relevant to understanding effects of BLP in developing lung. The growth-promoting effects of BLP in the gut and pancreas in vivo may be mediated in part via release of cholecystokinin (CCK) and/or gastrin (39, 42). Neuroregulatory effects of GRP derived from thyroidal C cells may include stimulation of calcitonin secretion (1) and thyroid hormone secretion (3), in contrast to calcitonin and calcitonin gene–related peptide (CGRP), which inhibit thyroid hormone secretion (3). The BLP-related peptide neuromedin B (NMB) (Fig. 11.1) has indirect effects on thyroid function via direct actions on the release of thyroid-stimulating hormone (TSH) that vary depending on the thyroid status of the animal (56).

Bombesin-like peptide was the first neuropeptide localized to NE cells in human fetal lung in 1978 by Wharton et al., with the highest tissue levels detected by

1. BOMBESIN (BLP) FAMILY

	1 ... 14
Bombesin	pGlu-Gln-Arg-Leu-*Gly-Asn*-Gln-*Trp-Ala-Val-Gly-His-Leu-Met*-NH_2
GRP 14-27	-Met-Tyr-Pro-Arg-*Gly-Asn*-His-*Trp-Ala-Val-Gly-His-Leu-Met*-NH_2

2. RANATENSIN (RN) FAMILY

	1 ... 11
RN-C	pGlu-Val-Pro-*Trp-Ala*-Val-*Gly-His-Phe-Met*-NH_2
Neuromedin B (NMB)	Gly-Asn-Leu-*Trp-Ala*-Thr-*Gly-His-Phe-Met*-NH_2

3. PHYLLOLITORIN (PL) FAMILY

	1 ... 9
Leu^8-PL (L8PL)	p*Glu-Leu-Trp-Ala-Val-Gly-Ser*-Leu-*Met*-NH_2
Phe^8-PL (P8PL)	p*Glu-Leu-Trp-Ala-Val-Gly-Ser*-Phe-*Met*-NH_2

Fig. 11.1 Key C-terminal amino acid differences (underlined) between the three major groups of bombesin-like peptides and related peptides (36).

radioimmunoassay (RIA) in human fetal lung (92). BLP appears in human pulmonary neuroendocrine cells (PNECs) as soon as the cells are detectable at 8–9 weeks gestation (72). Peak relative numbers of BLP-positive PNECs occur at about mid-gestation in human fetal lung, which is the time of maximal GRP gene expression. Bombesin-like peptide is also at high levels in many SCLCs (82). Several groups have studied the function of BLP in normal and neoplastic cell proliferation. It was shown to be a potent mitogen for murine Swiss 3T3 fibroblasts, normal adult human bronchial epithelial cells, and SCLC cell lines (82). Unstimulated growth of BLP-responsive and BLP-producing SCLC lines can be blocked either in culture or in nude mice by monoclonal antibodies (mAbs) to bombesin, indicating the operation of an autocrine feedback loop. Multiple BLP receptor–specific antagonists have been demonstrated to inhibit growth of SCLC cell lines (43).

Shipp et al. (63) demonstrated that the cell surface metalloendopeptidase CD10/neutral endopeptidase 24.11 (CD10/NEP, common acute lymphoblastic leukemia antigen, CALLA) can hydrolyze BLP. The growth of BLP-responsive SCLCs was inhibited by CD10/NEP and potentiated by CD10/NEP inhibition. A specific BLP receptor antagonist inhibited SCLC colony formation resulting from the addition of either phosphoramidon or bombesin. These data indicate that CD10/NEP inhibition led to effectively increased levels of endogenous BLP which then acted in an autocrine fashion to promote clonal SCLC growth. In addition to SCLCs, the proliferation of normal human bronchial epithelium and many non-small-cell carcinomas (NSCLCs) can be regulated by CD10/NEP inhibition (18). These responses are likely to be mediated by both BLP/GRP-preferring and NMB-preferring receptors, which have been cloned (8).

Considering the abundance of BLP in PNECs, the high number of PNECs in human fetal lung, and the potentially important role of BLP as a growth factor in lung development, Spindel et al. began to study GRP gene expression in human fetal lung

(72) using a cDNA spanning most of the proGRP cDNA that had been cloned from a human pulmonary carcinoid tumor. The GRP mRNAs were first detectable in fetal lung at 9–10 weeks gestation, plateaued at levels 25-fold higher than in adult lungs from 16 to ~30 weeks, coinciding with the pseudoglandular and canalicular periods of lung development, and then declined to near adult levels by 34 weeks gestation. Using in situ hybridization, we demonstrated transient expression of GRP mRNAs in PNECs (from 9 weeks gestation to ~22 weeks) in a proximal-to-distal fashion in parallel with the growth of fetal airways (72). In contrast, BLP immunostaining was detectable at 9.5 weeks gestation and remained elevated until several months after birth. A direct comparison of in situ hybridization and immunohistochemical studies in serial sections showed that (*1*) GRP mRNA and BLP peptide consistently colocalized in mid-gestation fetal lung; (*2*) only at 9.5 weeks gestation were there ~20% more cells detected by in situ hybridization than by BLP immunostaining, suggesting that a lag period might occur between the time of initial GRP gene transcription and processing of proGRP via cleavage and amidation into mature GRP; and (*3*) in neonatal lung, many cells containing BLP immunostaining no longer contained detectable GRP mRNA. At least part of this dissociation between GRP mRNA and BLP peptide could be due to storage of GRP peptide in dense-core granules of resting PNECs. However, we cannot exclude the possibility that GRP is not the only pulmonary BLP and that another mammalian BLP-like peptide gene may be expressed in the perinatal period, such as a mammalian phyllolitorin analog (33).

My major interest was to pursue the functional relevance of BLP in fetal lung development, using three distinct experimental approaches: (*1*) administration of exogenous BLP (79); (*2*) treatment with a well-characterized blocking monoclonal antibody (2A11) to BLP (79, 80); and (*3*) potentiation of tissue levels of endogenous BLP by blocking peptide degradation by CD10/NEP inhibition (32, 81). To facilitate these investigations, my colleagues and I used mice, which provided a readily available, cost-effective, well-characterized, and rapid assay system for screening effects on mammalian lung development. Bombesin-like peptide was detected in fetal murine lung between embryonic day 16 (e16) and neonatal day 3, which is similar to elevated BLP levels in human fetal lung from mid-gestation to the early neonatal period (13, 72, 82). The GRP mRNA was detected as early as e16 in fetal murine lung using Northern blot analyses of poly$(A)^+$ RNA, with peak expression occurring just before birth (79), and levels dropping off substantially after birth (79). Thus, mice demonstrate transient expression of the GRP gene, analogous to what was observed in human fetal lung. Although at first glance this appears to be a different time course of expression in mice versus humans, it is quite similar according to the chronology of major developmental events. Thus, peak GRP gene expression most closely coincides with the onset of surfactant synthesis and type II pneumocyte maturation, which occurs over the last 2 days before birth in the mouse, but the last half of human fetal gestation. Classic experiments by Buckingham and Avery analyzed type II pneumocyte differentiation and surfactant production first in mice and found surface-active material at the highest levels during the two days prior to birth (10).

The three experimental systems we have used to analyze mammalian lung development are (*1*) fetal murine lung in organ culture, to provide a rapid screening tool for assessing effects of peptides on cell proliferation and differentiation; (*2*) fetal murine lung in utero, to specifically address questions related to placental peptide transfer and type II pneumocyte maturational effects in vivo and hence potential clinical applicability; and (*3*) human fetal lung in organ culture, which provides the gold standard for understanding human fetal lung development with the ultimate goal of clinical usefulness in the prevention of respiratory distress syndrome (RDS) and/or bronchopulmonary dysplasia (BPD) in premature infants.

In the first series of experiments, exogenous bombesin was administered to cultured human fetal lung and fetal murine lung both in utero and in organ cultures (79). We determined that bombesin does cross the placenta when administered in utero. Increased parameters of both growth and lung organ maturation were observed. Growth, or pulmonary cell proliferation, was evaluated using ^{3}H-thymidine incorporation into acid-precipitable nuclear DNA, normalized for DNA content; total DNA and protein content per lung; and nuclear autoradiography following ^{3}H-thymidine administration in vivo. There were significant dose-dependent increases in ^{3}H-thymidine incorporation following in utero bombesin administration on both e17 and e18, which occurred together with elevated total protein and total DNA per lung. Tissue autoradiography demonstrated increased labeling of mesenchymal cells as well as epithelial cells in airways and primitive alveoli, indicating a broad-ranging proliferative effect. These data are consistent with bombesin being a direct growth factor for bronchial epithelial cells and pulmonary fibroblasts. Maturation, or type II cell differentiation, was assessed by ^{3}H-choline incorporation into saturated phosphatidylcholine (SPC), the rate-limiting step in surfactant phospholipid synthesis, normalized for protein content; total SPC content per lung; and electron microscopy for glycogen, which disappears with epithelial cell differentiation, and for content of lamellar bodies (LBs), one of the major morphological manifestations of pulmonary surfactant. Bombesin treatment in utero induced significant dose-dependent elevations in ^{3}H-choline uptake and total SPC content per lung, which was evident only on e18. Ultrastructurally, there was a dose-dependent increase in the number of cells containing LB (differentiated type II cells) on e18, but there was no difference in the number of LBs per type II cell. These data suggest that total surfactant production per cell was comparable, but that there was an effect of bombesin on type II cell differentiation and/or proliferation. However, it was unknown whether the effect on type II cells was direct or required an intermediary cell such as a fibroblast to be observed, such as via FPF (55).The effects on ^{3}H-thymidine and ^{3}H-choline uptake that we observed appeared to be dissociable, with the choline effect being observed only on e18 in utero; this suggests that the cell proliferation and differentiation responses may occur by independent mechanisms. It is unlikely that the bombesin effects in utero were mediated by endogenous glucocorticoids because there was no difference in fetal mouse serum corticosterone levels. Finally, the same effects on thymidine and choline incorporation were observed in both human and murine fetal lung organ cultures, and the effects of bombesin were blocked by a specific anti-bombesin monoclonal antibody (2A11), indicating that at least part of the in utero effect was mediated by bombesin acting directly on fetal lung. The effect of bombesin on human fetal lung was comparable in magnitude to that observed with peak concentrations of dexamethasone (10 nM) in the same cultured lung.

In the second series of experiments, anti-BLP monoclonal antibody 2A11 was used to test for blocking function of endogenous BLP. First, 2A11 (IgG_1) alone blocked fetal murine lung automaturation in serum-free lung organ cultures by ~60% compared with control cultures incubated with only an irrelevant IgG_1 (MOPC) as assessed by choline incorporation ($P < 0.001$) (79); there was no effect of 2A11 on thymidine incorporation in the same cultures. We then tested the effect of 2A11 on fetal lung maturation in utero and observed a dose-dependent inhibition of lung maturation on e18 (up to ~35% inhibition) as assessed by choline uptake consistent with the prior observation of a BLP-induced maturational effect on e18 in utero (80). Again, there was no effect pf 2A11 on thymidine incorporation on e18, suggesting that other lung growth factors may compensate if endogenous BLP levels drop substantially.

In the third series of experiments, our aim was to raise the tissue levels of endogenous BLP by inhibiting their degradation and then to test for specific effects that could in turn be blocked by specific BLP receptor antagonists. We chose to potentiate endogenous tissue levels of BLP by inhibiting BLP degradation using CD10/NEP, which hydrolyzes a number of naturally occurring peptides (62), including substance P, neurotensin, endothelin, and BLP (9). First, we used immunoperoxidase and in situ hybridization analyses to localize CD10/NEP and its mRNAs to human fetal airway epithelial cells, including PNECs (63, 81). Especially high levels of CD10/NEP were present on undifferentiated airway epithelial cells and airway-associated mesenchyme including smooth muscle in the older fetuses (81), which are likely targets for BLP. CD10/NEP gene expression occurs during the same developmental window as GRP in both human fetal (81) and murine fetal lung (32). In human fetal lung organ culture, CD10/NEP inhibition by either of two chemically dissimilar agents (SCH32615 and phosphoramidon) resulted in more than a doubling of ^{3}H-thymidine incorporation, which was completely prevented by treatment with a highly specific BLP receptor antagonist, [Leu^{13}-psi(CH_2NH) Leu^{14}]bombesin (L13BN) (81). These experiments support a role for endogenous BLP in mediating cell proliferation in human fetal lung early in the second trimester.

To specifically address questions of effects on lung organ maturation, we extended our experiments on CD10/NEP inhibition to the mouse in utero, which was made feasible by the availability of a long-acting CD10/NEP inhibitor that could be administered to laboratory animals in vivo. We demonstrated CD10/NEP mRNA in fetal murine lung from e15 to e18 (32). CD10/NEP inhibition by SCH32615 given in utero from e12 to e14 resulted in significantly increased thymidine uptake only from e15 to e18, which is consistent with an effect corresponding to the time course of CD10/NEP mRNA expression. Similar to treatment with exogenous BLP,

CD10/NEP inhibition from e15 to e17 in utero was found to elevate parameters of fetal lung growth and maturation on e18, increasing incorporation of ^{3}H-thymidine into nuclear DNA and ^{3}H-choline incorporation into saturated phosphatidylcholine in organ culture. Tissue autoradiography for nuclear labeling by ^{3}H-thymidine demonstrated significantly increased labeling of type II pneumocytes (K. King and M. Sunday, unpublished data). Ultrastructural evidence showed a trend toward increased relative numbers of type II cells (defined as lamellar body–containing cells) in primitive alveoli and a dose-dependent significant decrease in the number of lamellar bodies per type II cell consistent with surfactant secretion. Finally a fivefold increase in levels of surfactant apoprotein A transcripts ($P < 0.05$) was found (32). The effects on proliferation and type II cell differentiation were completely blocked by a BLP receptor–specific antagonist, [D-Phe^{12},Leu^{14}]bombesin, suggesting that CD10/NEP modulates fetal lung development mediated by endogenous BLP. The lack of an effect with BLP receptor antagonists given alone either in human fetal lung organ cultures (81) or in mice in utero (32) could be related to partial agonist function of the antagonists counteracting any inhibitory effects, or it could indicate the presence of novel, as yet undiscovered BLP receptors.

Other laboratories have demonstrated similar enhancement of lung growth and maturational events by BLP (4, 16, 38, 71). In 1992 Fraslon and Bourbon (16) (see Chap. 4) demonstrated that < 1 nM GRP stimulated proliferation of isolated e19.5 fetal rat type II cells as assessed by total DNA content and thymidine incorporation. Gastrin-releasing peptide at 10 nM or more was inhibitory for growth of both type II cells and fibroblasts, which is consistent with GRP receptor down-regulation. Furthermore, 10 nM GRP stimulated ^{3}H-choline incorporation into surfactant phospholipids, which is consistent with observations in utero and in lung organ cultures (79). These data suggest that BLP can directly stimulate type II cell surfactant synthesis, although trace contamination with fibroblasts in the primary type II cell cultures cannot be ruled out.

Asokananthan and Cake (4) have confirmed and extended these studies by demonstrating that BLP stimulates surfactant phospholipid secretion from cultured e19 fetal rat type II cells. Furthermore, GRP-enhanced surfactant secretion was blocked by specific inhibitors of protein kinase C and the calcium/calmodulin-dependent protein kinase, but not at all by inhibitors of protein kinase A. These observations indicate that the signal transduction mechanism in type II cells involves intracellular calcium and protein kinase C, similar to what has been observed in 3T3 fibroblasts (57).

Bombesin-like peptide might also function as an autocrine differentiation factor for pulmonary NE cells. Cutz and co-workers (71) found that GRP stimulated an increase in numbers of 5HT^{+} cells in fetal rabbit PNEC cultures, without any effect on thymidine labeling of these cells. These results are consistent with recruitment of immature cells not yet expressing the full PNEC phenotype. Gastrin-releasing peptide did stimulate proliferation of non-PNECs, predominantly mesenchymal cells, in the same cultures (71). Consistent with these observations are results from studies by Wang et al., who subsequently used in situ hybridization to localize GRP receptor transcripts in both epithelial cells and mesenchymal cells, mainly in the distal airway epithelial tubes and surrounding mesenchyme; proximal airways showed decreased signal (89). These results are consistent with our localization of CD10/NEP transcripts and protein to the smallest undifferentiated airways and surrounding mesenchyme (81), because CD10/NEP functions at the cell surface by hydrolyzing peptides in the vicinity of their cognate receptors (62).

Li et al. have carried out functional investigations of BLP-induced proliferation in fetal rhesus monkey lung (38). These monkeys express the GRP gene in lung at mid-gestation, as determined by Northern blot analyses, similar to human fetal lung (72), indicating that this might be a good animal model for direct comparison to human fetal lung development. The GRP receptors are expressed with a similar time course, as shown by RNAse protection analyses, with GRP receptor mRNAs localized primarily to airway epithelium. These results differ somewhat from in situ hybridization studies in other laboratories analyzing fetal human (89), rat (88), and mouse (33) lung that have localized GRP receptor mRNAs at the highest levels in airway-associated mesenchyme. However, Cutz et al. (89) did identify low levels of GRP receptor mRNAs in the epithelium as well as in the non-airway-associated mesenchyme, thus supporting all of the published in situ studies. Li et al. (38) also localized GRP mRNAs to airway epithelium of the smallest budding airways as well as to NE cells, but BLP or proGRP immunostaining was undetectable. This result is intriguing and would agree with studies in the laboratories of Warburton (95) and Sunday (23) demonstrating CGRP and PGP 9.5 together with the Clara cell marker CC10 in undifferentiated airway epithelium, which supports the concept of totipotential airway epithelial precursor cells. Li et al. also carried out functional studies with 1-mm cubes of fetal monkey lung in organ culture for 5 days. The addition of bombesin (either 1 nM or 10 nM) significantly increased DNA synthesis in airway epithelial cells, as determined by BrdU labeling, and apparently significantly increased the airway size and number.

We have also addressed the question of involvement of BLP in branching morphogenesis of embryonic murine lung buds (33). Pulmonary NE cells are known to be localized predominantly at airway branch points. In our prior work, we showed that GRP and GRP mRNAs occurred in well-differentiated PNECs exclusively in branching human fetal airways. Using RT-PCR analyses, we found that GRP and GRP receptor genes are expressed in fetal mouse lung as early as e12, when lung buds are beginning to branch. By in situ hybridization, GRP receptor transcripts were at the highest levels in mesenchymal cells at cleft regions of branching airways and blood vessels. To explore the possibility that BLP might play a role in branching morphogenesis, e12 lung buds were cultured for 48 h in serum-free medium. In the presence of 0.10–10 μm bombesin, branching was augmented compared with controls cultured in media alone, with a peak at 1 μm ($P < 0.005$). The specific bombesin receptor antagonist [Leu^{13}-psi(CH$_2$NH)Leu^{14}] bombesin (L13BN) completely abolished bombesin-induced branching. A bombesin-related peptide, [Leu^{8}]-phyllolitorin (L8PL), similarly increased branching and also augmented thymidine incorporation in lung buds. These observations suggest that BLP secreted by undifferentiated airway epithelial cells could contribute to lung branching morphogenesis. Furthermore, components of branch points such as fibronectin might induce pulmonary NE cell differentiation as part of a positive feedback loop, which could account in part for the high prevalence of these cells at branch points. Fibronectin, which is known to be abundant at branch points, induces GRP gene expression in H82, an undifferentiated SCLC cell line. Similarly, Aguayo et al. (2) independently identified bombesin/GRP-preferring receptors in e13 murine lung and observed a trend toward increased murine branching morphogenesis, with 1 to 100 nM bombesin in serum-containing media.

Mechanisms for BLP-induced branching are likely to be similar for epithelial and vascular systems and include altered cell adhesion and/or cell motility, and/or differential cell proliferation (20, 91). Bombesin-like peptide could also alter epithelial cell migration. Bombesin has been reported to stimulate chemotaxis of macrophages and SCLC cell lines (59). Bombesin-like peptide could trigger the release of a soluble branching factor from pulmonary mesenchymal cells, which could act secondarily to promote branching.

Calcitonin Gene–Related Peptide and Calcitonin

In the lung, calcitonin gene–related peptide (CGRP) occurs in intrapulmonary sensory nerves (7, 73), undifferentiated airway epithelium (95), and serous glands of the trachea (5) as well as in pulmonary NE cells (73); calcitonin is found only in pulmonary NE cells (75). Calcitonin gene–related peptide is derived from the same gene as calcitonin by alternative splicing (73), but is preferentially expressed by pulmonary NE cells early in fetal lung development in both rodents (87) and humans (29). Most functional analyses have focussed on CGRP as a potential growth factor in the lung. It is likely to be responsible in part for the growth-promoting effects of neuroepithelial bodies (NEBs) on non-NE airway epithelial cells (27). White et al. (93) have also carried out analyses of normal adult guinea pig tracheal epithelium showing significant effects of exogenous CGRP on cell proliferation. All of these growth effects were blocked by a specific CGRP receptor antagonist in a dose-dependent fashion.

Calcitonin gene–related peptide and calcitonin receptors may also be involved in the modulation of growth processes. In NE cell lines, calcitonin mRNA is lowest and CGRP is highest during rapid growth (50), apparently by reversible alterations in alternative RNA-processing patterns dependent on growth conditions in vitro. Similarly, high CGRP levels in developing pulmonary NE cells early in ontogeny may be linked to the rapid growth phase of lung development, with calcitonin becoming more prevalent only when pulmonary NE cells are fully differentiated (75). The precise roles for CGRP and calcitonin in developing fetal lung remain to be established.

To make matters more complicated, additive, synergistic, or antagonistic effects might occur between CGRP, calcitonin, and BLP, especially because all three of these peptides are contained in the same neurosecretory granules (74). Stahlman and Gray (74) have suggested that these three peptides could act in concert, or perhaps one peptide may act in a paracrine role (e.g., on bronchial or bronchiolar smooth muscle) with the second peptide acting in an autocrine fashion on the parent cell (e.g., in the regulation of granule production or release). In analyses of smooth-muscle contraction–induced BLP and substance P in guinea pigs in vivo (19), CGRP and/or calcitonin were able to effectively inhibit increases in airway tone. It was suggested that CGRP and/or calcitonin could prevent airway smooth muscle contraction by interfering with BLP- or substance P–induced changes in intracellular calcium concentration (19).

Enkephalins, Corticotropin, and Corticotropin Releasing Hormone

Leu-enkephalin is expressed by pulmonary NE cells in postnatal lung of infants with chronic lung disease (75). Leu-enkephalin is an opioid peptide that could function to regulate growth processes induced by BLP or other peptides in developing lung. In the gastrointestinal tract, met-enkephalin and beta-endorphin effectively antagonized gut-contracting effects of BLP (97). Opioid peptides mediate growth inhibitory effects on human lung cancer cell lines, both SCLC and NSCLC,which can be reversed by nicotine (44). The opioid peptide beta-endorphin is synthesized as part of a larger molecule, proopiomelanocortin (POMC), which also gives rise to corticotropin by proteolytic cleavage. Corticotropin, a 39 amino acid peptide, and POMC-derived peptides, including beta-endorphin, are absent from normal fetal or adult human lung but have been localized to rare pulmonary NE cells in postnatal lung from infants with chronic lung disease (75). Corticotropin and GRP immunoreactivities have been localized to distinct pulmonary NE cell subpopulations (82).

It is possible that corticotropin and corticotropin-releasing hormone (CRH) from lung, brain, and/or pituitary could have direct effects on lung neuromuscular development, cell differentiation, and/or proliferation, and/or have indirect effects on fetal lung development via increased endogenous glucocorticoid production. Corticotropin-releasing hormone, produced in the hypothalamus and cerebral cortex, is a key regulator of the mammalian stress response mediated via the hypothalamic-pituitary-adrenal axis, stimulating the release of corticotropin from the pituitary. Corticotropin, in turn, stimulates the adrenal cortex to produce glucocorticoids, which mediate adaptive responses to stress. Like corticotropin, CRH is produced in fetal lung (31). Although the cell of origin has not been definitively identified, CRH mRNAs are transiently expressed from e12.5 to e17.5 in the region of the branching bronchioles, corresponding to the late pseudoglandular and early canalicular phases of lung development (31).

To define the importance of CRH in development, Muglia et al. (49) constructed CRH knockout mice, all of which demonstrate a fetal glucocorticoid requirement for lung maturation. Homozygous CRH-deficient mice born to heterozygous mothers have no detectable abnormalities, despite evidence of impaired adrenal response to stress (49). Matings between CRH-deficient mice result in apparently normal pregnancies, but after a full gestation, the progeny all die within the first day of life despite a normal external appearance. Histologically, CRH-deficient newborn lungs have thickened alveolar septae and fewer alveolae compared with wild-type lungs, and surfactant apoprotein B (SP-B) mRNA levels are decreased (49). Treatment of pregnant homozygous females with glucocorticoids completely reversed the abnormal lung architecture and SPB deficiency in homozygous deficient mice from homozygous matings, resulting in the production of viable litters that survived without subsequent postnatal glucocorticoid treatment. Essentially identical observations have been made in a glucocorticoid receptor knockout mouse (60). These observations indicate an absolute requirement for glucocorticoids in the lung during fetal rather than postnatal life, which is consistent with in vivo and in vitro studies showing the ability of glucocorticoids to promote lung maturation (68).

Pulmonary Nerve Fiber Peptides: Tachykinins and Vasoactive Intestinal Peptide

Tachykinins substance P, neurokinin A, and neuropeptide K are all derived from a single preprotachykinin gene by alternative splicing of seven exons (73) and have been studied most extensively as potential bronchoconstrictor peptides involved in asthma. Together with CGRP, the tachykinins are the major peptides expressed in sensory nerves. In addition, substance P has been demonstrated in human pulmonary NE cells, both isolated pulmonary NE cells and NEBs, especially in fetal lung (17). The presence of substance P–positive cytoplasmic processes that interdigitate with the other epithelial cells suggests that these cells might have a paracrine influence on neighboring cells. The inhibition of growth of SCLC and NSCLC cell lines by substance P analogues (11) also suggests that substance P could modulate lung epithelial cell proliferation.

Vasoactive intestinal peptide (VIP) is localized to the parasympathetic nerves of the lung (73), and has been studied as a bronchodilator peptide implicated in the pathophysiology of asthma. It acts as a potent growth factor for several cell types in cultured postimplantation mouse embryos via multiple vasoactive intestinal peptide (VIP) receptors (21). After a 4-h incubation, VIP stimulates growth, increasing somite number, embryonic volume, DNA and protein content, and number of cells in S-phase (21); a VIP antagonist modulates the effects on growth, completely suppressing VIP-stimulated mitosis in the brain but only decreasing growth by about 40% in non-neuronal tissues. The same antagonist is highly effective at inhibiting growth of NSCLCs, for which VIP can act as an autocrine growth factor (48). Vasoactive intestinal peptide also elevates intracellular cAMP and increases the secretion rate of BLP from SCLC cell lines (34). Vasoactive intestinal peptide might function as a growth and/or differentiation factor through inducing BLP secretion in fetal lung.

A WORKING HYPOTHESIS

Much remains to be learned about the interactions between multiple bioactive peptides produced by different cell types during both lung development and lung injury. There are numerous growth factors and cytokines to consider that could modulate cell proliferation, differentiation, secretion, and/or receptor function. Many of the neuropeptides listed in Table 11.1 are not discussed in this review because there is little or no information available pertaining to specific roles in lung development. However, it is clear from cumulative observations that there is significant functional redundancy of bioactive peptides in developing lung, as would be expected for an organ whose function is so critical for postnatal survival. Figure 11.2 summarizes several bioactive peptides currently recognized as key players in lung development. It should also be noted that during branching morphogenesis (~e11 to e14 in the mouse), there is production of multiple bioactive peptides including CGRP and probably BLPs by undifferentiated epithelial cells (23, 95). The processes involved in stimulation of branching are likely to include altered cell adhesion, migration, differential cell proliferation, and apoptosis. The striking complete lack of branching in the FGF receptor dominant-negative transgenic mouse (54) suggests that bFGF could be a more critical player in branching morphogenesis than the other peptides. Also of interest is the dissociation between branching and growth observed in these mice lacking FGF signaling (54). We observed a dissociation between cell proliferation and branching morphogenesis with BLP (33). It is possible that the major effect of all of these peptides is to induce the release of a branching factor (as yet unidentified) from the mesenchyme of embryonic lung buds. Around e14 to e16, epithelial cell

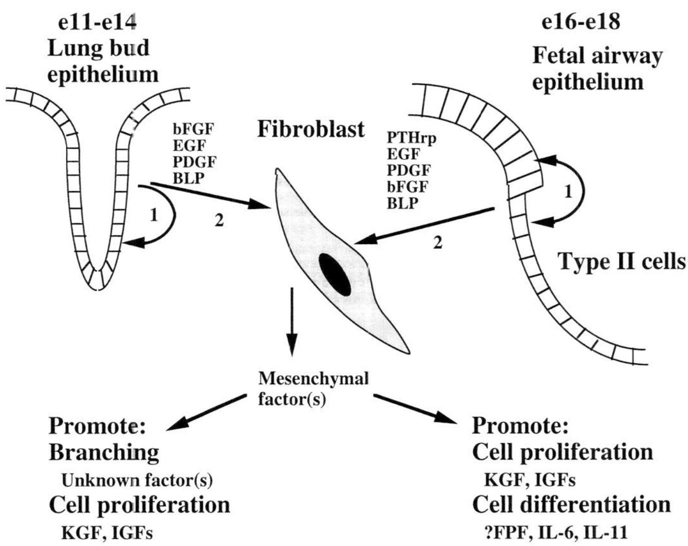

Fig. 11.2 Bioactive peptides and windows of lung development. In developing murine lung buds et e11 to e14, the peptides EGF, PDGF, bFGF, and BLP act to promote branching morphogenesis, probably via both direct effects on cell adhesion, migration, and proliferation, and indirect effects via mesenchymal factors that have yet to be identified. At e16 to e18, the bioactive peptides EGF, PDGF, bFGF, and PTHrp are produced by non-NE epithelial cells in developing lung; BLP and CGRP are synthesized and secreted by NE and epithelial cells, but are localized as clusters or isolated cells, with a predominance at branch points.

differentiation begins as defined morphologically, immunocytochemically, and functionally (10, 95). Again, effects of these diverse peptides on cell proliferation and/or differentiation could be both direct and indirect, inducing the release of mesenchymal factor(s) such as FPF, IL-6, or IL-11. In addition, bioactive peptide growth factors produced by the mesenchyme include KGF and IGFs. Figure 11.2 is purposely simplified to highlight the similarities between different bioactive peptides with regard to the ultimate effects on developing fetal lung. Key questions remaining to be answered include: what is the mesenchymal-derived branching factor? Is the same factor also able to induce type II cell differentiation in fetal lung during the canalicular phase, or is a distinct factor implicated for maturational events? Is there any purpose in utero for localization of NE cells at branch points, or is this simply a consequence of the induction of NE cells by components of branch points, such as fibronectin (33)? The answers to these questions will depend on a more complete understanding of the basic mechanisms of cell differentiation.

REFERENCES

1. Abe, Y., A. Kanamori, Y. Yajima, and T. Kameya. Increase in cytoplasmic Ca^{2+} and stimulation of calcitonin secretion from human medullary thyroid carcinoma cells by the gastrin-releasing peptide. *Biochem. Biophys. Res. Commun.* 185: 833–838, 1992.
2. Aguayo, S.M., W.E. Schuyler, J.J. Murtagh, and J. Roman. Regulation of lung branching morphogenesis by bombesin-like peptides and neutral endopeptidase. *Am. J. Respir. Cell Mol. Biol.* 10: 635–642, 1994.
3. Ahren, B. Regulatory peptides in the thyroid gland—a review on their localization and function. *Acta Endocrinol.* 124: 225–232, 1991.
4. Asokananthan, N. and M.H. Cake. Stimulation of surfactant lipid secretion from fetal type II pneumocytes by gastrin-releasing peptide. *Am. J. Physiol.* 270: L331–L337, 1996.
5. Baluk, P., J.A. Nadel, and D.M. McDonald. Calcitonin gene-related peptide in secretory granules of serous cells in the rat tracheal epithelium. *Am. J. Respir. Cell Mol. Biol.* 8: 446–453, 1993.
6. Baraniuk, J.N., P.B. Silver, J.D. Lundgren, P. Cole, M.A. Kaliner, and P.J. Barnes. Bombesin stimulates human nasal mucous and serous cell secretion in vivo. *Am. J. Physiol.* 262: L48–52, 1992.
7. Barnes, P.J. Cytokines as mediators of chronic asthma. *Am. J. Respir. Crit. Care Med.* 150: S42–S49, 1994.
8. Battey, J. and E. Wada. Two distinct receptor subtypes for mammalian bombesin-like peptides. *Trends Neurosci.* 14: 524–528, 1991.
9. Blau, H.M. and D. Baltimore. Differentiation requires continuous regulation. *J. Cell Biol.* 112: 781–783, 1991.
10. Buckingham, S. and M.E. Avery. Time of appearance of lung surfactant in the fetal mouse. *Nature* 193: 688–689, 1962.
11. Bunn, P.A., D. Chan, J. Stewart, L. Gera, R. Tolley, P. Jewett, M. Tagawa, C. Alford, T. Mochzuki, and N. Yanaihara. Effects of neuropeptide analogues on calcium flux and proliferation in lung cancer cell lines. *Cancer Res.* 54: 3602–3610, 1994.
12. Caniggia, I., J. Lui, R. Han, S. Buch, K. Funa, K. Tanswell, and M. Post. Fetal lung epithelial

cells express receptors for platelet-derived growth factor. *Am. J. Respir. Cell Mol. Biol.* 9: 54–63, 1993.

13. Cho, T., W. Chan, and E. Cutz. Distribution and frequency of neuroepithelial bodies in post-natal rabbit lung: quantitative study with monoclonal antibody against serotonin. *Cell Tissue Res.* 255: 353–362, 1989.
14. Floros, J., H.C. Nielsen, and J.S. Torday. Dihydrotestosterone blocks fetal lung fibroblast-pneumonocyte factor at a pretranslational level. *J. Biol. Chem.* 262: 13592–13598, 1987.
15. Flowe, K.M., T.H. Welling, and M.W. Mulholland. Gastrin-releasing peptide stimulation of amylase release from rat pancreatic lobules involves intrapancreatic neurons. *Pancreas* 9: 513–517, 1994.
16. Fraslon, C. and J.R. Bourbon. Comparison of effects of epidermal and insulin-like growth factors, gastrin releasing peptide and retinoic acid on fetal lung cell growth and maturation in vitro. *Biochim. Biophysica Acta* 1123: 65–75, 1992.
17. Gallego, R., T. Garcia-Caballero, E. Roson, and A. Beiras. Neuroendocrine cells of the human lung express substance-P-like immunoreactivity. *Acta Anat.* 139: 278–282, 1990.
18. Ganju, R.K., M.E. Sunday, D.G. Tsarwhas, A. Card, and M.A. Shipp. The expression of CD10/NEP in non-small cell lung carcinomas: relationship to cellular proliferation. *J. Clin. Invest.* 94: 1784–1791, 1994.
19. Gatto, C., R.C. Lussky, L.W. Erickson, K.J. Berg, J.D. Wobken, and D.E. Johnson. Calcitonin and CGRP block bombesin- and substance P–induced increases in airway tone. *J. Appl. Physiol.* 66: 573–577, 1989.
20. Goldin, G.V. and L.A. Opperman. Induction of supernumerary tracheal buds and the stimulation of DNA synthesis in the embryonic chick lung and trachea by epidermal growth factor. *J. Embryol. Exp. Morphol.* 60: 235–243, 1980.
21. Gressens, P., J.M. Hill, I. Gozes, M. Fridkin, and D.E. Brenneman. Growth factor function of vasoactive intestinal peptide in whole cultured mouse embryos. *Nature* 362: 155, 1993.
22. Gross, I., S.A. Rooney, D.A. Smart, J.B. Warshaw, J.F. Sissom, S.B. Hoath, and D.W. Dynia. Influence of epidermal growth factor on fetal rat lung development in vitro. *Pediatr. Res.* 20: 473–477, 1986.
23. Haley, K., J. Drazen, R. Osathanondh, and M.E. Sunday. Comparison of the ontogeny of protein gene product 9.5, chromogranin A and proliferating cell nuclear antigen in human fetal lung . *Microsc. Res. Tech.* 37: 62–68, 1996.
24. Han, R.N.N., J. Liu, A.K. Tanswell, and M. Post. Expression of basic fibroblast growth factor and receptor: immunolocalization studies in developing rat fetal lung. *Pediatr. Res.* 31: 435–440, 1992.
25. Han, R.N.N., C. Mawdsley, P. Souza, A.K. Tanswell, and M. Post. Platelet-derived growth factors and growth-related genes in rat lung. III. Immunolocalization during fetal development. *Pediatr. Res.* 31: 323–329, 1992.
26. Haynesworth, S.E., M.A. Baber, and A.I. Caplan. Cytokine expression by human marrow–derived mesenchymal progenitor cells in vitro: effects of dexamethasone and IL-1 alpha. *J. Cell. Physiol.* 166: 585–592, 1996.
27. Hoyt, R.F., Jr., S.P. Sorokin, E.M. McDowell, and N.A. McNelly. Neuroepithelial bodies and growth of the airway epithelium in developing hamster lung. *Anat. Rec.* 236: 15–22, 1993.
28. Johnson, M.D., M.E. Gray, G. Carpenter, R.B. Pepinsky, and M.T. Stalhman. Ontogeny of epidermal growth factor receptor and lipocortin-1 in fetal and neonatal human lungs. *Hum. Pathol.* 21: 182–191, 1990.

29. Johnson, M.D., M.E. Gray, and M.T. Stahlman. Calcitonin gene-related peptide in human fetal lung and in neonatal lung disease. *J. Histochem. Cytochem.* 36: 199–204, 1988.
30. Karaplis, A.C., A. Luz, J. Glowacki, R.T. Bronson, V.L.J. Tybulewicz, H.M. Kronenberg, and R.C. Mulligan. Lethal skeletal dysplasia from targeted disruption of the parathyroid hormone-related peptide gene. *Genes Dev.* 8: 277–289, 1994.
31. Keegan, C.E., J.P. Herman, I.J. Karolyi, K.S. O'Shea, S.A. Camper, and A.F. Seasholtz. Differential expression of corticotropin-releasing hormone in developing mouse embryos and adult brain. *Endocrinology* 134: 2547–2555, 1994.
32. King, K.A., J. Hua, J.S. Torday, J.M. Drazen, S.A. Graham, M.A. Shipp and M.E. Sunday. CD10/neutral endopeptidase regulates fetal lung growth and maturation in utero by potentiating endogenous bombesin-like peptides. *J. Clin. Invest.* 91: 1969–1973, 1993.
33. King, K.A., J.S. Torday, and M.E. Sunday. Bombesin and [leu8]phyllolitorin promote fetal mouse lung branching morphogenesis via a specific receptor-mediated mechanism. *Proc. Natl. Acad. Sci. USA* 92: 4357–4361, 1995.
34. Korman, L.Y., D.N. Carney, M.L. Citron, and T.W. Moody. Secretin/vasoactive intestinal peptide-stimulated secretion of bombesin/gastrin releasing peptide from human small cell carcinoma of the lung. *Cancer Res.* 46: 1214–1218, 1986.
35. Kramer, S., F.H. Reynolds, JR., M. Castillo, D.M. Valenzuela, M. Thorikay, and J.M. Sorvillo. Immunological identification and distribution of parathyroid hormone-related protein polypeptides in normal and malignant tissues. *Endocrinology* 128: 1927–1937, 1991.
36. Lazarus, L.H., W.E. Wilson, G. Gaudino, B.J. Irons, and A. Guglietta. Evolutionary relationship between nonmammalian and mammalian peptides. *Peptides* 6: 295–307, 1985.
37. Lee, K., J.D. Deeds, and G.V. Segre. Expression of parathyroid hormone–related peptide and its receptor messenger ribonucleic acids during fetal development of rats. *Endocrinology* 136: 453–463, 1995.
38. Li, K., S.R. Nagalla, and E.R. Spindel. A rhesus monkey model to characterize the role of gastrin-releasing peptide (GRP) in lung development. *J. Clin. Invest.* 94: 1605–1615, 1994.
39. Liehr, R.M., S. Rosewicz, R.D. Reidelberger, and T.E. Solomon. Direct vs. indirect effects of bombesin on pancreatic growth. *Digestion* 46: 202–207, 1990.
40. Liu, J.P., J. Baker, A.S. Perkins, E.J. Robertson, and A. Efstratiadis. Mice carrying null mutations of the genes encoding insulin-like growth factor (IGF-1) and type 1 IGF receptor (IGF1R). *Cell* 75: 59–72, 1993.
41. Liu, M., J. Liu, S. Buch, K. Tanswell, and M. Post. Antisense oligonucleotides for PDGF-B and its receptor inhibit mechanical strain-induced fetal lung cell growth. *Am. Physiol. Soc.* L178–L184, 1995.
42. Lu, L. and C.D. Logsdon. CCK, bombesin, and carbachol stimulate c-*fos*, c-*jun*, and c-*myc* oncogene expression in rat pancreatic acini. *Am. J. Physiol.* 263: G327–332, 1992.
43. Mahmoud, S., J. Staley, J. Taylor, A. Bogden, J.P. Moreau, D. Coy, I. Avis, F. Cuttitta, J.L. Mulshine, and T.W. Moody. [$Psi^{13,14}$] bombesin analogues inhibit growth of small cell lung cancer in vitro and in vivo. *Cancer Res.* 51: 1798–1802, 1991.
44. Maneckjee, R. and J.D. Minna. Opioid and nicotine receptors affect growth regulation of human lung cancer cell lines. *Proc. Natl. Acad. Sci. USA* 87: 3294–3298, 1990.
45. Masui, A., N. Kato, T. Itoshima, K. Tsunashima, T. Nakajima, and N. Yanaihara. Scratching behavior induced by bombesin-related peptides. Comparison of bombesin, gastrin-releasing peptide and phyllolitorins. *Eur. J. Pharmacol.* 238: 297–301, 1993.

45a. McDonald, T.J. H. Jornvall, G. Nilsson, M. Vagne, M. Ghatei, S.R. Bloom, and V. Mutt. Characterization of a gastrin-releasing peptide from porcine non-antral gastric tissue. *Biochem. Biophys. Res. Commun.* 90: 227–233.

46. Miettinen, P.J., J.E. Berger, J. Meneses, Y. Phung, R.A. Pedersen, Z. Werb, and R. Derynck. Epithelial immaturity and multiorgan failure in mice lacking epidermal growth factor receptor. *Nature* 376: 337–341, 1995.

47. Moats-Staats, B.M., W.A. Price, L. Xu, W. Jarvis, and A.D. Stiles. Regulation of the insulin-like growth factor system during normal rat lung development. *Am. J. Respir. Cell Mol. Biol.* 12: 56–64, 1995.

48. Moody, T.W., F. Zia, M. Draoui, D.E. Brenneman, M. Fridkin, A. Davidson, and I. Gozes. A vasoactive intestinal peptide antagonist inhibits non-small cell lung cancer growth. *Proc. Natl. Acad. Sci. USA* 90: 4345–4349, 1993.

49. Muglia, L., L. Jacobson, P. Dikkes, and J. Majzoub. Corticotropin-releasing hormone deficiency reveals major fetal but not adult glucocorticoid need. *Nature* 373: 427–432, 1995.

50. Nelkin, B.D., K.Y. Chen, A. De Bustros, B.A. Roos, and S.B. Baylin. Changes in calcitonin gene RNA processing during growth of a human medullary thyroid carcinoma cell line. *Cancer Res.* 49: 6949–6952, 1989.

51. Nielsen, H.C. Androgen receptors influence the production of pulmonary surfactant in the testicular feminization mouse fetus. *J. Clin. Invest.* 76: 177–181, 1985.

52. Nunez, J.S. and J.S. Torday. Fetal rat lung type II cells and fibroblasts actively recruit surfactant substrate. *J. Nutrition* 125: 1639S–1644S, 1995.

53. Panos, R.J., J.S. Rubin, S.A. Aaronson, and R.J. Mason. Keratinocyte growth factor and hepatocyte growth factor/scatter factor are heparin-binding growth factors for alveolar type II cells in fibroblast-conditioned medium. *J. Clin. Invest.* 92: 969–977, 1993.

54. Peters, K., S. Werner, X. Liao, S. Wert, J. Whitsett, and L. Williams. Targeted expression of a dominant negative FGF receptor blocks branching morphogenesis and epithelial differentiation of the mouse lung. *EMBO J.* 13: 3296–3301, 1994.

55. Post, M., A. Barsoumian, and B.T. Smith. The cellular mechanism of glucocorticoid acceleration of fetal lung maturation: fibroblast-pneumonocyte factor stimulates cholinephosphate cytidylyltransferase activity. *J. Biol. Chem.* 261: 2179–2184, 1986.

56. Rettori, V., C.C. Pazos-Moura, E.G. Moura, J. Polak, and S.M. McCann. Role of neuromedin B in control of the release of thyrotropin in hypothyroid and hyperthyroid rats. *Proc. Natl. Acad. Sci. USA* 89: 3035–3039, 1992.

57. Rozengurt, E. Early signals in the mitogenic response. *Science* 234: 161–166, 1986.

58. Rubin, L., O. Kifor, J. Hua, E.M. Brown, and J.S. Torday. Parathyroid hormone (PTH) and PTH-related protein stimulate surfactant phospholipid synthesis in fetal rat lung, apparently by a mesenchymal-epithelial mechanism. *Biochim. Biophys. Acta* 1223: 91–100, 1994.

59. Ruff, M., E. Schiffmann, V. Terranova, and C.B. Pert. Neuropeptides are chemoattractants for human tumor cells and monocytes: a possible mechanism for metastasis. *Clin. Immunol. Immunopathol* 37: 387–396, 1985.

60. Schmid, W., T.J. Cole, J.A. Blendy, and G. Schutz. Molecular genetic analysis of glucocorticoid signalling in development. *J. Steroid Biochem. Mol. Biol.* 53: 33–35, 1995.

61. Sen, N. and M.H. Cake. Enhancement of disaturated phosphatidylcholine synthesis by epidermal growth factor in cultured fetal lung cells involves a fibroblast–epithelial cell interaction. *Am. J. Respir. Cell Mol. Biol.* 5: 337–343, 1991.

62. Shipp, M.A., G.B. Stefano, B. Scharrer, and E.L. Reinherz. CD10 (CALLA, common acute

lymphoblastic leukemia antigen)/neutral endopeptidase 24.11 (NEP, "enkephalinase"): molecular structure and role in regulating met-enkephalin mediated inflammatory responses. *Adv. Neuroimmunol.* 1: 139–149, 1991.

63. Shipp, M.A., G.E. Tarr, C.-Y. Chen, S.N. Switzer, L.B. Hersh, H. Stein, M.E. Sunday, and E.L. Reinherz. CD10/NEP hydrolyzes bombesin-like peptides and regulates the growth of small cell carcinomas of the lung. *Proc. Natl. Acad. Sci. USA* 88: 10662–10666, 1991.
64. Shoyab, M., G.D. Plowman, V.L. McDonald, J.G. Bradley, and G.J. Todaro. Structure and function of human amphiregulin: a member of the epidermal growth factor family. *Science* 243: 1074–1076, 1989.
65. Sibilia, M. and E.F. Wagner. Strain-dependent epithelial defects in mice lacking the EGF receptor [published erratum appears in Science 269: 909]. *Science* 269: 234–238, 1995.
66. Simonet, W.S., M.L. Derose, N. Bucay, H.Q. Nguyen, S.E. Wert, L. Zhou, T.R. Ulich, A. Thomason, D.M. Danilenko, and J.A. Whitsett. Pulmonary malformation in transgenic mice expressing human keratinocyte growth factor in the lung. *Proc. Natl. Acad. Sci. USA* 92: 12461–12465, 1995.
67. Smith, B.T. Lung maturation in the fetal rat: acceleration by injection of fibroblast-pneumonocyte factor. *Science* 204: 1094–1095, 1979.
68. Smith, B.T. and M. Post. The influence of hormones on fetal lung development. In: *Maternal-Fetal Endocrinology,* edited by D. Tulchinsky, and A.B. Little. Philadelphia: W.B. Saunders, 1994, p. 365–378.
69. Souza, P., M. Kuliszewski, J. Wang, I. Tseu, A.K. Tanswell, and M. Post. PDGF-AA and its receptor influence early lung branching via an epithelial–mesenchymal interaction. *Development* 121: 2559–2567, 1995.
70. Souza, P., L. Sedlackova, M. Kuliszewski, J. Wang, J. Liu, I. Tseu, M. Liu, A.K. Tanswell, and M. Post. Antisense oligodeoxynucleotides targeting PDGF-B mRNA inbibit cell proliferation during embryonic rat lung development. *Development* 120: 2163–2173, 1994.
71. Spiers, V., E. Bienkowski, V. Wong, and E. Cutz. Paracrine effects of bombesin/gastrin-releasing peptide and other growth factors on pulmonary neuroendocrine cells in vitro. *Anat. Rec.* 236: 53–61, 1993.
72. Spindel, E.R., M.E. Sunday, H. Hofler, H.J. Wolfe, J.F. Habener, and W.W. Chin. Transient elevation of mRNAs encoding gastrin-releasing peptide (GRP), a putative pulmonary growth factor, in human fetal lung. *J. Clin. Invest.* 80: 1172–1179, 1987.
73. Springall, D.R., S.R. Bloom, and J.M. Polak. Neural, endocrine, and endothelial regulatory peptides. In: *The Lung: Scientific Foundations,* edited by R.G. Crystal, J.B. West, P.J. Barnes, N.S. Cherniak, and E.R. Weibel. New York: Raven Press, 1991, p. 69–90.
74. Stahlman, M.T. and M.E. Gray. Colocalization of peptide hormones in neuroendocrine cells of human fetal and newborn lungs: an electron microscopic study. *Anat. Rec.* 236: 206–212, 1993.
75. Stahlman, M.T., A.G. Kasselberg, D.N. Orth, and M.E. Gray. Ontogeny of neuroendocrine cells in human fetal lung: II. An immunohistochemical study. *Lab. Invest.* 52: 52–60, 1985.
76. Stahlman, M.T., D.N. Orth, and M.E. Gray. Immunocytochemical localization of epidermal growth factor in the developing human respiratory system and in acute and chronic lung disease in the neonate. *Lab. Invest.* 60: 539–547, 1989.
77. Stiles, A.D. and A.J. D'Ercole. The insulin-like growth factors and the lung. *Am. J. Respir. Cell Mol. Biol.* 3: 93–100, 1990.
78. Strandjord, T.P., J.G. Clark, W.A. Hodson, R.A. Schmidt, and D.K. Madtes. Expression of

transforming growth factor-α in mid-gestation human fetal lung. *Am. J. Respir. Cell Mol. Biol.* 8: 266–272, 1993.

79. Sunday, M.E., J. Hua, H.B. Dai, A. Nusrat, and J.S. Torday. Bombesin increases fetal lung growth and maturation in utero and in organ culture. *Am. J. Respir. Cell Mol. Biol.* 3: 199–205, 1990.
80. Sunday, M.E., J. Hua, B. Reyes, H. Masui, and J.S. Torday. Anti-bombesin antibodies modulate fetal mouse lung growth and maturation in utero and in organ cultures. *Anat. Rec.* 236: 25–32, 1993.
81. Sunday, M.E., J. Hua, J. Torday, B. Reyes, and M.A. Shipp. CD10/neutral endopeptidase 24.11 in developing human fetal lung: patterns of expression and modulation of peptide-mediated proliferation. *J. Clin. Invest.* 90: 2517–2525, 1992.
82. Sunday, M.E., L.M. Kaplan, E. Motoyama, W.W. Chin, and E.R. Spindel. Biology of disease: gastrin-releasing peptide (mammalian bombesin) gene expression in health and disease. *Lab. Invest.* 59: 5–24, 1988.
83. Threadgill, D.W., A.A. Dlugosz, L.A. Hansen, T. Tennenbaum, U. Lichti, D. Yee, C. Lamantia, T. Mourton, K. Herrup, and R.C. Harris. Targeted disruption of mouse EGF receptor: effect of genetic background on mutant phenotype. *Science* 269: 230–234, 1995.
84. Torday, J., J. Hua, and R. Slavin. Metabolism and fate of neutral lipids of fetal lung fibroblast origin. *Biochim. Biophys. Acta* 1254: 198–206, 1995.
85. Torday, J.S. Dihydrotestosterone inhibits fibroblast-pneumonocyte factor mediated synthesis of saturated phosphatidylcholine by fetal rat lung cells. *Biochim. Biophys. Acta* 835: 23–28, 1985.
86. Torday, J.S. and S. Kourembanas. Fetal rat lung fibroblasts produce a TGFbeta homolog that blocks alveolar type II cell maturation. *Dev. Biol.* 139: 35–41, 1990.
87. Wada, C., C. Hashimoto, T. Kameya, K. Yamaguchi, and M. Ono. Developmentally regulated expression of the calcitonin gene related peptide (CGRP) in rat lung endocrine cells. *Virchows Arch. B. Cell Pathol.* 55: 217–223, 1988.
88. Wada, E., J. Battey, and S. Wray. Bombesin receptor gene expression in rat embryos: transient GRP-R gene expression in the posterior pituitary. *Mol. Cell. Neurosci.* 4: 13–24, 1993.
89. Wang, D., H. Yeger, and E. Cutz. Expression of gastrin releasing peptide receptor gene in developing lung. *Am. J. Respir. Cell Mol. Biol.* 14: 409–416, 1996.
90. Wang, J., M. Kuliszewski, W. Yee, L. Sedlackova, J. Xu, I. Tseu, and M. Post. Cloning and expression of glucocorticoid-induced genes in fetal rat lung fibroblasts: transforming growth factor-β3. *J. Biol. Chem.* 270: 2722–2728, 1995.
91. Warburton, D., R. Seth, L. Shum, P.G. Horcher, F.L. Hall, Z. Werb and H.C. Slavkin. Epigenetic role of epidermal growth factor expression and signalling in embryonic mouse lung morphogenesis. *Dev. Biol.* 149: 123–133, 1992.
92. Wharton, J., J.M. Polak, S.R. Bloom, M.A. Ghatei, E. Solcia, M.R. Brown, and A.G.E. Pearse. Bombesin-like immunoreactivity in the lung. *Nature* 273: 769–770, 1978.
93. White, S.R., M.B. Hershenson, K.S. Sigrist, A. Zimmermann, and J. Solway. Proliferation of guinea pig tracheal epithelial cells induced by calcitonin gene-related peptide. *Am. J. Respir. Cell Mol. Biol.* 8: 592–596, 1993.
94. Whitsett, J.A., T.E. Weaver, M.A. Lieberman, J.C. Clark, and C. Daugherty. Differential effects of epidermal growth factor and transforming growth factor-beta on synthesis of Mr = 35,000 surfactant associated protein in fetal lung. *J. Biol. Chem.* 262: 7908–7913, 1987.

95. Wuenschell, C.W., M.E. Sunday, G. Singh, P. Minoo, H.C. Slavkin, and D. Warburton. Embryonic mouse lung epithelial progenitor cells co-express immunohistochemical markers of diverse mature cell lineages. *J. Histochem. Cytochem.* 44: 113–123, 1996.
96. Yasui, S., A. Nagai, A. Oohira, M. Iwashita, and K. Konno. Effects of anti-mouse EGF antiserum on prenatal lung development in fetal mice. *Pediatr. Pulmonol.* 15: 251–256, 1993.
97. Zetler, G. Antagonism of the gut-contracting effects of bombesin and neurotensin by opioid peptides, morphine, atropine or tetrodotoxin. *Pharmacology* 21: 348–354, 1980.

chapter 12

TRANSGENIC MODELS OF LUNG DEVELOPMENT AND DISEASE

Thomas R. Korfhagen and Jeffrey A. Whitsett

FORMATION of the lung requires the ordered control of cell proliferation and differentiation that are mediated by a myriad of autocrine and paracrine signals. Intracellular signaling controls cellular proliferation, migration, differentiation, and matrix deposition through complex networks of growth factors and their receptors. Growth factor signaling through interactions among specific cell surface receptors, in turn, controls gene expression. While in vitro cellular and biochemical studies are useful for identifying molecular detail of signaling pathways and control of gene expression, in vivo studies are useful in further defining precise molecular events controlling formation of the lung. The complex intracellular and intercellular events involved in normal lung development are thought to be recapitulated in recovery from lung injury, underscoring the importance of deciphering the complex pathways regulating pulmonary morphogenesis. This chapter focuses on studies of critical molecular pathways regulating the growth and differentiation of the respiratory epithelium using transgenic mouse models in vivo.

TRANSGENIC MODELING

Transgenic technology involves methods for mutating the genome in intact animals. Mutations can elicit gain or loss of physiologic function. This chapter reviews the most widely used methodologies for introducing mutations that affect respiratory function (Table 12.1). Although transgenic models can be produced in a variety of species, mice have been most widely used for research purposes. Mice have a number

Table 12.1 Comparison of Transgenic Models

Transgenic Model	*Mechanism*	*Outcome*
Gain of function: transgenes	DNA inserts randomly; levels of expression vary with position effects	Phenotype usually detectable in heterozygotes and homozygotes
Loss of function: gene targeting	DNA inserts at a specific locus; generates a null mutation	Phenotype often detectable only in homozygotes
Loss of function: dominant/negative	DNA inserts randomly: levels of expression vary with position effects	Requires high level expression to block function; may be active in heterozygotes or homozygotes

of practical advantages for transgenic studies. Their small size reduces cost of housing and their relative fecundity, and extensive knowledge of mouse genetics, husbandry, and reproductive biology permits rapid generation and analysis of animals needed for experimental purposes. Although the mouse may differ in some physiologic parameters from other species, principles derived from mouse models can be readily applied to larger animals or humans.

Gain of Function

Most gain-of-function studies are performed by introducing a transgene into fertilized mouse eggs. A typical transgene consists of a promoter, a cDNA or minigene encoding the desired gene of interest, and transcription termination sequences. The double-stranded DNA of the transgene is directly microinjected into the male pronucleus of recently fertilized mouse eggs. The microinjection requires micromanipulators and mechanical injectors and is performed under direct vision via light microscopy. Injected oocytes are transferred to the uterine horn of surrogate dams where they implant and undergo normal growth and development. After microinjection, 20%–30% of the offspring bear the inserted transgene, usually inserted in a single position in the mouse genome. The offspring, termed founders, are bred, transmitting the transgene to their offspring, thereby producing founder transgenic lines. Inserted transgenes are usually arranged as concatamers in a head-to-tail manner, with copy numbers varying from less than one to hundreds. Because insertion of the transgenic DNA occurs randomly, transgenes may occasionally interrupt other genes, creating insertional mutations. Sometimes these mutants disrupt normal development, confounding the analysis of the phenotype produced by the transgene. Levels of transgene expression may be influenced by other *cis*-active elements located near the site of insertion. Alternatively, the transgene may be relatively inactive because of its random insertion into inactive chromatin domains. Either of these influences is termed a *position effect*. It may be necessary to analyze multiple transgenic founder lines to discriminate experimental artifacts resulting from insertional mutations from the influence of the protein derived from the inserted transgene.

Since the sites of integration and copy numbers may influence the level of transgene expression, analysis of independent transgenic founder lines, varying in levels of transgene expression, is important in assessing the biological outcome of the experiment. Transgenic offspring are generally identified in the first weeks of life using Southern blot techniques, or polymerase chain reaction (PCR), with probes specific for the inserted gene. Transgenes generated by this methodology are often active in heterozygotes, although transgenic offspring can usually be bred to homozygosity. In some experiments, mice are maintained as inbred strains to minimize heterogeneity of phenotype due to genetic background (Table 12.1).

Transcriptional Control and Design of Transgenes

Expression of eukaryotic genes is controlled primarily at the level of gene transcription. *Cis*-acting elements are functional regions of genomic DNA that bind nuclear proteins. Interaction between *trans*-acting nuclear proteins and *cis*-active sites alters the structure of DNA near the start site of transcription, making it more accessible to RNA polymerase II, enhancing the synthesis of a primary RNA transcript. *Cis*-active elements may include proximal promoter elements, generally located near the start of transcription and often including CCAAT or TATA sequences and other ubiquitous *cis*-active sites that interact with nuclear proteins to regulate gene transcription. Enhancers are *cis*-active elements that act independently of position or orientation to regulate the level of transcription. Although often located near the start site of transcription, enhancers may be located within the gene or even at great distances from the locus. Complex interactions between enhancers and promoters provide the correct temporal–spatial signals required to control mRNA production. There is an increasingly complex array of nuclear transcription factors that are being identified that interact with *cis*-active sites to enhance or inhibit transcription of genes in eukaryotes.

Enhancer and promoter elements and associated *trans*-acting nuclear proteins that regulate respiratory epithelial cell gene expression have recently been identified. *Cis*-active elements from the human surfactant protein-C (SP-C) gene have been widely used to generate transgenic mice in studies of lung development (42). Examples of such transgene constructs are presented in Figure 12.1.

Lung Development and Developmental Expression of SP-C Transgenes

Organogenesis requires interactions of epithelial- and mesenchymal-derived cells and matrix to control cellular proliferation, migration, adhesion, and differentiation (3). Wessels (41) and recently Shannon (35) used tissue recombination experiments, wherein proximal and distal epithelium and mesenchyme were exchanged, to prove that the underlying mesenchyme is required for normal lung epithelial cell differentiation. Although these studies demonstrate the significance of epithelial–mesenchymal interactions ex vivo, transgenic studies are needed to decipher the molecular signals in vivo. Budding of the foregut endoderm into the surrounding mesenchyme initiates lung development on day 9–10 of an 18- to 21-day gestation. The initial buds undergo branching morphogenesis associated with concomitant differentiation

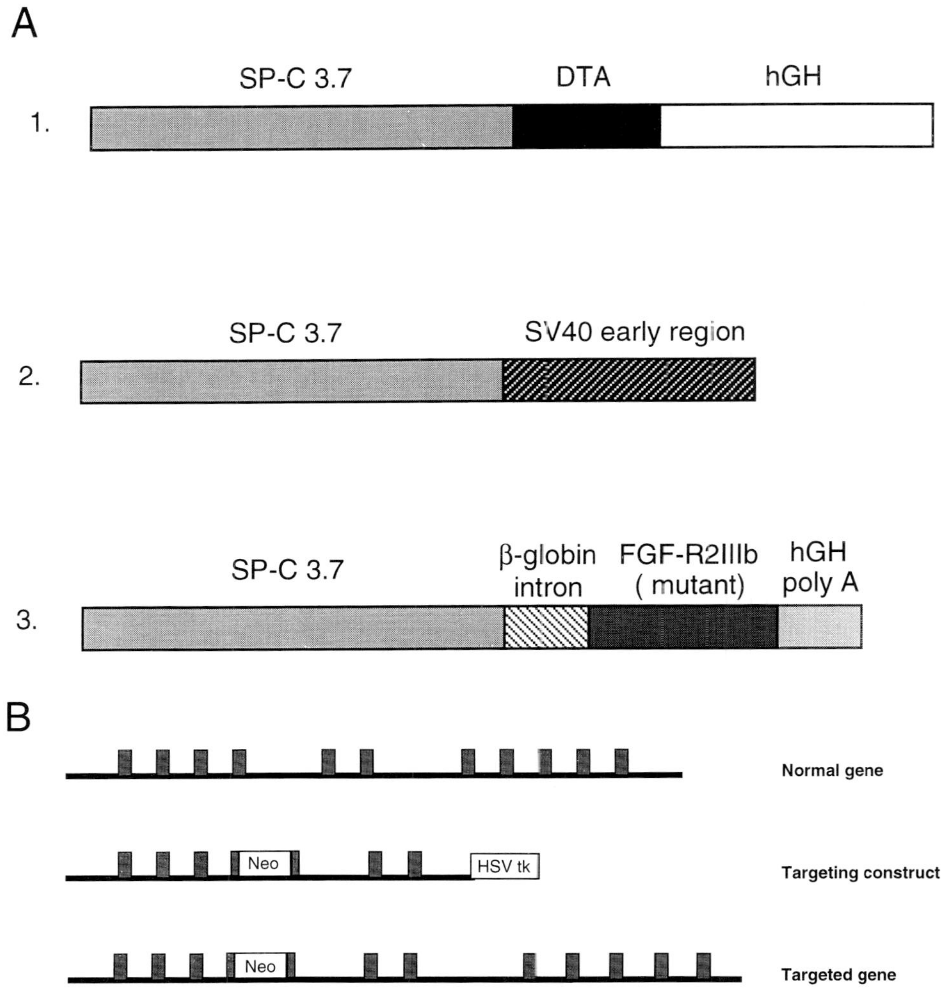

Fig. 12.1 Schematic representation of transgene constructs. (*A*) *1.* SP-C-DTA: The gene encoding bacterial diphtheria toxin A (*DTA*) was cloned downstream of the human 3.7 SP-C gene promoter/enhancer sequences (*SP-C 3.7*). A portion of the human growth hormone gene was cloned to provide correct splicing and termination sequences (*hGH*) (25). *2.* SP-C-T antigen: The SV40 early region encoding the large T antigen and correct splicing and termination signals was cloned downstream of SP-C 3.7 (44). *3.* SP-C-FGF-R2 IIIb (mutant): a kinase domain truncated region of human FGF-R2 IIIb [*FGF-R2 IIIb* (*mutant*)] was cloned downstream of SP-C 3.7. Intron and poly A addition sequences were cloned from the β-globin gene (*β-globin intron*) or from the human growth hormone gene (*hGH poly A*) to provide correct splicing and termination signals (31). (*B*) Schematic representation of targeting strategy to generate SP-B-deficient mice (9). A portion of the normal mouse SP-B gene (normal gene) was used to construct the targeting construct. The bacterial neomycin-resistance gene (*Neo*) was cloned into the fourth exon. The herpes simplex virus thymidine kinase gene (*HSV-tk*) was cloned downstream of exon 6. The targeting construct recombined by homologous recombination with the normal gene to replace exon 4 with the disrupted fourth exon (targeted gene). The HSV-tk gene was lost in the recombination event. The targeted gene was confirmed by Southern blot analysis and homozygous mice lacked SP-B (9).

of the epithelium and mesenchyme to form the conducting airways and terminal gas exchange region necessary for respiration at birth (36). The morphologic features typical of distinct stages in lung development are shared across many species. Four distinct stages of lung morphogenesis are recognized and termed the *pseudoglandular, canalicular, saccular* (prenatal), and *alveolar* phases (postnatal). Mice are born in the saccular phase rapidly initiating alveolarization by day 2 postnatally. The endogenous SP-C gene is expressed very early in the respiratory epithelium and is expressed exclusively in type II cells and the alveolus of the adult lung (13, 40). Thus the regulatory region of the SP-C gene was considered ideal for generating transgenic mice in which genes or cDNAs could be directed to the respiratory epithelium throughout development.

Studies with the bacterial CAT reporter gene were used to determine the developmental spatial and temporal pattern of expression of human SP-C-derived transgenes in transgenic mice. Approximately 3.7 kb of the 5′-flanking region, including the endogenous transcription start site, contained enhancer and promoter sequences that directed gene expression exclusively in lung epithelial cells and not in other cells or organs. Expression of SP-C-CAT transgenes was first detected in the lung buds on gestation day 10, during the early pseudoglandular period (Fig. 12.2). Expression was confined to the developing distal respiratory epithelium throughout the prenatal period. During postnatal alveolarization and in the adult, transgene expression was detected in bronchiolar epithelial and in type II alveolar epithelial cells (40). The 3.7 SP-C kb human enhancer/promoter sequences were subject to positional effects, leading to transgenic mouse lines that express distinct levels of CAT activity. Offspring from each transgenic line inherit lung cell–specific expression and the level of expression typical of that line and pass the transgene to their offspring.

Cell Ablation: Identification of Progenitor Cells—SP-C-DTA Mice

The temporal and spatial appearance of progenitor cells of the distal epithelium were studied by producing mice expressing the diphtheria toxin A (DTA) gene under control of the surfactant protein C gene promoter (Fig. 12.1). DTA inhibits protein synthesis within cells by a process of ADP-ribosylation of elongation factor-2. Cell death occurs with even low-level DTA expression ablating the cell and causing loss of descendant cells (11). The more severely affected SP-C-DTA transgenic mice died immediately postnatally as they failed to expand their lungs at birth, so analysis was confined to founder mice. The most severely affected lungs lacked development of type II or type I cells; the lungs of one founder consisted of two saccules lined by an immature cuboidal epithelium, and they lacked normal mesenchymal tissues but had morphologically normal trachea (25). The transgenic model demonstrated that progenitor cells of the distal lung parenchyma are committed early in lung development, and distinct subsets of proximal (tracheal) and distal respiratory cells are differentiated along distinct pathways as early as the SP-C promoter is expressed in the pseudoglandular period. The structural features of the lungs from SP-C-DTA mice support the concept that growth and differentiation of pulmonary mesenchyme require interactions with the developing respiratory epithelium.

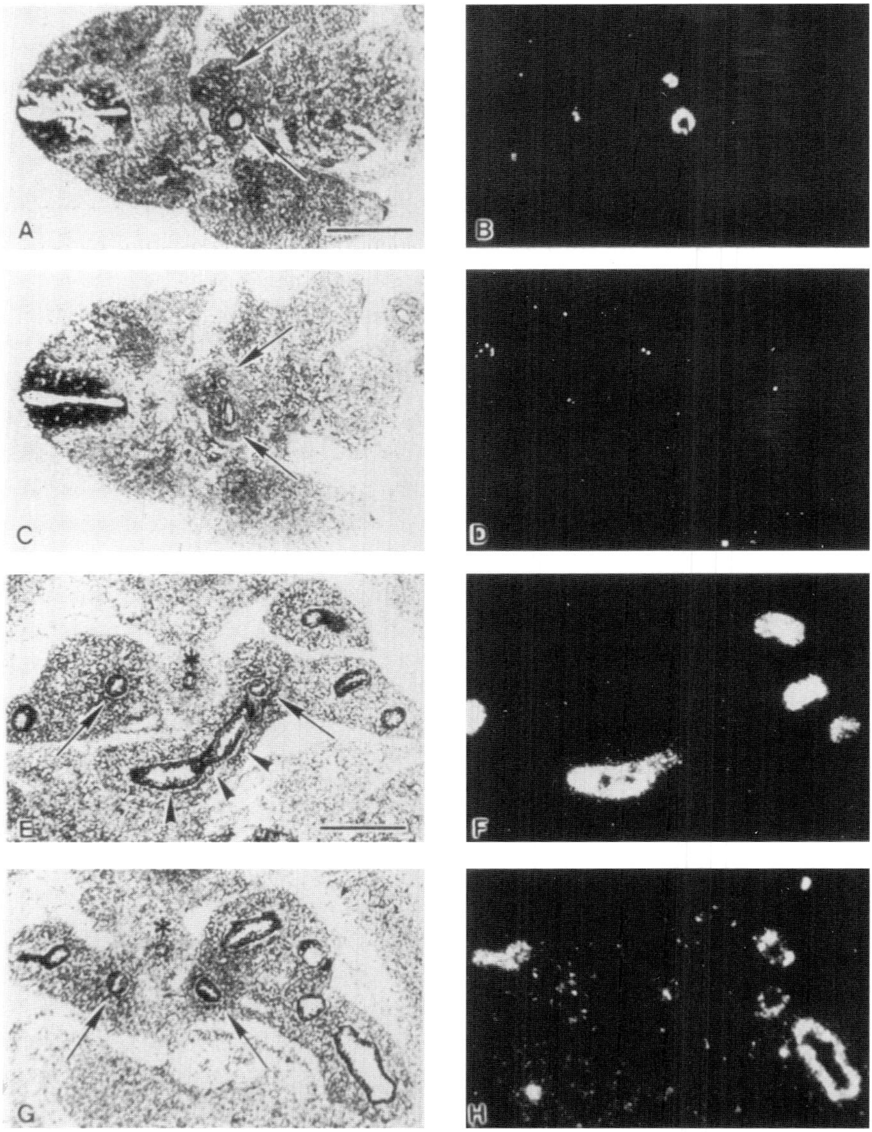

Fig. 12.2 SP-C transgene expression in the developing lung. To determine the spatial and temporal expression of SP-C transgenes in the developing lungs, SP-C-CAT transgenic mice were generated. In situ hybridization was used to determine the cellular sites of transgene expression with the CAT probe. The cellular sites of expression of the mouse SP-C transgene were detected by in situ hybridization with a probe for the mouse SP-C gene. The left column shows bright-field photomicrographs corresponding to the dark-field micrographs (right column) showing in situ signals. Mid-thoracic sections of gestation day 10 fetal mice (*A–D*) contained lung buds (*arrow*) that were positive for the CAT transgene (*B*) but not the endogenous SP-C gene (*D*). The transgene was expressed earlier in development than the endogenous mouse SP-C gene. Mid-thoracic sections of gestation day 11 fetal mice (*E-H*) contained more extensive branching tubules (*arrows*) that were positive for both the CAT transgene (*F*) and the endogenous SP-C gene (*H*). *Arrowheads* mark a developing secondary bronchus. The transgene overlapped expression of the endogenous SP-C in the distal epithelium from gestational day 11 to birth (40). Bar = 250 μm. *Asterisk* designates the esophagus. [Used by permission (40).]

Lung Tumors Formed in SP-C T Antigen Transgenic Mice

Wikenheiser et al. used gain-of-function transgenic studies to generate lung tumors (44). The human SP-C promoter was used to drive expression of SV40 large T antigen in transgenic mice (Fig. 12.1). Mice expressing the SP-C-T antigen mRNA developed pulmonary tumors during the postnatal period (Fig. 12.3). The morphology of the tumors was typical of pulmonary adenocarcinoma consisting of papillary, lepidic, and solid tumor types. In vivo, most of the tumor cells expressed CCSP (Clara cell secretory protein), a marker of bronchiolar epithelial cells. Some tumor cells expressed SP-C, a marker of type II cells; however, cells expressing both SP-C and CCSP were not readily detected (44, 46). Clonal cell lines (termed *mouse lung epithelial cells* or MLE cells) were produced from the SP-C-T antigen tumors (45). In vitro, MLE cells expressed a variable pattern of respiratory epithelial cell–specific mRNAs, including SP-A, SP-B, and SP-C but not CCSP. SP-A and SP-B are normally synthesized by both bronchiolar epithelial and type II cells. When MLE-15 cells were used to produce tumors in nude mice, most of the cells expressed CCSP but not SP-C (46). In vitro, MLE-15 cells expressed SP-C, -A, and -B but not CCSP. Thus expression of marker genes by MLE-15 cells varied with culture conditions, demonstrating the pluripotency of MLE cell differentiation along bronchiolar and alveolar pathways. Gene expression by MLE cells was controlled by the environmental milieu in which the cells were grown.

Loss of Function: Dominant/Negative Transgenes

Loss of gene function in vivo can be achieved by the insertion of a transgene encoding a gene product that acts in a dominant-negative manner to inhibit or reduce the function of a specific gene product. For example, receptor tyrosine kinases are widely studied systems in which dominant-negative mutations can be used to disrupt receptor-mediated signalling in vivo. Studies of the epidermal growth factor receptor (EGFR) have been used to decipher the molecular mechanism of dominant-negative activity (14, 18, 34). Tyrosine kinase receptors contain distinct extracellular ligand-binding, transmembrane, and intracellular kinase domains. Ligand binding induces receptor dimerization that is required for autophosphorylation and subsequent signal transduction. Deletion of the intracellular domain of tyrosine kinase–dependent receptors produces a membrane-bound receptor capable of ligand binding but lacking kinase activity. When the wild-type receptor dimerizes with a mutated receptor, both kinase activity and signal transduction are inhibited. The interaction of the dominant-negative molecule with the normal one generally requires high-level expression to increase the likelihood of forming a wild-type mutant dimer. This system has an advantage over gene targeting (described later in this chapter) in that loss of function can be readily generated in subsets of cells rather than in all cells in the mouse (Table 12.1).

Role of the Fibroblast Growth Factor Receptor System in Lung Morphogenesis: SP-C-FGF-R (mutant) Transgenic Mice

Since epithelial–mesenchymal interactions are known to be critical in normal lung development, growth factors produced by mesenchyme are likely to provide critical

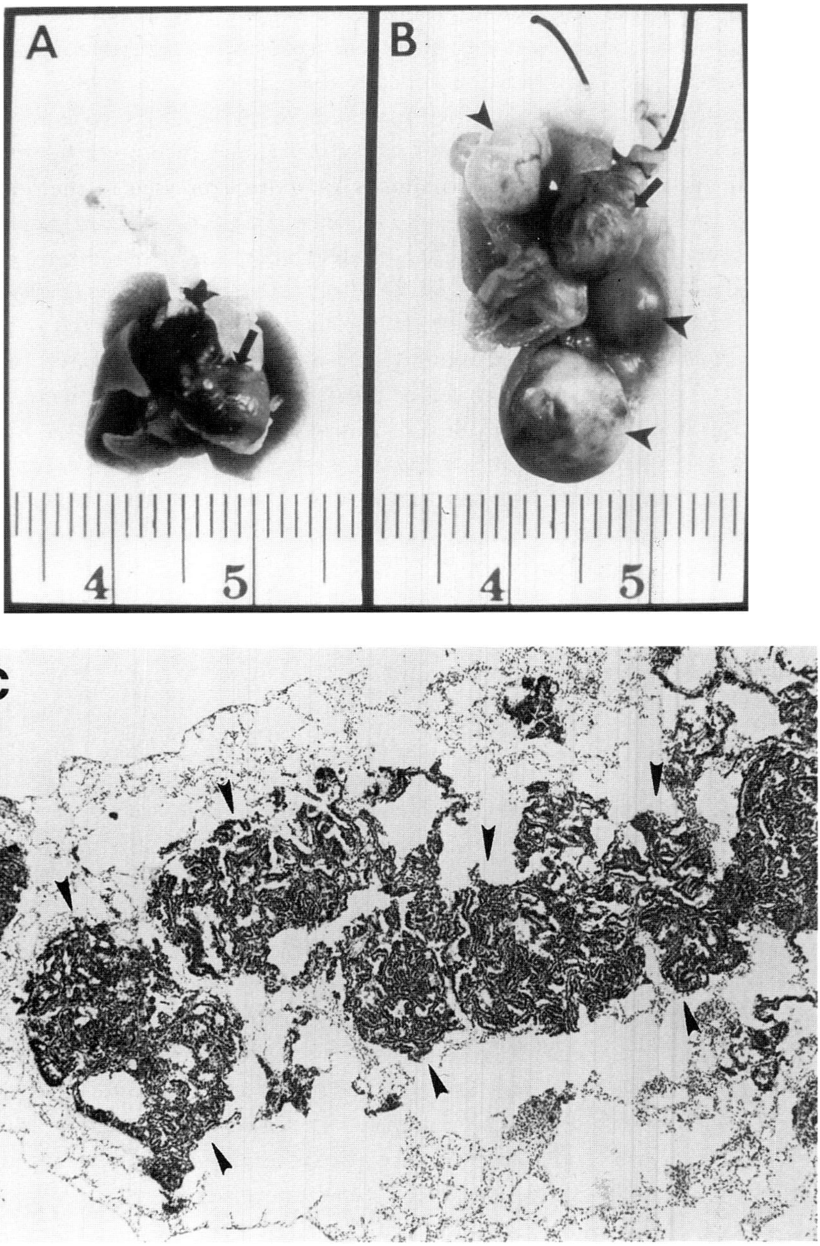

Fig. 12.3 SP-C-T antigen transgenic mice. To generate a model of lung epithelial tumorigenesis, transgenic mice were generated expressing SV40 large T antigen under control of the human SP-C promoter/enhancer (SP-C-T antigen) (44). Lungs of adult normal mice (*A*) were smaller than lungs of SP-C-T antigen mice (*B*). Hearts (*arrow*) were unaffected. Tumor nodules (*arrowheads*) were readily apparent in the SP-C-T antigen transgenics. Sections of transgenic lungs (*C*) revealed pulmonary adenocarcinomas (*arrowheads*). Mouse lung epithelial cells were cloned from tumor nodules [A and B used by permission (44).].

signals required for epithelial cell proliferation and differentiation associated with branching morphogenesis of the lung. While a variety of polypeptide hormones influence epithelial cell proliferation and expression of differentiation markers in vitro (23, 27), recent studies support an important role of the fibroblast growth factor receptors and ligands, acidic FGF, FGF-10, and keratinocyte growth factor (KGF). Acidic FGF (FGF-I), KGF (FGF-VII), and FGF-10 are expressed in the developing pulmonary mesenchyme (2, 12, 26). The FGF receptor (FGF-R2) is expressed at high levels in developing respiratory epithelial cells throughout prenatal lung morphogenesis (32). The FGF receptors are tyrosine kinases. Ligand binding causes dimerization and autophosphorylation of the cytoplasmic domain of the receptor, leading to an activation signal that alters proliferation and differentiation of cells. Null mutations in FGF receptors are often lethal early in embryonic development, prior to lung formation, making it impossible to study lung development in these mice. The role of FGF receptor signaling in lung development in vivo was determined by lung cell–specific expression of a dominant-negative FGF receptor in the developing respiratory epithelium (31). The receptor FGF-R2 IIIb was mutated by deletion of a major portion of the intracytoplasmic domain (Fig. 12.1). Since this receptor mediates FGF-I and VII signaling, cells expressing the mutant have signaling reduced or blocked from both growth factors. Transgenic mice expressing the mutated FGF-R2 under control of the 3.7 kb SP-C promoter/enhancer succumbed in the immediate perinatal period from respiratory distress. The lungs of the SP-C-FGF-R (mutant) transgenic mice consisted of a normal-appearing trachea and mainstem bronchi that ended in blind sacs. Pulmonary parenchyma, bronchioles, and alveolar regions were entirely lacking in some of the mice (Fig. 12.4). Expression of cell markers typical of the respiratory epithelium in the proximal airway, e.g., CCSP, were expressed in the bronchiolar epithelium of the mice bearing the mutated FGF receptor. Mesenchymal-derived components were also lacking in the lungs of the severely affected mice, further supporting the concept that epithelial–mesenchymal interactions are required for pulmonary morphogenesis. Expression of the FGF-R2b dominant-negative transgene blocked proliferation of a subset of progenitor cells distinct from those that form the trachea and bronchi. These findings support the observations made in the cell ablation studies in the SP-C-DTA transgenic mice, supporting the concept that progenitor cells of the respiratory epithelium are committed to distinct proximal and distal lineages early in the pseudoglandular period of lung development and signaling through FGF-R2b is required for development.

Transcriptional Control of Lung-specific Genes

With the recognition that formation of the pulmonary parenchyma is initiated by a small subset of epithelial cells during embryonic lung development, it has become of increasing interest to identify the genes controlling respiratory epithelial cell growth and differentiation. A typical molecular approach is to identify the *cis*- and *trans*-acting factors of lung cell specific differentiation genes and to identify the *cis* and *trans* control of transcriptional proteins that regulate differentiation genes. This

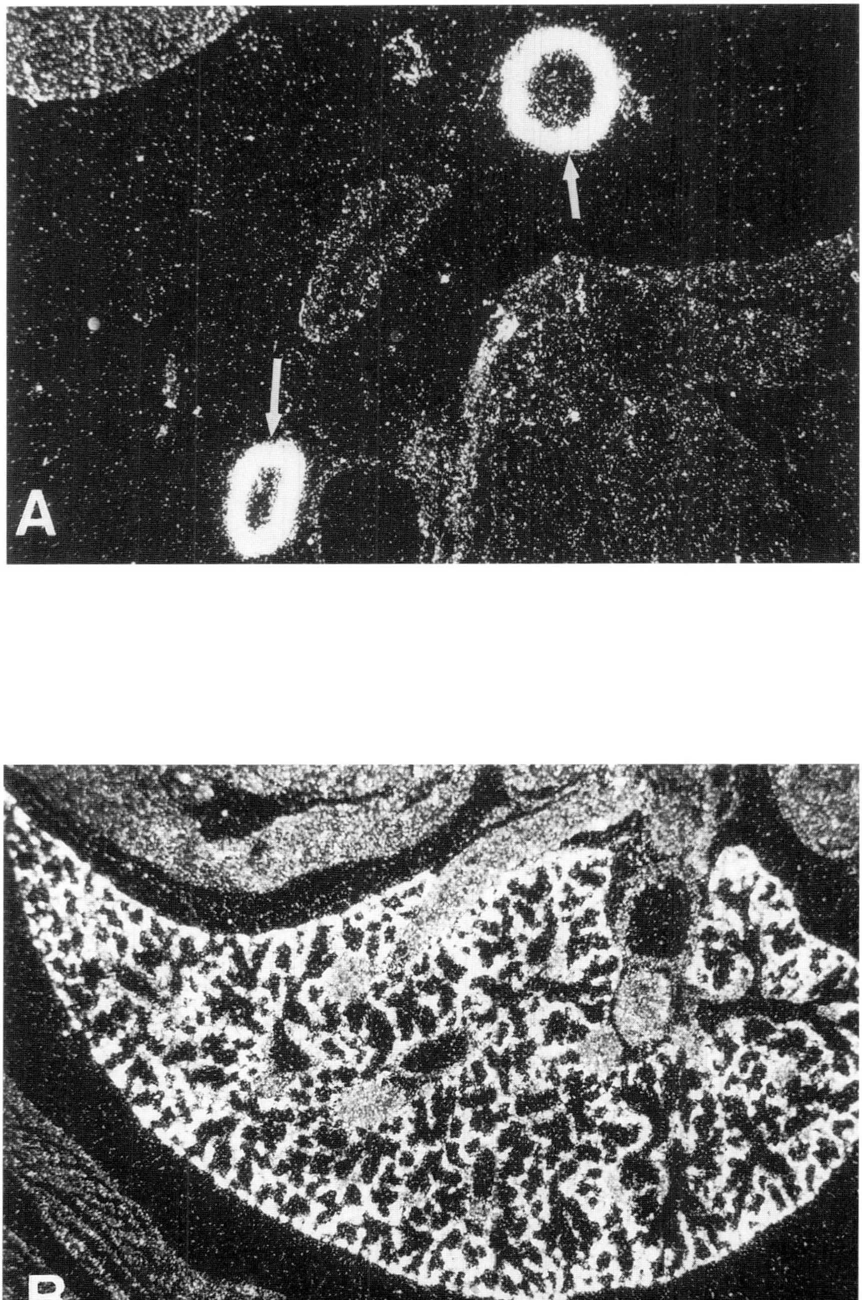
A
B

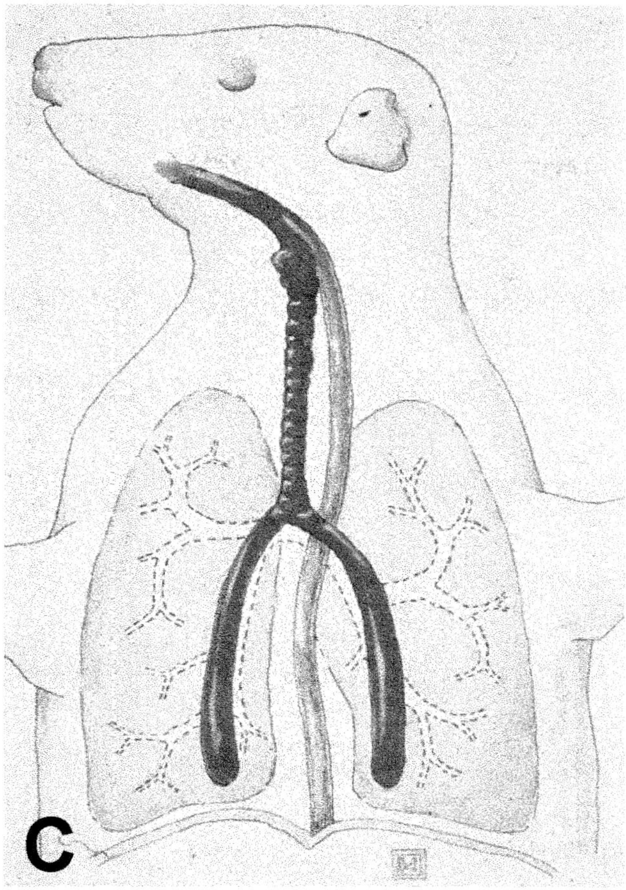

Fig. 12.4 Lungs of SP-C-FGF-R2 IIIb (mutant) mice. To determine whether signaling through the FGF-R2 IIIb receptor was critical for normal lung development, Peters et al. (31) used a dominant-negative FGF receptor to block normal signaling. The FGF-R2 IIIb receptor was deleted for the intracytoplasmic domains [FGF-R2 IIIb (mutant)] and used to generate transgenic mice with the human SP-C promoter/enhancer [SP-C-FGF-R2 IIIb (mutant)]. SP-C-FGF-R2 IIIb (mutant) mice succumbed at term. A transverse section at mid-chest contained only bronchial tubes (*A*) (facing page). The bronchial tubes were identified by in situ hybridization with the CCSP cDNA (*arrow*). A transverse mid-chest section of a normal term mouse reveals normal lung (*B*) (facing page) identified by in situ hybridization with SP-C cDNA. The residual lung tissue of an SP-C-FGF-R2 IIIb (mutant) contained a trachea, two blind ending bronchi, but no distal epithelial cells or mesenchymal derivatives (*C*). [C was used by permission (31).]

approach has been useful in deciphering hierarchies of genes regulating differentiation and gene expression of many tissues including the lung.

Surfactant proteins A, B, and C (SP-A, SP-B, SP-C) are expressed exclusively in the lung epithelium. SP-A provides innate immunity and protection of surfactant from protein inactivation (24, 28, 33, 37, 47). SP-B and SP-C are hydrophobic proteins required for surfactant function by affecting structure and function of lipid bilayers and facilitating surface activity of phospholipids (17, 21, 30, 39). SP-B and SP-C are first detected in the developing epithelium of the pseudoglandular period, while SP-A is first detected in the developing epithelium of the canalicular period. In the adult, SP-A and SP-B are expressed in bronchiolar and type II cells whereas SP-C is expressed exclusively in type II cells. Studies in vitro of the transcriptional control of SP-A, -B, and -C genes have led to identification of the hierarchy of gene expression controlling lung cell differentiation.

The SP-B Gene as a Model of Respiratory Epithelial Cell Gene Expression

Transcriptional control of the SP-B gene served as a useful paradigm in elucidating transcriptional control of genes expressed selectively in the respiratory epithelium. In the adult lung, SP-B is expressed in nonciliated bronchiolar and alveolar type II cells. Initial identification of the transcriptional control regions of the SP-B gene was accomplished by the use of human pulmonary adenocarcinoma cells (H441 cells) in vitro. Using cell transfection, DNAse I footprint and electrophoretic mobility shift assays (EMSA), *trans*-active proteins, and *cis*-active sequences of the human SP-B gene promoter controlling gene transcription were identified. DNAse footprint analyses demonstrated two protected sites, SP-B-f1 and SP-B-f2, unique to H441 extracts. Three nonspecific protected sites were detected in both HeLa and H441 extracts, designated SP-B-f3 to f5. The latter sites contained consensus *cis*-active binding sequences for CAAT box proteins, SP-1 and AP-1, respectively. The AP-1 site was contained within the coding sequence of the SP-B gene. Using transfection analyses in H441 cells *cis*-active sequences (containing all five sites) between nucleotide positions –218 and +41 were required for full basal promoter activity. Deletion of the AP-1 site (SP-B-f5) in the coding sequences between +7 and +39 reduced transcriptional activity to nearly background levels. Deletion of either SP-B-f1 or f2 sites, unique to H441 cells, also markedly diminished transcriptional activity, indicating that cooperation of each of these sites and *trans*-active proteins is required for full transcriptional activity (4). Using EMSA, the *trans*-active factors HNF-3α and β bound to SP-B-f2 and thyroid transcription factor-1 (TTF-1) bound to SP-B-f1. Both HNF-3 and TTF-1 transactivated SP-B but transactivation was greater with TTF-1 (5). Cell-specific control of the basal promoter of the human SP-B gene required complex interactions of five *cis*-active binding sites with the ubiquitous *trans*-active proteins, SP-1, CAAT box proteins, and AP-1, and proteins selectively expressed in the developing foregut endoderm, HNF-3α and β and TTF-1.

In the human SP-B gene, sequences between positions –439 and –331 acted as an enhancer increasing the transcriptional activity of the basal promoter. Three distinct binding sites for TTF-1 were identified within this enhancer. Mutation of each of these sites independently or in combination prevented TTF-1 binding and reduced transcriptional activity in cell transfections with TTF-1 (48). The human SP-B gene is regulated by both ubiquitous and cell-specific *trans*-active proteins binding to enhancer and basal promoter *cis*-active sequences which, in combination, lead to cell-specific transcriptional control of the SP-B gene.

A Central Role for TTF-1 in Regulation of Lung Gene Expression

TTF-1 is a 38 kDa nuclear protein containing a consensus homeobox domain and a 17 amino acid domain identifying it as a member of the Nkx2 family of transcription factors. TTF-1 regulates expression of the thyroid-specific thyroperoxidase, thyroglobulin, and thyrotropin receptor genes in addition to lung-specific genes (8, 10). Co-transfection of TTF-1 expression vectors with other lung-specific promoters of the SP-A, SP-C, and CCSP genes demonstrated that TTF-1 transactivates each of these genes (5–7, 19, 20). TTF-1 is produced in the developing respiratory epithelium from the early pseudoglandular stages of lung development and in the distal epithelium and type II cells of the adult. This pattern overlaps the cellular expression pattern of the surfactant genes (Fig. 12.5) (49). To date, TTF-1 is the only transcription factor known to commonly regulate all of the known lung-specific genes. Co-localization, timing of expression, and transactivation of surfactant protein genes by TTF-1 demonstrates the central role of TTF-1 as a molecular regulator in the developing lung.

Loss of Function: Gene Targeting

Gene targeting is used to generate a null mutation eliminating expression of the mouse gene at its chromosomal locus. A targeting construct replaces the normal gene and produces a mutation in the mouse genome that inhibits production of the gene product. Generally, targeting constructs consist of a cloned gene wherein a portion has been replaced with a minigene that produces bacterial neomycin phosphotransferase, conferring resistance to the toxic neomycin analog, G418. The construct is designed so that the mutated gene cannot produce a normal gene product. The targeting construct is electroporated into embryonic stem (ES) cells. These cells are pluripotent cells maintained in an undifferentiated state in vitro by controlling media conditions. The targeting construct inserts into a single site in the ES cell genome by homologous recombination. Embryonic stem cells bearing the mutated gene are selected during culture in G418 because of resistance conferred by the neomycin-resistance gene. As with injected transgenes, most targeting genes insert randomly in the ES cell genome and not by homologous recombination. To further facilitate selection of the desired ES cells, in which the targeting construct has inserted by homologous recombination into the normal allele, the targeting construct often contains a second selectable marker—for example, herpes virus thymidine kinase (HSV-tk) gene. The construct is designed so that when homologous recombination occurs, the targeting construct loses the HSV-tk gene and is not killed by ganciclovir. If the targeting construct is inserted randomly, the HSV-tk gene is retained.

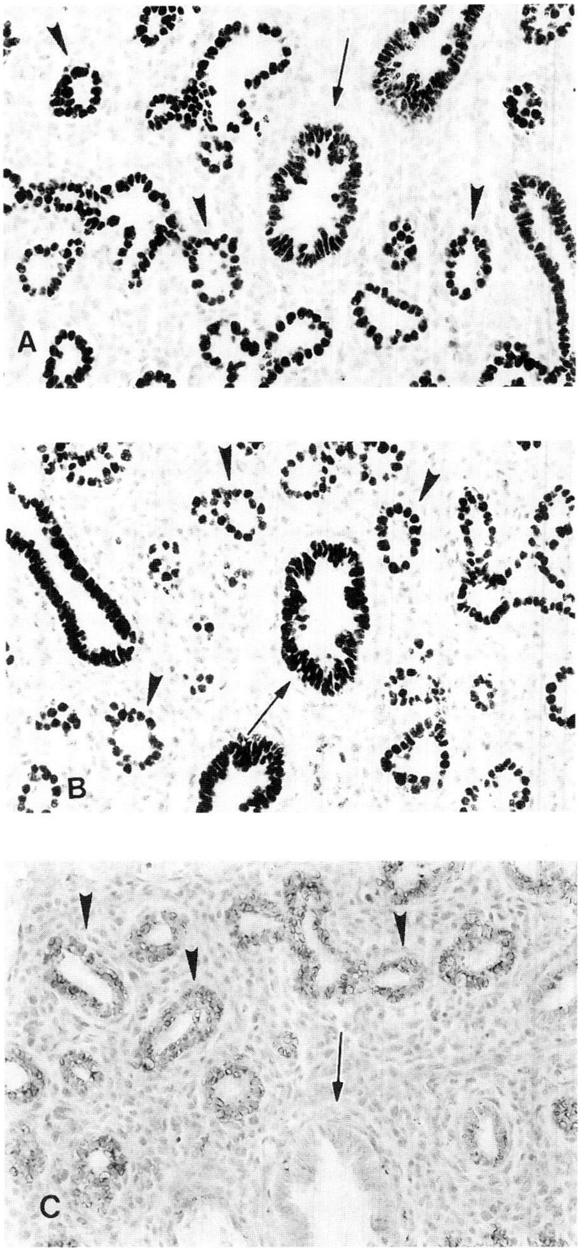

Fig. 12.5 Co–expression of HNF-3β, TTF-1, and SP-C in the developing lung. To determine if HNF-3β, TTF–1, and SP-C were expressed in the same sets of developing lung epithelial cells, sections of gestation day 15 fetal mouse lungs were immunostained for TTF-1 (*A*), HNF-3β (*B*), and SP-C (C). HNF-3β and TTF-1 are identified in developing proximal (*arrows*) and distal (*arrowheads*) epithelial cells. SP-C is expressed only in developing distal epithelium. Co-localization studies support the role of TTF-1 and HNF-3β as transcriptional regulators in the developing lung epithelium.

To select for correctly targeted ES cells after electroporation, cells are grown in media containing G418 and the nucleoside analog, ganciclovir. The presence of the neomycin gene confers resistance to G418 and HSV-tk confers sensitivity to ganciclovir. The ES cells with a random insertion will contain both the neomycin gene and HSV-tk gene and do not survive selection. In contrast, the correctly targeted cell, in which the neomycin gene is retained as part of the mutated allele, and the HSV-tk is lost during the recombination event, survives. Correctly targeted ES clones are confirmed by restriction mapping with Southern blot and/or PCR analysis. Genetically altered ES cells are then cloned and reinjected into mouse blastocysts that are reimplanted in pseudopregnant female mice. Offspring bearing the targeted cells are identified by inheritance of distinct coat color genes used to distinguish contributions from the ES cells in contrast to the injected host blastocysts. When genetically altered ES cells contribute to the germ-line cells of chimeric male mice, the sperm of the offspring contains the targeted gene. The targeted gene can be transferred through breeding (germ-line transmission), producing heterozygous and ultimately, homozygous offspring. Homozygous mice are usually null mutants and each cell of the targeted mouse lacks the targeted gene product. The insertion site can be engineered to create mutations of biological interest that will be expressed under control of the transcriptional regulation of the endogenous gene. The use of this technology in lung research has been reviewed recently (42).

TTF-1 Gene–Targeted Mice

The in vitro studies of TTF-1 gene–targeted mice have demonstrated the central role of TTF-1 in control of lung-specific surfactant protein genes. To directly determine the role of TTF-1 in vivo, a null mutation of the TTF-1 locus was generated by gene targeting in mice. Lungs from TTF-1 gene–targeted mice failed to form distal alveolar, bronchiolar, or mesenchymal lung structures (22) but did maintain proximal conducting airway structures. The gene-targeted mice provide critical data confirming the in vitro data that TTF-1 is a central transcriptional regulator of lung cell differentiation in vivo. The morphology of the lungs of the TTF-1 gene–targeted mice correlate with the morphology of the SP-C-DTA cell–ablated mice and the SP-C-FGF-R2 dominant-negative mice in that all three transgenic models fail to form distal lung structures. Signaling through the FGF-R2 receptor and expression of TTF-1 are critical molecular events in development of the distal lung.

Transcriptional Regulation of the TTF-1 Gene and HNF-3β Gene Targeted Mice

With the identification of TTF-1 as a common molecular regulator of lung cell differentiation, the human TTF-1 gene was cloned to determine the transcriptional mechanisms regulating its expression. Five hundred and fifty base pairs of the 5′-flanking region of the human gene directed lung cell–selective expression (15). Two *cis*-active sites at nucleotide position –135 to –124 and –14 to –3 bound lung cell nuclear proteins. These *cis*-active sites were transactivated by the foregut-derived HNF-3β, and the importance of these sites was confirmed by mutating the sequences to reduce

HNF-3β binding (16). HNF-3β was first recognized as a regulator of liver-specific gene transcription. Gene-targeted mice lacking HNF-3β have multiple anomalies in all germ layers and fail to develop foregut endoderm or its derivatives, including the lung (1). HNF-3β precedes expression of TTF-1 and may serve as a transcriptional regulator of the TTF-1 gene. Loss-of-function studies with gene-targeted mice demonstrate that both transcription factors, HNF-3β and TTF-1, regulate lung-specific gene expression and are required for morphogenesis of the lung.

Hierarchal Control of Gene Expression in Lung Development

HNF-3β regulates TTF-1 gene expression and SP-B expression in lung cells, TTF-1 in turn transactivates the lung-specific genes SP-A, -B, and -C and CCSP. The correct spatial–temporal expression of each of the lung-specific genes requires combinatorial interactions among TTF-1, HNF-3 family members, and other nuclear transcription proteins.

SP-B Gene–Targeted Mice: A Model of Lung Disease

Transgenic technology has also been used to determine the role of the surfactant protein genes in lung development and to model human diseases. Surfactant is required for perinatal adaptation of the lung to air breathing. SP-B is critical for the normal structure of surfactant lipid bilayers and facilitation of normal surface activity of the surfactant phospholipids in vitro (17, 21, 30, 39). Deficiency of SP-B has been associated with respiratory distress in premature infants, adult respiratory distress syndrome (ARDS), and in infants with hereditary SP-B deficiency (see ref. 43 for review). To generate a mouse model of SP-B deficiency, gene targeting was used to generate a null mutation (Fig. 12.1). Homozygous SP-B-deficient mice died of respiratory failure at birth (9). Type II cells in the gene-targeted mice lacked lamellar bodies, which are the normal secretory granules containing surfactant. Tubular myelin (the morphologic form of surfactant) was deficient in alveoli of SP-B knockout mice. Abnormalities of surfactant protein C processing were also detected. Lungs of SP-B-deficient mice produced an abnormally processed precursor of SP-C. The lethal phenotype of the SP-B knockout mice was similar to the findings in human infants with genetic SP-B deficiency (29). Human SP-B deficiency causes lethal respiratory distress following birth and is inherited as an autosomal recessive trait. Lungs of newborn infants with SP-B deficiency develop a form of alveolar proteinosis in which aberrantly processed proSP-C fragments accumulate (29, 38). Type II cells from SP-B deficient infants and mice lack lamellar bodies and fail to produce tubular myelin, the abundant extracellular form of surfactant in the air space. The SP-B knockout mouse provides a model for studying the role of SP-B in lung function or for the design of new therapies for surfactant deficiency.

SUMMARY

Transgenic technology involving gain of function or loss of function have confirmed that distal cell development initiates in the pseudoglandular period and requires FGF signaling. Loss-of-function studies using gene targeting support a role of HNF-3 family members and TTF-1 in regulating expression of surfactant protein genes and lung morphogenesis. Gene targeting has also been used to produce a transgenic mouse model of SP-B deficiency. Increasing sophistication in transgenic technology, through which genes can be regulated in a spatial and temporal manner, will continue to provide important insight into molecular regulators of the pathogenesis of pulmonary disease and lung development.

REFERENCES

1. Ang, S.L. and J. Rossant. HNF-3β is essential for node and notochord formation in mouse development. *Cell* 78: 561–574, 1994.
2. Bellusci, S., Grindley, J., Emoto, H., Itoh, N., and Hogan, B. Fibroblast growth factor 10 (FGF-10) and branching morphogenesis in the embryonic mouse lung. *Development* 124: 4867–4868, 1997.
3. Bernfield, M. Developmental biology: preventive medicine for neonatology. *Pediatr. Res.* 27: S21–S27, 1990.
4. Bohinski, R.J., J.A. Huffman, J.A. Whitsett, and D.L. Lattier. *Cis*-active elements controlling lung cell–specific expression of human pulmonary surfactant protein-B gene. *J. Biol. Chem.* 268: 11160–11166, 1993.
5. Bohinski, R.J., and J.A. Whitsett. Surfactant protein B gene promoter directs lung-specific gene expression and contains a complex nuclear protein binding site for thyroid transcription factor TTF-1 and hepatocyte nuclear factor 3. *Pediatr. Res.* 35: 326A, 1994.
6. Bruno, M.D., R.J. Bohinski, K.M. Huelsman, J.A. Whitsett, and T.R. Korfhagen. Lung cell specific expression of the murine surfactant protein A gene is mediated by interactions between the SP-A promoter and thyroid transcription factor-1. *J. Biol. Chem.* 270: 6531–6536, 1995.
7. Bruno, M.D., K.A. Huelsman, I. Fink, J.A. Whitsett, and T.R. Korfhagen. Transcriptional control of the mouse SP-A gene. *Am. J. Respir. Crit. Care Med.* A299, 1996.
8. Civitareale, D., R. Lonigro, A.J. Sinclair, and R. DiLauro. A thyroid specific nuclear protein essential for tissue specific expression of the thyroglobulin promoter. *EMBO J.* 8: 2573–2542, 1989.
9. Clark, J.C., S.E. Wert, C.J. Bachurski, M.T. Stahlman, B.R. Stripp, T.E. Weaver, and J.A. Whitsett. Targeted disruption of the surfactant protein B gene disrupts surfactant homeostasis, causing respiratory failure in newborn mice. *Proc. Natl. Acad. Sci. USA* 92: 7794–7798, 1995.
10. Damante, G., D. Fabbro, L. Pellizzari, D. Civitareale, S. Guazzi, M. Polycarpou-Schwartz, S. Cauci, F. Quadrifoglio, S. Formisano, and R. Di Lauro. Sequence-specific DNA recognition by the thyroid transcription factor-1 homeodomain. *Nucl. Acids Res.* 22: 3075–3083, 1994.
11. Evans, G.A. Dissecting mouse development with toxigenics. *Gene Dev.* 3: 259–263, 1989.
12. Fu, Y., M.P. Spirito, Z.X. Yu, S. Biro, J. Sasse, J. Lei, V.J. Ferrans, S.E. Epstein, and W. Casscells. Acidic fibroblast growth factor in the developing rat embryo. *J. Cell Biol.* 114: 1261–1273, 1991.
13. Glasser, S.W., T.R. Korfhagen, M.D. Bruno, C. Dey, and J.A. Whitsett. Structure and expression of the pulmonary surfactant protein-SP-C gene in the mouse. *J. Biol. Chem.* 265: 21986–21991, 1990.

14. Honegger, A.M., A. Schmidt, A. Ullrich, and J. Schlessinger. Evidence for epidermal growth factor (EGF)-induced intermolecular autophosphorylation of the EGF receptors in living cells. *Mol. Cell. Biol.* 10: 4035–4044, 1990.
15. Ikeda, K., J.C. Clark, J.R. Shaw-White, M.T. Stahlman, C.J. Boutell, and J.A. Whitsett. Gene structure and expression of human thyroid transcription factor-1 in respiratory epithelial cells. *J. Biol. Chem.* 270: 8108–8114, 1995.
16. Ikeda, K., J.R. Shaw-White, S.E. Wert, and J.A. Whitsett. Hepatocyte nuclear factor 3 activates transcription of thyroid transcription factor 1 in respiratory epithelial cells. *Mol. Cell. Biol.* 16: 3626–3636, 1996.
17. Johansson, J., T. Curstedt, and B. Robertson. The proteins of the surfactant system. *Eur. Respir. J.* 7: 372–391, 1994.
18. Kashles, O., Y. Yarden, R. Fischer, A. Ullrich, and J. Schlessinger. A dominant negative mutation suppresses the function of normal epidermal growth factor receptors by heterodimerization. *Mol. Cell. Biol.* 11: 1454–1463, 1991.
19. Kelly, S.E., C.J. Bachurski, M.S. Burhans, and S.W. Glasser. *Cis*-acting sequences involved in basal regulation of the SP-C promoter flank the TTF-1 responsive elements. *Am. J. Respir. Crit. Care Med.* A299, 1996.
20. Kelly, S.E., C.J. Bachurski, M.S. Burhans, and S.W. Glasser. Transcription of the lung-specific surfactant protein C gene is mediated by thyroid transcription factor-1. *J. Biol. Chem.* 271: 6881–6888, 1996.
21. Keough, K.M.W. Physical chemistry of pulmonary surfactant in the terminal air spaces. In: *Pulmonary Surfactant: From Molecular Biology to Clinical Practice,* edited by B. Robertson, L.M.G. van Golde, and J.J. Baatenburg. Amsterdam: Elsevier, 1992, p. 109–164.
22. Kimura, S., Y. Hara, T. Pineau, P. Fernandez-Salguero, C.H. Fox, J.M. Ward, and F.J. Gonzalez. The T/ebp null mouse: thyroid specific enhancer-binding protein is essential for the organogenesis of the thyroid, lung, ventral forebrain, and pituitary. *Genes Dev.* 10: 60–69, 1996.
23. King, R.J., M.B. Jones, and P. Minoo. Regulation of lung cell proliferation by polypeptide growth factors. *Am. J. Physiol.* 257 (*Lung Cell. Mol. Physiol. 1*): L23–L38, 1989.
24. Korfhagen, T.R., M.D. Bruno, G.F. Ross, K.M. Huelsman, M. Ikegami, A.H. Jobe, S.E. Wert, B.R. Stripp, R.E. Morris, S.W. Glasser, C.J. Bachurski, H.S. Iwamoto, and J.A. Whitsett. Altered surfactant function and structure in SP-A gene targeted mice. *Proc. Natl. Acad. Sci. USA* 93: 9594–9599, 1996.
25. Korfhagen, T.R., S.W. Glasser, S.E. Wert, M.D. Bruno, C.C. Daugherty, J.D. McNeish, J.L. Stock, S.S. Potter, and J.A. Whitsett. *Cis*-acting sequences from a human surfactant protein gene confer pulmonary-specific gene expression in transgenic mice. *Proc. Natl. Acad. Sci. USA* 87: 6122–6126, 1990.
26. Mason, I.J., F. Fuller-Pace, R. Smith, and C. Dickson. FGF-7 (keratinocyte growth factor) expression during mouse development suggests roles in myogenesis, forebrain regionalization and epithelial-mesenchymal interactions. *Mech. Dev.* 45: 15–30, 1994.
27. McGowan, S.E. Extracellular matrix and the regulation of lung development and repair. *FASEB J.* 6: 2895–2904, 1992.
28. McIntosh, J.C., S. Mervin-Blake, E. Conner, and J.R. Wright. Surfactant protein A protects growing cells and reduces TNF-α activity from LPS-stimulated macrophages. *Am. J. Physiol.* 271 (*Lung Cell. Mol. Physiol. 15*): L310–L319, 1996.
29. Nogee, L.M., G. Garnier, H.C. Dietz, L. Singer, A.M. Murphy, D.E. deMello, and H.R.

Colten. A mutation in the surfactant protein B gene responsible for fatal neonatal respiratory disease in multiple kindreds. *J. Clin. Invest.* 93: 1860–1863, 1994.

30. Notter, R.H. Physical chemistry and physiological activity of pulmonary surfactant. In: *Surfactant Replacement Therapy*, edited by D.L. Shapiro and R.H. Notter. New York: Alan R. Liss, 1989, p. 19–70.
31. Peters, K., S. Werner, X. Liao, S. Wert, J. Whitsett, and L. Williams. Targeted expression of a dominant negative FGF receptor blocks branching morphogenesis and epithelial differentiation of the mouse lung. *EMBO J.* 13: 3296–3301, 1994.
32. Peters, K.G., S. Werner, G. Chen, and L.T. Williams. Two FGF receptor genes are differentially expressed in epithelial and mesenchymal tissues during limb formation and organogenesis in the mouse. *Development* 114: 233–243, 1992.
33. Pison, U., M. Max, A. Neuendank, S. Weißbach, and S. Pietschmann. Host defense capacities of pulmonary sufactant: evidence for 'non-surfactant' functions of the surfactant system. *Eur. J. Clin. Invest.* 24: 586–599, 1994.
34. Redemann, N., B. Holzmann, T. von Rüden, E.F. Wagner, J. Schlessinger, and A. Ullrich. Anti-oncogenic activity of signalling-defective epidermal growth factor receptor mutants. *Mol. Cell. Biol.* 12: 491–498, 1992.
35. Shannon, J.M. Induction of alveolar type II cell differentiation in fetal tracheal epithelium by grafted distal lung mesencyme. *Dev. Biol.* 166: 600–614, 1994.
36. Ten Have-Opbroek, A.A.W. The development of the lung in mammals: an analysis of concepts and findings. *Am. J. Anat.* 162: 201–219, 1981.
37. van Iwaarden, F., B. Welmers, J. Verhoef, H.P. Haagsman, and L.M.G. van Golde. Pulmonary surfactant protein A enhances the host-defense mechanism of rat alveolar macrophages. *Am. J. Respir. Cell. Mol. Biol.* 2: 91–98, 1990.
38. Vorbroker, D.K., S.A. Profitt, L.M. Nogee, and J.A. Whitsett. Aberrant processing of surfactant protein C in hereditary SP-B deficiency. *Am. J. Physiol.* 268 (*Lung Cell. Mol. Physiol.* 12): L647–L656, 1995.
39. Weaver, T.E. and J.A. Whitsett. Function and regulation of expression of pulmonary surfactant-associated proteins. *Biochem. J.* 273: 249–264, 1991.
40. Wert, S.E., S.W. Glasser, T.R. Korfhagen, and J.A. Whitsett. Transcriptional elements from the human SP-C gene direct expression in the primordial respiratory epithelium of transgenic mice. *Dev. Biol.* 156: 426–443, 1993.
41. Wessells, N.K. Mammalian lung development: interactions in formation and morphogenesis of tracheal buds. *J. Exp. Zool.* 175: 455–466, 1970.
42. Whitsett, J.A., and C. Gerard. Transgenic mice for study of pulmonary disease. In: *The Lung: Scientific Foundations*, edited by R.G. Crystal and J.B. West. Philadelphia: Lippincott-Raven Publishers, 1997, p. 383–393.
43. Whitsett, J.A., L.M. Nogee, T.E. Weaver, and A.D. Horowitz. Human surfactant protein B structure, function, regulation and genetic disease. *Physiol. Rev.* 75: 749–757, 1995.
44. Wikenheiser, K.A., J.C. Clark, R.I. Linnoila, M.T. Stahlman, and J.A. Whitsett. Simian virus-40 large T-antigen directed by transcriptional elements of the human surfactant protein-C gene produces pulmonary adenocarcinomas in transgenic mice. *Cancer Res.* 52: 5342–5352, 1992.
45. Wikenheiser, K.A., D.K. Vorbroker, W.R. Rice, J.C. Clark, C.J. Bachurski, H.K. Oie, and J.A. Whitsett. Production of immortalized distal respiratory epithelial cell lines from surfactant protein C/simian virus 40 large T antigen transgenic mice. *Proc. Natl. Acad. Sci. USA* 90: 11029–11033, 1993.

46. Wikenheiser, K.A., and J.A. Whitsett. Tumor progression and cellular differentiation of pulmonary adenocarcinomas in SV40 large T antigen transgenic mice. *Am. J. Respir. Cell Mol. Biol.* 16: 713–723, 1997.

47. Wright, J.R. Immunomodulatory functions of surfactant. *Semin. Respir. Crit. Care Med.* 16: 61–68, 1995.

48. Yan, C., Z. Sever, and J.A. Whitsett. Upstream enhancer activity in the human surfactant protein B gene is mediated by thyroid transcription factor 1. *J. Biol. Chem.* 270: 24852–24857, 1995.

49. Zhou, L., L. Lim, R.H. Costa, and J.A. Whitsett. Thyroid transcription factor-1, hepatocyte nuclear factor-3β, surfactant protein B, C, and Clara cell secretory protein in developing mouse lung. *J. Histochem. Cytochem.* 44: 1183–1193, 1996.

chapter 13

NUTRITIONAL ASPECTS OF LUNG DEVELOPMENT

Masendu Kalenga, Claude Gaultier, and Peter H. Burri

THE relationship between nutrition and the respiratory system has been extensively explored during the last two decades, especially the potentially deleterious effects of inadequate nutrition on lung structure and function. It is of special concern that in several clinical conditions undernutrition occurs during the most critical periods of normal lung restructuring. Nutritional perturbations are likely to interfere with cellular and extracellular functions, which in turn may impair lung growth and development and may eventually predispose to chronic lung diseases. Conversely, pulmonary diseases may increase nutritional requirements and also impede adequate nutrition supply.

For obvious reasons, our knowledge of nutrition-related pulmonary alterations is mainly based on animal experiments. The most information comes from rodents, whose normal lung growth and development have been widely studied. This chapter reviews current knowledge of the role of nutrition in lung development, mainly based on the consequences of inadequate nutrition. It focuses primarily on alterations that develop during the periods of most accelerated remodeling of the gas exchange compartment, that is, late in gestation and early in the postnatal period. Although lung development has to be considered essentially as a continuum, antenatal and postnatal periods will be reviewed separately because of differences in nutritional pathophysiology between the two periods. Results in experimental animals are discussed before reviewing available information from humans.

NUTRITION AND PRENATAL LUNG MATURATION

Animal Studies

Fetal lung metabolism dramatically increases near term (as suggested by a greater requirement in nutritional substrates) when glucose oxidation serves as the most important source of energy fuel (36, 68). Glucose also acts, at least in part, by regulating gene expression of the metabolic pathways of various biochemical components of the lung, especially of proteins (16, 54). Dietary lipids are also critical at this period as fatty acids play an essential role in the structural and functional dynamics of fetal lung cells toward maturation (85). Thus, providing nutritional substrates in sufficient amounts during the last third of gestation is crucial.

The effects of antenatal undernutrition on the developing lung have been analyzed in various ways. Curle and Adamson examined the effects of maternal starvation on the fetal rat lung by depriving rats of solid food from gestational day 13 until parturition (19). They observed 25% stillbirths and a 25% mortality rate within the 3 days after birth. At birth, lungs of starved fetuses were much smaller than those of fetuses from mothers given normal rations. Morphological and histochemical studies indicated that prenatal malnutrition is associated with delayed cytodifferentiation of epithelial cells. In particular, there is glycogen retention in type II pneumocytes and a reduction in acid phosphatase activity, indicating that the expected increase in cellular metabolism did not occur. Accordingly, evidence has been reported that antenatal undernutrition negatively interferes with pulmonary surfactant production. In newborn animals from mothers starved during late gestation, lung hypoplasia is characteristically associated with a decrease in lung phospholipid content (25, 34, 50). Importantly, disaturated phosphatidylcholine (DSPC), the major surface active component, decreases in surfactant fraction most among rat pups from mothers fed a protein-poor diet throughout gestation (34). Although the functional significance of this nutrition-related surfactant depletion has not yet been established, it has been shown that lung extracts from malnourished rat fetuses had an increase in minimal surface tension (25).

The effects of prenatal underfeeding on the formation of terminal air spaces varies with both animal species and timing of malnutrition. Young rats whose mothers were subjected to food restriction during late gestation have been shown to achieve quite normal alveolization when examined at 2 weeks of age (19). The bulk formation of alveoli in this species is essentially a postnatal phenomenon. In guinea pigs, whose alveolar maturation is accomplished before birth (49), maternal food restriction during the last third of pregnancy caused fetal lung hypoplasia with significantly decreased alveolization (48). This appears to be the reason for increased perinatal mortality. Normal feeding after birth resulted in almost complete catch-up growth. However, morphometric analyses revealed that prenatally starved animals still had significantly reduced volume and surface area of parenchymal components as adults, even though the morphological aspect was normal.

Lipids, have been shown to be crucial to fetal lung development. Rat pups from mothers fed fat-free (58) or essential fatty acid–deficient diets (1, 17) suffer from retarded lung growth with delayed maturation as judged by decreased lung DSPC. A further role of lipids in early lung development is protection against oxidant-induced lung injury. Feeding pregnant rats with diets enriched in polyunsaturated fatty acids (PUFA) have been shown to provide better tolerance to hyperoxia for newborn rats (80). In particular, consumption of a PUFA-rich diet was associated with less pulmonary injury than that associated with a low-PUFA diet. One speculation is that intracellular PUFA could scavenge excess oxygen free radicals and prevent their interaction with critical membrane PUFA (78).

In addition to macronutrients, vitamins and minerals play an important role in fetal lung maturation. For example, vitamin A is an essential factor in the regulation of type II pneumocyte proliferation and in the incorporation of choline in DSPC (91). Conversely, prenatal hypervitaminosis A has been shown to cause thickening of septal walls with atelectasis in fetal lung parenchyma (59). Similarly, many trace elements, including selenium, are involved in fetal and neonatal lung development. Selenium deficiency during gestation up to postnatal day 4 may result in lung growth retardation with septal attenuation (47). Because selenium-dependent glutathione-oxydase was not affected however, it was hypothesized that the protective effects of selenium are independent of the anti-oxidant system. These observations illustrate how important vitamins and minerals are to lung development and how difficult it may be to interpret nutrition-related changes. Indeed, a lack of macronutritients is inevitably accompanied by a deficiency in specific key micronutritients.

Human Observations

The impact of prenatal undernutrition on human lung development has never been examined in any systematic manner. One form of fetal malnutrition is intrauterine growth retardation (UIGR) that results in newborns small for their respective gestational age. Among many other etiopathogenic factors, poor maternal nutrition is one common cause of fetal growth retardation (82). Postmortem studies have shown that lungs of IUGR infants were lighter than expected for body weight but their alveolar development was appropriate for gestational age (33). In clinical practice, it has been recognized for many years that growth-retarded infants have less risk of developing neonatal respiratory distress syndrome (RDS) than normal growth infants of similar gestational age (66). One possible explanation for this relative protection is that the stress generated by placental insufficiency stimulates the release of corticosteroids from maternal or fetal adrenal glands, resulting in accelerated structural and functional maturation of the fetal lung.

Interestingly, Olowe and Akinkugbe found that Nigerian fetuses achieved the same lecithin/sphingomyelin (L/S) ratios as for white fetuses in San Diego approximately 1 week earlier (62). One speculation was that accelerated maturation in Nigerian infants could be related to the higher palmitic acid content of maternal dietary fat (61). However, this hypothesis must be tempered as there are many other studies showing that black premature infants are much less likely to develop RDS

(29, 37). Rather than being an effect of diet composition, the observed variations could be related to possible biological differences between blacks and whites in the timing of lung maturation (69). Additionally, failure to take into account many confounding maternal factors that are likely to influence fetal lung maturation such as pregnancy complications, socioeconomic conditions, physical activity, and nutritional status, may lead to misinterpretation. All these factors could have contributed to the difference in L/S ratios among Nigerian and San Diego fetuses. It is noteworthy that poor nutrition has been associated with increased serum corticosteroids (2). These considerations, along with the lack of systematic clinical studies, make it difficult to compare human observations with those in experimental animals regarding the impact of nutritional disorders on lung maturation.

Fetal malnutrition may eventually impede growth of conducting airways. This has been suggested by British studies analyzing the relationship between birth weight and respiratory function. Forced expiratory volume in 0.75 sec ($FEV_{0.75}$) and maximum expiratory flow at different levels of forced vital capacity were found to be lower than expected for height in 7-year-old children who were <2000 g at birth (14). Although premature and full-term small-for-gestational-age babies were not dissociated, it was surprising that alterations in respiratory function were independent of neonatal pulmonary illness. Quite similar findings were reported in adults over 59 years of age in whom low birth weight was associated with a significantly decreased FEV_1 even after adjustment for other confounding factors such as height, age, smoking habits, and social class (5). In addition, lower birth weight and weight at 1 year appeared to increase the death rate for chronic obstructive airway disease in adulthood. More significantly, in children aged 5 to 11 years who had a low birth weight, impairment in respiratory function (low FEV_1) was found to be unrelated to gestational age (71). Impaired lung function in relationship with low birth weight has also been reported in adult Indians (80b). These data suggest that fetal undernutrition is associated with a permanent reduction of the dimensions of airways, eventually predisposing to chronic obstructive pulmonary disease. Because the formation of conducting airways is largely completed before the end of gestation, the cause of IUGR is likely an early event.

On the basis of these observations it appears that maternal and fetal nutrition may influence fetal lung growth and development. In humans, it is unknown how much the gas exchange compartment can be affected structurally and functionally by undernutrition experienced before birth. Importantly, it seems that tissue maturation takes priority over nonspecific lung growth.

NUTRITION AND EARLY POSTNATAL LUNG REMODELING

In most mammalian species, including human, the lung parenchyma still undergoes dramatic changes during the early postnatal period (11). In the rat model, one of most studied species, these critical modifications occur during the first 3 postnatal weeks (10, 12), referred to as the neonatal period. This includes not only significant growth but also several structural and functional changes, such as the formation of alveoli and maturation of the capillary network (see Chap. 5), and the accumulation of connective tissue (see Chap. 2). Importantly, the implementation of efficient surfactant synthesis and of various functions like antioxidant and antimicrobial activities rely on alveolar maturation. All these processes can be affected by inadequate postnatal nutrition.

Animal Studies

Lung Growth

The pioneering study by Winick and Noble remains a good reference regarding the deleterious effects of early postnatal malnutrition (89). They studied rats underfed for 3 weeks during one of the following periods: birth to day 21, or suckling period (18 instead of 9 pups per litter); day 21 to day 42; and day 42 to day 63 (1/2 ration); each restriction period was followed by normal feeding up to day 133. The most severe effects were observed after neonatal undernutrition: lung weight, DNA, and protein at day 21 was approximately 45% lower than in age-matched controls. Since the lung protein-to-DNA ratio remained normal, it was concluded that cell replication was reduced, but lung cells were of normal dimensions. In contrast, lung DNA and protein content were normal in rats underfed beyond the neonatal period. Importantly, after a 16-week period of refeeding, neonatally underfed rats still exhibited 32% lower lung weight and DNA than to age-matched controls. Neonatal underfeeding appeared to permanently impair the most intensive phase of cell replication that occurs in the rat lung during the first 2 weeks of life (88). The mechanisms that underlie failure to catch-up lung growth following early malnutrition and refeeding are certainly complex. Obviously, most developmental biological processes are essentially time regulated, mostly via hormonal control. Persistently inadequate protein biosynthesis and cytoplasmic growth after malnutrition occurring during early life may be related to a permanent alteration in the homeostasis of insulin (83) and in the production of growth factors (18).

Various types of nutritional deficiency can affect lung growth. Kwashiorkor is a common presentation of early childhood malnutrition in which inadequate protein supply is the primary factor. This condition can be experimentally induced by feeding animals with protein-poor diets ad libitum (23), a nutritional model referred to as protein restriction. It is disappointing that rats subjected to protein restriction spontaneously reduce their food intake and thus consume less glucose, fat, vitamins, and minerals, all of which are essential for lung development. The pulmonary consequences of neonatal protein restriction were studied using a progressive restriction model (41). The casein concentrations of diets were 15% (control diet) from birth to day 7, 12% from day 8 to day 14, and 8% thereafter until day 49. Weaning was accomplished at day 21 and animals were sacrificed and their lungs analyzed at day 49. Lung weight and DNA content were approximately 40% less in protein-restricted rats than in control rats. Unlike in the study by Winick and Noble, lungs of protein-restricted rats had a 24% lower protein concentration and a 20% decrease in protein-to-DNA ratio than in lungs of controls. Clearly, protein restriction with neonatal start was particularly deleterious, as lung cells were not only fewer but also smaller.

Architecture of Lung Parenchyma

A study by Das (21) has provided strong evidence that severe nutritional deprivation early during life may compromise normal postnatal rearrangement of the lung parenchyma. Lungs of rat pups starved twice for 24 hr (mother withdrawal) on postnatal days 1 and 5 and otherwise receiving normal lactation remained smaller (52% less weight) with delayed alveolar development at day 14 (still large terminal air spaces with thicker walls) than age-matched rats receiving normal lactation. In this model, the severity of starvation at the period of massive septation of saccules may have permanently blunted the normal process of alveolar formation. Less stressful models of milk restriction (in which the litter size was 18 instead of 10 for the control group) do not seem to affect normal alveolization as adequate saccule septation at day 14 can be accomplished despite a 40% restriction in lung growth (52).

Further evidence of the relative preservation of lung maturation has been recently provided in a study using prolonged protein restriction with subsequent nutritional rehabilitation (42, 43). In one group, early protein restriction was applied: rats were exposed to an 8% casein diet from birth to postnatal day 49. Some animals were then refed the control diet (18% casein) for 11 weeks. Lung growth, as indicated by postfixation volume, was reduced by 33% and 42% at days 21 and 49, respectively, compared with control animals. Figure 13.1 shows the morphological appearance of the lung parenchyma at different ages. In protein-deficient rats at day 21 (compare Fig. 13.1b with 13.1a), it appeared that normal steps of postnatal maturation of lung parenchyma, i.e., alveolization and microvascular maturation, proceeded independently of the limited growth of the thoracic cage. At day 49 (compare Fig. 13.1d with 13.1c), except for an obvious reduction in septal thickness, alveolization remained quite normal, without septal disruption. After refeeding, normal morphology was restored (compare Fig. 13.1f with 13.1e).

Morphometric analysis indicated that volume and surface densities of different parenchymal components were preserved during early protein restriction, so that in absolute terms the reduction in various parameters, including alveolar surface area, was proportional to that in lung volume. Refeeding resulted in a striking lung regrowth in previously malnourished rats, but there was still an approximately 20% reduction in lung volume as well as in volume and surface areas of different parenchymal components. The pulmonary diffusion capacity of oxygen remained nonetheless essentially adapted to body weight. It was remarkable that despite an early start and a long duration of protein restriction resulting in severe growth retardation, only minimal and reversible alterations in the architecture of lung parenchyma were observed. Thus more severe protein restriction (4% casein) is required to induce more pronounced parenchymal damage (55).

It is remarkable that in rats restricted in protein intake over the entire period

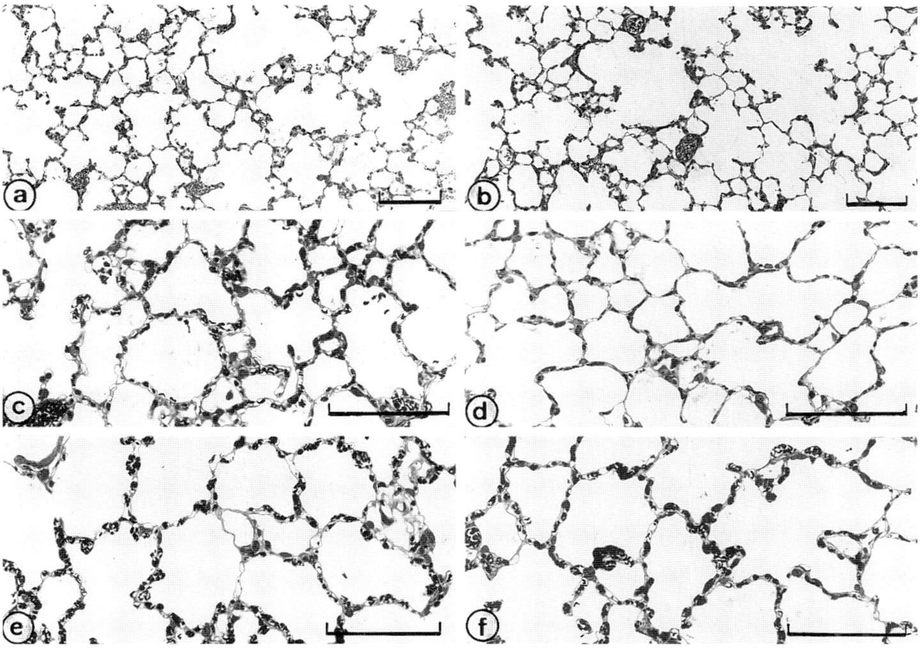

Fig. 13.1 Light photomicrographs of lung parenchyma in rats subjected to early protein restriction and then refed a normal diet after day 49 compared with age-matched controls. Day 21: (*a*) control rats; (*b*) protein-restricted rats. Normal alveolization with a well matured aspect was observed in malnourished rats. Their alveoli tended to be smaller than that of controls (bar = 100 μm). Day 49: (*c*) control rats; (*d*) protein-restricted rats. There was still an aspect of normal alveolization, but in malnourished rats, alveolar septa appeared thinner and elongated. No alveolar disruption was observed (bar = 100 μm). Day 126 (after refeeding): (*e*) control rats; (*f*) previously protein-restricted rats. The morphology of the lung parenchyma appears normal in previously malnourished rats (bar = 100 μm). [From Kalenga et al. (43), with permission.].

of intensive lung growth, refeeding after 7 weeks postnatal resulted in a greater parenchymal tissue proliferation than that expected at similar age in rats raised in normal conditions. Normal morphological appearance and normal volume and surface densities of parenchymal components suggest that adjustments during catch-up lung growth involve substantial formation of new alveoli. Whether this implies a re-activation of septation mechanisms is unknown

In an interesting series of publications, Sahebjami and colleagues reported the effects of starvation on lung biochemistry and ultrastructure in mature rats (73-77). The most significant finding was an emphysema-like aspect in adult rats losing about 30% of their initial weight (76, 77). One week of refeeding could not restore normal architecture of the parenchyma. Using similar food restriction, "nutritional emphysema" has been induced by Kerr and co-workers in young rats (45). Others have observed an alveolar enlargement without septal disruption in adult rats treated in a similar manner (35). It appears that severe nutritional depletion can be associated with structural disorganization of lung parenchyma, possibly resulting in emphysema. The finding that starvation may amplify alveolar injury produced by elastase (75) or hyperoxia (28) provides further evidence of the deleterious effects of severe malnutrition on the gas exchange compartment. The exact mechanisms governing these nutrition-related structural changes are in dispute. Both decreased accumulation and increased breakdown of connective tissue have been advocated, but none has received clear demonstration. Interestingly, severe starvation does not induce emphysema-like changes in hamsters (44) or in obese rats (72), probably because of much lower connective tissue turnover in hamsters than in rats and higher fat stores in obese rats.

Lung Biochemistry

One important function of alveolar cells after birth is the synthesis and release of pulmonary surfactant by type II pneumocytes. It has long been recognized that postnatal food deprivation negatively influences the metabolism of surfactant, at least quantitatively (7, 20, 30, 32, 50, 73). Possible mechanisms involved in this metabolic change include the reduction in energetic substrates and in key enzymes necessary for the synthesis of phospholipids (32). There is no available information about alterations in surfactant amount and composition, including possible adaptive mechanisms, in response to inadequate nutrition during early postnatal life.

Alterations induced by protein-energy malnutrition in the developing lung also comprise modifications in extracellular matrix proteins, mainly collagen and elastin. In the growing rat lung, while collagen content increases linearly, which stabilizes alveolar walls, lung elastin concentration peaks between postnatal days 12 and 20 and is associated with an increase in tissue recoil (57). Because of the conjunction between intensive elastin accumulation and massive alveolization marked by the constant presence of elastic fibers at the tip of newly forming alveoli, it has been hypothesized that elastic fibers probably serve as anchoring cables during saccule septation (10). Underfeeding has been shown to impair both collagen and elastin accumulation in the growing lung (41, 53, 74), with neonatal undernutrition triggering a greater reduction in elastin (41). The delayed alveolization due to severe nutritional deprivation during the lactation period is associated with a decreased intraseptal accumulation of elastin (21). In contrast, most studies suggest that moderate nutritional deficiency occurring after the neonatal period is less deleterious to the metabolism of elastin. Weanling rats restricted in protein (6, 55) or fed one-third the normal daily food consumption (45, 74) for 3 to 4 weeks show a substantial increase in lung elastin concentration, with lung collagen concentration remaining within normal range.

It is easily imaginable that the unavailability of proteins and energetic substrates during malnutrition may negatively affect the metabolism of lung elastin and collagen. Also, the decrease in lung lysyl oxidase activity during starvation (51) suggests that post-translational modifications of collagen and elastin fibers, notably the formation of inter- and intramolecular cross-links, may be inadequate. In addition, other associated deficiencies could affect both the quality and the quantity of structural proteins. The production of desmosine, an intermolecular cross-link of elastin, has been shown to be impaired by a selective deprivation in vitamin B-6 (56) or in copper (60). Likewise, collagen synthesized in the absence of vitamin C is insufficiently hydroxylated and consequently, less stable (46). Similarly, the increased lung distensibility in rats deficient in vitamin D (31) is presumably linked to a defective synthesis or conformation of connective tissue elements.

Characterization of lung mechanical consequences of nutrition-induced alterations in lung biochemistry usually refers to the analysis of air or saline pressure-volume (P-V) curves. Most investigators have used excised lungs. Although differences exist among reported results, the most characteristic finding in lungs of malnourished rats is an increase in recoil pressure during air-filling (40, 41, 75, 76). Figure 13.2a illustrates this increase, which is commonly attributed to an increase in alveolar surface forces resulting from surfactant depletion. In adult rats, reduction in lung surfactant content and subsequent mechanical changes may be restored by nutritional rehabilitation (73, 76). The P-V curves obtained with saline provide information on the elasticity of lung tissue (86). Early protein restriction affecting the neonatal phase of elastin accumulation (39) is associated with a decrease in lung

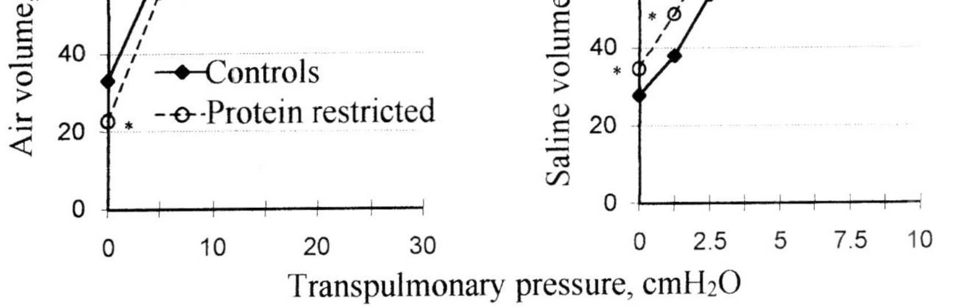

Fig. 13.2 Deflation pressure-volume (P-V) curves in rats subjected to protein restriction during the neonatal period (delayed restriction model) compared with age-matched controls. (*a*) Air-filling: lung volumes were expressed as percentage of volume at 30 cm H_2O. The P-V curve of protein-deficient rats shifted upward and to the left. (*b*) Saline-filling: lung volumes were expressed as percentage of volume at 10 cm H_2O. In protein-deficient rats the curve shifted upward and to the left. *P<0.005. [From Kalenga and Henquin (41), with permission.]

tissue recoil (41, 50), whereas protein restriction starting after this critical phase causes a rise in lung elastin concentration, the result being an increase in lung recoil (55). Figure 13.2b presents the pattern of lung recoil reduction following protein restriction begun during the neonatal period. In weanling or adult rats, a decrease in lung recoil has been observed when underfeeding was associated with a reduction in lung elastin concentration (53) or with emphysematous changes comprising a disorganization of elastic fibers (77). The physiological significance of these findings and their long-term consequences have yet to be established.

Some observations related to the stability of lung connective tissue during protein-energy malnutrition are intriguing. Less severe structural changes were observed during nutritional emphysema, when the diet of food-restricted rats was free of proteins (45). It was suggested that the lung connective tissue may have acquired more structural stability. This speculation is based on a previous report showing that dermal collagen fibers from protein-restricted rats were less soluble than those from rats fed a normal diet (3). Similarly, the pressure at the point of lung rupture, which increases in correlation with lung collagen accumulation (57), has been shown to be higher in malnourished rats, both with air and saline inflation (40, 41). Again, the mechanisms behind these observations need to be clarified, especially with regard to lung growth and development.

Human Observations

A typical example in neonatology in which nutrition plays a critical role in postnatal lung remodeling is that of tiny premature infants, particularly those born before 30 weeks of gestational age. Their structurally and functionally immature respiratory system suddenly has to cope with the gas-exchange function, which often implies use of aggressive interventions such as oxygenotherapy and artificial ventilation. Lung immaturity, barotrauma, oxygen toxicity, inflammation, and infection predispose to pulmonary injury that may lead to chronic lung disease, whose major form is bronchopulmonary dysplasia (BPD). Because of poor nutritional intake, increased energy expenditure (90), and poor intestinal absorption (67), many infants with respiratory disease undergo periods of inadequate nutrition with resulting growth failure. It is now well recognized that inadequate nutrition plays an amplifying role in the development of BPD (79). As mentioned earlier, lack of nutritional substrates may impede cellular growth and differentiation, surfactant synthesis, inactivation of free radicals, and post-injury repair (27). Eventually, poor nutrition may also contribute to tissue breakdown.

Characteristically, lung parenchyma of long-standing BPD presents an emphysematous-like aspect (81). This parenchymal damage is associated with alteration in structural biochemistry, mainly in lung elastin. In infants who develop BPD, elastin degradation products have been found in greater amount during the first few days, and thereafter in lower quantity than in age-matched infants recovering without sequelae (9). There is speculation that in BPD-prone infants, a first phase of increased elastolysis is followed by decreased elastosynthesis, possibly because of inadequate nutrition. Obviously, it is difficult to establish the specific role of undernutrition among many other etiopathogenic factors. However, on the basis of above data, maintenance of adequate nutrition should be one main target in the management of premature infants with respiratory disease. Provision of nutrients in sufficient amounts, particularly calories, enhances lung repair as indicated by the resulting improved BPD outcome (79).

On the basis of experimental observations, many clinical trials have been conducted to evaluate the possible protective effect of specific nutrients in infants at risk of BPD. Early provision of essential fatty acids is one nutritional intervention that can benefit lung restructuring in very low birth-weight infants. It is noteworthy that low plasma levels of linoleic acid have been reported in small premature babies (26). Furthermore, tracheal aspirate in RDS infants at risk of BPD was found to have significantly lower levels of linoleic acid than in RDS infants not developing BPD, suggesting that supplementation with essential fatty acids could be a valuable protective intervention. Unfortunately, no definitive conclusion can be drawn as conflicting results have been reached with early use of PUFA-rich lipids in very low birth-weight premature infants (78). Further investigation is needed to clarify this issue.

Similarly, the protective effect of supplementation with vitamins and trace elements has not yet been well established. Vitamin A has received particular attention because of its role in differentiation and maintenance of the integrity of epithelial cells (91). Infants with RDS who develop BPD have been shown to have lower serum vitamin A than age-matched infants who did not develop BPD, although this finding could be related to feeding practice (15). Accordingly, some authors have shown that early supplementation of premature babies with vitamin A reduces the incidence and severity of BPD (63, 70). However, other investigators were unable to demonstrate such an effect of vitamin A (64).

In addition to being an important factor in infants with respiratory disorders, malnutrition is by far the most important cause of morbidity and mortality among preschool children in developing countries (22). At this age, the still-restructuring lung may be sensitive to various nutritional deficiencies. However, our knowledge of nutrition-related respiratory disorders at this stage of life is limited. Except for the well-known increased risk for pulmonary infections (38, 84), little has been reported on the effects of childhood malnutrition on lung growth and development. In an older study, Emerson and Green (24) reported that malnutrition (7.5% below normal weight for height) does not affect lung vital capacity in children of ages 7 to 15 years. It is clear that this study included only children with a small nutritional deficit. Decreased peak flow rates in relationship with poor nutrition have been repeatedly shown in both children (13, 65) and adults (62b) who do not have respiratory disease, suggesting a qualitative effect of malnutrition on lung development. This hypothesis, however, is confounded by the fact that respiratory muscle weakness due to poor nutrition may reduce patient capacity to properly perform forced expiration. In this way, decreased flow rates have been reported in nutrition-depleted adults patients suffering from nonrespiratory disease (4). Interestingly, peak expiratory rates have been found to be slightly increased in stunted schoolchildren (65).

Because dwarfing is associated with greater sitting height relative to the total height, these children should have relatively greater thoracic cages.

Pulmonary changes associated with adult malnutrition are worth mentioning as they have inspired many experimental studies. The most striking findings are from Jewish physicians in the Warsaw Ghetto during World War II (87). They described a "syndrome of the atony of the lung" that was characterized by hyperaerated lungs and decreased diaphragmatic excursions during severe malnutrition. More significantly, histopathological studies revealed emphysematous changes that were also found in lungs of many subjects <40 years of age. An observation supported by experimental nutritional emphysema discussed above. The implication of these findings has not yet been systematically explored with respect to childhood malnutrition. In one postmortem survey, only 1 out of 151 cases of childhood protein-energy malnutrition was found to have emphysema, but no further details were provided (8). To address this issue properly, more systematic investigations with specifically targeted histological analyses need to be conducted.

In sum, inadequate nutrition early during postnatal life may be associated with various adverse effects on the growing lung. In animals, the importance of observed alterations depends on a number of factors including animal species and the severity of nutritional deficiency.

CONCLUSIONS

The data reviewed above provide substantial evidence that nutrition plays a critical role in the regulation of various processes of lung restructuring. In particular, experimental studies have shown how deleterious malnutrition can be when it is experienced during the period of intensive lung growth. Alterations concern the most critical functions involved in parenchymal maturation like epithelial cell replication and differentiation, surfactant production, and connective tissue synthesis. Although long-term functional consequences of early malnutrition still need to be determined, it may be that structural maturation of the gas-exchange compartment is better preserved than nonspecific lung growth. Obviously, persistent controversies and many unanswered questions indicate how far we are from a detailed understanding of the effects of inadequate nutrition on specific steps of cellular metabolism and intercellular functions. This is also applicable to the mechanisms underlying growth reactivation after refeeding. These fields represent an important direction for future investigation, which must take into account both normal and pathological conditions with reference to clinical conditions. Here, the role of biological mediators, including growth factors, needs exploration.

Because data obtained from experimental animals cannot be readily extrapolated to human beings, more systematic clinical observations are needed. Further investigation should be done to more precisely determine the potential benefits from nutritional interventions such as supplementation of specific key nutrients to prevent or treat infant chronic lung disease and its complications. Clinical observations should also focus on the possibility of interactions between early undernutrition, notably IUGR and preschool protein-energy malnutrition, and specific or nonspecific chronic lung disease during adulthood.

REFERENCES

1. Alam, S.Q. and B.S. Alam. Lung surfactant and fatty acid composition of lung tissue and lavage of rats fed diets containing different lipids. *Lipids* 19: 38–43, 1984.
2. Alleyne, G.A.O., D. Halliday, and J.C. Waterlow. Chemical composition of organs of children who died of malnutrition. *Br. J. Nutr.* 23: 783–790, 1967.
3. Anasuya, A. and B.S. Narasinga Rao. Relationship between body collagen and urinary hydroxyproline excretion in young rats fed a low-protein or a low-calorie diet. *Br. J. Nutr.* 24: 97–107, 1970.
4. Arora, N.S. and D.F. Rochester. Respiratory muscle strength and maximal voluntary ventilation in undernourished patients. *Am. Rev. Respir. Dis.* 126: 5–8, 1982.
5. Barker, D.J.P., K.M. Godfrey, G. Fall, C. Osmond, P.D. Winter, and S.O. Shaheen. Relation of birth weight and childhood respiratory infection to adult lung function and death from chronic obstructive airways disease. *Br. Med. J.* 303: 671–675, 1991.
6. Blankenship, J.W., B. Chase McKinney, P.J. Roos, and L.B. Sandberg. Quantitation of lung elastin and collagen in protein and essential fatty acid malnourished rats. *Connect. Tissue Res.* 29: 311–318, 1993.
7. Brown, L.A.S, A.S. Bliss, and W.J. Longmore. Effects of nutritional status on the lung surfactant system: food deprivation and caloric restriction. *Exp. Lung Res.* 6: 133–147, 1984.
8. Brown, R.E. Pediatric post-mortem survey in Uganda. *Trop. Geogr. Med.* 17: 289–300, 1965.
9. Bruce, M.C., K.E. Wedig, N. Jentoft, R.J. Martin, P.W. Cheny, T.F. Boat, and A. Fanaroff. Altered urinary excretion of elastin-links in premature infants who develop bronchopulmonary dysplasia. *Am. Rev. Respir. Dis.* 131: 568–572, 1985.
10. Burri, P.H. The postnatal growth of the rat lung III. Morphology. *Anat. Rec.* 180: 77–98, 1974.
11. Burri P.H. Postnatal development and growth. In: *The Lung. Scientific Foundations,* 2nd ed., edited by R.G. Crystal, J.B. West, E.R. Weibel, and P.J. Barnes. Philadelphia: Lippincott-Raven, p. 701–714, 1997.
12. Burri, P.H., J. Dbaly, and E.R. Weibel. The postnatal growth of the rat lung I. Morphometry. *Anat. Rec.* 178: 711–730, 1974.
13. Carswell, P., J. Hellier, P.S.E.G Harland, and R.H. Meakins. Peak expiratory flow rate and malnutrition. *Trans. R. Soc. Trop. Med. Hyg.* 74: 814, 1980.
14. Chan, K.N., C.M. Noble-Jamieson, A. Elliman, E.M. Bryan, and M. Silverman. Lung function in children of low birth weight. *Arch. Dis. Child.* 64: 817–820,1989.
15. Chan, V., A. Greenough, P. Cheesman, and H. Gamsu. Vitamin A level and feeding practice in neonates with and without chronic lung disease. *J. Perinat. Med.* 21: 205–210, 1993.
16. Clarke, S.D. and S. Abraham. Gene expression: nutrient control of pre- and posttranscriptional events. *FASEB. J.* 6: 3146–3152, 1992.
17. Clarke, S.D., L. Benjamin, and S.D. Phinney. Fetal growth and fetal lung phospholipid content in rats fed safflower oil, manhaden oil, or hydrogenated coconut oil. *Am. J. Nutr.* 47: 828–835, 1988.

18. Crace, C.J., I. Swenne, D.J. Hill, and R.D. Milner. Tissue and serum insulin-like growth factor (IGF I) concentrations in rats subjected to temporary protein-energy malnutrition early in life. *Ups. J. Med. Sci.* 96: 17–22, 1991.
19. Curle, D.C. and Y.R. Adamson. Retarded development of neonatal rat lung by maternal malnutrition. *J. Histochem. Cytochem.* 26: 401–408, 1978.
20. D'Amours, R., L. Clerch, and D. Massaro. Food deprivation and surfactant in adult rats. *J. Appl. Physiol.* 42: 88–92, 1977.
21. Das, R.M. The effects of intermittent starvation on lung development in suckling rats. *Am. J. Pathol.* 117: 326–332, 1984.
22. de Onis, M., C. Monteiro, J. Akré, and G. Clugston. The world-wide magnitude of protein-energy malnutrition: an overview from the WHO global database on child growth. *Bull. World Health Organ.* 71: 703–712, 1993.
23. Edozien, J.C. Experimental Kwashiorkor and marasmus. *Nature* 220: 917–919, 1968.
24. Emerson, P.W. and H. Green. Vital capacity of the lungs of children. *Am. J. Dis. Child.* 22: 202–211, 1921.
25. Faridy, E.E. Effect of maternal malnutrition on surface activity of fetal lungs in rats. *J. Appl. Physiol.* 39: 535–540, 1975.
26. Farrell, P.M., G.R. Gutcher, M. Palata, and D. DeMets. Essential fatty acid deficiency in premature infants. *Am. J. Nutr.* 48: 220–229, 1988.
27. Frank, L. Antioxidants, nutrition, and bronchopulmonary dysplasia. *Clin. Perinatol.* 19: 541–561, 1992.
28. Frank, L. and E. Groseclose. Oxygen toxicity in newborn rats: the adverse effects of undernutrition. *J. Appl. Physiol.* 55: 1248–1255, 1982.
29. Fujikura, T. and L.A. Froelick. The influence of race and other factors on pulmonary hyaline membranes. *Am. J. Obstet. Gynecol.* 95: 572–578, 1966.
30. Gail, D.B., G. Massaro, and D. Massaro. Influences of fasting on the lung. *J. Appl. Physiol.* 42: 88–92, 1977.
31. Gaultier, C., A. Harf, N. Balmain, P. Cuisinier-Gleizes, and H. Mathieu. Lung mechanics in rachitic rats. *Am. Rev. Respir. Dis.* 130: 1108–1110, 1984.
32. Gross, I., I. Ilic, C.M. Wilson, and S.A. Rooney. The influence of postnatal nutritional deprivation on phospholipid content of developing rat lung. *Biochim. Biophys. Acta* 441: 412–422, 1976.
33. Gruenwald, P. Chronic fetal distress and placental insufficiency. *Biol. Neonate* 5: 215, 1963.
34. Guarner, V., C. Tordet C., and J.R. Bourbon. Effects of maternal protein-calorie malnutrition on the phospholipid composition of surfactant isolated from fetal and neonatal rat lungs. Compensation by inositol and lipid supplementation. *Pediatr. Res.* 31: 629–635, 1992.
35. Harkema, J.R., J.L. Mauderly, R.E. Gregory, and J.A. Pickerell A. Comparison of starvation and elastase models of emphysema in the rat. *Am. Rev. Respir. Dis.* 129: 584–591, 1984.
36. Hamosh, M., M.R. Simon, D.K. Mullon, and P. Hamosh. Metabolic activity of developing rat lung. *Biol. Neonate* 39: 117–126,1981.
37. Hulsey, T.C., G.R. Alexander, P.Y. Robillard, D.J. Annibale, and A. Keenan. Hyaline membrane disease: the role of ethnicity and maternal risk characteristics. *Am. J. Obstet. Gynecol.* 168: 572–576, 1993.
38. James, J.W. Longitudinal study of the morbidity of diarrheal and respiratory infections in malnourished children. *Am. J. Clin. Nutr.* 25: 690–694, 1972

39. Kalenga, M. and Y. Eeckhout. Effects of protein deprivation from the neonatal period on lung collagen and elastin in the rat. *Pediatr. Res.* 26: 125–127, 1989.
40. Kalenga, M. and J.C. Henquin. Alteration of lung mechanics by protein-calorie malnutrition in weaned rats. *Respir. Physiol.* 68: 29–39, 1987.
41. Kalenga, M. and J.C. Henquin. Protein deprivation from the neonatal period impairs lung development in the rat. *Pediatr. Res.* 21: 45–49, 1987.
42. Kalenga, M., S.A. Tschanz, and P.H. Burri. Protein deficiency and the growing rat lung. I. Nutritional findings and related lung volume. *Pediatr. Res.* 37: 783–788, 1995.
43. Kalenga, M., S.A. Tschanz, and P.H. Burri. Protein deficiency and the growing rat lung. II. Morphometric analysis and morphology. *Pediatr. Res.* 37: 789–795, 1995.
44. Karlinsky, J.B., R.H. Goldstein, B. Ojserkis, and J.L. Snider. Lung mechanics and connective tissue levels in starvation-induced emphysema in hamsters. *Am. J. Physiol.* 251: R282–R288, 1986.
45. Kerr, J.S., D.J. Riley, S. Lanza-Jacoby, R.A. Berg, H.C. Spilker, S.Y. Yu, and N.H. Edelman. Nutritional emphysema in the rat: influence of protein depletion and impaired lung growth. *Am. Rev. Respir. Dis.* 131: 644–650, 1985.
46. Kietly, C.A., I. Hopkinson, and M.E. Grant. The collagen family: structure, assembly and organisation in the extracellular matrix. In: *Connective Tissue and its Heritable Disorders*, edited by P.M. Royce and B. Steinmann. New York: Wiley-Liss, p. 103–147, 1993.
47. Kim, H.Y., M.F. Picciano, M.A. Wallig, and J.A. Milner. The role of selenium in the development of neonatal rat lung. *Pediatr. Res.* 29: 440–445, 1991.
48. Lechner, A.J. Perinatal age determines the severity of retarded lung development induced by starvation. *Am. Rev. Respir. Dis.* 131: 638–643, 1985.
49. Lechner, A.J. and N. Banchero. Advanced pulmonary development in new-born guinea pigs (*Cavia porcellus*). *Am. J. Anat.* 163: 235–246, 1982.
50. Lechner, A.J., D.C. Winston, and J.E. Bauman. Lung mechanics, cellularity and surfactant after prenatal starvation in guinea pigs. *J. Appl. Physiol.* 60: 1610–1614, 1986.
51. Madia, A.M., S.J. Rozovski, and H.M. Kagan. Changes in lung lysyl oxidase activity in streptozotocin diabetes and starvation. *Biochim. Biophys. Acta* 585: 481–487, 1979.
52. Massaro, D., N. Teich, S. Maxwell, G.D. Massaro, and P. Whitney. Postnatal development of alveoli. Regulation and evidence for a critical period in rats. *J. Clin. Invest.* 76: 1297–1305, 1985.
53. Matsui, R., R.H. Goldstein, K. Mihal, J.S. Brody, M.P. Steele, and A. Fine. Type I collagen formation in rat type II alveolar cells immortalised by viral gene products. *Thorax* 49: 201–206, 1994.
54. Muona, P., J. Peltonen, S. Jaakkola, and J. Uitto. Increased matrix gene expression by glucose in rat neural connective tissue cells in culture. *Diabetes* 40: 605–611, 1991.
55. Myers, B.A., M.A. Dubick, J. Gerreits, R.B. Rucker, A.C. Jackson, K.M. Reiser, S.M. Williams, and J.A. Last. Protein deficiency: effects on lung mechanics and the accumulation of collagen and elastin in the rat lung. *J. Nutr.* 113: 2308–2315, 1983.
56. Myers, B.A., M.A. Dubick, R.D. Reynolds, and R.B. Bucker. Effect of vitamin B-6 (pyridoxine) deficiency on lung elastin cross-linking in perinatal and weanling rat pups. *Biochem. J.* 229: 153–160, 1985.
57. Nardell, E.A. and J.S. Brody. Determinants of mechanical properties of rat lung during postnatal development. *J. Appl. Physiol.* 53: 140–148, 1982.
58. Nelson, G.H., J.C. McPherson, L. Perling, and R. Ciechan. The effect of maternal dietary fat on fetal pulmonary maturation in rats. *Am. J. Obstet. Gynecol.* 138: 466, 1980.

59. Newman, L.M. and E.M. Johnson. Characterization of morphological and physiological abnormalities following fetal hypervitaminosis A exposure in the rat. *Teratology* 21: 58A, 1980.
60. O'Dell, B., K.H. Kilburn, W.N. McKenze, and R.J. Thurston. The lung of the copper-deficient rat: a model for developmental emphysema. *Am. J. Pathol.* 91: 413–432, 1978.
61. Okoh, O., R. Grosspietzsch, and L. von Klitzing. Hat die Ernahrugsgewohnhit mit hohem Anteil an Palmol (Palmitinaure) Einfluss auf die niedrige Atemnotsyndromrate in Nigeria? *Monatschr. Kinderheikd.* 127: 669, 1979.
62. Olowe, S.A. and A. Akinkubge. Amniotic fluid lecithin/sphengomyelin ratio: comparison between an African and a North American community. *Pediatrics* 62: 38–43, 1978.
62b. Ong, T.J., A. Mehta, S. Ogston, and S. Mukhopadhyay. Prediction of lung function in the inadequately nourished. *Arch. Dis. Child.* 79: 18–21, 1998.
63. Papagoroufalis, C., M. Cairis, E. Pantazatou, C.H. Megreli, M. Xanthou. A trial of vitamin A supplementation for the prevention of bronchopulmonary dysplasia BPD in very low birthweight (VLBW) infants. *Pediatr. Res.* 23: 518A, 1988.
64. Pearson, E., C. Bose, T. Snidow, L. Parson, T. Young, G. Bose, and A. Stiles. Trial of vitamin A supplementation in very low birth weight infants at risk for bronchopulmonary dysplasia. *J. Pediatr.* 121: 420–427, 1992.
65. Primhak, R. and F.S. Coates. Malnutrition and peak expiratory flow rate. *Eur. Respir. J.* 1: 801–803, 1988.
66. Procianoy, R.S., J.A. Garcia-Prats, J.M. Adams, A. Silvers, and A.J. Rudolph. Hyaline membrane disease and intraventicular hemorrhage in small for gestational age infants. *Arch. Dis. Child.* 55: 502–505, 1980.
67. Reimers, K.J., S.J. Carlson, and K.A. Lombard. Nutritional management of infants with bronchopulmonary dysplasia. *Nutr. Clin Pract.* 7: 127–32, 1992.
68. Rhoades, R.A. and D.A. Ryder. Fetal lung metabolism: response to maternal fasting. *Biochim. Biophys. Acta* 663: 621–629, 1981.
69. Richardson, D.K. and J.S. Torday. Racial differences in predictive value of the lecithin/sphengomyelin ratio. *Am. J. Obstet. Gynecol.* 170: 1273–1278, 1994.
70. Robbins, S.T. and A.B. Fletcher. Early vs. delayed vitamin A supplementation in very-low-birth-weight infants. *J. Parenter. Enter. Nutr.* 17: 220–225, 1993.
71. Rona, R.J., M.C. Gulliford, and S. Chinn. Effects of prematurity and intrauterine growth on respiratory health and lung function in childhood. *Br. Med. J.* 306: 817–820, 1993.
72. Sahebjami, H. Effects of food deprivation on experimental emphysema in obese rats. *Exp. Lung Res.* 18: 675–686, 1992.
73. Sahebjami, H. and J. MacGee. Effects of starvation on lung biochemistry in rats. *Am. Rev. Respir. Dis.* 126: 483–487, 1982.
74. Sahebjami, H. and J. MacGee. Effects of starvation on lung mechanics and biochemistry in young and old rats. *J. Appl. Physiol.* 58: 778–784, 1985.
75. Sahebjami, H. and C.L. Vassalo. Influence of starvation in enzyme-induced emphysema. *J. Appl. Physiol.* 49: 284–288, 1978.
76. Sahebjami, H. and C.L. Vassalo. Effects of starvation and refeeding on lung mechanics and morphometry. *Am. Rev. Respir. Dis.* 119: 443–451, 1979.
77. Sahebjami, H. and J.A. Wirman. Emphysema-like changes in the lungs of starved rats. *Am. Rev. Respir. Dis.* 124: 619–624, 1981.
78. Sosenko, I.R. Do polyunsaturated fatty acids protect against oxidant-induced lung damage? *J. Nutr.* 125: 1652S–1656S, 1995.

79. Sosenko, I.R. and L. Frank. Nutritional influences on lung development and protection against chronic lung disease. *Semin. Perinatol.* 15: 462–468, 1991.
80. Sosenko, I.R., S.M. Inni, and L. Frank. Polyunsaturated fatty acid and protection of newborn rats from oxygen toxicity. *J. Pediatr.* 112: 630–637, 1988.
80b. Stein, C.E., K. Kumaran, C.H. Fall, S.O. Shaheen, C. Osmond, and D.J. Barker. Relation of fetal growth to adult lung function in south India. *Thorax* 1997 52: 895–899, 1997.
81. Stocker, J.T. Pathological features of long standing "healed" bronchopulmonary dysplasia. *Hum. Pathol.* 17: 943–961, 1986.
82. Susser, M.B. Prenatal nutrition, birthweight, and psychological development: an overview of experiments, quasi-experiments, and natural experiments in the past decade. *Am. J. Clin. Nutr.* 34: 784–803, 1981.
83. Swenne, I., C.J. Crace, and R.D.G. Milner. Persistent impairment of insulin secretory response to glucose in adult rats after limited period of protein-calorie malnutrition early in life. *Diabetes* 36: 454–458, 1987.
84. Tupasi T., N.V. Mangubat, M.E.S. Sunico, D.M. Magdangal, E.E. Navarro, Z.A. Leonor, S. Lupisan, F. Medalla, and M.G Lucero. Malnutrition and acute respiratory tract infections in Filipino children. *Rev. Infect. Dis.* 12: S1047–S1054, 1990.
85. Viscardi, R.M. Role of fatty acids in lung development. *J. Nutr.* 125: 1645S–1651S, 1995.
86. von Neergaard, K. Neue Auffassungen über einen Grundbegriff der Atemmechanik. Die Retraktionskraft der Lunge, abhängig von der Oberflächenspannung in den Alveolen. *Z. Gesamte Exp. Med.* 66: 373–394, 1929.
87. Winick, M. *Hunger Disease: Studies by Jewish Physicians in the Warsaw Ghetto.* New York: John Wiley and Sons, 1979.
88. Winick, M. and A. Noble. Quantitative changes in DNA, RNA and protein during prenatal and postnatal growth in the rat. *Dev. Biol.* 12: 451– 466, 1965.
89. Winick, M. and A. Noble. Cellular response in rats during malnutrition at various ages. *J. Nutr.* 89: 300–306, 1966.
90. Yeh, T.F, D.A. McClean, O.A. Ajayi, and R.S. Pildes. Metabolic rate and energy balance in infants with bronchopulmonary dysplasia. *J. Pediatr.* 114: 448–51.
91. Zachman, R.D. Role of vitamin A in lung development. *J. Nutr.* 125: 1634S–1638S, 1995.

chapter 14

PULMONARY HYPOPLASIA: ROLE OF MECHANICAL FACTORS IN PRENATAL LUNG GROWTH

Richard Harding and Cheryl Albuquerque

PULMONARY hypoplasia is a term used to describe lungs that are sufficiently restricted in growth such that their ability to exchange respiratory gases is impaired; however, hypoplastic lungs are usually not simply small but are also structurally abnormal or immature. It is now recognized that fetal lung hypoplasia rarely occurs in isolation and is usually associated with other intrauterine abnormalities. This chapter considers how such abnormalities result in lung hypoplasia, and how lung structure and function are affected. For further information, the reader is directed to reviews of lung hypoplasia and the control of fetal lung growth (34, 42, 48, 62, 78, 90, 96, 139, 149, 163, 168).

DEFINITION OF LUNG HYPOPLASIA

Central to any discussion of lung hypoplasia is its definition. As a graded and variable phenomenon, lung hypoplasia is difficult to define precisely, and can have multiple definitions depending on the stage of development at which the lung is examined and what parameters are measured. Hypoplasia of an organ or tissue can be defined as its "incomplete development or underdevelopment" (32). Lung hypoplasia is commonly considered to be a statistically significant reduction in the amount of lung tissue present at autopsy, and this may be quantified as a reduction in the expected tissue weight (wet or dry) or total number of lung cells (or total amount of DNA); these values are usually expressed in relation to body weight. By convention, modern usage is such that a *hypoplastic* tissue should contain fewer cells, not a similar number of smaller cells (i.e., hypotrophy), but this distinction is often not made. In the clinical setting, lung hypoplasia in the fetus or newborn infant is often recognized only at autopsy and it is usually assumed that the lung hypoplasia was a causal factor in death. A convenient and widely used definition of lung hypoplasia is based on the ratio of (wet) lung weight to body weight (LBWR); reduced lung DNA content or reduced numbers of alveoli are often used as supporting evidence. In infants dying earlier than at 28 weeks of gestation, a value of LBWR of ≤0.015 has been used, and in infants of more than 28 weeks' gestation a value of ≤0.012 is used (7, 113); for comparison, LBWR in healthy neonates is 0.018 ± 0.003 (7).

IN VIVO DETECTION OF LUNG HYPOPLASIA

Fetal Detection

With the advent of noninvasive imaging techniques, there have been numerous studies aimed at detecting or predicting lung hypoplasia in the fetus in utero. Most studies have used ultrasonographic techniques to obtain fetal dimensions that reflect the size of the lungs (42). Several methods have been proposed to predict pulmonary hypoplasia, but it is apparent that no single method has acceptable diagnostic accuracy. Although lung tissue may be visualized if high-resolution equipment is used, most studies have focused on reduced chest size as a predictor of pulmonary hypoplasia (25).

Thoracic circumference was one of the first indices used to predict pulmonary hypoplasia; this followed the demonstration in normal fetuses of a linear relationship between chest dimensions, heart growth, and gestational age (124). In four of six cases in which the thoracic contents were mainly lung and heart, the chest circumference was highly predictive of pulmonary hypoplasia. The thoracic circumference was obtained in an axial section through the fetal thorax at the level of the four-chamber view of the heart (124). In contrast, another study found that thoracic circumference had a low sensitivity for the diagnosis of lung hypoplasia and was inferior to other methods (166).

The ratio of thoracic-to-abdominal circumferences has been used to diagnose pulmonary hypoplasia; this ratio is constant (at 0.89 ± 0.12, 2 SD) throughout gestation and values of ≤ 0.77 are consistent with pulmonary hypoplasia (25). The accuracy of this ratio has been tested in 16 pregnancies complicated by rupture of membranes before 26 weeks (28). Six fetuses met the diagnostic criteria for pulmonary hypoplasia (LWBW ratio <0.012); prior to delivery, all had thoracic-to-abdominal circumference ratios of more than 2 SDs below the mean for gestational age and all died immediately after delivery. In cases in which the fetal abdomen is altered in size, as with obstructive uropathies and diaphragmatic hernia, the ratio of chest circumference to femur length has been used (40).

In the presence of pleural effusions, a lung:thoracic ratio has been used to identify pulmonary hypoplasia (23). A coronal section of the fetal thorax at the level of the lung hilus enabled the measurement of distance from the hilus to the thoracic wall; in all four cases with pulmonary hypoplasia, the lung:thoracic ratio was <0.6. Lung length was used to predict pulmonary hypoplasia in 20 pregnancies with rupture of membranes at <25 weeks' gestation and >1 week duration (143); the authors reported 92% sensitivity and 100% specificity. Lung length was measured in a sagittal view from the apex of the lung to the dome of the diaphragm during apnea. Another view is a plane through the long axis of the fetal thorax from the superior end of the sternum to the level of the diaphragm or the inferior surface of the heart (25).

Breathing-related modulation of blood flow velocity in the ductus arteriosus has been used to determine pregnancies at risk for pulmonary hypoplasia (165). However, this test does not distinguish between lethal and nonlethal forms of pulmonary hypoplasia and has limitations in clinical practice. Another method that has been recently described employs Doppler techniques to visualize fetal pulmonary arterial flow velocity (95); in this study, an abnormal waveform was associated with postmortem evidence of pulmonary hypoplasia.

Postnatal Detection

Neonates with pulmonary hypoplasia have a small chest circumference and, because of respiratory insufficiency, require prolonged ventilatory support. These cases are often complicated by persistent pulmonary hypertension and air leak syndromes such as multiple pneumothoraces and pulmonary interstitial emphysema. Pulmonary hypertension with subsequent persistence of fetal circulation and right-to-left shunting frequently occurs secondary to incomplete development of the distal pulmonary vasculature (144, 162). Among live-born infants, the diagnosis of pulmonary hypoplasia is made by radiological criteria, which include small, well-aerated lungs with downward sloping ribs and diaphragmatic elevation to the seventh rib; these signs are usually accompanied by cyanosis, tachypnea, hypoxia, and acidosis (94, 161). A bell-shaped chest on X-ray is suggestive, but not obligatory, for the diagnosis of pulmonary hypoplasia.

INCIDENCE OF PULMONARY HYPOPLASIA

The incidence of pulmonary hypoplasia in the general population ranges from 11 to 14 per 10,000 births (91, 163) and the perinatal mortality rate in affected infants is 70% (162). The presence of lung hypoplasia in fetal and neonatal autopsies has been documented in a number of studies over the last 4 decades. In postnatal deaths it is assumed that lung hypoplasia, if present, contributed to death. When lung hypoplasia has been identified on the basis of a low LBWR in "perinatal" autopsies, its incidence ranges from 5% (51) to 22% (79) (Table 14.1). In an autopsy series of live-born infants dying within the first postnatal week over a 15-year period, an 18% incidence of lung hypoplasia was found (113). Although overall neonatal mortality

Table 14.1 Incidence of Lung Hypoplasia in "Perinatal" Autopsies

Age at autopsy	*No. Examined*	*No. cases*	*Incidence (%)*	*Years*	*Reference*
Birth–2 days	2000	93	4.9	—	(51)
Newborn	756	77	10.2	1968–78	(129)
Perinatal	165	13	7.9	1970–72	(159)
Perinatal	709	49	11.7	1976–83	(91)
Perinatal	235	34	14.5	1979–82	(171)
18 weeks g.a. to 2 years	113	25	22	1987–90	(79)
Fetuses > 20 weeks	248	(31)	12.5	2 years	(48)
Neonates	—	—	16	2 years	(48)
Stillborn and up to 28 days postnatal	1377	134	9.7	—	(120)
Neonates < 7 days	419	77	18	1971–85	(113)

g.a., gestational age.

fell significantly during this period, the incidence of lung hypoplasia did not change; thus, over the study period (1971–1985) it became proportionately a more common cause of neonatal mortality (113).

ANOMALIES ASSOCIATED WITH LUNG HYPOPLASIA.

Most cases of fetal lung hypoplasia are associated with one or more intrauterine factors that could lead to impaired lung development. Only 5%–10% of cases appear to be primary or idiopathic, in that no abnormality other than lung hypoplasia can be identified (48, 129); this amounts to an incidence of 0.8 –1.6 per 10,000 births (161). In these cases, a genetic basis is possible as genetic abnormalities have been detected (129) and a familial occurrence has been recognized (48).

A wide range of intrauterine anomalies are associated with fetal lung hypoplasia. These have provided important clues as to the causes of deficits in fetal lung growth and to the conditions necessary for normal lung growth. Anomalies associated with pulmonary hypoplasia have been grouped into seven categories (149): renal and urinary tract anomalies, amniotic fluid aberrations unrelated to the urinary system, diaphragmatic hernia, hydrops fetalis, skeletal and neuromuscular pathologies, central nervous system anomalies, and other conditions causing compression of the fetal thorax (pleural effusion, fetal hydrothorax, chylothorax, and intrathoracic masses). The most common cause of abnormal thoracic wall development, and one of the most common causes of fetal lung hypoplasia, is congenital diaphragmatic hernia (CDH) (129). In the absence of a closure defect, the diaphragm may be affected by abnormal development or function of its muscle (e.g., neuropathies or muscular dystrophies), leading to diaphragmatic eventration (i.e., elevation of the dome of the diaphragm). The structural development of the rib cage may be affected by conditions that affect bone or cartilage growth, leading to skeletal dysplasia; these include congenital scoliosis, certain types of dwarfism, and osteogenesis imperfecta. A number of abnormalities grouped together as "space-occupying lesions" can reduce the intrathoracic volume available for lung growth; such lesions include intrathoracic cysts, chylothorax or intrapleural effusion of fluid, pericardial effusion, and neuroblastoma (149). Hydrops fetalis (immunological and nonimmunological) results in the accumulation of fluid in the thorax and in one survey was the most common finding associated with lung hypoplasia (120).

Congenital Diaphragmatic Hernia

The incidence of CDH has been estimated as 1/3000 to 1/5000 live births (22). The diaphragm (i.e., the pleuroperitoneal membrane) normally "closes" at 45–50 days after ovulation. As a result of incomplete closure, abdominal contents are able to enter the thorax (22). Although the diaphragmatic defect is usually unilateral, most often affecting the left side, both lungs can be affected. As a result of the hernia and entry of abdominal viscera into the thorax, a mediastinal shift often occurs; as well as affecting the contralateral lung, this may interfere with swallowing, resulting in polyhydramnios.

Postnatal survival of infants with CDH is approximately 50% (138). Of 83 fetuses with isolated CDH diagnosed before 25 weeks gestation, 60% died despite optimal postnatal care (68). The clinical course of infants with isolated CDH depends on the degree of pulmonary hypoplasia which, in turn, depends on the timing of onset of herniation during development, the volume of viscera herniated, and the duration of herniation. The long-term outcome for infants with CDH who survive the neonatal period is dependent on the severity of pulmonary hypoplasia, the degree of bronchopulmonary dysplasia resulting from chronic ventilatory support, and associated anomalies. There is a high incidence of neurological problems in children with CDH and complications such as sensorineural hearing loss, seizures, and developmental delay are seen in 20% to 30% of patients (106).

Congenital Cystic Adenomatoid Malformation of the Lung

Congenital cystic adenomatoid malformation of the lung (CCAM) is caused by a failure of the maturation of bronchiolar structures and occurs at the 5th or 6th week of gestation, during the pseudoglandular stage of lung development (155). This abnormality is characterized by the conglomeration of multiple cystic areas within the lung tissue. The lesion is unilobar in 80%–95% of cases and bilateral in about 2% of cases.

Three major types of CCAM lesion have been identified, based on their pathologic characteristics (155). Type I lesions account for 50% of cases and consist of single or multiple cysts lined by ciliated pseudostratified epithelium; these cysts are large (3–10 cm) and few in number. In type II lesions, the cysts are <1 cm in size, lined by ciliated cuboidal to columnar epithelium and are associated with other anomalies of the kidneys or gastrointestinal tract. Type III lesions are large and noncystic and there is a poorer prognosis. Prenatal surgical intervention has been used to remove CCAM, allowing normal lung growth in utero (69).

Primary Fetal Hydrothorax

Primary fetal hydrothorax (PFHT) occurs in about 1 in 15,000 pregnancies (105). The effusions may be clinically benign, but ~50% will cause fetal or neonatal death, usually secondary to pulmonary hypoplasia with or without associated hydrops. Pathognomic in the antenatal detection of pleural effusions is the ultrasonic demonstration of an echo-free area between the lung, chest wall, and diaphragm. The severity of primary fetal hydrothorax ranges from clinically insignificant to intrathoracic compression that results in lethal pulmonary hypoplasia or hydropic stillbirth; the overall mortality of fetuses with PFHT has been reported to be 53% (105).

The aim of management of fetuses with PFHT is prevention of pulmonary hypoplasia while allowing the fetus to reach a gestational age at which it can be safely delivered in a nonhydropic state. The development of a mediastinal shift, significant lung compression, or hydrops fetalis prior to 35 weeks' gestation justifies prenatal drainage under ultrasound guidance to prevent pulmonary hypoplasia (3, 17, 18). After 35 weeks' gestation, pleural drainage may facilitate neonatal resuscitation if performed immediately prior to delivery.

Nonimmune Hydrops Fetalis

Hydrops fetalis (immunological and nonimmunological) results in the accumulation of fluid in the thorax and in one survey was the most common finding associated with lung hypoplasia (120). Nonimmune hydrops fetalis (NIHF) is defined as generalized edema of soft tissue, with or without effusions in serous cavities, with no hematological evidence of isoimmunization. These changes are readily identifiable by ultrasound but they are not specific for determining the etiology, which may involve many factors. The overall mortality in NIHF remains high at 75%–95%, with pulmonary hypoplasia being the most common cause of neonatal death, irrespective of underlying etiology (23, 49).

Reduced Amniotic Fluid Volume

The association between pulmonary hypoplasia and oligohydramnios was first observed in infants with bilateral renal agenesis (132). Abnormalities that result in reduced or absent fetal urine formation include bilateral renal agenesis and renal dysplasia, and those that restrict urinary flow into the amniotic sac, including agenesis or stenoses or the ureters or urethra, urethral valve, and obstruction of the bladder outlet. Fetuses with prolonged leakage of amniotic fluid are also at risk for developing pulmonary hypoplasia. It is likely that lung hypoplasia is a result of physical restraint of the fetus as compression deformities of the extremities and facies are highly correlated with lethal pulmonary hypoplasia (144). We believe that, as explained later, lung hypoplasia may result from an exaggerated flexion of the fetal trunk due to reduced uterine dimensions. (Fig. 14.1).

Following prolonged premature rupture of membranes, the incidence of clinical or autopsy diagnosed pulmonary hypoplasia ranges from 5% to 60% (13, 114, 125,

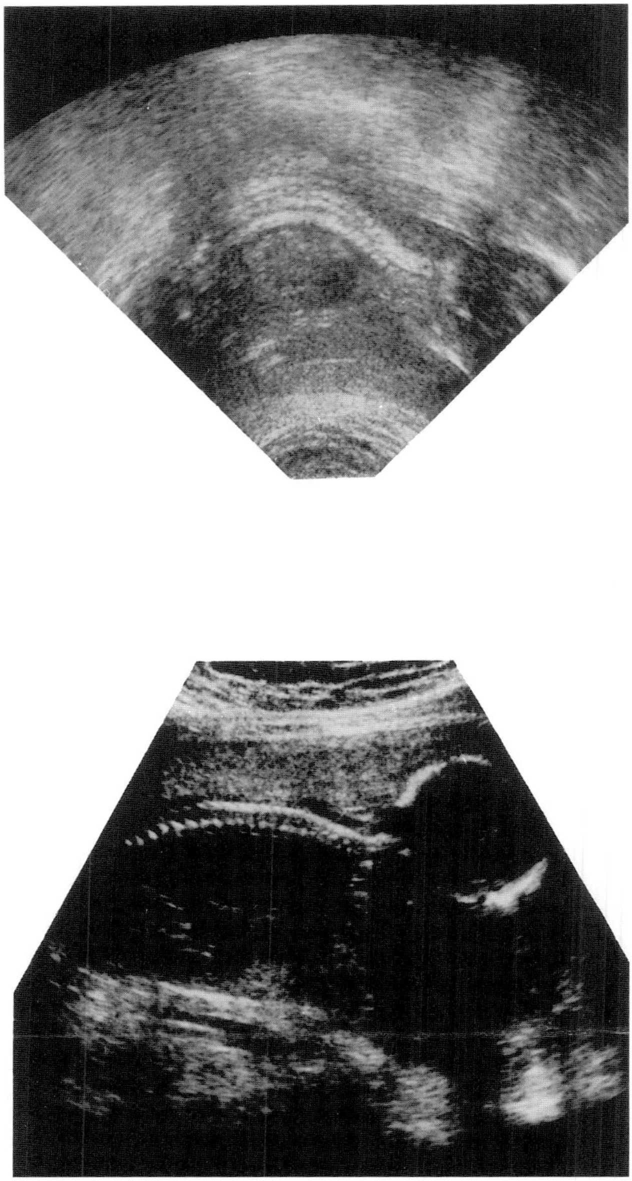

Fig. 14.1 Ultrasound images of human fetuses at approximately 18 weeks of gestation, showing the spinal column and head. In each, the head is to the right and the dorsum is uppermost. The upper panel shows a fetus in the presence of oligohydramnios and the lower panel shows a fetus with a normal volume of amniotic fluid. Note the increased degree of spinal flexion in the fetus with oligohydramnios.

143, 162). The reasons for the large differences in reported rates include the subjective nature of clinical criteria used to diagnose pulmonary hypoplasia, different rates of autopsies in nonsurvivors, and different autopsy criteria. It is apparent that earlier gestational age at rupture of membranes is associated with increased risk of pulmonary hypoplasia; this condition was more likely if membrane rupture occurred before 24 weeks than if it occurred after 25 weeks (143). In patients with premature rupture of membranes at <25 weeks, an incidence of 5% has been reported (114). The extent of pulmonary hypoplasia is dependent upon the degree of oligohydramnios, its duration, and the gestational age and stage of lung development at which the oligohydramnios occurred (125).

There appear to be no management schemes that will prevent the sequelae of prolonged oligohydramnios, although fluid has been instilled into the amniotic sac in an attempt to reverse oligohydramnios and lung hypoplasia (80). Because the duration of membrane rupture is not an independent risk factor for pulmonary hypoplasia, delivery at any given gestational age to try to prevent pulmonary hypoplasia is not indicated. Prenatal diagnosis of an underlying disorder that may lead to pulmonary hypoplasia is a requisite for consideration of in utero treatment. In utero shunting of bilateral obstructive uropathies, involving the placement of vesicoamniotic shunts, has been reported (137). Due to the high incidence of catheter clogging, displacement, or associated risk of chorioamnionitis, vesicoamniotic shunts are not satisfactory for long-term fetal urinary tract decompression.

Neural Abnormalities

Abnormalities of the nervous system, including defects in the central nervous system or phrenic nerves, are less commonly associated with lung hypoplasia than abnormalities of thoracic or amniotic fluids. Phrenic nerve agenesis may be associated with impaired development of the diaphragmatic muscle and can allow diaphragmatic eventration. Central neural defects associated with lung hypoplasia include anencephaly, microcephaly, and encephalocoele; such defects are likely to be associated with the absence of normal fetal breathing movements that are necessary for normal lung development (33). Pulmonary hypoplasia occurs in fetuses with neuromuscular abnormalities leading to prolonged immobility, such as Pena Shokeir syndrome (fetal akinesia sequence) (130), and this has been confirmed in an animal study (109).

Other Causes of Lung Hypoplasia

A number of apparently unrelated causes of fetal lung hypoplasia have been identified in experimental animals. These include maternal ethanol consumption in rats (81), maternal exposure to cigarette smoke in guinea pigs (27), and ectopic gestation in rats (110). There is also evidence that intrauterine growth restriction, in which the fetus is both undernourished and hypoxemic, may cause lung hypoplasia (107), although there is other evidence to the contrary (136). In this regard, it is of interest that maternal undernutrition, as well as early postnatal undernutrition, can adversely affect lung growth (44, 55, 97). It is possible that some of these factors may account for so-called primary lung hypoplasia.

A Common mechanism Underlying Induction of Lung Hypoplasia?

There is abundant experimental and clinical evidence that, in the fetus, the mean level of lung expansion (i.e., luminal volume) plays an important role in determining the rate of lung growth and defining pulmonary architecture (62, 88, 89). A common feature of the intrauterine abnormalities associated with lung hypoplasia is that they all have the potential to cause a prolonged reduction in the mean level of expansion of the fetal lungs. Such a reduction in lung expansion, if sustained, would be expected to cause lung hypoplasia. There is also evidence that nutritional and metabolic, and perhaps endocrine, factors can contribute to fetal lung hypoplasia. It is possible that these may also act via adverse effects on lung liquid dynamics and lung expansion. As suggested by Wigglesworth in 1987 (168), a critical factor in fetal lung growth seems to be the retention of an adequate volume of luminal liquid within the lungs.

STRUCTURAL ALTERATIONS IN HYPOPLASTIC LUNGS

Measurements of DNA content of hypoplastic lungs, identified on the basis of low LBWR, have shown that these lungs contain a reduced number of cells (170). Hypoplastic lungs also have a reduced volume when inflated at a pressure of 45.5 cm H_2O (75). Such lungs are not simply small, but show evidence of structural immaturity that is probably a result of prolonged periods of pulmonary underexpansion during fetal life. As discussed below, many of the structural alterations seen in hypoplastic lungs can be reproduced experimentally by reducing the mean level of lung expansion for extended periods. The range and degree of morphological changes observed in hypoplastic lungs depend on many factors, such as the extent of the reduction in lung growth, at what stage of lung development it began, how long the causative factors existed, and the stage of development at which the lungs were examined.

Airway Branching

A reduced number of airway generations has been described in hypoplastic lungs resulting from CDH (87), rhesus immunization (24), and renal agenesis and dysplasia (75). Similar findings were made in hypoplastic lungs associated with a wide range of causative factors (120), and comparable alterations in lung structure have been seen in oligohydramnios-induced lung hypoplasia in nonhuman primates (74) and rabbits (175). The major effect is a reduced number of smaller airways (bronchioli), which develop later than the larger airways. A reduction in bronchiolar branching would be expected to reduce the number of acini (terminal respiratory units) and hence the number of alveoli (or terminal sacs) and the total surface area available for gas exchange. The degree of reduction in airway branching likely depends on the onset and duration of the anomaly that produced lung hypoplasia, and the degree of reduction of lung expansion.

Alveolar Number

Estimates of alveolar number are usually obtained using the radial alveolar count (35). Several studies have shown hypoplastic lungs to contain fewer alveoli or terminal sacs, indicating an impairment of alveolar development (7, 75, 120, 135, 162). In experimental studies in which lung hypoplasia was induced by oligohydramnios or spinal cord transection, there was a reduced number of alveoli (74, 175).

Thickness of Air–Blood Barrier

In normal lungs the separation between "capillary blood" and "alveolar air" becomes reduced during fetal development, declining from 2.12 μm at 30 weeks to 1.27 μm at 40 weeks (120); a further reduction in this distance occurs during development, reaching adult values of 0.2–0.5 μm. In severely hypoplastic lungs, the air–blood interface may be thicker than expected (120).

Elastic Tissue

In normal human lungs, the appearance of elastin occurs relatively late in lung development, such that elastin content at 40 weeks is almost five times that at 20 weeks (120). In hypoplastic lungs, there is evidence of reduced elastin formation (52), which would be expected to alter their mechanical properties.

Epithelial Maturation

In hypoplastic lungs associated with oligohydramnios, evidence of epithelial structural immaturity has been reported (172). It was found that in the peripheral parts of the acinus, the lungs contained narrow, simple tubules lined by cuboidal epithelium (172); this is typical of an earlier stage of lung development, and is suggestive of delayed or arrested epithelial maturation (168). A developmental delay is supported by the observation that the ratio of lamellar body area to epithelial cell area was found to be decreased in hypoplastic lungs (120). Evidence of a developmental delay in alveolar epithelial cell maturation has also been obtained in rat and ovine models of CDH (20, 133).

Pulmonary Surfactant

In normal lung development, the phospholipid (and hence surfactant) content increases with gestation (43). The phospholipid content (mg phospholipid/mg DNA, an index of pulmonary surfactant content per lung cell) was found to be reduced in hypoplastic lungs, except in those associated with oligohydramnios (172). A similar finding of a reduced pulmonary content of disaturated phosphatidylcholine (DSPC) was made in most cases of lung hypoplasia studied recently (120).

In rabbits, lung hypoplasia has been induced by shunting amniotic fluid into the maternal peritoneal cavity so as to cause oligohydramnios. The hypoplastic lungs contained increased concentrations of total phospholipids, phosphatidylcholine (PC), and DSPC and a greater lecithin:sphingomyelin (L/S) ratio than control lungs (73, 175). However, another study in rabbits showed that the density of surfactant protein-A (SP-A)-containing type II cells was reduced in hypoplastic lungs (6). Functionally, hypoplastic lungs of fetal rabbits appeared to be more mature, as evidenced by increased stability during pressure-volume manipulations (85). In fetal guinea pigs (26) and rats (12) exposed to oligohydramnios, it was found that hypoplastic lungs had unaltered amounts of DSPC per gram of lung tissue compared with controls, indicating that epithelial maturation was unaffected. Thus, at present there appears to be no clear relation between lung hypoplasia and the development of pulmonary surfactant production.

Vascular Development

Infants born with hypoplastic lungs often show evidence of persistent pulmonary hypertension, which is apparently due, in part, to an attenuated pulmonary vascular bed (115). For example, the hypoplastic lungs of infants who died following CDH contain fewer blood vessels per lung unit (98), resulting in a reduction in the total cross-sectional area of the pulmonary vascular bed. In another study of hypoplastic lungs, a reduction in the number of pulmonary arteries was observed, and in some cases (associated with renal agenesis) arterial wall thickness was reduced (75). Other studies have shown increased amounts of muscle in the pulmonary arteries of hypoplastic fetal lungs and that the muscle extends to precapillary vessels, which in normal lungs, are not muscularized (19, 98). There is evidence that overconstriction of pulmonary vessels may be involved in persistent pulmonary hypertension of the newborn, possibly as a result of diminished activity of intrinsic vasodilator mechanisms (115).

EFFECTS OF LUNG HYPOPLASIA ON POSTNATAL LUNG FUNCTION

As a graded phenomenon, lung hypoplasia can cause varying degrees of respiratory compromise in the newborn, ranging from fatal asphyxia, to acute or subacute respiratory insufficiency, to only mild, transient respiratory symptoms. It is possible that mild or asymptomatic forms of lung hypoplasia may not be detected. In the case of preterm infants, lung hypoplasia may be associated with lung immaturity (i.e., epithelial immaturity and surfactant deficiency), which may compound the effects of reduced lung size. In this way, lung hypoplasia may exacerbate the respiratory distress syndrome.

There are few published studies of lung function following nonfatal lung hypoplasia; most of these are on survivors of CDH. Although respiratory function may appear to return to normal in infancy (93), there is both functional (36) and structural (76, 164) evidence that defects can persist, at least into childhood. Indeed, it is apparent that impaired lung development during fetal life can have a sustained impact upon respiratory health, as there may be permanent alterations in lung architecture (56). For example, it seems likely that "catch-up" growth in hypoplastic lungs occurs mainly by alveolar enlargement rather than by increased airway and alveolar numbers, which may lead to emphysematous changes in the lungs and later airflow limitation (36).

In a study of postnatal respiratory function in lambs exposed to oligohydramnios during fetal life, it was found that, although lung hypoplasia was still present 4 weeks after birth, lung function at rest appeared normal (82). The major alteration was a persistent reduction in respiratory system compliance, which was attributable to a stiff chest wall. This suggests that conventional tests of lung function may not be reliable indicators of nonlethal lung hypoplasia and that impaired lung growth can impact upon the development of the chest wall.

CONTROL OF LUNG EXPANSION IN THE FETUS

During fetal life, pulmonary epithelial cells actively and continually secrete a liquid (127) that has a unique and quite stable composition (1). This liquid, known as fetal lung liquid, flows from its site of secretion, along the bronchial tree into the trachea, larynx, and pharynx, and from there it either passes into the amniotic sac or is swallowed by the fetus (61). Thus, the "air spaces" of the fetal lung normally contain this unique liquid, and not amniotic fluid as was once thought. In fetal sheep, the rate of lung liquid production increases from about 2 ml/h/kg of body weight near mid-gestation (127) to about 4 ml/h/kg close to term (62); it is likely that the age-related increase in the rate of secretion is due to increased luminal surface area. The volume of liquid within the "air spaces" of the ovine fetal lung increases during this period from approximately 1 ml (<5 ml/kg body weight) at mid-gestation to 150–200 ml (45–50 ml/kg) by full term (78) (Fig. 14.2). Data on lung liquid production rates and volume are not available for the human fetus. Studies in fetal sheep have shown that fetal lung liquid production and volume are independently controlled, production being largely under the influence of metabolic and endocrine factors while volume is primarily influenced by physical factors, in particular the transpulmonary pressure gradient and the resistance of the upper respiratory tract (Fig. 14.3).

Experimentally, the luminal volume of the fetal lungs is usually measured by indicator dilution methods (78); this volume can be considered analogous to the functional residual capacity (FRC) of the air-filled lung in that it is the basal, or resting, volume. [In the fetus, lung liquid volume is not significantly altered by individual breathing movements, as "tidal volume" is usually <2 ml (57)]. Although it is

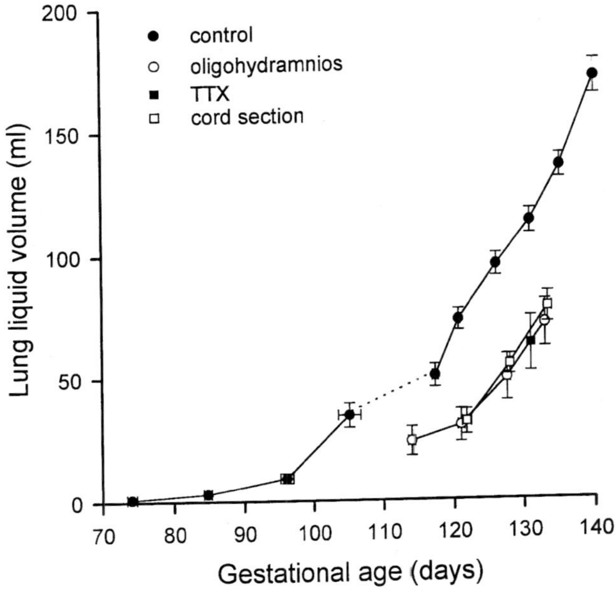

Fig, 14.2 Changes in lung liquid volume, obtained by indicator dilution techniques during the latter half of gestation in fetal sheep, showing influence of oligohydramnios (*open circles*) (29) and abolition of fetal breathing movements by either spinal cord transection [*open squares,* (64)] or tetrodotoxin-induced blockade of conduction in phrenic nerves [*filled square,* (108)]. Data from normal fetal sheep are shown by *filled circles;* data from fetuses <110 days' gestation were obtained from Olver et al. (127) and data from older fetuses are from studies by Harding and Hooper (62, 78).

often stated that the level of lung expansion (i.e., lung liquid volume) in the fetus during late gestation is similar to the FRC of the neonate (116, 157), recent studies in large numbers of healthy fetal sheep have shown that, by term, fetal lung liquid volume is considerably greater than FRC in the postnatal lamb (45–50 ml/kg vs. 25–30 ml/kg) (62, 78). The high level of lung expansion in the late-gestation fetus may be explained by the considerable attenuation of lung parenchymal tissue that has occurred by this stage of development, owing to the formation of large numbers of terminal sacs and alveoli, together with a low level of lung recoil (due to the absence of an air–liquid interface) and the existence of mechanisms that actively oppose the escape of lung liquid. A reduction in luminal volume at birth is to be expected because, as luminal liquid is replaced by air, an air–liquid interface is created within the alveoli and lung recoil is greatly increased, as indicated by a decrease (relative to atmospheric pressure) in intrapleural pressure (8).

Under normal intrauterine conditions, the mean level of fetal lung expansion (i.e., lung liquid volume) is considerably greater than the static relaxation volume of the lungs, the latter volume being that observed when the lungs are allowed to passively equilibrate with the chest wall (62). In late-gestation fetal sheep, lung liquid

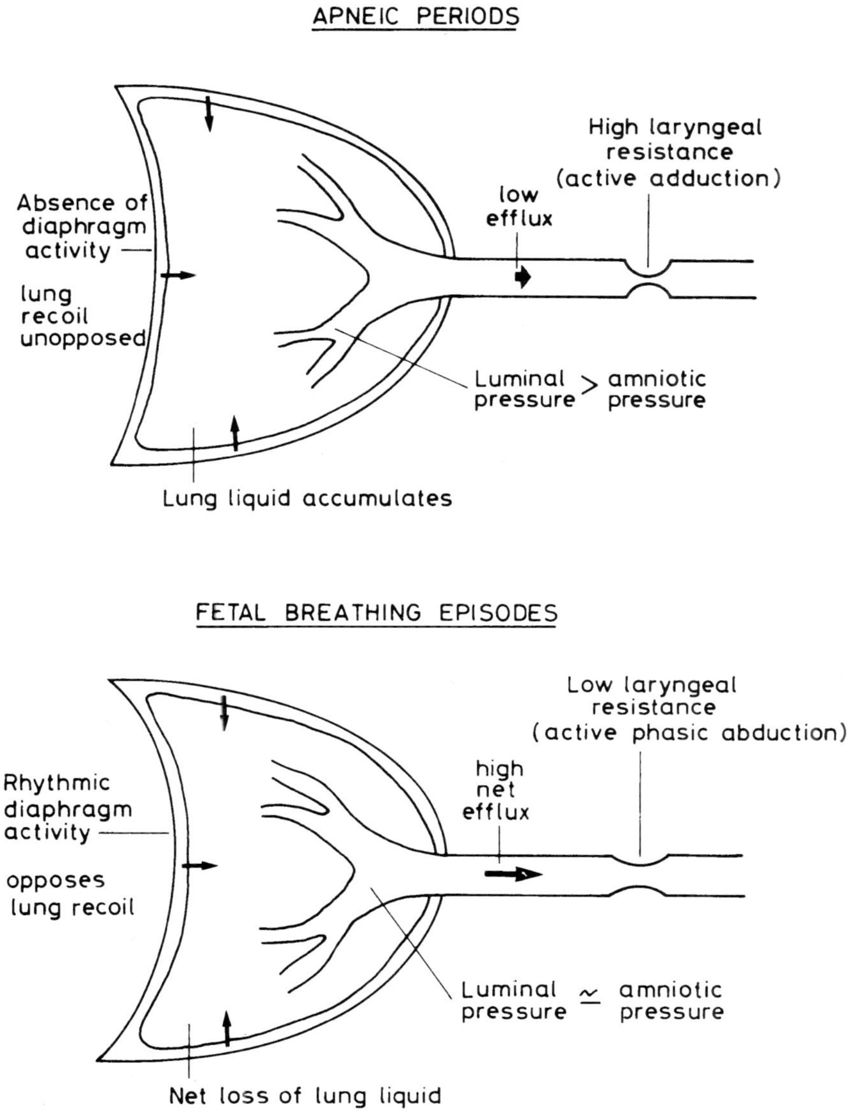

Figure 14.3 Schematic depiction of mechanisms involved in the regulation of lung liquid flow and hence lung expansion in the late-gestation ovine fetus during periods when there are no fetal breathing movements (i.e., apnea, *upper diagram*) and during episodes of fetal breathing (*lower diagram*). During "apnea," lung recoil is opposed by high resistance of the upper respiratory tract (larynx), thereby retaining lung liquid and creating a supra-amniotic pressure in the lung luminal liquid; the diaphragm does not contribute to opposition of lung recoil. During fetal breathing episodes, there is increased efflux of lung liquid due to a reduced upper "airway" resistance in the presence of lung recoil pressure; lung recoil is partially opposed by rhythmic contraction of the diaphragm. [From R. Harding and S.B. Hooper, 1996, with permission from the *Journal of Applied Physiology* (62).]

volume was reduced from 105 ml (~39 ml/kg) to 68 ml (~23 ml/kg) when the lungs were allowed to passively equilibrate with the chest wall [(108) Fig. 14.4]. This reduction in volume demonstrates that the fetal lungs have an effective elastic recoil, which must be opposed in the intact fetus so as to maintain the lungs in an expanded state.

Studies in late-gestation fetal sheep show that two factors are particularly important for opposing the escape of lung liquid and maintaining lung expansion; these are fetal breathing movements (64, 108) and the resistance of the upper respiratory tract (principally the larynx) [(59, 60, 108) Figs. 14.3 and 14.4]. During episodes of fetal breathing movements, the resistance of the upper respiratory tract is reduced (due to rhythmic laryngeal dilation) and lung liquid flows from the lungs at a greater rate than during intervening periods of fetal "apnea" when the resistance of the upper respiratory tract is increased (due to sustained laryngeal constriction) (59, 60, 67). In the absence of rhythmic diaphragmatic contractions during fetal breathing episodes, the efflux of lung liquid would be increased, leading to a loss of lung

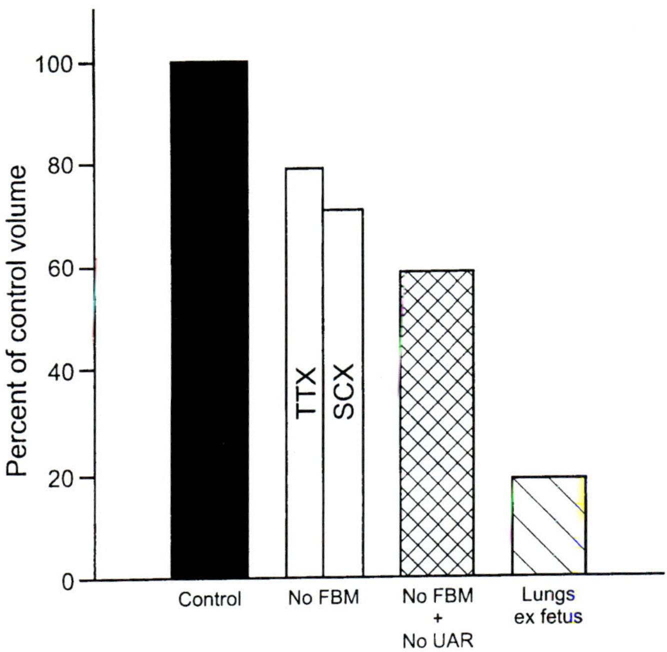

Figure 14.4 Effects on lung liquid volume in late-gestation fetal sheep of removing the influence of fetal breathing movements alone (*No FBM, open columns*), by tetrodotoxin-blockade of conduction in phrenic nerves (*TTX*), and by cervical spinal transection (*SCX*), the effects of combined abolition of fetal breathing and upper respiratory tract (*No FBM + No UAR, cross-hatched bar*) and removal of lungs from fetus (*Lungs ex-fetus, hatched bar*). Data are compared with mean value obtained from normal fetal sheep in utero (*filled bar*). [From R. Harding and S.B. Hooper, 1996, with permission from the *Journal of Applied Physiology*).]

expansion. Thus, it is evident that the ability of fetal breathing to maintain lung liquid volume is the principal means by which fetal breathing facilitates lung growth, rather than the small variations in lung dimensions that fetal breathing movements induce (58, 66).

ROLE OF LUNG DISTENSION IN CONTROL OF LUNG GROWTH

Experimentally it has been shown that prolonged alterations in the degree to which the fetal lungs are expanded by their luminal liquid induce corresponding changes in the growth and structural maturation of lung tissue. Thus, any factor that interferes with the ability of the fetal lungs to remain expanded will eventually lead to lung hypoplasia. Abnormalities that induce lung hypoplasia may do so by interfering with fetal breathing movements or by reducing their efficacy in opposing lung recoil, or they may interfere with the ability of the fetal lungs to expand to their normal volume.

Effects of Reduced Lung Expansion

Sustained reductions in the level of fetal lung expansion result in hypoplasia and structural immaturity of the lungs; this has been demonstrated in fetal sheep in which lung liquid has been allowed to escape under gravity via a tracheal catheter (4, 77, 112). Affected lungs are not only hypoplastic (i.e., reduced numbers of cells) but have thicker interalveolar walls and less potential air space (4). In fetal sheep, 7 days of pulmonary underexpansion is sufficient to reduce pulmonary DNA synthesis rates but insufficient to produce measurable reductions in pulmonary DNA content (77). The results of these studies indicate that during fetal life, an appropriate degree of lung expansion with luminal liquid is essential for normal lung growth. Indeed, it is apparent that prolonged underdistension of fetal lungs during the latter half of gestation (e.g., 20 days) can effectively abolish further lung growth (112).

Effects of Increased Lung Expansion

Overexpansion of the fetal lungs can be induced experimentally by obstruction of the fetal trachea. Under these conditions, lung liquid secretion continues until the luminal pressure increases to a level (~5 mmHg) that is sufficient to inhibit further secretion (78, 122). In fetal sheep during late gestation, lung liquid volume can increase approximately threefold after 7 days of tracheal obstruction (122), and increased DNA synthesis is measurable by 2 days (84, 122). Prolonged pulmonary overexpansion, induced in the fetus by tracheal obstruction, leads to pulmonary hyperplasia and enhanced structural maturation (e.g., thinning of interalveolar walls) (4, 77, 112). Similar findings have been shown in human fetuses with congenital obstruction of the upper respiratory tract (72, 148, 173). Recent evidence has indicated that lung distension may also be an important determinant of lung growth after birth; the lungs of weanling ferrets exposed to a distending pressure of 6 cm H_2O for 2 weeks showed increases in volume and DNA and protein content (176).

How Is Lung Hypoplasia Caused?

Congenital Diaphragmatic Hernia

Congenital diaphragmatic hernia affects the fetal lung in two ways; first, it allows the lung on the affected side to remain in a recoiled state, and second, it allows abdominal viscera to enter the thoracic cavity. Thus, the commonly stated explanation of lung hypoplasia associated with CDH, namely lung compression by intrathoracic abdominal viscera entering the thorax, appears to be oversimplistic. Although it is evident that abdominal viscera do occupy space within the fetal thorax, this may not be the primary causative factor. It seems most likely that the lung on the side of the diaphragmatic defect fails to grow initially because this defect has resulted in the abolition of any opposition to the lung's inherent tendency to recoil (i.e., the lung is able to collapse). In essence, the situation is analogous to a unilateral pneumothorax postnatally, except that the recoil pressure of the fetal lung (because it is liquid filled) is smaller than that of the postnatal lung. Thus in CDH, the fetal lung fails to grow because it cannot be maintained in an expanded state; in the case of unilateral CDH, this could also affect the contralateral lung, as the mediastinum (which is highly compliant) would be able to move toward that lung under the influence of its elastic properties. The entry of abdominal viscera into the thoracic space created by the hypoplastic lung is likely to be a secondary event and may result in further lung collapse owing to the compressive effects of enlarging abdominal viscera. It has been suggested that fetal intestines may become trapped in the thorax at diaphragm closure and that the expansion of these may compress the lungs (129).

Intrathoracic Fluid and Masses

A number of abnormalities grouped together as "space-occupying lesions" can reduce the volume within the thorax; these include intrathoracic cysts, chylothorax or intrapleural effusion of fluid, pericardial effusion, and neuroblastoma (149). Space-occupying lesions, cysts, and intrathoracic fluid are recognized causes of fetal lung hypoplasia because they prevent the lungs from expanding (168). If fluid is drained from the fetal chest with specialized catheters, lung growth can be restored, leading to normal lung function after birth (17, 18).

Skeletomuscular Abnormalities

Abnormalities of the spine and rib cage may, like intrathoracic fluid, result in lung hypoplasia by reducing the intrathoracic space available to the growing lungs. The structural development of the rib cage may be affected by conditions that affect bone or cartilage growth, leading to skeletal dysplasia; these include congenital scoliosis, certain types of dwarfism, and osteogenesis imperfecta. The net effect of these is a reduced intrathoracic volume, possibly combined with an increase in chest wall compliance.

Neurological Abnormalities

The maintenance of a high level of lung expansion, which is essential for normal growth of the fetal lungs, is dependent upon fetal breathing movements. Fetal breathing can be impaired by central or peripheral neural defects. Central neural defects associated with lung hypoplasia include anencephaly, microcephaly, and encephalocoele; defects such as these are likely to be associated with the absence of normal fetal breathing movements and hence play a causal role in lung hypoplasia (33). Phrenic nerve agenesis would result in a reduced thoracic volume due to an inability of the diaphragm to resist lung recoil.

Experimentally, bilateral section of the phrenic nerves, which abolishes diaphragmatic muscular activity and causes diaphragmatic atrophy (38, 47, 152), has been shown to result in lung hypoplasia (5, 9, 38, 119). However, in these experiments it is not possible to attribute lung hypoplasia to the abolition of fetal breathing, as atrophy of the diaphragm could contribute to a reduced ability of the lung to remain expanded. More refined experiments have shown that the abolition of fetal breathing movements, while avoiding diaphragmatic atrophy (via spinal cord transection above the phrenic motoneurons), results in lung hypoplasia (64, 100, 169). The lung hypoplasia can be attributed to a sustained reduction in the mean level of lung expansion resulting from reduced opposition to lung recoil [(64, 108) Fig. 14.2 and 14.4).

It is possible that interference with the control of laryngeal muscle activity may affect fetal lung growth, as these muscles play an important role in regulating the flow of liquid to and from the lungs. Section of the recurrent laryngeal nerves causes an increase in the rate of fluid leaving the lungs during periods of fetal "apnea" (67); functional bypass of the upper respiratory tract has a similar effect (60). However, we know of no clinical evidence that laryngeal or upper respiratory defects are related to lung hypoplasia. Experimentally, bypass of the upper respiratory tract (by the creation of a tracheoamniotic shunt) leads to lung hypoplasia in fetal sheep (37); however, the effects varied in different lobes. This variation could be related to the unusual patterns of tracheal flow that occur in the presence of a tracheoamniotic shunt. It has been found that a substantial influx of fluid (rather than the normal efflux) occurs during episodes of fetal breathing movements, and an accelerated rate of efflux occurs during intervening apneic periods (60).

Oligohydramnios

This also leads to a reduction in thoracic volume. The experimental induction of oligohydramnios, by draining amniotic fluid, causes a reduction in fetal lung expansion (i.e., reduced lung liquid volume) (29, 63, 147) which, if prolonged, leads to lung hypoplasia (29) (Fig. 14.1). This reduction in fetal lung expansion occurs within 48 h and is reversed when amniotic fluid volume is restored (63, 147). A reduced lung liquid volume apparently occurs as result of increased flexion of the fetal trunk, which is caused by the reduction in uterine volume (45, 63) (Fig. 14.1). Increased trunk flexion reduces lung volume by causing an increase in abdominal pressure, which in turn causes an upward displacement of the diaphragm (63) and a reduction in thoracic dimensions (65) (Fig. 14.5); a reduction in lung volume can also be induced postnatally by trunk flexion. If the reduction in lung expansion associated with oligohydramnios is prevented, by obstruction of the fetal trachea, then lung hypoplasia does not occur (2).

An absence of fetal breathing movements in the presence of oligohydramnios has been reported in cases of premature membrane rupture (141), and there is some evidence that the lack of fetal breathing may exacerbate the lung hypoplasia (14–16, 50, 142). Such an effect is plausible, as animal studies have shown that both fetal breathing and a normal amount of amniotic fluid are necessary for normal lung growth in the fetus. In such cases, it is unlikely that the lack of amniotic fluid per se

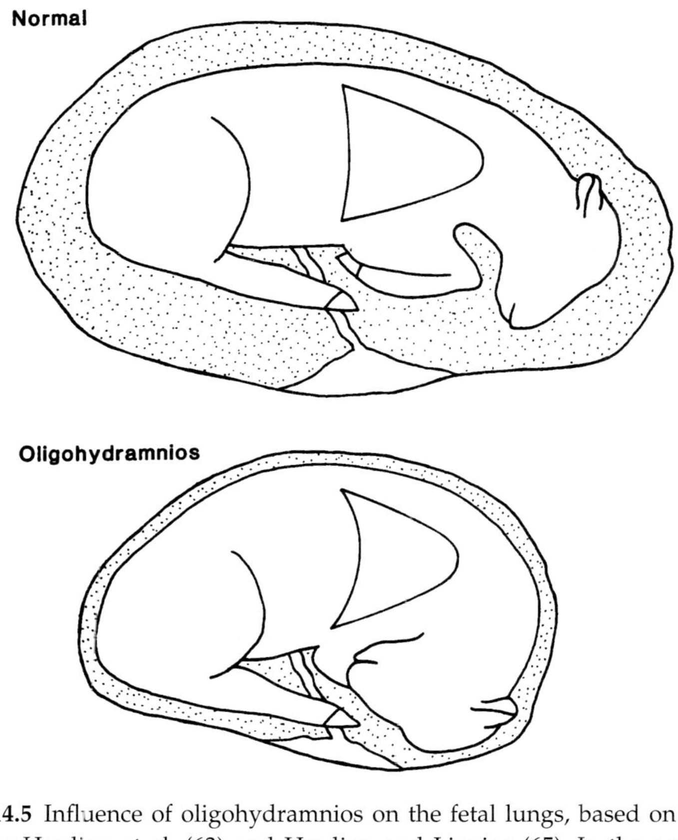

Figure 14.5 Influence of oligohydramnios on the fetal lungs, based on data obtained by Harding et al. (63) and Harding and Liggins (65). In the presence of oligohydramnios, the fetal trunk is increasingly flexed owing to a reduction in uterine volume. Spinal flexion increases abdominal pressure, elevating the diaphragm. At the same time, transverse and dorsoventral thoracic dimensions are reduced.

leads to the inhibition of fetal breathing activity, as several studies in fetal sheep have shown that drainage of amniotic fluid does not affect the incidence of fetal breathing (30, 63, 111, 147). Thus, it is not unexpected that the replacement of amniotic fluid in oligohydramnios cases does not increase the incidence of fetal breathing movements (39). In the presence of premature membrane rupture, particularly if infection is present, it is possible that other factors, such as the release of cytokines, inhibit fetal breathing movements.

LUNG GROWTH AND TISSUE STRESS: UNDERLYING MECHANISMS

It is apparent that the mean level of lung expansion has a profound influence on lung tissue growth and structural maturation, and that this effect is exerted at a local level. However, the processes by which tissue stress is transduced into a growth response are not yet clear. The lung is one of many soft, elastic tissues that are affected by physical factors such as tissue stress, and clues as to transduction mechanisms operating in the lungs may be obtained from other tissues. Other soft elastic tissues in which growth and/or cellular differentiation are known to be affected by mechanical stress include skeletal and smooth muscle (10, 41, 46) vascular endothelial cells (160), periodontal epithelial cells (21), and skin (117, 153).

It is possible that increased tissue growth in response to mechanical stress is mediated by cellular distortion, via deformation of the extracellular matrix and cytoskeleton, leading to cellular hypertrophy or cell division (134, 140). In the fetal lung, there is evidence that cellular hypertrophy precedes, and may stimulate, mitosis when tissue stress is increased (122). It has been suggested that mechanical stimuli may lead to increased synthesis and release of chemical mediators that can stimulate cell division, affect the cellular phenotype, or alter cellular metabolic activity. The fetal lung can synthesize a range of substances with the capacity to stimulate cell division or to promote cellular differentiation. Peptide growth factors detected in the developing lung and that may be involved in regulating cell division and differentiation include insulin-like growth factors (IGFs) I and II (167), gastrin-releasing peptide (99), fibroblast growth factor (53), platelet-derived growth factor (PDGF) (54), transforming growth factor alpha (92), epidermal growth factor (156), and fibroblast-pneumonocyte growth factor (150). It has also been suggested that interleukin-1 and -2 may be implicated in lung growth (86).

There are few in vivo experiments that have explored the role of growth factors during early development. In fetal sheep, pulmonary IGF-ll expression was significantly increased when lung growth was stimulated by increased distension (77) and decreased when lung growth was retarded by decreased distension (64, 77). The increased lung tissue growth induced by partial pneumonectomy in rats was accompanied by increased tissue levels of IGF-I (154). In rabbits subjected to partial lung resection followed by increased growth of remaining lung tissue, there was an increase in blood levels of a substance that resembled IGF-II and stimulated the growth of type II epithelial cells in vitro (151). Observations such as these suggest that IGFs may play a paracrine role in mediating the lung growth response to increased mechanical stress.

In vitro studies, in which rhythmic stretching aimed at simulating the effects of fetal breathing movements was applied to organotypic cultures of lung cells, have shown that growth-promoting substances are released; these stimulated DNA synthesis, but the effects were restricted to epithelial cells (103). In similar in vitro experiments, the expression of mRNA for PDGF was increased by repetitive stretching of lung tissue, and this effect was blocked by antisense oligonucleotides for PDGF and its receptor (101).

There has been considerable interest in the second messenger systems that mediate stretch-induced cell growth and mitosis. It has been shown that cellular levels of cAMP and cAMP-dependent protein kinase are increased in remaining, and growing, lung tissue following partial pneumonectomy (123, 145). Mechanical stimulation of lung cell growth in vitro led to increased activity of protein kinase C (102). Intracellular movement of calcium may also play a role in the transduction process leading to increased lung growth, at least in epithelial cells. Stretching cultures of pulmonary epithelial (type II) cells causes increased influx of Ca into these cells (104, 146, 174), presumably via stretch-sensitive Ca channels. When stretch-activated channels are blocked in rat lung cells in vitro, both the influx of Ca and increase in DNA synthesis, which normally occur during rhythmic stretching, are inhibited (104). Further evidence for a role of intracellular Ca in the pulmonary growth response is that levels of the Ca-dependent regulatory protein calmodulin were increased in lung tissue during the growth response that followed partial pneumonectomy. Furthermore, this growth response was inhibited by the calmodulin antagonist trifluoperazine (126).

In Utero Reversal of Lung Hypoplasia by Increased Lung Expansion

Because fetal lung hypoplasia, or the associated intrauterine abnormalities, can be recognized by imaging techniques, attempts have been made to eliminate the predisposing factors or, if the cause cannot be eliminated, to stimulate lung growth in utero. In recent years, there has been interest in stimulating the growth of hypoplastic lungs by obstructing the trachea in utero. Animal studies have shown that tracheal obstruction expands the lungs by the continued production of lung liquid, thereby stimulating lung growth and structural maturation. This has been shown to occur in the presence of lung hypoplasia following experimental CDH (31, 71) or prolonged drainage of lung liquid (121). Animal experiments on the effects of tracheal obstruction using an intratracheal balloon have indicated that this approach may be beneficial in the treatment of lung hypoplasia (11, 70), and clinical trials have been conducted with some success (68, 118). A potential problem associated with the use of tracheal obstruction to reverse lung hypoplasia is that it may inhibit the production of pulmonary surfactant (83, 128, 131). There is evidence from a rat model of CDH that glucocorticoid treatment, in the absence of tracheal obstruction, may benefit lung development (158), but this has yet to be confirmed in a large animal model. If effective, this approach may overcome some of the difficulties associated with tracheal obstruction, although it seems likely that concomitant tracheal obstruction may be necessary. Another potential problem associated with tracheal obstruction is the enlargement of existing alveoli, which may lead to later structural and functional deficiencies of the lungs. It is clear that further studies of the long-term effects of tracheal obstruction are needed before this can become regarded as an effective prenatal treatment for lung hypoplasia.

REFERENCES

1. Adamson, T.M., R.D.H. Boyd, H.S. Platt, and L.B. Strang. Composition of alveolar liquid in the foetal lamb. *J. Physiol.* 204: 159–168, 1969.
2. Adzick, N.S., M.R. Harrison, P.L. Glick, R.L. Villa, and W. Finkbeiner. Experimental pulmonary hypoplasia and oligohydramnios: relative contributions of lung fluid and fetal breathing movements. *J. Pediatr. Surg.* 19: 658–665, 1984.
3. Aguirre, O.A., B.E. Finley, L.E. Ridgway, T.L. Bennett, and T.A. Cowles. Resolution of unilateral fetal hydrothorax with associated non-immune hydrops after intrauterine thoracentesis. *Ultrasound Obstet. Gynecol.* 5: 346–348, 1995.
4. Alcorn, D., T.M. Adamson, T.F. Lambert, J.E. Maloney, B.C. Ritchie, and P.M. Robinson. Morphological effects of chronic tracheal ligation and drainage in the fetal lamb lung. *J. Anat.* 123: 649–660, 1977.
5. Alcorn, D., T.M. Adamson, J.E. Maloney, and P.M. Robinson. Morphological effects of chronic bilateral phrenectomy or vagotomy in the fetal lamb lung. *J. Anat.* 130: 683–695, 1980.
6. Asabe, K., N.Toki, S. Hashimoto, S. Suita, and K. Sueishi. An immunohistochemical study of the expression of surfactant apoprotein in the hypoplastic lung of rabbit fetuses induced by oligohydramnios. *Am. J. Pathol.* 145: 631–639, 1994.
7. Askenazi, S.S. and M. Perlman. Pulmonary hypoplasia: lung weight and radial alveolar count as critical diagnosis. *Arch. Dis. Child.* 54: 614–618, 1979.
8. Avery, M.E. and C.D. Cook. Volume-pressure relationships of lungs and thorax in fetal, newborn, and adult goats. *J. Appl. Physiol.* 16: 1034–1038, 1961.
9. Bamford, O.S., A. Rivera, T. Tadalan, and W. Ellis. Effects of in utero phrenic nerve section on the development of collagen and elastin in lamb lungs. *Am. Rev. Respir. Dis.* 146: 1202–1205, 1992.
10. Baskin, L., P.S. Howard, and E. Macarak. Effect of physical forces on bladder smooth muscle and urothelium. *J. Urol.* 150: 601–607, 1993.
11. Bealer, J.F., E.D. Skarsgard, M.H. Hedrick, M. Meuli, K.J. Vanderwall, A.W. Flake, N.S. Adzick, and M.R. Harrison. The "PLUG" odyssey; adventures in experimental fetal tracheal occlusion. *J. Pediatr. Surg.* 30: 361–365, 1995.
12. Blachford, K.G. and W.M. Thurlbeck. Lung growth and maturation in experimental oligohydramnios in the rat. *Pediatr. Pulmonol.* 3: 328–333, 1987.
13. Blott, M. and A. Greenough. Neonatal outcome after prolonged rupture of the membranes starting in the second trimester. *Arch. Dis. Child.* 63: 1146–1150, 1988.
14. Blott, M. and A. Greenough. Oligohydramnios in the second trimester of pregnancy, fetal breathing and normal lung growth. *Early Hum. Dev.* 17: 37–40, 1988.

15. Blott, M., A. Greenough, K.H. Nicolaides, and S. Campbell. The ultrasonographic assessment of the fetal thorax and fetal breathing movements in the prediction of pulmonary hypoplasia. *Early Hum. Dev.* 21: 143–151, 1990.
16. Blott, M., A. Greenough, K.H. Nicolaides, G. Moscoso, D. Gibb, and S. Campbell. Fetal breathing movements as predictor of favourable pregnancy outcome after oligohydramnios due to membrane rupture in second trimester. *Lancet* 2: 129–131, 1987.
17. Blott, M., K.H. Nicolaides, and A. Greenough. Pleuroamniotic shunting for decompression of fetal pleural effusions. *Obstet. Gynecol.* 71: 798–800, 1988.
18. Blott, M., K.H. Nicolaides, and A. Greenough. Postnatal respiratory function after chronic drainage of fetal pulmonary cyst. *Am. J. Obstet. Gynecol.* 159: 858–859, 1988.
19. Bohn, D., M. Tamura, D. Perrin, G. Barker, and M. Rabinovitch. Ventilatory predictors of pulmonary hypoplasia in congenital diaphragmatic hernia, confirmed by morphologic assessment. *J. Pediatr.* 111: 423–431, 1987.
20. Brandsma, A.E., D. Tibboel, T.M. Vulto, J. Egberts, and A.T. Have-Opbroek. Ultrastructural features of alveolar epithelial cells in the late fetal pulmonary acinus: a comparison between normal and hypoplastic lungs using a rat model of pulmonary hypoplasia and congenital diaphragmatic hernia. *Microsc. Res. Tech.* 26: 389–399, 1993.
21. Brunette, D.M. Mechanical stretching increases the number of epithelial cells synthesizing DNA in culture. *J. Cell. Sci.* 69: 35–45, 1984.
22. Butler, N. and A.E. Claireaux. Congenital diaphragmatic hernia as a cause of perinatal mortality. *Lancet* 1: 659–663, 1962.
23. Castillo, R.A., L.D. Devoe, H.A. Hadi, S. Martin, and D. Geist. Nonimmune hydrops fetalis: clinical experience and factors related to a poor outcome. *Am. J. Obstet. Gynecol.* 155: 812–816, 1986.
24. Chamberlain, D., A. Hislop, E. Hey, and L. Reid. Pulmonary hypoplasia in babies with severe rhesus isoimmunisation: a quantitative study. *J. Pathol.* 122: 43–52, 1977.
25. Chitkara, U., J. Rosenburg, F.A. Chervenak, G.S. Berkowitz, R. Levine, R.M. Fagerstrom, B. Walker, and R.L. Berkowitz. Prenatal sonographic assessment of the fetal thorax: normal values. *Am. J. Obstet. Gynecol.* 156: 1069–1074, 1987.
26. Collins, M.H., A. C. Moessinger, and J. Kleinerman. Fetal lung hypoplasia. In: *CRC Handbook of Animal Models of Pulmonary Disease,* edited by J.O. Cantor. Boca Raton, FL: CRC Press, 1989, p. 129–157.
27. Collins, M.H., A.C. Moessinger, J. Kleinerman, J. Bassi, P. Rosso, A.H. Collins, L.S. James, and W.A. Blanc. Fetal lung hypoplasia associated with maternal smoking: a morphometric analysis. *Pediatr. Res.* 19: 408–412, 1985.
28. D'Alton, M., B. Mercer, E. Riddick, and D. Dudley. Serial thoracic versus abdominal circumference ratios for the prediction of pulmonary hypoplasia in premature rupture of the membranes remote from term. *Am. J. Obstet. Gynecol.* 166: 658–663, 1992.
29. Dickson, K.A. and R. Harding. Decline in lung liquid volume and secretion rate during oligohydramnios in fetal sheep. *J. Appl. Physiol.* 67: 2401–2407, 1989.
30. Dickson, K.A. and R. Harding. Fetal breathing and pressures in the trachea and amniotic sac during oligohydramnios in sheep. *J. Appl. Physiol.* 70: 293–299, 1991.
31. DiFiore, J.W., D.O. Fauza, R. Slavin, C.A. Peters, J.C. Fackler, and J.M. Wilson. Experimental fetal tracheal ligation reverses the structural and physiological effects of pulmonary hypoplasia in congenital diaphragmatic hernia. *J. Pediatr. Surg.* 29: 248–257, 1994.
32. Dorland, W.A.N. (ed.). *Dorland's Illustrated Medical Dictionary*. Philadelphia: W.B. Saunders, 1988.

33. Dornan, J.C., J.W. K. Ritchie, and C. Meban. Fetal breathing movements and lung maturation in the congenitally abnormal human fetus. *J. Dev. Physiol.* 6: 367–375, 1984.
34. Editorial. Breath of life. *Lancet* 1: 305–306, 1989.
35. Emery, J.L. and A. Mithal. The number of alveoli in the terminal respiratory unit of man during late intra-uterine life and childhood. *Ach. Dis. Child.* 35: 544–547, 1960.
36. Falconer, A.R., R.A. Brown, P. Helms, T. Gordon, and J.A. Baron. Pulmonary sequelae in survivors of congenital diaphragmatic hernia. *Thorax* 45: 126–129, 1990.
37. Fewell, J.E., A.A. Hislop, J.A. Kitterman, and P. Johnson. Effect of tracheostomy on lung development in fetal lambs. *J. Appl. Physiol.* 55: 1103–1108, 1983.
38. Fewell, J.E., C.C. Lee, and J.A. Kitterman. Effects of phrenic nerve section on the respiratory system of fetal lambs. *J. Appl. Physiol.* 51: 293–297, 1981.
39. Fisk, N.M., D.G. Talbert, U. Nicolini, J. Vaughan, and C.H. Rodeck. Fetal breathing movements in oligohydramnios are not increased by amnioinfusion. *Br. J. Obstet. Gynaecol.* 99: 464–468, 1992.
40. Fong, K., A. Ohlsson, and A. Zalev. Fetal thoracic circumference: a prospective cross-sectional study with real time ultrasound. *Am. J. Obstet. Gynecol.* 158: 1154–1160, 1988.
41. Fortado, C.M. and J.G. Barnett. Effects of inhibiting DNA synthesis with hydroxyurea on stretch-induced skeletal muscle growth. *Exp. Neurol.* 87: 487–494, 1985.
42. Fox, H.E. and S.S. Badalian. Ultrasound prediction of fetal pulmonary hypoplasia in pregnancies complicated by oligohydramnios and in cases of congenital diaphragmatic hernia: a review. *Am. J. Perinatol.* 11: 104–108, 1994.
43. Froh, D.K. and P.L. Ballard. Fetal lung maturation. In: *Textbook of Fetal Physiology.* edited by G.D. Thorburn and R. Harding. Oxford: Oxford University Press, 1994, p. 168–185.
44. Gaultier, C. Malnutrition and lung growth. *Pediatr. Pulmonol.* 10: 278–286, 1991.
45. Gembruch, U. and M. Hansmann. Artificial instillation of amniotic fluid as a new technique for the diagnostic evaluation of cases of oligohydramnios. *Prenat. Diagn.* 8: 33–35, 1988.
46. Goldspink, D.F., V.M. Cox, S.K. Smith, L.A. Eaves, N.J. Osbaldeston, D.M. Lee, and D. Mantle. Muscle growth in response to mechanical stimuli. *Am. J. Physiol.* 268: E288–E297, 1995.
47. Goldstein, J.D. and L.M. Reid. Pulmonary hypoplasia resulting from phrenic nerve agenesis and diaphragmatic amyoplasia. *J. Pediatr.* 97: 282–287, 1980.
48. Gould, S.J. Pulmonary hypoplasia, hyaline membrane disease and chronic lung disease. In: *Fetus and Neonate: Breathing,* edited by M.A. Hanson, J.A.D. Spencer, C.H. Rodeck, and D. Walters. Cambridge: University of Cambridge Press, 1994, p. 214–236.
49. Graves, G.R. and X.X. Baskett. Nonimmune hydrops fetalis: antenatal diagnosis and management. *Am. J. Obstet. Gynecol.* 148: 563–565, 1984.
50. Greenough, A., M. Blott, K. Nicolaides, and S. Campbell. Interpretation of fetal breathing movements in oligohydramnios due to membrane rupture. *Lancet* 2: 182–183, 1988.
51. Gruenwald, P. Hypoplasia of the lungs. *J. Mt. Sinai Hosp.* 24: 913–919, 1957.
52. Haidar, A., T.A. Ryder, and J.S. Wigglesworth. Failure of elastin development in hypoplastic lungs associated with oligohydramnios: an electronmicroscopic study. *Histopathology* 18: 471–473, 1991.
53. Han, R.N.N., J. Liu, A.K. Tanswell, and M. Post. Expression of basic fibroblast growth factor and receptor: immunolocalization studies in developing rat fetal lung. *Pediatr. Res.* 31: 435–440, 1992.
54. Han, R.N.N., C. Mawdsley, P. Souza, A.K. Tanswell, and M. Post. Platelet-derived growth

factors and growth-related genes in rat lung. III. Immunolocalization during fetal development. *Pediatr. Res.* 31: 323–329, 1992.

55. Harding, J.E. and B.M. Johnston. Nutrition and fetal growth. *Reprod. Fertil. Dev.* 7: 539–547, 1995.
56. Harding, R. Sustained alterations in postnatal respiratory function following sub-optimal intra-uterine conditions. *Reprod. Fertil. Dev.* 7: 431–441, 1995.
57. Harding, R. Fetal breathing movements. In: *The Lung: Scientific Foundations*, edited by R. G. Crystal, J.B. West, E.R. Weibel, and P.J. Barnes. Philadelphia: Lipincott-Raven, 1997, p. 2093–2103.
58. Harding, R. Fetal pulmonary development: the role of respiratory movements. *Equine Vet. J.* (Suppl.) 24: 32–39, 1997.
59. Harding, R., A.D. Bocking, and J.N. Sigger. Upper airway resistances in fetal sheep: the influence of breathing activity. *J. Appl. Physiol.* 60: 160–165, 1986.
60. Harding, R., A.D. Bocking, and J.N. Sigger. Influence of upper respiratory tract on liquid flow to and from fetal lungs. *J. Appl. Physiol.* 61: 68–74, 1986.
61. Harding, R., A.D. Bocking, J.N. Sigger, and P.J.D. Wickham. Composition and volume of fluid swallowed by fetal sheep. *Q. J. Exp. Physiol.* 69: 487–495, 1984.
62. Harding, R. and S.B. Hooper. Regulation of lung expansion and lung growth before birth. *J. Appl. Physiol.* 81: 209–224, 1996.
63. Harding, R., S.B. Hooper, and K.A. Dickson. A mechanism leading to reduced lung hypoplasia in fetal sheep during oligohydramnios. *Am. J. Obstet. Gynecol.* 163: 1904–1913, 1990.
64. Harding, R., S.B. Hooper, and V.K. Han. Abolition of fetal breathing movements by spinal cord transection leads to reductions in fetal pulmonary expansion, growth and IGF-II gene expression. *Pediatr. Res.* 34: 148–153, 1993.
65. Harding, R. and G.C. Liggins. The influence of oligohydramnios on thoracic dimensions of fetal sheep. *J. Dev. Physiol.* 16: 355–361, 1991.
66. Harding, R. and G.C. Liggins. Changes in thoracic dimensions induced by breathing movements in fetal sheep. *Reprod. Fertil. Dev.* 8: 117–124, 1996.
67. Harding, R., J.N. Sigger, P.J.D. Wickham, and A.D. Bocking. The regulation of flow of pulmonary fluid in fetal sheep. *Respir. Physiol.* 57: 47–59, 1984.
68. Harrison, M.R., N.S. Adzick, A.W. Flake, R.W. Jennings, J.M. Estes, T.E. MacGilliviray, J.T. Cheuh, and J.D. Goldberg. Correction of congenital diaphragmatic hernia VI: Hard-earned lessons. *J. Pediatr. Surg.* 28: 1411–1418, 1993.
69. Harrison, M.R., N.S. Adzick, R.W. Jennings, B.W. Duncan, M.A. Rosen, R.A. Filly, J.D. Goldberg, and A.A. deLorimier. Antenatal intervention for congenital cystic adenomatoid malformation. *Lancet* II: 965–967, 1990.
70. Hashim, E., J.M. Laberge, M.F. Chen, and E.W. Quillen. Reversible tracheal obstruction in the fetal sheep: effects on tracheal fluid pressure and lung growth. *J. Pediatr. Surg.* 30: 1172–1177, 1995.
71. Hedrick, M.H., J.M. Estes, K.M. Sullivan, J.F. Bealer, J.A. Kitterman, A.W. Flake, N.S. Adzick, and M.R. Harrison. Plug the lung until it grows (PLUG): a new method to treat congenital diaphragmatic hernia in utero. *J. Pediatr. Surg.* 29: 612–617, 1994.
72. Hedrick, M.H., M.M. Fero, R.A. Filly, A.W. Flake, M.R. Harrison, and N.S. Adzick. Congenital high airway obstruction syndrome (CHAOS): a potential for perinatal intervention. *J. Pediatr. Surg.* 29: 271–274, 1994.
73. Higuchi, M., T. Kato, H. Yoshino, K. Matsuda, K. Gotoh, H. Hirano, K. Koyana, and M.

Maki. The influence of experimentally produced oligohydramnios on lung growth and pulmonary surfactant content in fetal rabbits. *J. Dev. Physiol.* 16: 223–227, 1991.

74. Hislop, A., D.V.I. Fairweather, R.J. Blackwell, and S. Howard. The effect of amniocentesis and drainage of amniotic fluid on lung development in *Macaca fascicularis*. *Br. J. Obstet. Gynaecol.* 91: 835–842, 1984.
75. Hislop, A., E. Hey, and L. Reid. The lungs in congenital bilateral renal agenesis and dysplasia. *Arch. Dis. Child.* 54: 32–38, 1979.
76. Hislop, A. and L. Reid. Persistent hypoplasia of the lung after repair of congenital diaphragmatic hernia. *Thorax* 31: 450–455, 1976.
77. Hooper, S.B., V.K. M. Han, and R. Harding. Changes in lung expansion alter pulmonary DNA synthesis and IGF-II gene expression in fetal sheep. *Am. J. Physiol.* (*Lung Cell. Mol. Physiol.*) 265: L403–L409, 1993.
78. Hooper, S.B. and R. Harding. Fetal lung liquid: a major determinant of the growth and functional development of the fetal lung. *Clin. Exp. Pharmacol. Physiol.* 22: 235–247, 1995.
79. Husain, A.N. and R.G. Hessel. Neonatal pulmonary hypoplasia: an autopsy study of 25 cases. *Pediatr. Pathol.* 13: 475–478, 1993.
80. Imanaka, M., S. Ogita, and T. Sugawa. Saline solution amnioinfusion for oligohydramnios after premature rupture of the membranes. *Am. J. Obstet. Gynecol.* 161: 102–106, 1989.
81. Inselman, L.S., S.E. Fisher, H. Spencer, and M. Atkinson. Effect of intrauterine ethanol exposure on fetal lung growth. *Pediatr. Res.* 19: 12–14, 1985.
82. Jakubowska, A.E., K. Billings, D.P. Johns, S.B. Hooper, and R. Harding. Respiratory function in lambs following prolonged oligohydramnios during late gestation. *Pediatr. Res.* 34: 611–617, 1993.
83. Joe, P., L.D. Wallen, C.J. Chapin, C.H. Lee, L. Allen, V.K. Han, L.G. Dobbs, S. Hawgood, and J.A. Kitterman. Effects of mechanical factors on growth and maturation of the lung in fetal sheep. *Am. J. Physiol.* (*Lung Cell. Mol. Physiol.*) 272: L95–L105, 1997.
84. Keramidaris, E., S.B. Hooper, and R. Harding. Effect of gestational age on the increase in fetal lung growth following tracheal obstruction. *Exp. Lung Res.* 22: 283–298, 1996.
85. King, J.C., W. Mitzner, A.B. Butterfield, and J.T. Queenan. Effect of induced oligohydramnios on fetal lung development. *Am. J. Obstet. Gynecol.* 154: 823–830, 1986.
86. King, R.J., M.B. Jones, and P. Minoo. Regulation of lung cell proliferation by polypeptide growth factors. *Am. J. Physiol.* (*Lung Cell. Mol. Physiol.*) 257: L23–L38, 1989.
87. Kitagawa, M., A. Hislop, E.A. Boyden, and L. Reid. Lung hypoplasia in congenital diaphragmatic hernia: a quantitative study of airway, artery and alveolar development. *Br. J. Surg.* 58: 342–346, 1971.
88. Kitterman, J.A. Physical factors and fetal lung growth. In: *Respiratory Control and Lung Development in the Fetus and Newborn,* edited by B.M. Johnston and P.D. Gluckman. Ithaca: Perinatology Press, 1986, pp. 63–85.
89. Kitterman, J.A. Physiological factors in fetal lung growth. *Can. J. Physiol. Pharmacol.* 66: 1122–1128, 1988.
90. Kitterman, J.A. The effects of mechanical forces on fetal lung growth. *Clin. Perinatol.* 23: 727–740, 1996.
91. Knox, W.F. and A.J. Barson. Pulmonary hypoplasia in a regional perinatal unit. *Early Hum. Dev.* 14: 33–42, 1986.
92. Kubiak, J., M.M. Mitra, A.R. Steve, J.D. Hunt, P. Davies, and B.R. Pitt. Transforming growth factor-α gene expression in late-gestation fetal rat lung. *Pediatr. Res.* 31: 286–290, 1992.

93 Landau, L.I., P.D. Phelan, G.L. Gillam, E. Coombs, and H.R. Noblett. Respiratory function after repair of congenital diaphragmatic hernia. *Arch. Dis. Child.* 52: 282–286, 1977.

94. Langer, R. and H.J. Kaufman. Primary (isolated) bilateral pulmonary hypoplasia: a comparative study of radiologic findings and autopsy results. *Pediatr. Radiol.* 16: 175–179, 1986.

95. Laudy, J.A.M., J.L.J. Gaillard, J.N.V.D. Anker, D. Tibboel, and J.W. Wladimiroff. Doppler ultrasound imaging: a new technique to detect lung hypoplasia before birth? *Ultrasound Obstet. Gynecol.* 7: 189–192, 1996.

96. Lauria, M.R., B. Gonik, and R. Romero. Pulmonary hypoplasia: pathogenesis, diagnosis and antenatal prediction. *Obstet. Gynecol.* 86: 466–475, 1995.

97. Lechner, A.J. Perinatal age determines the severity of retarded lung development induced by starvation. *Am. Rev. Respir. Dis.* 131: 638–643, 1985.

98. Levin, D.L. Morphologic analysis of the pulmonary vascular bed in congenital left-sided diaphragmatic hernia. *J. Pediatr.* 92: 805–809, 1978.

99. Li, K., S.R. Nagalla, and E.R. Spindel. A rhesus monkey model to characterize the role of gastrin-releasing peptide (GRP) in lung development. Evidence for stimulation of airway growth. *J. Clin. Invest.* 94: 1605–1615, 1994.

100. Liggins, G.C., G.A. Vilos, G.A. Campos, J.A. Kitterman, and C.H. Lee. The effect of spinal cord transection on lung development in fetal sheep. *J. Dev. Physiol.* 3: 267–274, 1981.

101. Liu, M., J. Liu, S. Buch, A.K. Tanswell, and M. Post. Antisense oligonucleotides for PDGF-B and its receptor inhibit mechanical strain-induced fetal lung cell growth. *Am. J. Physiol. (Lung Cell. Mol. Physiol.)* 269: L178–L184, 1995.

102. Liu, M., J. Xu, J. Liu, M.E. Kraw, A.K. Tanswell, and M. Post. Mechanical strain-enhanced fetal lung cell proliferation is mediated by phospholipase C and D and protein kinase C. *Am. J. Physiol. (Lung Cell. Mol. Physiol.)* 268: L729–L738, 1995.

103. Liu, M., J. Xu, A.K. Tanswell, and M. Post. Stretch-induced growth-promoting activities stimulate fetal rat lung epithelial cell proliferation. *Exp. Lung Res.* 19: 505–517, 1993.

104. Liu, M., J. Xu, A.K. Tanswell, and M. Post. Inhibition of mechanical strain-induced fetal rat lung cell proliferation by Gadolinium, a stretch-activated channel blocker. *J. Cell Physiol.* 161: 501–507, 1994.

105. Longaker, M.T., J.M. Laberge, J. Dansereau, J.C. Langer, T.M. Crombleholme, P.W. Callen, M.S. Golbus, and M.R. Harrison. Primary fetal hydrothorax: natural history and management. *J. Pediatr. Surg.* 24: 573–576, 1989.

106. Lund, D.P., J. Mitchell, V. Kharasch, S. Quigley, M. Kuehn, and J.M. Wilson. Congenital diaphragmatic hernia: the hidden morbidity. *J. Pediatr. Surg.* 29: 258–264, 1994.

107. Maloney, J.E., G. Bowes, V. Brodecky, X. Dennett, M. Wilkinson, and A. Walker. Function of the future respiratory system in the growth retarded fetal sheep. *J. Develop. Physiol.* 4:279–297, 1982.

108. Miller, A.A., S.B. Hooper, and R. Harding. Role of fetal breathing movements in control of fetal lung distension. *J. Appl. Physiol.* 75: 2711–2717, 1993.

109. Moessinger, A.C. Fetal akinesia deformation sequence: an animal model. *Pediatrics* 7: 857–863, 1983.

110. Moessinger, A.C. Fetal lung growth in experimental utero-abdominal pregnancy. *Obstet. Gynecol.* 68: 675–678, 1986.

111. Moessinger, A.C., J.E. Fewell, R.I. Stark, M.H. Collins, S.S. Daniel, M. Singh, W.A. Blanc, J. Kleinerman, and L.S. James. Lung hypoplasia and breathing movements following oligohydramnios in fetal lambs. In: *The Physiological Development of the Fetus and Newborn.* edited by C.T. Jones and P. Nathanielsz. New York: Academic Press, 1985, p. 293–298.

112. Moessinger, A.C., R. Harding, T.M. Adamson, M. Singh, and G.T. Kiu. Role of lung fluid volume in growth and maturation of the fetal sheep lung. *J. Clin. Invest.* 86: 1270–1277, 1990.
113. Moessinger, A.C., A. Santiago, N.S. Paneth, H.R. Rey, W.A. Blanc, and J.M. Driscoll. Time trends in necropsy prevalence and birth prevalence of lung hypoplasia. *Pediatr. Perinat. Epidemiol.* 3: 421–431, 1989.
114. Morales, W.J. and T. Talley. Premature rupture of membranes at <25 weeks: a management dilemma. *Am. J. Obstet. Gynecol.* 168: 503–507, 1993.
115. Morin, F.C. and K.R. Stenmark. Persistent pulmonary hypertension of the newborn. *Am. J. Respir. Crit. Care Med.* 151: 2010–2032, 1995.
116. Mortola, J.P. Dynamics of breathing in newborn mammals. *Physiol. Rev.* 67: 187–243, 1987.
117. Mustoe, T.A., T.H. Bartell, and W.L. Garner. Physical, biomechanical, histologic, and biochemical effects of rapid versus conventional tissue expansion. *Plast. Reconstr. Surg.* 83: 687–691, 1989.
118. Mychaliska, G.B., K.M. Bullard, and M.R. Harrison. In utero management of congenital diaphragmatic hernia. *Clin. Perinatol.* 23: 823–841, 1996.
119. Nagai, A., W.M. Thurlbeck, A.H. Jansen, S. Ioffe, and V. Chernick. The effect of chronic biphrenectomy on lung growth and maturation in fetal lambs. *Am. Rev. Respir. Dis.* 137: 167–172, 1988.
120. Nakamura, Y., K. Harada, I. Yamamoto, Y. Uemura, K. Okamoto, S. Fukuda, and T. Hashimoto. Human pulmonary hypoplasia. *Achiv. Pathol. Lab. Med.* 116: 635–642, 1992.
121. Nardo, L., S.B. Hooper, and R. Harding. Lung hypoplasia can be reversed by short-term obstruction of the trachea in fetal sheep. *Pediatr. Res.* 38: 690–696, 1995.
122. Nardo, L., S.B. Hooper, and R. Harding. Stimulation of lung growth by tracheal obstruction in fetal sheep: relation to luminal pressure and lung liquid volume. *Pediatr. Res.* 43: 184–190, 1998.
123. Nijjar, M.S. and W.M. Thurlbeck. Alterations in enzymes related to adenosine 3′,5′-monophosphate during compensatory growth of rat lung. *Eur. J. Biochem.* 105: 403–407, 1980.
124. Nimrod, C.,D. Davies, S. Iwanicki, J. Harder, D. Persaud, and S. Nicholson. Ultrasound prediction of pulmonary hypoplasia. *Obstet. Gynecol.* 68: 495–498, 1986.
125. Nimrod, C., F. Varela-Gittings, G. Machin, D. Campbell, and R. Wesenberg. The effect of very prolonged membrane rupture on fetal development. *Am. J. Obstet. Gynecol.* 148: 540–543, 1984.
126. Ofulue, A.F., R. Matsui, and W.M. Thurlbeck. Role of calmodulin as an endogenous initiatory factor in compensatory lung growth after pneumonectomy. *Pediatr. Pulmonol.* 15: 145–150, 1993.
127. Olver, R.E., E.E. Schneeberger, and D.V. Walters. Epithelial solute permeability, ion transport and tight junction morphology in the developing lung of the fetal lamb. *J. Physiol.* 315: 395–412, 1981.
128. O'Toole, S., J.A. Sharma, H.L. Karamanoukian, B. Holm, R.G. Azizkhan, and P.L. Glick. Tracheal ligation does not correct the surfactant deficiency associated with congenital diaphragmatic hernia. *J. Pediatr. Surg.* 31: 546–550, 1996.
129. Page, D.V. and J.T. Stocker. Anomalies associated with pulmonary hypoplasia. *Am. Rev. Respir. Dis.* 125: 216–221, 1982.
130. Pena, S.D.J. and M.H.K. Shokeir. Syndrome of camptodactyly, multiple ankyloses, facial anomalies and pulmonary hypoplasia. *J. Pediatr.* 85: 373–374, 1974.

131. Piedboeuf, B., J.M. Laberge, M. Gamache, P. Petrov, S. Belanger, M.F. Chen, E. Hashim, G. Ghitulescu, and F. Possmayer. Deleterious effect of tracheal obstruction on type II pneumocytes in fetal sheep. *Pediatr. Res.* 41: 473–479, 1997.
132. Potter, E.L. Bilateral renal agenesis. *J. Pediatr.* 29: 68–76, 1946.
133. Pringle, K.C. Human fetal lung development and related animal models. *Clin. Obstet. Gynecol.* 29: 502–513, 1986.
134. Rannels, D.G. Role of physical forces in compensatory growth of the lung. *Am. J. Physiol. (Lung Cell. Mol. Physiol.)* 257: L179–L189, 1989.
135. Reale, F.R. and J.R. Esterly. Pulmonary hypoplasia: a morphometric study of the lungs of infants with diaphragmatic hernia, anencephaly, and renal malformations. *Pediatrics* 51: 91–96, 1973.
136. Rees, S., J. Ng, K. Dickson, T. Nicholas, and R. Harding. Growth retardation and the development of the respiratory system in fetal sheep. *Early Hum. Dev.* 26: 13–27, 1991.
137. Reuss, A., J.W. Valdimiroff, R.J. Scholtmeijer, P.A. Stewart, P.J. Sauer, and M.F. Niermeijer. Prenatal evaluation and outcome of fetal obstructive uropathies. *Prenat. Diagn.* 8: 93–102, 1988.
138. Reynolds, M., S.R. Luck, and R. Lappen. The "critical" neonate with congenital diaphragmatic hernia: a 21-year perspective. *J. Pediatr. Surg.* 19: 364–369, 1984.
139. Richards, D.S. Complications of prolonged PROM and oligohydramnios. *Clin. Obstet. Gynecol.* 34: 759–768, 1991.
140. Riley, D.J., D.E. Rannels, R.B. Low, L. Jensen, and T.P. Jacobs. Effect of physical forces on lung structure, function and metabolism. *Am. Rev. Respir. Dis.* 142: 910–914, 1990.
141. Roberts, A.B., I. Goldstein, R. Romero, and J.C. Hobbins. Fetal breathing movements after preterm premature rupture of membranes. *Am. J. Obstet. Gynecol.* 164: 821–825, 1991.
142. Roberts, A.B. and J. Mitchell. Pulmonary hypoplasia and fetal breathing in preterm premature rupture of membranes. *Early Hum. Dev.* 41: 27–37, 1995.
143. Roberts, A.B. and J.M. Mitchell. Direct ultrasonographic measurement of fetal lung length in normal pregnancies and pregnancies complicated by prolonged rupture of membranes. *Am. J. Obstet. Gynecol.* 163: 1560–1566, 1990.
144. Rotschild, A., E.W. Ling, M.L. Puterman, and D. Farquharson. Neonatal outcome after prolonged preterm rupture of the membranes. *Am. J. Obstet. Gynecol.* 162: 46–52, 1990.
145. Russo, L.A., S.R. Rannels, K.S. Laslow, and D.E. Rannels. Stretch-related changes in lung cAMP after partial pneumonectomy. *Am. J. Physiol.* 257: E261–E268, 1989.
146. Sanderson, M.J., A.C. Charles, and E.R. Dirksen. Mechanical stimulation and intercellular communication increases intracellular Ca^{2+} in epithelial cells. *Cell Regul.* 1: 585–596, 1990.
147. Savich, R.D., F.A. Guerra, C.C. Lee, J.F. Padbury, and J.A. Kitterman. Effects of acute oligohydramnios on respiratory system of fetal sheep. *J. Appl. Physiol.* 73: 610–617, 1992.
148. Scurry, J.P., T.M. Adamson, and L.J. Cussen. Fetal lung growth in laryngeal atresia and tracheal agenesis. *Aust. Paediatr. J.* 25: 47–51, 1989.
149. Sherer, D.M., J.M. Davis, and J.R.J. Woods. Pulmonary hypoplasia: a review. *Obstet. Gynecol. Surv.* 45: 792–803, 1990.
150. Smith, B.T. and M. Post. Fibroblast-pneumonocyte factor. *Am. J. Physiol. (Lung Cell. Mol. Physiol.)* 257: L174–L178, 1989.
151. Smith, B.T., M. Post, and A.D. Stiles. Paracrine regulation of lung growth and matura-

tion: the substrate of normal functional development. In: *Abnormal Functional Development of the Heart, Lungs, and Kidneys: Approaches to Functional Teratology.* New York: Alan R. Liss, 1983, p. 135–141.

152. Somasundaram, K. and K. Prathap. The effect of intrauterine phrenic nerve division on the development of the lungs and diaphragm in fetal rabbits. *Aust. N. Z. J. Surg.* 45: 308–309, 1975.
153. Squier, C.A. The stretching of mouse skin in vivo: effect of epidermal proliferation and thickness. *J. Appl. Physiol.* 58: 452–458, 1985.
154. Stiles, A.D., I.R. Sosenko, B.T. Smith, and A.J. D'Ercole. Rapid rise in pulmonary somatomedin-C (SMC) levels in the regenerating lung. *Pediatr. Res.* 17: 391A,1993.
155. Stocker, J.T., J.E.R. Madewell, and R.M. Drake. Congential cystic adenomatoid malformation of the lung: classification and morphological spectrum. *Hum. Pathol.* 8: 155–171, 1977.
156. Strandjord, T.P., J.G. Clark, and D.K. Madtes. Expression of TGF-alpha, EGF, and EGF receptor in fetal rat lung. *Am. J. Physiol.* (*Lung Cell. Mol. Physiol.*) 267: L384–L389, 1994.
157. Strang, L.B. Fetal lung liquid: secretion and reabsorption. *Physiol. Rev.* 71: 991–1016, 1991.
158. Suen, H.C., K.D. Bloch, and P.K. Donahoe. Antenatal glucocorticoid corrects pulmonary immaturity in experimentally induced congenital diaphragmatic hernia in rats. *Pediatr. Res.* 523–529, 1994.
159. Sultana, Z., V.H. Talib, S.D. Patil, M.S. Deshpande, and K.D. Sharma. Hypoplasia of the lungs in the newborn. *Indian J. Pediatr.* 40: 419–421, 1973.
160. Sumpio, B.E., A.J. Banes, L.G. Levin, and G. Johnson. Mechanical stress stimulates aortic endothelial cells to proliferate. *J. Vasc. Surg.* 6: 252–256, 1987.
161. Swischuk, L.E., C.J. Richardson, M.M. Nichols, and M.J. Ingman. Primary pulmonary hypoplasia in the neonate. *J. Pediatr.* 95: 573–577, 1979.
162. Thibeault, D.W., E.C. Beatty, R.T. Hall, S.K. Bowen, and D.H. O'Niell. Neonatal pulmonary hypoplasia with premature rupture of fetal membranes and oligohydramnios. *J. Pediatr.* 107: 273–277, 1985.
163. Thurlbeck, W.M. Prematurity and the developing lung. *Clin. Perinatol.* 19: 497–519, 1992.
164. Thurlbeck, W.M., K. Kida, C. Langston, M.J. Cowan, J.A. Kitterman, W. Tooley, and H. Bryan. Postnatal lung growth after repair of diaphragmatic hernia. *Thorax* 34: 338–343, 1979.
165. Van Eyck, J., K. Van Mooren, and J.W. Wladimiroff. Ductus arteriosus flow velocity modulation by fetal breathing movements as a measure of fetal lung development. *Am. J. Obstet. Gynecol.* 163: 558–566, 1990.
166. Vintzileos, A.M., W.A. Campbell, J.F. Rodis, D.J. Nochimson, M.G. Pinette, and B.M. Petrikovsky. Comparison of six different ultrasonographic methods for predicting lethal fetal pulmonary hypoplasia. *Am. J. Obstet. Gynecol.* 161: 606–612, 1989.
167. Wallen, L.D. and V.K. Han. Spatial and temporal distribution of insulin-like growth factors I and II during development of rat lung. *Am. J. Physiol.* (*Lung Cell. Mol. Physiol.*) 267: L531–L542, 1994.
168. Wigglesworth, J.S. Pathology of the lung in the fetus and neonate, with particular reference to problems of growth and maturation. *Histopathology* 11: 671–689, 1987.
169. Wigglesworth, J.S. and R. Desai. Effects on lung growth of cervical cord section in the rabbit fetus. *Early Hum. Dev.* 3: 51–65, 1979.

170. Wigglesworth, J.S. and R. Desai. Use of DNA estimation for growth assessment in normal and hypoplastic fetal lungs. *Arch. Dis. Child.* 56: 601–605, 1981.
171. Wigglesworth, J.S. and R. Desai. Is fetal respiratory function a major determinant of perinatal survival? *Lancet* 1: 264–267, 1982.
172. Wigglesworth, J.S., R. Desai, and P. Guerrini. Fetal lung hypoplasia: biochemical and structural variations and their possible significance. *Arch. Dis. Child.* 56: 606–615, 1981.
173. Wigglesworth, J.S., R. Desai, and A.A. Hislop. Fetal lung growth in congenital laryngeal atresia. *Pediatr. Pathol.* 7: 515–525, 1987.
174. Wirtz, H.R.W. and L.G. Dobbs. Calcium mobilization and exocytosis after one mechanical stretch of lung epithelial cells. *Science* 250: 1266–1269, 1990.
175. Yoshimura, S., H. Masuzaki, K. Miura, H. Hayashi, H. Gotoh, and T. Ishimaru. The effects of oligohydramnios and cervical cord transection on lung growth in experimental pulmonary hypoplasia in rabbits. *Am. J. Obstet. Gynecol.* 177: 72–77, 1997.
176. Zhang, S., V. Garbutt, and J.T. McBride. Strain-induced growth of the immature lung. *J. Appl. Physiol.* 81: 1471–1476, 1996.

chapter 15

PULMONARY ANTIOXIDANT DEFENSE MECHANISMS

Ronald L. Morton and Carl W. White

PULMONARY injury due to hyperoxia generally is acknowledged to be an important element in the pathogenesis of bronchopulmonary dysplasia (BPD). With present management, most premature infants are not likely to develop this sometimes crippling or even fatal disorder. This probably relates to the relative pulmonary maturity and adequacy of antioxidative systems in most such patients. Nonetheless, the likelihood of BPD increases progressively at lower gestational ages, probably on account of the lung's structural and biochemical immaturity. Risk factors such as patent ductus arteriosus and late-onset sepsis may collaborate with oxidative stress to increase the likelihood of BPD.

PATHOGENIC EVENTS IN THE DEVELOPMENT OF OXYGEN TOXICITY

At the organ level, elevation of inspired oxygen tension carries with it the mixed blessing of decreased pulmonary artery pressure with increased blood flow to the lung. The latter increases the delivery of not only oxygen itself but also formed elements, including platelets, red blood cells, and inflammatory cells. Platelets and red blood cells contribute to the vascular congestion and eventual loss of pulmonary capillary surface area that results from exposure to hyperoxia (3, 21). As injury progresses, increased pulmonary blood flow also causes increased capillary filtration and favors the formation of pulmonary edema, a process already made more likely by prematurity.

As injury progresses, inflammatory cells have the additional capacity to release various proteolytic enzymes, reactive oxygen species, and various eicosanoid mediators. Again, at the whole organ level, the cellular composition of the lung changes in response to varying oxygen tensions in local microenvironments and to differing susceptibilities of individual lung cell types to hyperoxic injury. In the lung of adult animals, this results in a loss of endothelial and alveolar type I epithelial cells. Depending on the severity of injury, these damaged cells can be replaced by surviving or regenerating endothelial and epithelial type II cells. At the level of individual lung cells, increased oxygen tension results in the formation of increased concentrations of reactive products of oxygen, such as superoxide and hydrogen peroxide, at multiple sites (42). As oxygen and these products react with specific targets of oxidative injury, there is progressive impairment of respiration and a loss of energy production capacity. These result from the sequential and progressive loss of activities of aconitase (44), other tricarboxylic acid enzymes (44), and eventually, of mitochondrial cytochromes (4). Clearly, the quantities of energy required to perform work to maintain cell homeostasis and repair injury are increased during hyperoxic damage. In the lungs of premature infants, such work includes, but is not limited to, the movement of ions and fluid, the manufacture and delivery of pulmonary surfactant, regeneration of damaged cells, and lung growth. Despite these increased demands, the lung gradually fails in the performance of vital functions, resulting in early respiratory failure followed later by impaired and deranged lung growth.

Antioxidant defense really includes all of the defensive functions described above. These include the up-regulation of surfactant protein and of ion transport protein production as well as the gradual replacement of the alveolar epithelial surface with the apparently more oxygen-resistant type II cell. Also included are the up-regulation of various classical enzymatic and nonenzymatic antioxidants as well as the metabolic shifts that allow for continued energy production in the face of increased demand.

ROLE OF PREMATURITY: DEVELOPMENTAL FACTORS

In general, the development of the antioxidant enzyme system has shown parallels with that of the surfactant system. Frank and Sosenko (41) have argued that it is the response of the antioxidant enzyme systems to the hyperoxic challenge, rather than the absolute levels of antioxidants present at birth, that determines the outcome of such exposure. Nonetheless, the development of all the antioxidant enzymes is not coordinate; that is, all of the enzymes are not necessarily up-regulated concomitantly nor by the same oxidant, cytokine, or hormonal stimuli.

PERINATAL ANTIOXIDANT DEFENSE SYSTEMS

Developmental Aspects

The classical lung antioxidant enzymes (AOEs), including superoxide dismutase (SOD), glutathione peroxidase (GP) and reductase (GR), glucose-6-phosphate dehydrogenase (G6PDH), and catalase (CAT), have been extensively studied in the developing animal. These activities increase during the final 10%–20% of gestation in the lungs of rat, rabbit, hamster, guinea pig, and fetal lamb, and parallel the marked increases in surfactant production before birth (38, 40, 95). In fetal rat lung, absolute activities of mitochondrial MnSOD decrease during the final 20% of gestation. However, when normalized for the mitochondrial marker enzyme cytochrome oxidase, *manganese superoxide dismutase* (MnSOD) activity increases by three- to fourfold over this interval. In addition, MnSOD activity increases markedly with air or oxygen exposure after delivery, as does copper-zinc SOD (CuZnSOD) activity (87). Further evidence that lung antioxidant enzyme activities increase before birth comes from a study of immunoenzyme staining for the two forms of superoxide dismutase in fetal (late gestation day 18 to 20) and neonatal (day 22) rats. Staining for both CuZnSOD and MnSOD was more intense in the bronchiolar epithelium and alveolar wall of the neonatal than the fetal rat lung (1). Thus, in all species studied to date, there is an increase in the activities of the lung's classical antioxidant enzymes during late fetal development.

Neonatal Tolerance

In addition to the developmental increase in AOEs, most term animals exposed to hyperoxia for extended periods develop further adaptive increases in response to a high-oxygen environment (100% oxygen). One study compared the lung antioxidant enzyme response in neonatal rats to adult rats continuously exposed to >95% oxygen for 72 h. Neonatal rat lungs had significant increases in the activities of all AOEs measured (from 120% to 176% increases compared to air controls), whereas the adult rat lungs did not demonstrate any significant increase in the activities of SOD, GP, GR, or the level of glutathione (GSH). The neonatal rats also survived more than 5 days of hyperoxic exposure without any signs of respiratory distress, whereas all adult rats died within 3 days of exposure. Hence, for many species, the term neonatal animal is considerably more resistant to oxygen toxicity than the adult animal under hyperoxic conditions (101).

One factor in the acquisition of tolerance under hyperoxic conditions in neonatal animals may be the inducibility of AOEs. Neonatal full-term rabbits continuously exposed to >90% oxygen for 72 h showed marked increases in activities of classical antioxidant enzymes. However, premature rabbits did not increase antioxidant enzymes well and sustained more lung damage. Elevated lung lavage albumin concentrations and lung conjugated diene levels, the latter an indicator of lung lipid peroxidation, as well as greater morphologic damage, were noted in the preterm rabbit compared to the term animal (41). In contrast to the rabbit, the premature rat pup exposed to >95% oxygen for up to 14 days after birth had increased lung AOEs and improved survival from 7 to 9 days after hyperoxic exposure, with less evidence of lung edema compared to term neonates in this species (12).

In lesser mammals, a second factor that may influence the acquisition of neonatal tolerance to hyperoxia is the timing of weaning from a primarily high-fat milk diet to a high-carbohydrate diet. Neonatal rats continuously exposed to >95% oxygen for 7 days were separated into prematurely weaned (15- to 17-day-old) or normally weaned (24- to 25-day-old) groups. The survival rate of the prematurely weaned group was nearly twice that of the normally weaned group (78% vs. 41%). There was no difference in lung antioxidant enzyme activity (SOD, CAT, and GP) measured between the two groups studied. However, serum corticosterone and triiodothyronine levels were greater in the prematurely weaned animals, possibly implicating a role for hormonal influences on the development of hyperoxic tolerance around the time of weaning. On the other hand, this change in dietary substrates may have influenced acquisition of tolerance through other mechanisms. The hormonal, enzymatic, and/or other metabolic factors causing the protective effect of premature weaning remain poorly understood (35).

In summary, neonatal animals may develop greater tolerance to hyperoxia than adult animals. This neonatal tolerance to a high-oxygen environment may operate through several mechanisms, including the inducibility of the AOEs, differences in hormones and/or growth factors, and effects of different nutrient intakes. The phenomenon of hyperoxic tolerance in the premature animal is variable depending on the species studied, with the premature rabbit sustaining more damage and the premature rat less damage than their term counterparts. There may be limitations, however, in the pertinence of findings from rodents and other small mammals to the clinical situation of human premature infants.

Hormonal Influences

Often human mothers in preterm labor are treated with glucocorticoids prior to delivery. This treatment can diminish or prevent the sequelae of respiratory distress syndrome (RDS) in the neonate. Glucocorticoid pretreatment can induce the maturation of the surfactant system in the late fetal lung. The results of pretreatment with hormones [either dexamethasone (DEX) or thyroid-releasing hormone (TRH)] and hyperoxic exposure at birth upon the lung antioxidant system has been studied in several animal models.

The effects of prenatal treatment with glucocorticoids on the lung response to subsequent hyperoxic exposure has been studied in many species. Prenatal DEX treatment results in improved survival and decreased pathologic evidence of lung injury in term newborn rats exposed to hyperoxia (36, 54). On the other hand, the preterm rabbit does not increase lung antioxidant enzyme activities after antenatal DEX treatment and subsequent hyperoxic exposure at birth (86). However, dexamethasone increases lung AOE activities after hyperoxic exposure in the preterm guinea pig, but fails to affect survival in hyperoxia in this species (88). This finding suggests that the elevation of AOEs in response to hyperoxia may not be responsible for adaptation or may not be the sole cause of such adaptation.

The effects of thyroid hormones (prenatal treatment with TRH and DEX or TRH alone) on the inducibility of lung antioxidant enzymes have been explored. Prenatal treatment with TRH and DEX in term newborn rats actually depressed the late gestational rise in antioxidant enzymes (73). However, hormone-pretreated

(TRH and TRH + DEX) term newborn rats exposed to hyperoxia showed a normal antioxidant enzyme response (73). Nonetheless, there was decreased survival and increased lung injury in these animals (74). In contrast, *premature* rats after TRH + DEX pretreatment and 14 days of hyperoxic exposure (>95% O_2) showed increased survival in hyperoxia from days 3 to 7 compared to sham hormone-treated controls (10).

Another study examined the effect of the antithyroid drug, propylthiouracil (PTU). Term neonatal rats pretreated with PTU have improved survival (77% vs. 25% at day 14) compared to controls, as well as evidence of decreased acute lung injury in hyperoxia. Such an effect could be mediated through any of several possible mechanisms, including decreased metabolic demands and/or decreased oxygen consumption (75). Thyroid supplementation and inhibition, respectively, have previously been noted to decrease and increase survival of adult rats in hyperoxia.

In summary, the effect of glucocorticoid or thyroid hormone pretreatment in the neonatal animal upon subsequent hyperoxic survival varies, depending on the species studied and gestational age. The term newborn rat shows improved hyperoxic survival after DEX pretreatment, but decreased survival when pretreated with TRH and DEX. By contrast, the preterm rat has increased survival in hyperoxia from days 3 to 7 after TRH + DEX pretreatment. However, the preterm rabbit and guinea pig have decreased survival with DEX pretreatment and hyperoxic exposure.

Iron Metabolism

Since iron may contribute to lung damage through the Fenton and Haber-Weiss reactions producing hydroxyl radical, chelation therapy has been studied in relation to oxidant stress. In one model, iron chelators such as deferoxamine and the 21 amino steroid U74389F were studied in the newborn rat after hyperoxic exposure (32, 39). Treated pups showed less evidence of morphologic lung damage than controls and less inhibition of lung development by hyperoxia. However, when the effect of deferoxamine was evaluated in a premature baboon model for bronchopulmonary dysplasia, rapid lethal toxicity occurred during exposure of these animals to hyperoxia; death occurred after development of a shock-like state and cardiovascular collapse (25). Death was dose related, but it persisted even with marked dosage reduction in hyperoxia-treated prematures.

Recently, hyperoxia has been shown to cause rapid and profound inactivation of the Krebs cycle enzyme aconitase (44, 67b), an effect which appears to occur independently of superoxide production. Hyperoxia may be mediated directly by elevated concentrations of dioxygen rather than by reactive species (45). In cultured cells in which mitochondrial MnSOD expression was increased either by pretreatment with cytokines or by genetic means, progressive aconitase inhibition by hyperoxia was unchanged. In cultured cells, iron withholding by deferoxamine caused substantial impairment of the reactivation of aconitase and decreased basal aconitase activities of cells even under normal oxygenation (45). The toxic poison fluorocitrate, a potent inhibitor of aconitase, also caused rapid death through cardiovascular collapse when administered in the whole animal, and in cultured cells, it reproduced the impairments of respiration and growth caused by hyperoxia. These findings resemble those occurring somewhat more gradually in MnSOD knockout mice in which cardiovascular failure and death progress with the onset of air breathing in the neonatal period in association with diminished cardiac aconitase activity (62). Thus, elevation of oxygen tension and/or superoxide, diminished MnSOD activity, and withholding of iron may interact to produce failure of cellular function and death.

Withholding of iron caused by the actions of inflammatory cytokines such as interleukin (IL)-1 and tumor necrosis factor (TNF) may also impair the reactivation of aconitase during or after oxidative stress in lung cells (46). These findings may also have implications for the worsening of BPD in prematures caused by pulmonary infection, inflammation, and/or sepsis (20). Despite marked MnSOD upregulation in the lungs of infected and/or septic prematures (19a), oxidative stress, aconitase inhibition, and impairment of respiration could still progress through excessive iron withholding caused by cytokines.

The results of these studies indicate the complexities of iron metabolism under oxidant stress. Iron plays an important and beneficial role in the regulation and reactivation of aconitase (56), in the composition of succinate dehydrogenase (TCA cycle) and of multiple enzymes of the respiratory chain, as a required component for the antioxidant activity of the enzyme catalase, and as an essential co-factor allowing for cell growth in the lung. On the other hand, excessive release of iron from aconitase's iron-sulfur cluster and from other cellular sites may play a harmful role in catalyzing free-radical reactions such as those noted above and others (51a).

Proteins that transport and/or store iron may also be important in pulmonary antioxidant defense. For example, transferrin (TF) is a major iron transport protein that may have a protective function against lipid peroxidation by preventing excess iron accumulation in lung fluid. In the baboon and human, TF mRNA expression displays a distinct pattern of developmental regulation. Interestingly, the premature baboon has decreased expression of TF before birth, and this may contribute to increased susceptibility to hyperoxic lung damage (102).

Nutritional Effects: Importance of Thiols

Various forms of malnutrition or undernutrition can have deleterious effects on both antioxidant defenses and neonatal lung development. Frank and Groseclose (37) showed that the adverse effects of hyperoxia and undernutrition on the neonatal lung are additive.

The protein or amino acid composition of the diet can affect the response of the developing lung to hyperoxia. Adult rats fed a diet low in sulfur-containing amino acids develop more severe lung oxygen toxicity (27). In contrast, rats fed a diet supplemented with selenium or sulfur-containing amino acids have lower mortality when exposed to hyperoxia (32).

A recent study demonstrated the result of hyperoxic stress on circulating and lung sulfur amino acids in young mice (77). Plasma cysteine and methionine levels were found to decrease in mice exposed to hyperoxia in association with depletion of hepatic glutathione, but not protein stores. In addition, in pair-feeding studies, decreases in plasma cysteine were shown to be due to hyperoxia and not curtailment of food intake alone (77). In contrast, plasma methionine was directly related to food intake. In hyperoxia, lung reduced glutathione and cysteine were preserved, apparently at the expense of hepatic and circulating glutathione and cysteine reserves. Neither hepatic nor lung cystathionase activities were inhibited by hyperoxia. However, during hyperoxic exposure, a fivefold elevation in lung cystathionine levels, which occurred without changes in other sulfur amino acids or lung cystathionase activity and in the presence of ongoing oxidation of lung glutathione, suggested that the lung's transsulfuration pathway is activated by exposure to hyperoxia. Finally, additional findings in transgenic mice with elevated CuZnSOD activities in their tissues indicated that the increased demands for cysteine may have been related in part to toxic oxygen metabolites such as superoxide (97). Taken together, these findings suggest that oxidant stress, such as that induced by hyperoxic exposure, may cause increased demands for cysteine in the lung, which appear to be met both by use of hepatic and circulating stores and by new synthesis within the lung. The need for maintenance of lung reduced glutathione and other thiol-containing antioxidants may be one cause for this increased cysteine demand.

In a human study, both term and premature infants exposed to hyperoxia were found to have low plasma total cysteine. Infants who were ventilated with high concentrations of oxygen for respiratory failure, including that caused by persistent pulmonary hypertension of the newborn (PPHN) and hyaline membrane disease (HMD), had low plasma total cysteine levels compared to values found in cord blood from healthy infants, fasted infants not treated with supplemental oxygen, or healthy fed infants. Plasma levels of both methionine and cysteine tended to be even lower in premature infants with HMD, as suggested in numerous previous studies. Fasted infants with noncardiopulmonary illnesses also had decreased plasma methionine levels but maintained normal plasma cysteine levels. The decreases in plasma methionine levels appeared to be related primarily to nutritional deprivation, whereas the decreases in plasma cysteine could not be explained altogether by decreased intake. During the recovery of patients with PPHN, who were treated either conventionally or with extracorporeal membrane oxygenation (ECMO), their plasma cysteine and methionine levels increased through day 5, but not serine or glycine levels. Plasma cysteine levels increased more rapidly and to a higher value with ECMO therapy. This may have been due to a lowering of the inspired oxygen tension and presumably, of pulmonary oxidant stress, with the institution of ECMO, or alternatively, to increased substrate available in the larger blood volume of the ECMO circuit, or to both. Regardless, plasma total cysteine and methionine were low in both term and premature infants receiving high inspired oxygen concentrations for respiratory failure. Both oxidative stress and nutritional factors may have contributed to these abnormalties. Clinical recovery, lowering of inspired oxygen tension, and increased nutritional support were associated with increases in plasma sulfur amino acids (98). Taken together, these studies indicate that the demand for cysteine, which already appears to be an essential amino acid for premature infants, may be even more greatly increased in those treated for respiratory distress with high concentrations of oxygen.

GENETIC REGULATION OF ANTIOXIDANTS

Perinatal Animal

The regulation of antioxidant enzyme expression at the genetic level has been studied in the developing animal. In the prenatal period from days 19 to 22, CuZnSOD activity decreased and MnSOD activity remained constant, whereas CAT and GP activities progressively increased. Around the time of birth (prenatal day 22 to postnatal day 1) there was a slight increase in CuZnSOD activity, ending the prenatal decline, whereas MnSOD and CAT showed significant increases in activities, and GP showed a slight decline in activity, ending the prenatal increase. In the postnatal period from days 1 to 5, CuZnSOD and CAT activities progressively increased, MnSOD activity remained constant, and GP activity declined slightly (Fig. 15.1). The mRNA concentrations of the AOEs were measured in lungs from these same animals. During the prenatal period CuZnSOD and GP mRNA concentrations progressively decreased, whereas MnSOD mRNA remained constant and CAT mRNA increased. At birth (from prenatal day 22 to postnatal day 1) the concentrations of CuZnSOD and CAT mRNAs decreased by about 40% (a change opposite that seen in their activity) and the MnSOD mRNA level increased slightly (Fig. 15.2). The investigators concluded that the changes in the activities of these four AOEs in the prenatal period generally reflect the changes in their mRNA concentrations (9). However, absolute mRNA levels were hardly faithfully represented in AOE activities. Instead, most messages, except for MnSOD, tended to "re-set" themselves at lower levels, whereas most AOE activities, except for GP, re-set themselves at higher levels. These data clearly indicate the increasing importance of oxygen-dependent post-transcriptional mechanisms after birth (vide infra).

Several investigators have examined the level at which the different antioxidant enzymes are regulated during the perinatal period. Clerch and Massaro (17) found that after exposure of the newborn term rat to >95% oxygen, the concentrations of MnSOD and GP mRNAs increased and the increase in concentration of AOE mRNAs was associated with a prolongation of their half-lives. These investigators postulated that during the neonatal period, the level of regulation is at least partly post-transcriptional and involves increased stability of the mRNAs. Chen et al. (11) examined the effect of prenatal hormone treatments with TRH plus DEX on antioxidant enzyme gene regulation in the fetal rat lung. They found that the mRNA concentrations of the antioxidant enzymes studied (Mn and CuZn SOD, CAT, GP), decreased, but that the half-lives (stabilities) were unchanged. On this basis, they speculated that the level of genetic regulation is that of gene transcription in this setting.

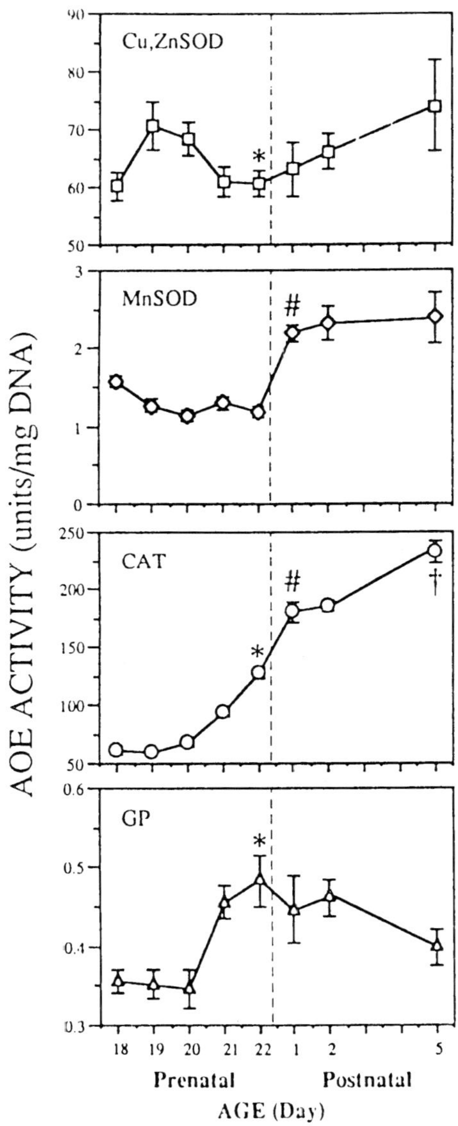

Fig. 15.1 Prenatal and postnatal developmental changes in rat lung antioxidant enzyme (AOE: CuZnSOD, MnSOD, CAT, and GP) activities. Values are mean plus or minus SEM. *P < 0.05 for prenatal day 22 vs. prenatal day 19. #P < 0.01 for postnatal day 1 vs. prenatal day 22. †P < 0.01 for postnatal day 5 vs. postnatal day 1. [From Chen and Frank (9), with permission.]

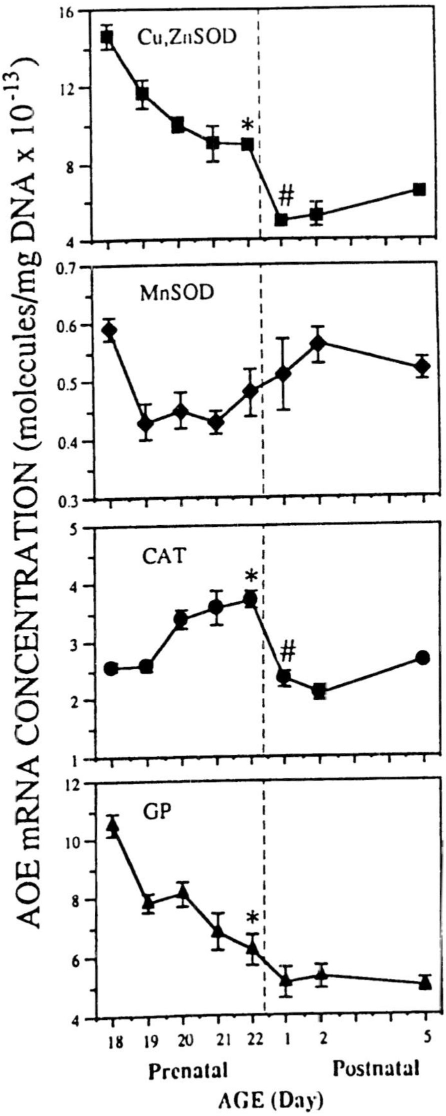

Fig. 15.2. Prenatal and postnatal developmental changes in concentration of rat lung antioxidant enzyme (AOE: CuZnSOD, MnSOD, CAT, GP) mRNA. Values are mean plus or minus SEM. *P < 0.05 for prenatal day 22 vs. prenatal day 19. #P < 0.01 for postnatal day 1 vs. prenatal day 22. [From Chen and Frank (9), with permission.]

The regulation of perinatal catalase gene expression has also been examined. In one study, Clerch and co-workers evaluated the effects of dexamethasone treatment and hyperoxia on catalase gene expression in rat lung during the perinatal period (15). After prenatal treatment with dexamethasone, the lung catalase mRNA concentration increased without a change in the half-life of its mRNA (stability). Upon exposure to hyperoxia, the half-life of catalase mRNA doubled without changing the rate of transcription. They concluded that catalase gene expression is regulated differently depending on the environmental conditions. During late gestation and after prenatal hormone treatment catalase is transcriptionally regulated, whereas after hyperoxic exposure catalase is regulated translationally. Several studies have examined the mechanisms through which the catalase enzyme is genetically regulated. In one study, a redox-sensitive protein that forms specific complexes with catalase mRNA was isolated (16). This protein may be important in the genetic regulation of catalase.

In summary, the genetic regulation of antioxidant enzymes in the lung of perinatal animals is a complex developmental phenomenon. In the perinatal rat lung, gradual increases in CAT and GP activities occur during late gestation, with rapid increases in MnSOD and CAT activities occurring at the time of birth. These changes in AOE activities generally parallel the changes seen in lung AOE mRNA concentrations before birth. The level at which regulation of antioxidant gene expression occurs has been shown to be, at least in part, translational in the neonatal animal exposed to hyperoxia and transcriptional in the neonatal animal pretreated with thyroid and glucocorticoid hormones.

Adult Animal

Clerch and Massaro have also examined the effect of hyperoxia on regulation of antioxidant gene expression in the adult rat lung. They induced tolerance to oxygen toxicity by pretreatment of the animals with endotoxin and found that after exposure to oxygen plus endotoxin for 48 h, both the concentration and stability of antioxidant enzyme mRNAs (MnSOD, CAT and GPX) increased (18). In another study, Iqbal and co-workers examined the effects of endotoxin pretreatment and hyperoxic exposure on CuZnSOD mRNA expression in adult rats. They found that after pretreatment with endotoxin the CuZnSOD mRNA increased by 45% after 48 h of air or >95% oxygen exposure. An additional 24 h of hyperoxic exposure was required to increase lung CuZnSOD mRNA in the rats exposed only to oxygen (51). In the study by Clerch and Massaro, the MnSOD mRNA concentration increased by 110% in the air + endotoxin–treated group relative to the air + saline–treated group, whereas in the study by Iqbal et al., the CuZnSOD mRNA concentration only increased by 45% between these same two respective groups after 48 h of exposure. In the studies in our laboratory (61), changes in MnSOD mRNA were even greater, whereas those in CuZnSOD mRNA were negligible, in lungs of rats treated with endotoxin and exposed to air or hyperoxia. This pattern is the same as that previously observed by Visner et al. in a rat lung epithelial-like cell line after treatment with endotoxin (94).

A study by Ho et al. (50) investigated the effects of sublethal hyperoxic stress

(85%) on lung MnSOD expression in adult rats over an exposure period of 14 days. They found an approximately 600% increase in MnSOD mRNA levels compared to air controls and a 400% increase in the rate of transcription of the MnSOD gene at day 3. The MnSOD protein increased by 640% and 520% at days 7 and 14, respectively, in rats exposed to hyperoxia compared to air-exposed control rats. Remarkably, the MnSOD enzyme-specific activity only increased by 70% and 120%, respectively, at days 7 and 14 of hyperoxic exposure relative to these air-exposed animals. From these studies, it appears that lung MnSOD genetic regulation occurs both at transcriptional *and* post-translational levels during adaptation to sublethal hyperoxia (50).

Mechanisms of Genetic Regulation

Some of the most detailed mechanistic studies to date on antioxidant enzyme gene regulation involve the enzymes CuZn and Mn superoxide dismutase. Several different mechanisms have been proposed regarding the genetic regulation of MnSOD. One mechanism involves the function of a redox-sensitive MnSOD mRNA-binding protein. In work by Fazzone et al. (30), a specific protein in rat lung which binds to the 3′-untranslated region of MnSOD mRNA and whose RNA-binding requires the presence of free sulfhydryl groups was isolated. These investigators found that this protein is developmentally regulated, being expressed more in the neonatal lung than in the adult.

Another area of recent progress in antioxidant gene regulation involves the glutathione-related enzyme gamma-glutamyl transferase (GGT). Joyce-Grady and co-workers (53) examined the differential gene expression in the perinatal and adult rat of three GGT mRNA transcripts and their promoters, and the effects of oxygen on these promoters. The GGT mRNA transcripts were found to be expressed at different time points in late gestation and early postnatal life. All three transcripts were present in the fetal lung, with GGT mRNA transcript II disappearing within 24 h and GGT mRNA transcript I being absent by day 10, leaving the adult pattern in which only transcript III is present. In addition, these investigators examined the presumed mechanisms causing this differential expression of the GGT gene. When rat alveolar type II cells in hypoxia were exposed to carbon monoxide, GGT mRNA II was suppressed. When the cells were exposed to hyperoxia, the GGT promoter III activated gene transcription. It was hypothesized that variations in oxygen tension were responsible for the regulation of each of these transcripts, with promoter II being under the control of a heme-dependent element and promoter III regulated by an oxygen response element within the gene (53).

SPECIFIC ANTIOXIDANTS

Glutathione and Thiols

Glutathione is a tripeptide composed of the amino acids glutamine, cysteine, and glycine. With the provision of these amino acids, two enzymes, gamma-glutamylcysteine synthetase (GCS) and glutathione synthase, are involved in the de novo synthesis of glutathione (GSH). GCS is an intracellular enzyme that is the initial, energy-dependent step in GSH synthesis. In mammals, separate cytoplasmic and mitochondrial pools of GSH exist. Mitochondria do not synthesize GSH; instead, they take it up from the cytoplasm. These systems are also ATP-dependent and inhibited by uncoupling oxidative phosphorylation. Elevation of cytosolic GSH may promote its mitochondrial uptake (67). Besides de novo synthesis, some cells can also produce glutathione by uptake from the extracellular environment. Gamma-glutamyl transpeptidase (GGT) is an additional membrane-bound enzyme that recycles extracellular GSH by cellular uptake, thereby providing substrates for resynthesis of GSH.

Oxidative Stress and Glutathione In Vitro

Several studies have examined the effects of oxidative stress on the GSH synthetic enzymes. In one study, pulmonary artery endothelial cells were subjected to oxidative stress after incubation with redox-cycling quinones (naphthoquinone or menadione). It was found that GSH almost doubled after 24 h of quinone exposure and that the enzymatic activity and mRNA content of GCS, the rate-limiting enzyme in GSH synthesis, increased (83). In a second study, investigators examined the effects of oxidative stress (menadione) on the enzyme gamma-glutamyl transpeptidase (GGT) in rat alveolar epithelial cells. Again, an elevation in the activity, protein content, and mRNA concentration of this enzyme was observed (58).

More recent studies evaluated the effects of acquired resistance to a sublethal oxidative stress (tert-butylhydroquinone) on GSH synthetic enzymes in rat alveolar epithelial-like (L2) cells. Levels of both enzymes, GCS and GGT, as well as intracellular GSH increased (64). However, the mechanisms responsible for the genetic regulation of these enzymatic changes were different. The increase in GCS mRNA was due to increased transcription, whereas the increase in GGT mRNA was due to decreased mRNA degradation (63).

In summary, these studies showed that under conditions of oxidative stress, pulmonary artery endothelial cells and pulmonary epithelial cells (alveolar type II cells) respond with increased de novo synthesis of GSH when expression of enzymes involved in both GSH synthesis and re-uptake is increased.

Hyperoxia and Glutathione

Glutathione may help protect neonatal lungs from oxygen injury. The effect of hyperoxia on GSH has been studied in several species and different cell lines. In cultured endothelial cells, hyperoxia increases uptake of GSH precursor amino acids (cystine and glutamate) and contributes to the adaptive increase in cell GSH (26). It is not clear that term or preterm neonates have the ability to increase lung GSH in response to hyperoxia. Species differences may occur. Term newborn rats exposed to hyperoxia increase their lung GSH content when exposed to hyperoxia, as do alveolar type II cells isolated from the lungs of such animals (55, 96). These results were not corrected for changes in protein content or cellular hypertrophy, which can occur during adaptation to hyperoxia. Such changes in GSH metabolism also occurred in rat and human fetal lung grown in explant culture. However, substrate availabilities may be considerably different in this system than in vivo. In an in vivo study in rats, the effects of hyperoxia on the enzyme GGT and GSH synthesis were investigated. After exposure of newborn rats to hyperoxic conditions, the lung mRNA expression, protein level, and enzyme activity of GGT were increased, as were the levels of GSH and protein-bound GSH (57). These in vivo data are in agreement with the findings described earlier from cultured cells. In contrast to rats, in term newborn sheep, lung GSH decreased from 235 ± 63 to 152 ± 25 nmol/mg DNA, while lung GSSG increased from 2.68 ± 0.42 to 4.97 ± 0.85 over 5 days of exposure to 95% oxygen. Glutathione reductase and total SOD activities also declined while gas exchange progressively worsened over this interval (48).

Less work had been done in epithelial cells from preterm animals. However, that which is available suggests that fetal GSH metabolism in hyperoxia may more closely resemble that of the term sheep than adult rat lung. In distal fetal rat lung epithelial cells, exposure to hyperoxia for 48 h caused a depletion of protein- and nonprotein-reduced thiols, which was preceded by cell DNA injury. Neither poly (ADP-ribose) polymerase activation nor ATP depletion were detected in association with these abnormalities. Depletion of nonprotein-reduced sulfhydryls with the specific inhibitor of GSH synthesis, buthionine sulfoximine (BSO), increased, whereas *N*-acetylcysteine prevented oxygen-mediated cytotoxicity. Thus, GSH appears to modulate hyperoxic damage to the distal epithelium of the premature rat lung in culture (14).

In summary, substrate availability plays an important role in determining the response of lung GSH to hyperoxia. Second, the adequacy of the lung GSH synthetic response in human prematures with RDS remains unknown but may also be dependent in part on nutritional support.

Glutathione Uptake

Recent studies have shown that glutathione can be taken up directly by lung epithelium and thereby reverse oxidant injury (2). Studies using a stable glutathione *S*-conjugate have shown that once taken up by the lung, GSH is concentrated in the alveolar type II cell. In additional studies of GSH uptake in rabbit alveolar type II cells from 24-h-old neonates, a 19-fold increase in GSH uptake and increased de novo GSH synthesis after hyperoxic or paraquat exposures were reported. This increased uptake of GSH was associated with protection from oxidative stress by hyperoxia or paraquat. Despite protection, fetal cells had a substantially lower GSH transport rate (6%) compared to neonatal cells, suggesting that developmental factors may be important (5). Hence, the premature lung may be dependent on GSH synthesis because of limited uptake potential.

Several studies have examined the effects of exogenous GSH during oxidative stress. In one study, Forman and Skelton (33) found that extracellular GSH significantly protected adult rat alveolar macrophages during hyperoxic exposure. Suppression of the respiratory burst stimulated by phorbol myristate acetate in these alveolar macrophages was used as a measure of toxicity. There was 43% burst suppression by oxygen alone versus 7% burst suppression in the presence of GSH, indicating a protective effect of exogenous GSH in these cells. A second study investigated the treatment of endothelial cells with exogenous GSH during oxidative stress (menadione) (8). Treatment with exogenous GSH prevented the loss of cellular GSH and ATP caused by this oxidative stress. It was proposed that exogenous GSH protects the cells by two mechanisms: first, GGT degrades extracellular GSH, thereby providing substrates for intracellular synthesis; second, GSH forms complexes with menadione and prevents menadione entrance into the cells. The potential relevance of these studies to the premature human newborn, however, is unknown.

Glutathione and Mitochondria

The mechanism of GSH protection from oxidative stress may involve its effects on mitochondrial function. In mice, administration of a GSH synthesis inhibitor causes mitochondrial abnormalities in lung endothelial cells and alveolar type II cells (67). In contrast, in hepatocytes, selective depletion of the mitochondrial GSH pool did not induce mitochondrial dysfunction under resting conditions. Nonetheless, under oxidative stress, cytotoxicity and death were potentiated (82). The nature of the mitochondrial impairment caused by GSH deficiency is not precisely known. Despite these suggestive data, Smith and Anderson found no association between lung mitochondrial GSH levels and susceptibility to hyperoxic lung damage in mice (85). In these studies, mice were exposed to 100% oxygen for 3 days and separated into fed versus non-fed groups. It was found that non-fed mice after hyperoxic exposure had lower total lung GSH levels and increased oxygen toxicity compared to fed mice. In addition, it was found that lung mitochondrial GSH levels were maintained despite decreased total lung GSH levels. Hence, the relative importance in lung of mitochondrial and cytoplasmic GSH pools in protection against hyperoxia and other oxidative stresses remains unsolved. However, interpretation of this study is confounded by deficiencies in other nutrients in the non-fed animals, which may have been of greater importance (vide infra).

In bacteria, glutathione also reactivates the critical mitochondrial matrix enzyme aconitase. Given that GSH is by far the most ubiquitous thiol reductant present in mammalian cells, where it is found at millimolar concentrations, GSH could be important in reactivation of oxidatively inactivated aconitase in the lung. In bacterial studies, an *E. coli* mutant deficient in GSH synthesis grew more slowly than the parent strain, and this effect was more pronounced with succinate, rather than glucose, as the carbon source. This GSH-deficient strain also had 25% lower aconitase activity than the parent when growing on either substrate, and aconitase activity was even lower when the bacterium was deficient in SOD. Adding GSH to the medium stimulated the growth of the deficient strain, and increased its aconitase activity, even in the presence of the protein synthesis inhibitor chloramphenicol. Dithiothreitol and 2-mercaptoethanol were considerably less potent than GSH in mediating these effects. In hyperbaric oxygen (4.2 atm), aconitase activity fell rapidly in the GSH-deficient and parent strains. However, aconitase reactivation, following discontinuation of such exposure, was considerably impaired in the GSH-deficient strain. Thus, it was concluded that GSH can facilitate aconitase reactivation by restoring ferrous iron transfer to the inactive [3FE-4S] cluster (43). The potential role of GSH in reactivating mammalian lung aconitase after hyperoxic inactivation remains uncertain. Although GSH may be involved in this function, other reducing systems could modulate aconitase activity independently.

Glutathione and Premature Humans

In preterm human infants, circulating GSH levels were quite low (2.4 ± 1.4 μM) in 23- to 33-week gestation newborns at birth relative to levels measured in adults (6–10 μM) (84). Plasma GSH levels declined with decreasing gestational age, whereas plasma GSSG levels increased. Both negative GSH and positive GSSG arteriovenous gradients across the lung were demonstrated, indicating that pulmonary uptake of GSH occurs in the newborn. Both in absolute terms and relative to total circulating GSH, uptake of GSH in the lung was considerably greater in the more premature group (23–33 weeks gestation) studied. These data suggest that at least some cell types in lungs of human prematures are able to take up GSH. However, it is unknown whether this mechanism is adequate to preserve and increase lung GSH during the oxidative stress of respiratory distress syndrome and its therapy.

In summary, available evidence suggests that plasma GSH is quite low in the premature human newborn, and tissue culture and animal data indicate that in the premature newborn, lung GSH may decline, rather than increase, in response to hyperoxia. The reasons for this response could be unavailability of precursor amino acid substrates, failure of their cellular uptake, failure of re-reduction of GSSG by the GSH redox system with cellular excretion, or a combination thereof. Glutathione uptake and/or synthetic systems could also be impaired. Most studies demonstrate that GSH is an important element of protection against oxidative stresses, including hyperoxia. Its importance may be related not only to its role in detoxification of peroxides through the GSH redox cycle but also to its function as a redox "buffer" through which it contributes to the maintenance of vital thiol groups within the cell.

Superoxide Dismutases

Mitochondrial manganese-containing superoxide dismutase (MnSOD) may be an especially important antioxidant because of the early insults that the mitochondria suffer during hyperoxia. In adult rats made tolerant to sublethal hyperoxia (85%), a relatively small increase (<50%) in cytosolic CuZnSOD occurs, but a much larger increase in mitochondrial MnSOD is associated with prolonged tolerance to hyperoxic lung damage and death (21). Interestingly, type II alveolar epithelial cell number, volume, and surface area increased maximally during the first week of hyperoxic adaptation. During the second week, considerably greater increases in MnSOD occurred. Despite adaptation to sublethal hyperoxia in adult rats, swollen abnormal mitochondria appear relatively early during oxygen-induced injury, whereas more bizarre, fused mitochondria become apparent during the second week (21). Because more than half of lung mitochondria are contained in epithelial type II cells, increases in MnSOD are likely related to both adaptive changes in lung cell populations and to its biochemical responses. In contrast to the oxygen-tolerant rat exposed to a lesser oxygen concentration, lung MnSOD activity decreased in the adult baboon exposed to 100% oxygen for up to 7 days when compared with air controls (19).

The ability of MnSOD to provide protection during hyperoxic exposure has been studied in transgenic mice. In one study, MnSOD-overexpressing transgenic mice were created that had fourfold elevation of MnSOD in mitochondria of selected pulmonary epithelial cells [Clara and type II alveolar cells; (100)]. The survival of these mice in hyperoxia at sea level pressures was increased by about 120 h, or about fivefold greater than what was observed in mice with constitutive overexpression of CuZnSOD, without alteration in MnSOD, throughout their cells and tissues (97, 99). These data suggest that in adult animals either (*1*) CuZnSOD activities in lung are already more nearly optimal, (*2*) increases in MnSOD expression are more important in adaptation, or (*3*) that both these statements are true.

Superoxide Dismutase and Prematures

Several studies have shown that expression of lung SODs is decreased in premature animals and infants with respiratory distress relative to those present after term gestation. In premature baboons, both lung CuZnSOD and MnSOD activities failed to increase during hyperoxic exposure relative to activities in lungs of fetal controls. A number of similar effects of oxygen, both on CuZnSOD and MnSOD expression, were noted in fetal peripheral lung cultured from premature baboons and exposed acutely (16 hr) to hyperoxia (67a).

The effect of hyperoxia on SOD activities was also striking in CuZnSOD and MnSOD proteins in human infants with respiratory distress. In a study using immunohistochemistry, CuZnSOD staining intensity increased 30-fold from weeks 16 through 38 of gestation, whereas MnSOD staining increased eightfold (29). Both SOD proteins were expressed at extremely low levels in the distal lung of oxygen-exposed premature RDS patients, apparently at lower levels than occur in fetuses of similar gestation. In addition, the lungs of one patient who survived long enough to develop bronchopulmonary dysplasia (BPD) showed continued expression of very low levels of CuZnSOD, whereas MnSOD had increased in a distribution consistent with alveolar type II cells as well as in other areas of the lung. Thus, the premature human appears to be deficient in both SOD proteins in lung, and their expression may be impaired during acute exposure to hyperoxia, unlike the known response of term newborns of many species.

Even the adequacy of the MnSOD response in the premature lung may still be in question. Clerch and co-workers also found that premature baboons (140 days gestation) increase MnSOD protein in lung tissue after 16 days of hyperoxic exposure [100% oxygen; (19a)]. It is unknown how rapidly this response occurred and to what extent the protein was active. Premature baboons with bacterial infection had a MnSOD response of much greater magnitude than those without infection. All available data suggest that lung of both primate and human prematures show increases in MnSOD protein in response to hyperoxic exposure. However, these increases in MnSOD may not be sufficiently rapid to be beneficial. In addition, the increased levels of protein expressed may not be active. In summarizing the primate and human studies, the persistently low CuZnSOD staining in the lungs of prematures is also of special interest.

Superoxide Dismutase and the Role of Cytokines

The role of cytokines in the protection of the lung from hyperoxic injury has been explored. After parenteral administration of the cytokines interleukin-1 (IL-1) and tumor necrosis factor (TNF) in adult rats, the mRNA, protein, and activity of MnSOD increased, whereas CuZnSOD mRNA and activity was unchanged following cytokines (61). A similar pattern, upregulation of MnSOD with no change in CuZnSOD expression, has been noted in protection of rats against hyperoxia afforded by intratracheal administration of TNF or IL-1 (89). Thus, a role for MnSOD in cytokine-mediated protection of the lung from hyperoxia has been postulated. Upregulation of MnSOD by inflammatory cytokines may be an important factor in MnSOD expression in the lungs of septic primates.

The role of the cytokines IL-1 and TNF and bacterial lipopolysaccharide (LPS) was initially examined to determine the induction of MnSOD mRNA in several lung cell lines. In both porcine and rat pulmonary artery endothelial cells (PAEC), treatment with LPS, TNF, or IL-1 resulted in induction of MnSOD mRNA but had no effect on CuZnSOD mRNA levels (92, 93). This effect could be blocked by actinomycin D, an RNA synthesis inhibitor, suggesting that this induction occurs at the transcriptional level. The role of the endogenous thiol reductant, thioredoxin, has been explored with regard to MnSOD gene regulation. In recent studies, it was observed that thiol-reducing agents can increase MnSOD mRNA, activity, and gene activation in human lung adenocarcinoma (A549) cells in association with activation of the transcription factor nuclear factor kappa B (NF-κB) (23). Along these lines, these authors also investigated the mechanism by which certain cytokines, IL1 and TNF-α can mediate MnSOD gene expression. They subjected a human lung cell line (A549) to treatment with several thiol-reducing or -oxidizing agents and then measured the effects on both NF-κB and MnSOD gene expression by these cytokines. They found that both these processes were activated by thiol-reducing agents but were inhibited by thiol-oxidizing and -alkylating agents. These findings suggest a strong association between NF-κB activation and MnSOD gene expression, and that reduced sulfhydryl groups are required for these responses (24).

Newer Antioxidants

Extracellular Superoxide Dismutase

Extracellular SOD (EC-SOD) is the most recently discovered member of the SOD family. It is a tetrameric protein (except in the rat where it is dimeric) with a molecular weight of 120,000, and it has been detected in human plasma, lymph, ascites, cerebrospinal fluid, and virtually every extracellular fluid. Extracellular SOD is present in all human tissues (65). The protein contains regions of amino acid sequence homology to CuZnSOD including the catalytic region. In lung, EC-SOD is located primarily in the extracellular matrix. Specifically, it is located in areas where there is a high density of type I collagen and other matrix elements, but not in areas rich in elastin or cartilage. The localization of EC-SOD to matrix appears to be conferred by its positively charged carboxyl-terminal heparin glycosaminoglycan-binding domain. In adult human lung, EC-SOD is located heavily around larger blood vessels and airways, with lesser quantities in the extracellular matrix around alveolar and capillary regions. Extracellular SOD is not present on endothelial cell surfaces of capillaries or on small muscular or large elastic vessels. Except for small amounts present in bronchial epithelial cells and type II epithelial cells, EC-SOD is confined to extracellular spaces in adult human lung (69). Potential differences in EC-SOD expression in the premature and term newborn lung relative to that of the adult have not yet been explored. The pharmacologic potential of EC-SOD to protect the lung against pulmonary oxygen toxicity is unknown. However, knockout mice lacking EC-SOD have exaggerated pulmonary inflammation and injury when exposed to hyperoxic environments or to ozone (6).

The human EC-SOD gene, located on chromosome 4, has been characterized. Tissue activities are disparately higher than mRNA in the lung, brain, and pancreas, suggesting that these tissues have enhanced binding affinity for the circulating protein or that their translation efficiencies are elevated (31). Intron 1 of the EC-SOD gene contains two antioxidant response elements (AREs). These are responsive to phenolic antioxidants that redox cycle as well as to hydrogen peroxide, and they exist in the NAD(P)H:quinone reductase gene and the 5′-untranslated portion of the rat glutathione A-transferase Ya gene (78). The functional aspects of EC-SOD gene expression, however, are not yet understood.

Nonetheless, it does appear that EC-SOD might have important modulatory functions related to the regulation of airway and or vascular tone in the lung. It is striking that EC-SOD shares many locations within the lung in common with, or adjacent to, cells that produce nitric oxide (NO). The rate of reaction of nitric oxide with superoxide is diffusion limited. From the initial discovery of NO as the endothelium-dependent relaxing factor (EDRF), it has been recognized that superoxide-dependent inactivation could be a key regulator of its activity. Addition of SOD to aqueous buffers greatly prolongs the biologic half-life of EDRF in physiologic experiments investigating vascular tone (47, 76). More recently, studies of transgenic mice expressing high levels of EC-SOD have demonstrated that EC-SOD expression can modulate vascular tone in the brain (70, 71). In a model for hyperbaric oxygen toxicity to the brain, EC-SOD overexpression in transgenic mice *enhanced* toxicity, whereas inhibition of EC-SOD and CuZnSOD with the nonspecific copper chelator diethlyldithiocarbamate diminished oxygen toxicity. These perhaps surprising results were made more understandable when it was found that inhibition of NO synthesis caused a similar protection against central nervous system (CNS) oxygen toxicity and eliminated the difference in sensitivity to this toxicity between the transgenic and nontransgenic mice. This is understandable since superoxide is the usual oxidant that eliminates biologically active NO via the formation of peroxynitrite and other species. In the situation of CNS O_2 toxicity, NO-mediated vasodilation must be a maladaptive response, resulting in increased oxygen delivery to the brain and increasing intracranial pressure by expanding the vascular compartment. Both factors would thereby enhance oxygen-dependent edema. In addition, NO could function directly as a neurotransmitter in the seizures that lead to death in CNS neurotoxicity of hyperbaric oxygen, and NO synthesis inhibition or detoxification should inhibit toxicity. In another model of brain injury due to cold, EC-SOD overexpression protected against injury. Nitric oxide synthesis inhibition also prevented injury and, in this situation, EC-SOD overexpression provided no additional protection. This suggests that superoxide and NO interact through a common mechanism, peroxynitrite formation, in bringing about injury (4a, 71). In a rat model of spontaneous systemic hypertension, intravenous administration of an SOD with high affinity for endothelial cell heparan sulfate was effective in lowering blood pressure (68). Within the lung, EC-SOD was highly localized to the surfaces of smooth muscle cells and in extracellular matrix surrounding blood vessels and airways. Taken together, these data regarding EC-SOD suggest that it may interact with nitric oxide in regulating vascular and possibly, airway tone. Increasingly it is recognized that pulmonary hypertension can be an important component of the respiratory distress syndrome during its initial phases as well as during its progression to BPD. Increased airway tone and reactivity may also be an important pathophysiologic factor during BPD evolution. Therefore, a better understanding of the biochemical interactions of NO and superoxide and of the molecular regulation of NO synthases and EC-SOD may improve knowledge of BPD pathophysiology. In addition to all these considerations, it is notable that EC-SOD is also localized in the vicinity of matrix proteins such as type I collagen. Collagen is susceptible to superoxide-dependent attack. In addition, superoxide can activate latent collagenases present in neutrophils. Collagen fragments produced via such mechanisms of degradation is chemotactic to neutrophils. Hence, EC-SOD could also act as an important anti-inflammatory agent by downregulating such mechanisms (69). Thus, EC-SOD could also play an important role in modulating inflammation during the evolution of BPD.

Extracellular SOD also could play other roles in modulating nitric oxide–mediated effects. In at least some cell types, its expression is upregulated by interferon gamma (IFN-γ), a feature it shares in common with inducible NO synthase (66). Because cytokines such as IFN-γ are upregulated in sepsis, such events could be relevant in premature infants at greatest risk of developing BPD.

Metallothionein

Metallothioneins are low-molecular-weight, cysteine-rich proteins whose antioxidant functions are incompletely understood. Regulation of intracellular metal ion homeostasis, with modification of the availability of these ions to participate in free radical reactions, is likely to be one important function of these proteins (72a). Alteration of metallothionein (MT) expression through genetic manipulation changes the susceptibility of both cultured cells and intact animals to various oxidative stresses. For example, MT knockout mice (homozygous null mutant animals) appear normal under basal conditions, but have exaggerated sensitivity in models of pulmonary oxygen toxicity and cadmium hepatotoxicity. Likewise, embryonic cells derived from these mice are more sensitive than those obtained from controls or heterozygotes to the toxicity of tert-butyl hydroperoxide or paraquat, and the former are more susceptible to apoptosis caused by a number of other stimuli (59). By contrast, expression of elevated levels of metallothionein decreased the sensitivity of NIH 3T3 cells to cytotoxic effects of t-butyl hydroperoxide (72a, 81), to DNA damage caused by NO and/or its derivative metabolites (80), and, in pulmonary endothelial cells in culture to hyperoxia (72a). Recent, elegant studies have shown that in pulmonary artery endothelial cells, overexpression of MT protects the cells from the toxic effects of hyperoxia at least in part by inhibition of the peroxidation of membrane phospholipids through a metal-independent pathway (72a). The mechanisms through which metallothionein functions as an antioxidant are not fully understood. Nonetheless, it is known that MT can inhibit lipid peroxidation, quench peroxyl radicals, reduce peroxynitrite, and form dinitrosyl iron sulfur complexes. Additional indirect evidence to suggest potential importance of MTs in antioxidant defense comes from studies of pulmonary oxygen toxicity in which MT gene expression is upregulated (72). Taken together, these studies indicate that MT can play an important role in defense against oxidative stress. However, the adequacy of the pulmonary MT response in the premature human is unknown.

Other Antioxidant Proteins

Another low-molecular-weight, thiol-containing protein, thioredoxin (TRX), is increasingly recognized as having important roles in antioxidant defense, signal transduction, and cell growth regulation. We have observed that TRX expression is markedly upregulated after premature or term birth, and that the stimulus responsible for this increased expression is oxygen (22). It appears that eventually TRX protein is also substantially increased by oxygen, although it is not yet clear whether early translation of TRX protein is impaired in the lung of the premature.

Another stress protein that can be induced by hyperoxia is heme oxygenase (HO), the rate-limiting step in bilirubin production. The net effect of this enzyme's action is the degradation of a pro-oxidant, heme, with the production of a potential antioxidant, bilirubin. Hence, HO induction could contribute to antioxidant defense. For example, a recent investigation demonstrated that HO-2 knockout mice exposed to hyperoxia have increased markers of oxidative stress and increased total lung iron accumulation during exposure to hyperoxia (28). Heme oxygenase gene expression is increased during adaptation of the newborn to hyperoxic stress, and the nature of HO's importance in such adaptation is currently being evaluated (28a). Likewise, recent elegant studies have begun to elucidate the complex mechanisms through which HO is upregulated in response to various oxidative stresses (13, 28, 60).

ENERGY METABOLISM IN OXYGEN TOXICITY AND HYPEROXIC TOLERANCE

It has been demonstrated, first in bacteria (43) and subsequently in mammalian lung cells and whole rat and baboon lungs, that the critical Krebs cycle enzyme aconitase is rapidly inactivated by elevated partial pressure of oxygen. In the lungs of premature baboons developing bronchopulmonary dysplasia (BPD) during 100% oxygen exposure, there is nearly complete loss of mitochondrial aconitase activity compared to lungs of those treated only with as-needed (PRN) oxygen who do not develop BPD (67b). Aconitase appears to be the enzyme most rapidly inactivated by hyperoxia, which is involved in energy metabolism. The enzyme possesses an iron-sulfur cluster that is susceptible to inactivation by a variety of oxidants including superoxide and peroxynitrite (7, 49), and by increased concentrations of dioxygen (O_2) itself, even at normobaric pressures. Although the consequences of such inactivation for cellular energy metabolism have not been completely elucidated, these findings do help to clarify a potential explanation for previous observations regarding metabolic events that occur in oxygen poisoning—namely, the decline in cellular respiration and increasing dependence on glycolysis for energy production.

In a cultured Chinese hamster ovary cell line (CHO-99) that was selected over a period of approximately 2 years to allow stable proliferation in 99% oxygen, a variety of metabolic changes that may contribute to these cells' adaptation have been detected. First, a number of antioxidant enzyme changes occurred; these included two- to fourfold increases in superoxide dismutases, catalase, and glutathione peroxidase. Likewise, the levels of reduced GSH increased in CHO-99 cells by more than fourfold, whereas GSSG levels did not significantly change (90). The relative volume of both mitochondria and peroxisomes increased substantially (91). In addition, the total ATP production through oxidative metabolism and glycolysis decreased by 36%, with that produced by oxidative phosphorylation decreasing by 52% and that due to glycolysis increasing fivefold (from 6% to 30%) (79). Similarly, lactate production increased fourfold in CHO-99 cells, relative to that for CHO-20 cells, in hyperoxia. Respiration rates in hyperoxia-adapted (CHO-99) cells growing in hyperoxia were approximately half that in air-adapted (CHO-20) cells growing in air. The steady-state ATP content of these cells decreased by 29% relative to their air-adapted controls. In addition, their adenylate energy charge also significantly decreased, further confirming the impairment of oxidative phosphorylation by hyperoxia. Activity of the hexose monophosphate shunt increased by approximately 50%, with absolute levels of NADPH increasing almost threefold and $NADPH/NADP^+$ ratios increasing almost twofold. Nonetheless, glucose-6-phosphate dehydrogenase, as assessed by activity assay, did not significantly increase in these cells, and these data suggested that the capacity for glucose metabolism through G6PD and the hexose monophosphate shunt was far from exceeded. In both air- and hyperoxia-adapted cells, only about 5% of the glucose consumed was metabolized through the hexose monophosphate shunt. Cyanide-resistant respiration, an indirect index of cellular production of reactive oxygen species, was elevated fourfold in CHO-99 cells, which suggests that a decrease in such production was not among the adaptive mechanisms. Likewise, diminished lipid peroxidation could not be detected in the CHO-99 cells (91). These studies point out the multiplicity of adaptive metabolic changes that can occur in cells under continuous hyperoxic stress and suggest that diverse strategies may be used to confer tolerance to such an insult. They also emphasize that metabolic changes pertinent to energy use and/or production may be especially pertinent to hyperoxic tolerance and that such changes may have been relatively overlooked in comparison to the attention given to the classical antioxidant enzymes in such protection.

In another transformed cell type, HeLa cells, these same investigators again developed an oxygen-resistant subclone by gradually increasing the ambient oxygen tension of the cells over approximately 21 months. Adaptations in energy production were again suggested to have occurred during the process. The authors observed that the mitochondria of the oxygen-adapted cells had a threefold greater mean profile area but were slightly decreased in number. Calculated mitochondrial volumes increased twofold in these cells, whereas the size of the oxygen- and air-adapted cells was not different. Although the mitochondrial matrix appeared less dense in the hyperoxia-adapted cells, there was observable structural damage. These changes resemble those occurring in lung mitochondria of rats adapted to hyperoxia (85% O_2) over prolonged periods (21). Respiration rates in hyperoxia-adapted cells decreased by about 40% in the hyperoxia-relative to air-adapted cells. However, the rates of cyanide-resistant respiration were almost identical in these two cell types. Hence, decreased cellular production of reactive oxygen species did not appear to contribute to tolerance. In contrast to the findings in CHO cells, these oxygen-adapted HeLa cells did not have increased activity of superoxide dismutases, catalase, or glutathione peroxidase, which suggests that such increases are dispensable in at least some cell types during oxygen adaptation. Likewise, the level of activity of G6PD was not related to the level of oxygen tolerance in these cells (52). Taken together, these studies provide evidence that adaptation of cellular energy metabolism alone, without changes in antioxidant defense systems (90, 91), can provide a substantial portion of the protection required for tolerance to hyperoxia.

SUMMARY

There is a surprising similarity between the changes in lung cellular composition that occur in the lungs of hyperoxia-adapted rats (21) and the histopathologic changes that resulting in the lungs of primates and infants affected by BPD (20). Among the morphologic features of oxygen-adapted rat lungs are a decrease in alveolar type I epithelial cells, capillary surface area, pulmonary vascular bed volume, and endothelial cell numbers, and an increase in numbers of inflammatory and interstitial cells along with increased volume of interstitial cells (21). Selection of these various cell types for survival and proliferation may reflect, at least in part, more favorable antioxidant profiles and/or bioenergetic capabilities in these cells, in addition to the effects of various growth factors. These changes all occur during normal adaptation to hyperoxia. However, in the premature human, many of these changes are likely to contribute to the pathophysiology of BPD.

In addition to these cellular changes, biochemical adaptation to pulmonary hyperoxic stress involves upregulation of numerous classes of proteins, including those of the classic and nonclassic antioxidant families, proteins involved in homeostasis of iron and transition metals, ion transport, connective tissue metabolism, surfactant proteins, and enzymes involved in energy metabolism. It is likely that each of these classes of proteins, as well as others yet to be discovered, are important in the adaptation process. The functions of, and interrelationships between, these various proteins are just beginning to be explored. It remains to be seen which critical proteins are deficient in the premature, and which, if any, can be augmented such that hyperoxic damage can be minimized and BPD thereby decreased.

REFERENCES

1. Asayama, K., H. Hayashibe, K. Dobashi, N. Uchida, M. Kobayashi, A. Kawaoi, and K. Kato. Immunohistochemical study on perinatal development of rat superoxide dismutases in lungs and kidneys. *Pediatr. Res.* 29: 487–491, 1991.
2. Bai, C., L.A. Brown, and D.P. Jones. Glutathione transport by type II cells, in perfused rat lung. *Am. J. Physiol.* 267: L447–L455, 1994.
3. Barry, B.D. and J.D. Crapo. Patterns of accumulation of platelets and neutrophils in rat lungs during exposure to 100% and 85% oxygen. *Am. Rev. Respir. Dis.* 132: 548–555, 1985.
4. Bassett, D.J.P., C.L. Elbon, and S.S. Reichenbaugh. Respiratory activity of lung mitochondria isolated from oxygen-exposed rats. *Am. J. Physiol.* 263: L1439–L1445, 1992.

4a. Beckman, J.S., T.W. Beckmen, J. Chen, P.A. Marshall, and B.A. Freeman. Apparent hydroxyl radical production by peroxynitrite: implications for endothelial injury from nitric oxide and superoxide. *Proc. Natl. Acad. Sci. USA* 87: 1620–1624, 1990.

5. Brown, L.A., C. Bai, and D.P. Jones. Glutathione protection in alveolar type II cells from fetal and neonatal rabbits. *Am. J. Physiol.* 262: L305–L312, 1992.
6. Carlsson. L.M., J. Jonsson, T. Edlund, and S.L. Marklund. Mice lacking extracellular superoxide dismutase are more sensitive to hyperoxia. *Proc. Natl. Acad. Sci. USA* 92: 6264–6268, 1995.
7. Castro. L., M. Rodriguez, and R. Radi. Aconitase is readily inactivated by peroxynitrite, but not by its precursor, nitric oxide. *J. Biol. Chem.* 269; 29409–29415, 1994.
8. Chang, M., M. Shi, and H.J. Forman. Exogenous glutathione protects endothelial cells from menadione toxicity. *Am. J. Physiol.* 262: L637–L643, 1992.
9. Chen, Y. and L. Frank. Differential gene expression of antioxidant enzymes in the perinatal rat lung. *Pediatr. Res.* 34: 27–31, 1993.
10. Chen, Y., I.R.S. Sosenko, and L. Frank. Positive regulation of pulmonary antioxidant enzyme gene expression by prenatal thyrotropin releasing hormone plus dexamethasone in premature rats exposed to hyperoxia. *Pediatr. Res.* 37: 611–616, 1995.
11. Chen Y., P.L. Whitney, and L. Frank. Negative regulation of antioxidant enzyme gene expression in the developing fetal rat lung by prenatal hormone treatments. *Pediatr. Res.* 33: 171–176, 1993.

12. Chen, Y., P.L. Whitney, and L. Frank. Comparative responses of premature versus full-term newborn rats to prolonged hyperoxia. Pediatr. Res. 35: 233–237, 1994.
13. Choi, A.M. and J. Alam. Heme oxygenase-1: function, regulation, and implication of a novel stress-inducible protein in oxidant-induced lung injury. *Am. J. Cell. Mol. Biol.* 15: 9–19, 1996.
14. Christie, N.A., A.S. Slutsky, B.A. Freeman, and A.K. Tanswell. Critical role for thiol, but not ATP depletion in 95% O_2-mediated injury in preterm pneumocytes in vitro. *Arch. Biochem. Biophys.* 313: 131–138, 1994.
15. Clerch, L.B., J. Iqbal, and D. Massaro. Perinatal rat lung catalase gene expression: influence of corticosteroid and hyperoxia. *Am J. Physiol.* 260: L428–L433, 1991.
16. Clerch, L.B. and D. Massaro. Oxidation-reduction sensitive binding of lung protein to rat catalase mRNA. *J. Biol. Chem.* 267: 2853–2855, 1992.
17. Clerch, L.B. and D. Massaro. Rat lung antioxidant enzymes: differences in perinatal gene expression and regulation. *Am J. Physiol.* 263: L466–L470, 1992.
18. Clerch, L.B. and D. Massaro. Tolerance of rats to hyperoxia. Lung antioxidant enzyme gene expression. *J. Clin. Invest.* 91: 499–508, 1993.
19. Clerch, L.B., D. Massaro, and A. Berkovich. Molecular mechanisms of antioxidant enzyme expression in lung during exposure to and recovery from hyperoxia. *Am. J. Physiol.* 274: L313–L319, 1998.
19a. Clerch, L.B., A.E. Wright, and J.J. Coalson. Lung manganese superoxide dismutase protein expression increases in the baboon model of bronchopulmonary dysplasia and is regulated at a posttranscriptional level. *Pediatr. Res.* 39: 253–258, 1996.
20. Coalson, J.J., V.T. Winter, D.R. Gerstmann, S. Idell, R.J. King, and R.A. deLemos. Pathophysiologic, morphometric, and biochemical studies of the premature baboon with bronchopulmonary dysplasia. *Am. Rev. Respir. Dis.* 192: 872–881, 1992.
21. Crapo. J.D., B.E. Barry, H.A. Foscue, and J. Shelburne. Structural and biochemical changes in rat lungs occurring during exposures to lethal and adaptive doses of oxygen. *Am. Rev. Respir. Dis.* 122: 123–143, 1980.
22. Das, K.C., X.-L. Guo, and C.W. White. Induction of the thioredoxin system in lungs of newborn primates by oxygen breathing at birth, during respiratory distress and during the evolution of bronchopulmonary dysplasia. *Am. J. Respir. Crit. Care Med.* 155: A18, 1997.
23. Das, K.C., Y. Lewis-Molock, and C.W. White. Activation of NF-κB and elevation of manganese superoxide dismutase gene expression by thiol reducing agents in lung adenocarcinoma (A549) cells. *Am. J. Physiol.* 269: L588–L602, 1995a.
24. Das, K.C., Y. Lewis-Molock, and C.W. White. Thiol modulation of TNF alpha and Il-1 induced MnSOD gene expression and activation of NF-kB. *Mol. Cell. Biochem.* 148: 45–57, 1995.
25. deLemos, R.A., R.J. Roberts, J.J. Coalson, J.A. deLemos, D.M. Null, Jr., and D.R. Gerstmann. Toxic effects associated with the administration of deferoxamine in the premature baboon with hyaline membrane disease. *Am. J. Dis. Child.* 144: 915–919, 1990.
26. Deneke, S.M., D.F. Baxter, D.T. Phelps, B.L. Fanburg. Increase in endothelial cell glutathione and precursor amino acid uptake by diethyl maleate and hyperoxia. *Am. J. Physiol.* 257: L265–L271, 1989.
27. Deneke, S.M., S.N. Gershoff, and B.L. Fanburg. Potentiation of oxygen toxicity in rats by dietary protein or amino acid deficiency. *J. Appl. Physiol.* 54: 147–151, 1983.
28. Dennery, P.A., D.R. Spitz, G. Yang, A. Tatarov, C.S. Lee, M.L. Shegog, and K.D. Poss.

Oxygen toxicity and iron accumulation in the lungs of mice lacking heme oxygenase-2. *J. Clin. Invest.* 101: 1001–1011, 1998.

28a. Dennery, P.A., H.E. Wong, K.J. Stridhar, P.A. Rodgers, J.E. Sim, and D.R. Spitz. Differences in basal and hyperoxia-associated HO expression in oxidant-resistant hamster fibroblasts. *Am. J. Physiol.* 271: L672–L679, 1996.

29. Dobashi, R., K. Asayama, H. Hayashibe, A. Munim, A. Kawaoi, M. Morikawa, and S. Nakazawa. Immunohistochemical study of copper-zinc and manganese superoxide dismutases in the lungs of human fetuses and newborn infants: developmental profiles and alterations in hyaline membrane disease and bronchopulmonary dysplasia. *Virchows Arch. A Pathol. Anat. Histopathol.* 423: 177–184, 1993.

30. Fazzone, H., A. Wangner, and L.B. Clerch. Rat lung contains a developmentally regulated MnSOD mRNA binding protein. *J. Clin. Invest.* 92: 1278–1281, 1993.

31. Folz, R.J., and J.D. Crapo. Extracellular superoxide dismutase (SOD3): tissue specific expression, genomic characterization, and computer-assisted sequence analysis of the human EC SOD gene. *Genomics* 22: 162–171, 1994.

32. Forman, H.J., E.I. Rotman, and A.B. Fisher. Roles of selenium and sulfur-containing amino acids in protection against oxygen toxicity. *Lab. Invest.* 2: 148–153, 1983.

33. Forman, H.J. and D.C. Skelton. Protection of alveolar macrophages from hyperoxia by gamma-glutamyl transpeptidase. *Am. J. Physiol.* 259: 1102–1107, 1990.

34. Frank, L. Hyperoxic inhibition of newborn rat lung development: protection by deferoxamine. *Free Radic. Biol. Med.* 11: 341–348, 1991.

35. Frank, L. Premature weaning of rat pups results in prolongation of neonatal tolerance to hyperoxia. *Pediatr. Res.* 29: 376–380, 1991.

36. Frank, L. Prenatal dexamethasone treatment improves survival of newborn rats during prolonged high oxygen exposure. *Pediatr. Res.* 32: 215–221, 1992.

37. Frank, L. and E. Groseclose. Oxygen toxicity in newborn rats: the adverse effects of undernutrition. *J. Appl. Physiol.* 53: 1248–1255, 1982.

38. Frank, L. and E.E. Groseclose. Preparation for birth into an O_2 rich environment: the antioxidant enzymes in the developing rabbit lung. *Pediatr. Res.* 18: 240–243, 1984.

39. Frank. L. and G.E. McLaughlin. Protection against acute and chronic hyperoxic inhibition of neonatal rat lung development with the 21-aminosteroid drug U74389F. *Pediatr. Res.* 33: 632–638, 1993.

40. Frank. L. and I.R.S. Sosenko. Prenatal development of lung antioxidant enzymes in four species. *J. Pediatr.* 110: 106–110, 1987.

41. Frank, L. and I.R.S. Sosenko. Failure of premature rabbits to increase antioxidant enzymes during hyperoxic exposure: increased susceptibility to pulmonary oxygen toxicity compared with term rabbits. *Pediatr. Res.* 29: 292–296, 1991.

42. Freeman, B.A. and J.D. Crapo. Biology of diseases: free radicals and tissue injury. *Lab. Invest.* 47: 412–426, 1981.

43. Gardner, P.R. and I. Fridovich. Effect of glutathione on aconitase in *Escherichia coli*. *Arch. Biochem. Biophys.* 301: 98–102, 1993.

44. Gardner, P.R., D.H. Nguyen, and C.W. White. Aconitase is a sensitive and critical target of oxygen poisoning in cultured mammalian cells and rat lungs. *Proc. Natl. Acad. Sci. USA* 91: 12248–12252, 1994.

45. Gardner, P.R., I. Raineri, L.B. Epstein, and C.W. White. Superoxide radical and iron modulate aconitase activity in mammalian cells. *J. Bicl. Chem.* 270: 13399–13405, 1995.

46. Gardner, P.R. and C.W. White. Failure of tumor necrosis factor and interleukin-1 to elicit

superoxide production in the mitochondrial matrices of mammalian cells. *Arch. Biochem. Biophys.* 334: 158–162, 1996.

47. Gryglewski, R.J., R.M.J. Palmer, and S. Moncada. Superoxide anion is involved in the breakdown of endothelium-derived relaxing factor. *Nature (Lond.)* 320: 454–446, 1986.
48. Hansen, T.N., C.V. Smith, A.L. Gest, H.W. Smith, and M. Giesler. Biochemical manifestations of oxygen toxicity in the newborn lamb. *Pediatr. Res.* 28: 613–617, 1990.
49. Hausladen, A. and I. Fridovich. Superoxide and peroxynitrite inactivate aconitases, but nitric oxide does not. *J. Biol. Chem.* 269: 29405–29408, 1994.
50. Ho, Y.S., M.S. Dey, and J.D. Crapo. Antioxidant enzyme expression in rat lungs during hyperoxia. *Am. J. Physiol.* 270: L810–L818, 1996.
51. Iqbal, J., L.B. Clerch, M.A. Hass, L. Frank, and D. Massaro. Endotoxin increases lung CuZn superoxide dismutase mRNMA: O_2 raises enzyme synthesis. *Am. J. Physiol.* 257: L161–L164, 1989.

51a. Keyer, K. and J.A. Imlay. Superoxide accelerates DNA damage by elevating free-iron levels. *Proc. Natl. Acad Sci. USA* 93: 13635–13640, 1996.

52. Joenje, H., J.J. Gille, A.B. Oostra, and P. Van der Valk. Some characteristics of hyperoxia-adapted HeLa cells. *Lab. Invest.* 52: 420–428, 1985.
53. Joyce-Grady, M., S.M. Oakes, D. Wuthrich, and Y. Laperche. Three alternative promoters of the rat gamma-glutamyl gene are active in developing lung and are differentially regulated by oxygen after birth. *J. Clin. Invest.* 97: 1774–1779, 1996.
54. Keeney, S.E., M.J. Mathews, and D.K. Rassin. Antioxidant enzyme responses to hyperoxia in preterm and term rats after prenatal dexamethasone administration. *Pediatr. Res.* 33: 177–180, 1993.
55. Kennedy, K.A. and N.L. Lane. Effect of in vivo hyperoxia on glutathione system in neonatal rat lung. *Exp. Lung Res.* 20: 73–83, 1994.
56. Kim, H.Y., T. LaVaute, K. Iwai, R.D. Klausner, and T.A. Rouault. Identification of a conserved and functional iron-responsive element in the 5′ untranslated region of mammalian mitochondrial aconitase. *J. Biol. Chem.* 271: 24226–24230, 1996.
57. Knickelbein, R.G., D.M. Ingbar, T. Seres, K. Snow, R.B. Johnston, Jr., O. Fayemi, F. Gumkowski, J.D. Jamieson, and J.B. Warshaw. Hyperoxia enhances expression of gamma-glutamyl transpeptidase and increases protein-*S*-glutathiolation in rat lung. *Am. J. Physiol.* 270: L115–L122, 1996.
58. Kugelman, A., H.A. Choy, R. Liu, M.M. Shi, E. Gozal, and H.J. Forman. Gamma-glutamyl transpeptidase is increased by oxidative stress in rat alveolar L2 epithelial cells. *Am. J. Respir. Cell Mol. Biol.* 11: 586–592, 1994.
59. Lazo, J.S., Y. Kondo, D. Dellapiazza, A.E. Michalska, K.H. Choo, and B.R. Pitt. Enhanced sensitivity to oxidative stress in cultured embryonic cells from transgenic mice deficient in metallothionein I and II genes. *J. Biol. Chem.* 270; 5506–5510, 1995.
60. Lee, P.J., J. Alam, G.W. Wiegand, and A.M. Choi. Overexpression of heme oxygenase-1 in human pulmonary epithelial cells results in growth arrest and increased resistance to hyperoxia. *Proc. Natl. Acad. Sci. USA* 93: 10393–10398, 1996.
61. Lewis-Molock, Y., K. Suzuki, N. Taniguchi, D.H. Nguyen, R.J. Mason, and C.W. White. Lung manganese superoxide dismutase increases during cytokine-mediated protection against pulmonary oxygen toxicity in rats. *Am. J. Respir. Cell. Mol. Biol.* 10: 133–140, 1994.
62. Li, Y., T.T. Huang, E.J. Carlson, S. Melov, P.C. Ursell, J.L. Olson, L.J. Noble, M.P. Yoshimura, C. Berger, and P.H. Chan. Dilated cardiomyopathy and neonatal lethality in mutant mice lacking manganese superoxide dismutase. *Nat. Genet.* 11: 376–381, 1995.

63. Liu, R.M., H. Hu, T.W. Robison, and H.J. Forman. Differential enhancement of gamma-glutamyl transpeptidase and gamma-glutamylcysteine synthetase by tert-butylhydroquinone in rat lung L2 cells. *Am. J. Respir. Cell Mol. Biol.* 14: 186–191, 1996.
64. Liu, R.M., H. Hu, T.W. Robison, and H.J. Forman. Increased gamma-glutamylcysteine synthetase and gamma-glutamyl transpeptidase activities enhance resistance of rat lung epithelial L2 cells to quinone toxicity. *Am. J. Respir. Cell Mol. Biol.* 14: 192–197, 1996.
65. Marklund, S.L. Properties of extracellular superoxide dismutase from human lung. *Biochemistry* 220: 269–272, 1984.
66. Marklund, S.L. Regulation by cytokines of extracellular superoxide dismutase and other superoxide dismutse isoenzymes in fibroblasts. *J. Biol. Chem.* 267: 6696–6701, 1992.
67. Martensson, J., J.C. Lai, and A. Meister. High-affinity transport of glutathione is part of a multi-component system essential for mitochondrial function. *Proc. Natl. Acad. Sci. USA* 86: 7185–7189, 1990.
67a. Morton, R.L., X.L. Guo, and C.W. White. Effect of oxygen on lung superoxide dismutase activities in premature baboons with bronchopulmonary dysplasia. *Am. J. Physiol.* (in press), 1998.
67b. Morton, R.L., D. Ikle, and C.W. White. Loss of lung mitochondrial activity due to hyperoxia in bronchopulmonary dysplasia in primates. *Am. J. Physiol.* 274: L127–L133, 1998.
68. Nakazono, K., N. Watanabe, K. Matsuno, J. Susaki, T. Sato, and N. Inoue. Does superoxide underlie the pathogenesis of hypertension? *Proc. Natl. Acad. Sci. USA* 88: 10045–10048, 1991.
69. Oury, T.D., L.Y. Chang, S.L. Marklund, B.J. Day, and J.D. Crapo. Immunocytochemical localization of extracellular superoxide dismutase in human lung. *Lab. Invest.* 70: 889–898, 1994.
70. Oury, T.D., Y.S. Ho, C.A. Piantadosi, and J.D. Crapo. Extracellular superoxide dismutase, nitric oxide, and central nervous system O_2 toxicity. *Proc. Natl. Acad. Sci. USA* 89: 9713–9719, 1992.
71. Oury, T.D., C.A. Piantadosi, and J.D. Crapo. Cold-induced brain edema in mice. Involvement of extracellular superoxide dismutase and nitric oxide. *J. Biol. Chem.* 268: 15394–15398, 1993.
72. Piedboeuf, B., C.J. Jonhston, R.H. Watkins, B.E. Hudak, J.S. Lazo, M.G. Cherian, and S. Horowitz. Increased expression of tissue inhibitor of metalloproteinases and metallothionein in murine lungs after hyperoxic exposure. *Am. J. Respir. Cell Mol. Biol.* 10: 123–132, 1994.
72a. Pitt, B.R., M. Schwarz, E.S. Woo, E. Yee, K. Wasserloos, S. Tran, W. Weng, R.J. Mannix, S.A. Watkins, Y.Y. Tyurina, V.A. Tyurin, V.E. Kagan, and J.S. Lazo. Overexpression of metallothionein decreases sensitivity of pulmonary endothelial cells to oxidant injury. *Am. J. Physiol.* 273: L856–L865, 1997.
73. Rodriguez, M.P., I.R. Sosenko, M.C. Antigua, and L. Frank. Prenatal hormone treatment with thyrotropin releasing hormone and with thyrotropin releasing hormone plus dexamethasone delays antioxidant enzyme maturation but does not inhibit a protective antioxidant enzyme response to hyperoxia in newborn rat lung. *Pediatr. Res.* 30: 522–527, 1991.
74. Rodriguez-Pierce, M., I.R.S. Sosenko, and L. Frank. Prenatal thyroid releasing hormone and throid releasing hormone plus dexamethasone lessen the survival of newborn rats during prolonged high O_2 exposure. *Pediatr. Res.* 32: 407–411, 1992.
75. Rodriguez-Pierce, M., I.R. Sosenko, P. Whitney, and L. Frank. Propylthiouracil treatment

decreases the susceptibility to oxygen radical-induced lung damage in newborn rats exposed to prolonged hyperoxia. *Pediatr. Res.* 35: 530–535, 1994.

76. Rubanyi, G.M. and P.M. Vanhoutte. Superoxide anions and hyperoxia inactivate endothelium-derived relaxing factor. *Am. J. Physiol.* 250: H822–H827, 1986.
77. Rusakow, L.S., C.W. White, and S.P. Stabler. O_2-induced changes in lung and storage pool thiols in mice: effect of superoxide dismutase. *J. Appl. Physiol.* 144: 911–915, 1993.
78. Rushmore, T.H., M.R. Morton, and C.B. Pickett. The antioxidant response element. *J. Biol. Chem.* 266: 11632–11639, 1991.
79. Schoonen, W.G.E.J., A.H. Wanamarta, J.M. Van der Kiel-van Moorsel, C. Jakobs, and H. Joenje. Respiratory failure and stimulation of glycolysis in Chinese hamster ovary cells exposed to normoxic hyperoxia. *J. Biol. Chem.* 265: 11118–11124, 1990.
80. Schwarz, M.A., J.S. Lazo, J.C. Yalowich, W.P. Allen, M. Whitmore, H.A. Bergonia, E. Tzeng, T.R. Billiar, P.D. Robbins, J.R. Lancaster, Jr., and B.R. Pitt. Metallothionein protects against the cytotoxic and DNA-damaging effects of nitric oxide. *Proc. Natl. Acad. Sci. USA* 92: 4452–4456, 1995.
81. Schwarz, M.A., J.S. Lazo, J.C. Yalowich, I. Reynolds, V.E. Kagan, V. Tyurin, Y.M. Kim, S.C. Watkins, and B.R. Pitt. Cytoplasmic metallothionein overexpression protects NIH 3T3 cells from tert-butyl hydroperoxide toxicity. *J. Biol. Chem.* 269: 15238–15243, 1994.
82. Shan, X.Q., T.Y. Aw, and D.P. Jones. Glutathione-dependent protection against oxidative injury. *Pharmacol. Ther.* 47: 67–71, 1990.
83. Shi, M.M., T. Iwamoto, and H.J. Forman. Gamma-glutamylcysteine synthetase and GSH increase in quinone-induced oxidative stress in BPAEC. *Am. J. Physiol.* 267: L414–L421, 1994.
84. Smith, C.V., T.N. Hansen, N.E. Martin, H.W. McMiken, and S.J. Elliott. Oxidant stress responses in premature infants during exposure to hyperoxia. *Pediatr. Res.* 125: 360–365, 1993.
85. Smith, L.J. and J. Anderson. Oxygen-induced lung damage. Relationship to lung mitochondrial glutathione levels. *Am. Rev. Respir. Dis.* 146: 1452–1457, 1992.
86. Sosenko, I.R.S., Y. Chen, L.T. Price, and L. Frank. Failure of premature rabbits to increase lung antioxidant enzyme activities after hyperoxic exposure: antioxidant enzyme gene expression and pharmacologic intervention with endotoxin and dexamethasone. *Pediatr. Res.* 37: 469–457, 1995.
87. Tanswell, A.K. and B.A. Freeman. Pulmonary antioxidant enzyme maturation in the fetal and neonatal rat: I. Developmental profiles. *Pediatr. Res.* 18: 584–587, 1984.
88. Town, G.I., G.J. Phillips, M. Landreau, J. Louden, S.T. Holgate and F.J. Kelly. Dexamethasone treatment fails to reduce hyperoxic lung injury in the premature guinea pig. *Biochem. Pharmacol.* 46: 1565–1572, 1993.
89. Tsan, M.F., J.E. White, C. Treanor, and J.B. Shaffer. Molecular basis for tumor necrosis factor–induced increase in pulmonary superoxide dismutase activities. *Am. J. Physiol.* 259: L506–L512, 1990.
90. Van der Valk, P., J.J. Gille, A.B. Oostra, E.W. Roubos, T. Siminia, and H. Joenje. Characterization of an oxygen-tolerant cell line derived from Chinese hamster ovary: antioxygenic enzyme levels and ultrastructural morphometry of peroxisomes and mitochondria. *Cell Tissue Res.* 239: 61–72, 1985.
91. Van der Valk, P., J.J. Gille, L.H. Van der Plas, J.F. Jongkind, A. Verkerk, A.W. Koning, and H. Joenje. Characterization of oxygen-tolerant chinese hamster ovary cells. II. Energy metabolism and antioxidant status. *Free Radic. Biol. Med.* 4: 345–356, 1988.

92. Visner, G.A., E.R. Block, I.M. Burr, and H.S. Nick. Regulation of manganese superoxide in porcine pulmonary artery endothelial cells. *Am. J. Physiol.* 260: L444–L449, 1991.
93. Visner G.A., S.E. Chesrown, J. Monnier, U.S. Ryan, and H.S. Nick. Regulation of manganese superoxide dismutase: Il-1 and TNF induction in pulmonary artery and microvascular endothelial cells. *Biochem. Biophys. Res. Commun.* 188: 453–462, 1992.
94. Visner, G.A., W.C. Dougall, J.M. Wilson, I.A. Burr, and H.S. Nick. Regulation of manganese superoxide dismutase by lipopolysaccharide, interleukin-1, and tumor necrosis factor. Role in the inflammatory response. *J. Biol. Chem.* 265: 2856–2864, 1990.
95. Walther, F.J., A.B. Wade, D. Warburton, and H.J. Forman. Ontogeny of antioxidant enzymes in fetal lamb lung. *Exp. Lung Res.* 17: 39–45, 1991.
96. Warshaw, J.B., C.W. Wilson, 3rd, K. Saito, and R.A. Prough. The responses of glutathione and antioxidant enzymes to hyperoxia in developing lung. *Pediatr. Res.* 19: 819–823, 1985.
97. White, C.W., D.H. Nguyen, K. Suzuki, N. Tanaguchi, L.S. Rusakow, K.B. Avraham, and Y. Groner. Expression of manganese superoxide dismutase is not altered in transgenic mice with elevated levels of copper-zinc superoxide dismutase. *Free Radic. Biol. Med.* 15: 629–636, 1993.
98. White, C.W., S.P. Stabler, R.H. Allen, S. Moreland, and A.A. Rosenberg. Plasma cysteine concentrations in infants with respiratory distress syndrome. *J. Pediatr.* 125: 769–777, 1994.
99. White, C.W., K.B. Avraham, P.F. Shanley, and Y. Groner. Transgenic mice with expression of elevated levels of copper-zinc superoxide dismutase in the lungs are resistant to pulmonary oxygen toxicity. *J. Clin. Invest.* 87: 2162–2168, 1991.
100. Wispé, J.R., B.B. Warner, J.C. Clark, C.R. Dey, J. Neuman, S.W. Glasser, J.D. Crapo, L.Y. Chang, and J.A. Whitsett. Human Mn-superoxide dismutase in pulmonary epithelial cells of transgenic mice confers protection from oxygen injury. *J. Biol. Chem.* 267: 23937–23941, 1992.
101. Yam, J., L. Frank, and R.J. Roberts. Oxygen toxicity: comparison of lung biochemical responses in neonatal and adult rats. *Pediatr. Res.* 12: 115–118, 1978.
102. Yang, F., W.E. Friedrichs, and J.J. Coalson. Regulation of transferrin gene expression during lung development and injury. *Am. J. Physiol.* 273: L417–426, 1997.

Grant support provided by the National Institutes of Health (NHLBI) HL52732 (CW), HL46481 (CW), HL52636 (CW) and HL07670 (RM). The authors also acknowledge the excellent technical assistance of Jacque Horvath.

chapter 16

LUNG DEVELOPMENT AFTER TRANSPLANTATION

Sheila G. Haworth and Alison A. Hislop

LUNG transplantation is now a therapeutic option for children with end-stage pulmonary parenchymal or vascular disease. En bloc heart-lung transplantation was pioneered by Reitz and colleagues and the first successful operation was carried out in 1981. Eventually, young patients were operated upon, who were generally adolescents with cystic fibrosis or the Eisenmenger syndrome. Successful single lung transplantation in adults with pulmonary fibrosis and emphysema and then in those with end-stage pulmonary vascular disease led to the extension of this technique to the pediatric age-group (43, 44). More recently, in children with pulmonary hypertensive congenital heart disease, single or bilateral sequential lung transplantation with intracardiac repair has become an acceptable alternative to heart-lung transplantation (2). The desperate lack of donor organs prompted the use of living related donor lobar lung transplantation in critically ill children (49). Using these different approaches, by 1997, 700 pediatric heart-lung and isolated lung transplantations had been carried out worldwide (32). The long-term outcome of the different procedures has not yet been compared, but the 2-year survival appears to be similar in bilateral lung and heart-lung transplantation, about 55%–60%. The incidence of rejection and bronchiolitis obliterans is not related to the indication for transplantation, or age (47). However, in a report on the St. Louis experience up to 1995, the patients transplanted at 3 years of age or less had a lower incidence of obliterative bronchiolitis than older pediatric cases (51).

The indications for transplantation in children tend to be different from those in adults. Cardiovascular diseases account for a greater proportion in children—30% as compared with 10%. The principle indications for transplantation during childhood fall under two categories: parenchymal lung disease and diseases of the pulmonary vasculature. Parenchymal lung disease includes cystic fibrosis and fibrosing lung diseases, such as idiopathic pulmonary fibrosis, interstitial pneumonitis, bronchopulmonary dysplasia, "adult" respiratory distress syndrome, and congenital abnormalities of lung development. Diseases of the pulmonary vasculature include primary pulmonary hypertension (plexogenic pulmonary arteriopathy and pulmonary veno-occlusive disease), pulmonary vascular disease co-existing with structural heart disease, pulmonary vein stenosis, and pulmonary vascular disease co-existing with parenchymal lung disease.

The effect of age on the outcome of lung transplantation is controversial. The figures from the International Registry indicate that long-term outcome may be worse in children less than 5 years of age (32). Another study reported that the outcome for children above 8 years of age is much like that of adults; those less than 8 years old fare less well (45). Other investigators reported that there was no difference in the outcome of children with cystic fibrosis transplanted who were older or younger than 10 years of age (1a, 60). In the recent, largest reported American series of children transplanted at 2 years of age or less, the hospital survival rate was 71%, which is no different from that seen in older patients (2). Sweet et al. (51) also reported 59% survival in patients up to 3 years old; this is not significantly different from the survival rate for older children. The short-term results are good, but the long-term implications for lung growth in these young patients is uncertain and a cause for concern.

LUNG GROWTH

Human Studies: What Do We Know?

Although the majority of children transplanted are still more than 10 years of age, increasingly, very young children of up to 2 years are being treated, particularly for pulmonary hypertensive congenital heart disease. In addition, lobar transplantation has been carried out in the neonatal period for children with congenital diaphragmatic hernia (49, 59). Lung development after transplantation will be determined by whether one or both lungs were transplanted, by the type and severity of disease in the contralateral lung following cadaveric unilateral lung transplantation, and in the residual lung tissue after living donor–related lobar transplantation. At least as important is the impact of postoperative disease, primarily obstructive bronchiolitis and infection. Age is the other major factor influencing subsequent lung growth. For all these reasons, few studies have been carried out to determine the growth of the transplanted lung and it is difficult to interpret much of the data that are available.

Guignon et al. (19) studied 16 patients transplanted at a mean age of 31.5 years and found that 1 year after transplantation, total lung capacity was within normal limits for age, including that of a child of 8 years at transplantation. Residual capacity was increased in cases transplanted for cystic fibrosis. The hyperinflation was thought to be due to structural adaptation of the transplanted lungs to fill the abnormal, expanded thoracic cage of the patient (19). The operative technique does not appear to influence subsequent lung growth. In a series of 51 patients (60), only 4 developed stenosis at the anastomotic site during the first year, and in these exceptional cases, stenosis was associated with the early development of obliterative bronchiolitis.

Most adults show a restrictive defect of lung volume, probably due to the deliberate selection of donors with smaller thoracic cavities than the recipient, but lungs do subsequently "size up" and "size down." It would be expected that the younger the donor the greater would be the likelihood of normal lung growth being compromised either by infection or rejection episodes. When a donor lung is transplanted into an older patient, the outcome will depend on whether the predominant influences on lung growth are intrinsic or originate in the recipient. These factors are not understood, and we also need to know if the lung will continue to grow normally if denervated. In humans, airway branching is complete during fetal life but airways continue to increase in size until the end of adolescence with a two- to threefold increase occurring between birth and adulthood (24). Up to half the adult number of alveoli are present at birth (30) and although the exact age at which alveolar multiplication ceases may vary, it is likely that all alveoli are present by 2–4 years of age (57, 64). Further growth is by increase in alveolar size. Thus, following transplantation in the first years of life, it seems likely that the alveolar number might not reach its full potential. Transplantation in older children probably compromises alveolar size and complexity. At all ages airway size and composition of the epithelium and airway wall can be affected by transplantation. The development of the pulmonary circulation follows that of the airways (27, 28) and any reduction in alveolar number will be accompanied by an equivalent reduction in alveolar vessels.

Experimental Studies

Since so little clinical information is available, experimental studies have been carried out in an attempt to determine the effect of transplantation on lung growth. Eight-week-old baboons underwent a left lung autotransplantation. At 13 weeks and 9 months of age, lung volume assessed by nitrogen washout and computer tomography indicated normal lung growth (54). After single left lung transplantation between neonatal piglets aged 8–10 weeks, computed tomography showed an increase in volume of both the allograft and the recipient contralateral lung with increase in airway diameter (20). If there was rejection of the transplanted single lung, there was excessive growth in the recipient, native contralateral lung of alveolar and airway surface area (38). However, in another study, autotransplantation or allotransplantation of a lobe in young piglets aged 10 weeks led to impaired airway but normal alveolar growth in the transplanted lobe as assessed by measuring a cross-sectioned area of airways in lung sections after 12 weeks of growth (36, 41).

Lung growth after transplantation has also been studied in the immature rat after unilateral lung transplantation, using quantitative morphormetric analysis. Using this model, both the response to transplantation and the effect of transplantation on the recipient's own right lung can be analyzed. Syngeneic (Lewis to Lewis) and allogeneic (Brown Norway to Lewis) transplants were carried out on immature rats aged 6 weeks. In the rat, as in the human, a large proportion of the respiratory region of the lung forms after birth and the transplantation studies were performed at an age when new alveoli were still being formed. The allogeneic transplants were treated with cyclosporin. When the animals were sacrificed after 6 months, the lung volume was measured, alveolar development was assessed by quantitative light microscopic techniques to determine the size and number of alveoli, and airway diameter was also measured. Analysis showed that the immature transplanted lung of both syngeneic and allogeneic animals continued to grow to a normal size (Fig. 16.1) by the formation of new alveoli, despite the presence of low-grade rejection activity in the immunosuppressed animals. The new structures were normally formed—the alveoli, the accompanying blood vessels, and the blood-gas barrier (Fig. 16.2). The structures were also appropriate in number and size for the age of the animal (26). There was no evidence of pulmonary hypertension. In a second study, using the same animal model (29), an immature lung was transplanted into an adult recipient rat and again the transplanted lung continued to grow, reaching its predicted adult number of alveoli in both the syngeneic and allogeneic transplants (Fig. 16.3). Thus

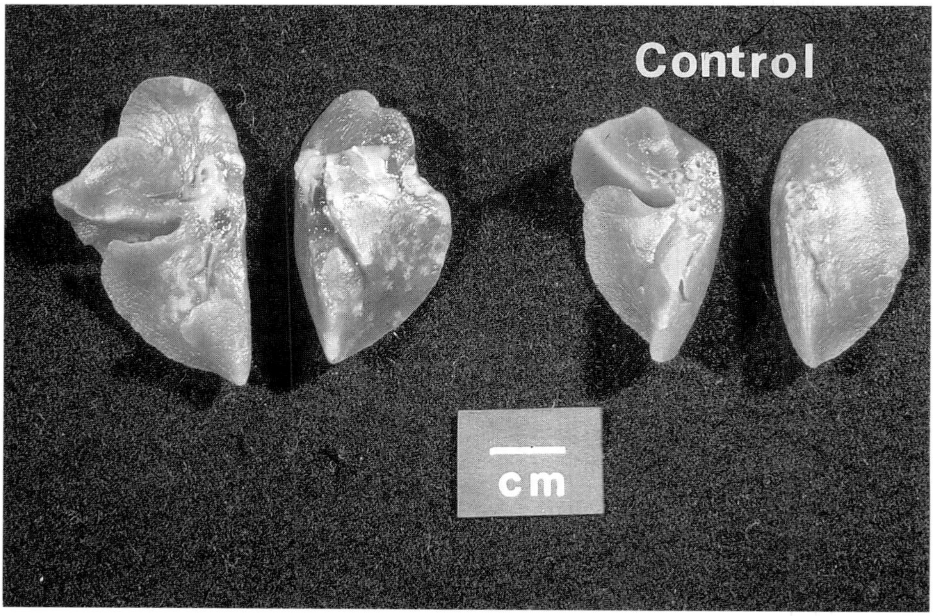

Fig. 16.1 Lungs of a Lewis rat 6 months after transplantation at 6 weeks of age with the left lung of another 6-week-old Lewis rat. For comparison, the lungs of a control Lewis rat aged 7.5 months are shown. The right native lung is much larger than the control right lung and the left lung has also increased in volume.

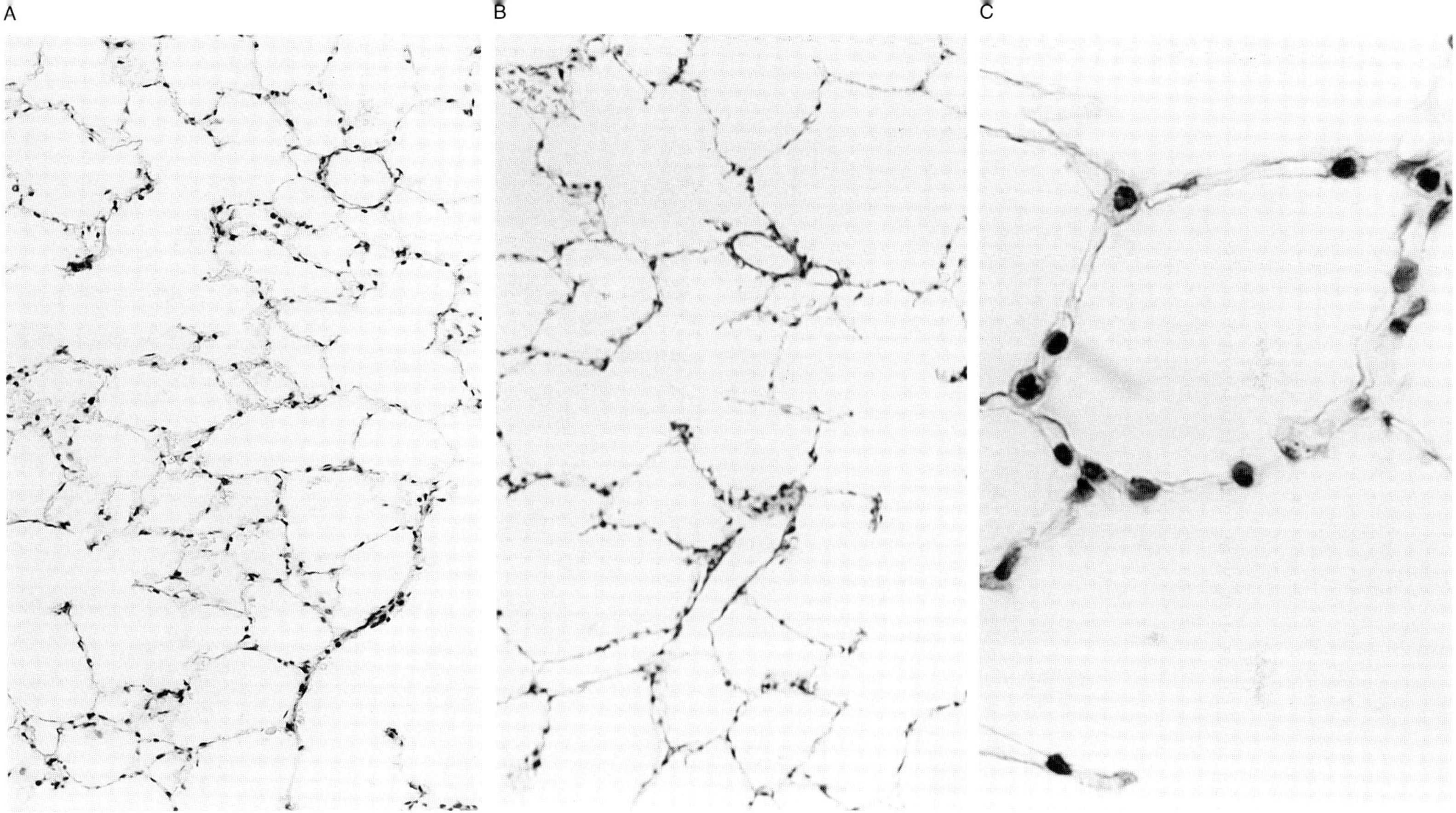

Fig. 16.2 Photomicrograph of the alveolar region of a control Brown Norway (BN) rat lung at 7.5 months (*A*) and a transplanted BN lung 6 months after transplantation at 6 weeks of age (*B*) (X 100). The lung architecture is normal in the transplanted lung but the alveoli are enlarged. The wall structure is normal in the BN transplanted lung (*C*) (X 400).

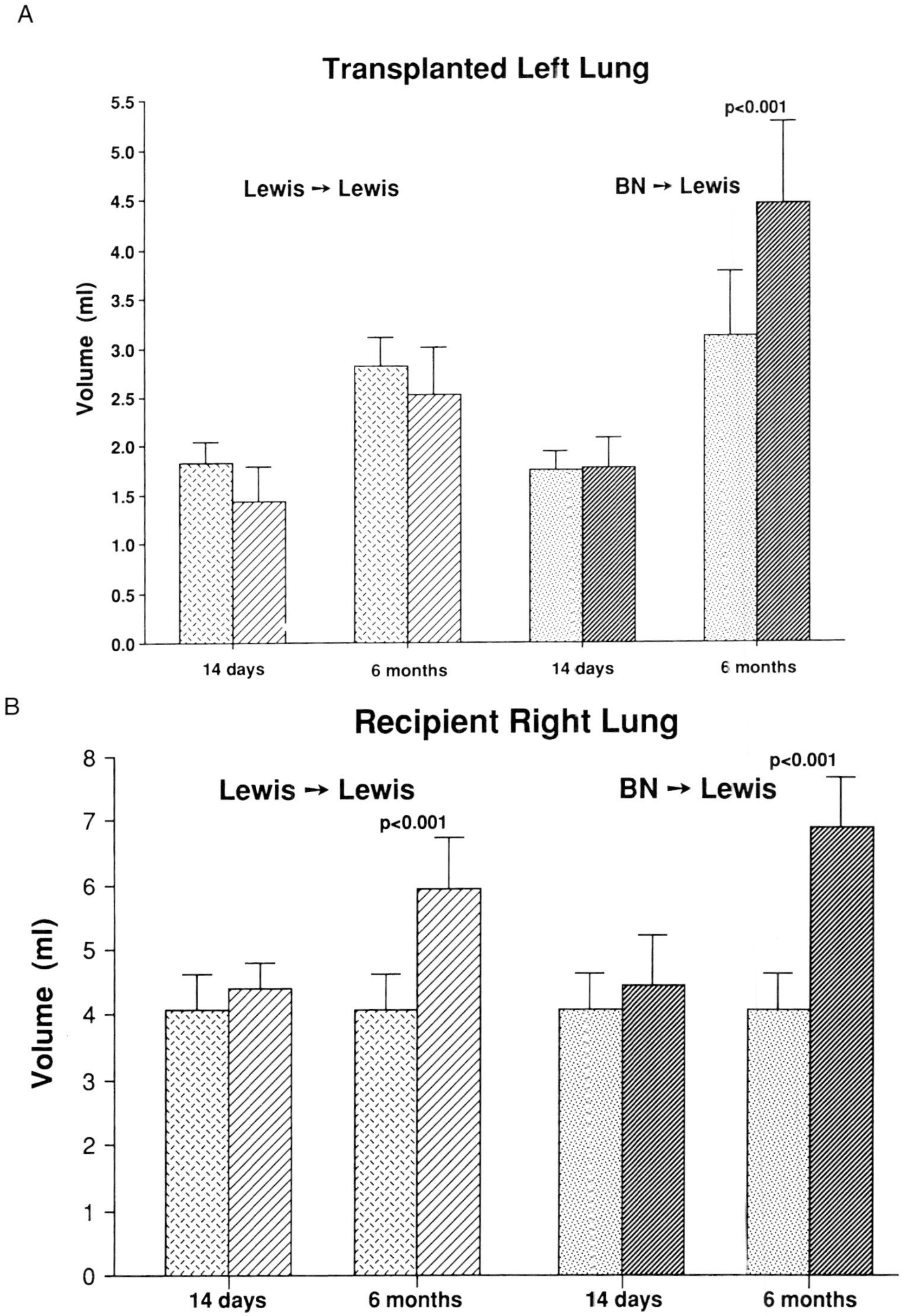

Fig. 16.3 Lung volume of A, transplanted left lung and B, recipient right lung (mean and SD) 14 days and 6 months after a lung from a 6-week-old donor (Lewis or BN rat) was transplanted into an adult Lewis rat. Control values left hand columns, transplant values right hand columns. After 6 months all lungs were normal or increased in volume. (C and D) Alveolar number and alveolar size

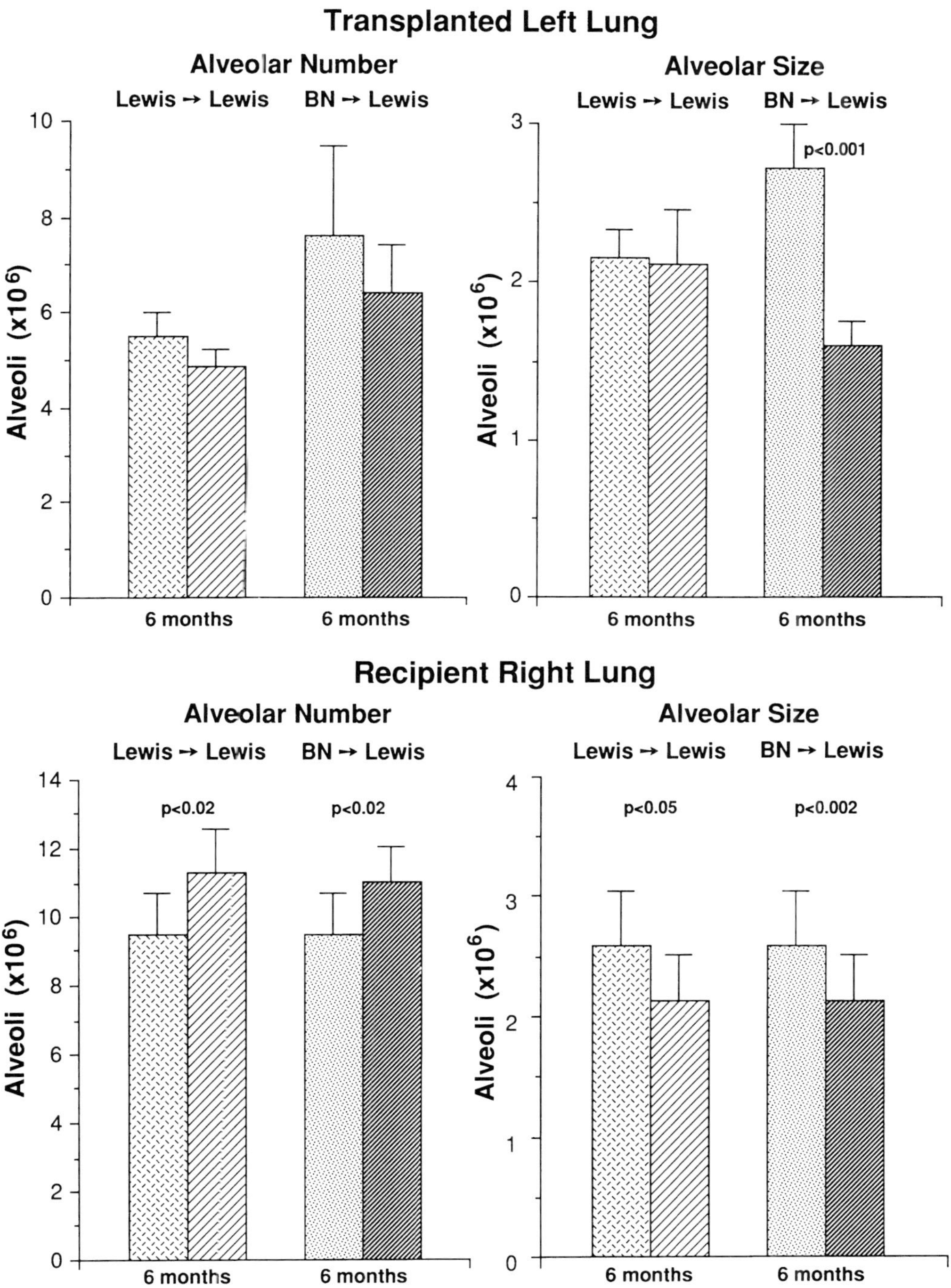

(alveoli/ml) for left transplanted and right recipient lung 6 months post transplant. Left lungs had a normal number of alveoli of normal size. Right lungs had an increased number of alveoli enlarged in size (decrease in number/ml) both contributing to the significant increase in lung volume. BN, Brown Norway.

transplantation into a mature host did not hamper the growth of the transplanted immature lung. The control of alveolar multiplication is poorly understood, but the continuation of alveolar multiplication seen in this denervated lung could be mediated by intrinsic neuropeptides. Intrinsic nerves containing neuropeptides are still present in both the human and rat lung after transplantation (48) and neuropeptides are known to have trophic functions (7).

There is much interest in the use of lobar or "reduced-size" adult lung transplants because of the shortage of donor organs in the pediatric age-group. Transplantation of an adult lobe into immature sheep, dogs, and piglets showed a good survival (1, 13, 39). Mature lobes from pigs aged 3 months transplanted into neonatal piglets (age 10–21 days) led post-operatively to preferential ventilation of the adult lobe because of its greater compliance (12). An outcome study on young piglets aged 8–10 weeks at operation and studied 12 weeks post-transplantation showed an increase in the adult transplanted lobar volume but no significant increase in alveolar number or size, suggesting growth of connective tissue and cellular components (37). Experimental studies have also been carried out in rats in which an adult Lewis cardiac lobe was transplanted into the left hemithorax of 6-week-old Lewis rats. Six months after lobar transplantation the lobe and the alveoli within it had increased in size (Fig. 16.4), but alveolar multiplication had not occurred and so the lobe appeared emphysematous (25). The results were thus different from those obtained after transplantation of an immature donor lung.

Experimental studies have shown that lung or lobar transplantation can disturb growth control in the contralateral, native lung of the recipient. When an immature left lung was transplanted into an immature rat (both syngeneic and allogeneic transplant) the number of alveoli in the native right lung was greater than normal only 2 weeks after transplantation and continued to increase, remaining greater than normal 6 months post-transplant (26). A similar response in the native lung occurred following syngeneic transplantation of an adult lobe into an immature rat, the contralateral lung showing an increase in lung volume and alveolar number 6 months later (25). Alveolar number was also increased in the native adult lung 6 months after transplantation of an immature lobe into an adult rat (syngeneic and allogeneic) (29). Such an increase in lung growth could have been compensatory, in both immature and adult recipients, because the right cardiac lobe was always resected during the operative procedure and in the adult recipients, the transplanted left lung was obviously smaller than the excised lung. However, the average difference between the recipient and donor left lung volume at the time of transplantation was only 0.8 ml, and the increase in volume of the right lung 6 months after transplantation was 2–3 ml. Previous studies have shown that the compensatory growth that occurs when one or two lobes of the right lung are removed from a young animal is not excessive and results in a lung of normal volume for age (8, 46). After a left pneumonectomy, the right lung grows rapidly by increasing cell number and then alveolar structures until the total volume is sufficient to replace the resected tissue (3). In our studies on the transplanted rat lung, the right lung volume alone was similar to the total lung volume of normal animals. These observations suggest

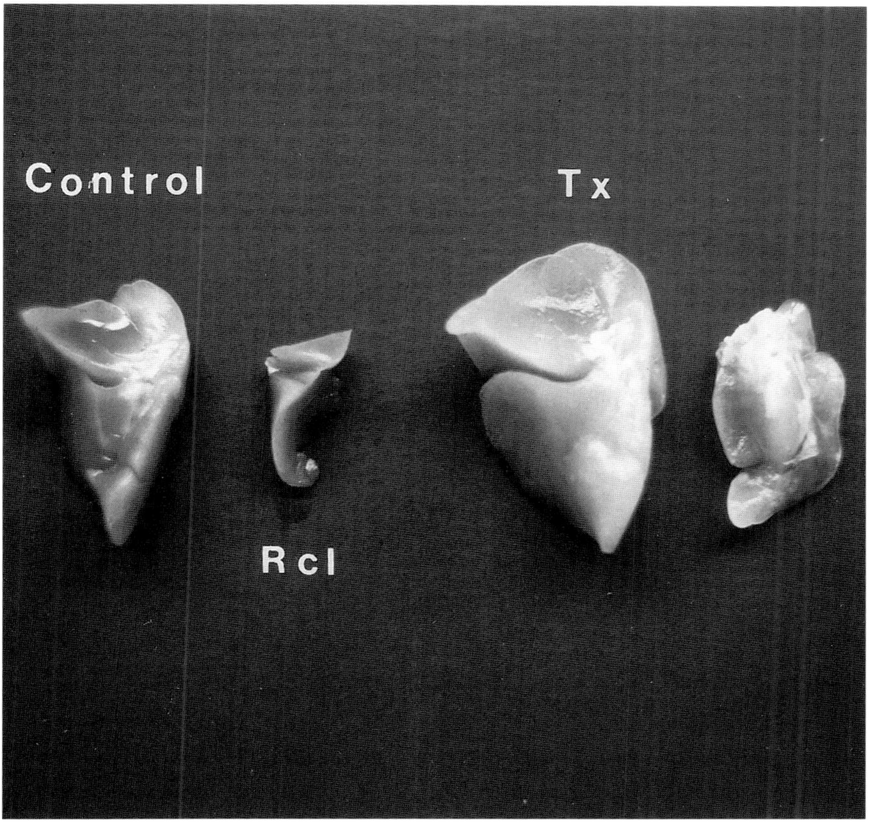

Fig. 16.4 Lungs of a Lewis rat 6 months after transplantation (T*x*) of a mature cardiac lobe into the left hemithorax of an immature rat. The right lung is enlarged. The transplanted cardiac lobe is also larger, and has changed in shape in comparison with the normal (control) right cardiac lobe (*Rcl*) of the same age.

that after transplantation, the right lung does not sense the presence of the denervated left lung. It is surprising that the right lung was not prevented from growing by the physical presence of the left lung since when inert material was left in the thorax after pneumonectomy in adult mice, the contralateral lung did not grow as rapidly as after pneumonectomy alone (4). In adult rats, post-pneumonectomy compensatory overgrowth is by increase in size of alveoli rather than number (5); this was also true of growing rats aged 6 weeks in studies from this laboratory in which young rats had undergone cardiac lobectomy (46). However, in a recent study after left lung pneumonectomy in 6-week-old rats, we found that the increase in volume was due to a combined increase in number and size of alveoli (25). Similarly, Holmes and Thurlbeck (31) found that when pneumonectomy was carried out in 4-week-old rats, the remaining lung grew by alveolar multiplication, but it grew by increase in alveolar size when the pneumonectomy was carried out at 12 week of age. Following pneumonectomy in young rabbits, the remaining lung increased in size because of alveolar multiplication (9). These findings imply that there is a critical time period during postnatal development when alveolar multiplication will occur. In a study on the long-term outcome of penumonectomy in 6 to 10-week-old dogs, Davies et al. (14) found that the remaining young lung grew by an increase in alveolar number, but the final number achieved after 5 years did not exceed the normal adult number of alveoli for that lung, even though lung volume was increased.

By contrast, in our transplantation studies on rats, the increase in volume of the contralateral recipient lung of both juvenile and adult animals was caused by an increase in alveolar number that exceeded the normal, in addition to the abnormal increase in alveolar size. The mechanisms responsible for these changes are unknown. But transplantation, with its attendant preservation time, may stimulate excessive growth, since, in animals receiving an allogeneic transplant in which the lung atrophied soon after operation, effectively producing a pneumonectomy, the remaining right lung enlarged by excessive alveolar multiplication (26). This was a much greater response than was seen after a standard pneumonectomy. Other studies also showed that the overgrowth of the right lung could only be explained in terms of transplantation and was not due either to denervation or to inadvertent narrowing of the airway or to vascular stenosis of the transplanted left lung, causing a disproportionate flow to the right lung (46). In both growing and adult recipients, the increase in right lung volume was seen after both syngeneic and allogeneic transplants, suggesting that this is not an immune response.

Thus it appears that the presence of a transplanted growing lung with its own intrinsic growth factors causes inappropriate stimulation of growth of any existing immature lung tissue or restimulates the growth of an adult contralateral lung, suggesting inappropriate epithelial and mesenchymal responses. In vitro studies suggest that proliferation of cultured epithelial cells involves activation by insulin-like growth factor-1 (IGF-1) or by epidermal growth factor (EGF) functioning with transforming growth factor α (TGF-α) (34). Optimal growth of tracheobronchial epithelial cells depends on the presence of EGF and TGF-α in the medium (55). These cells also synthesize and secrete TGF-α such that there is a degree of autoregulation (34). Epidermal growth factor also accelerates maturation of the alveolar epithelium (50). By contrast, TGF-β is a powerful inhibitor of epithelial cell multiplication (35), but its presence leads to an increase in protein synthesis (16). It appears that the balance between TGF-β and TGF-α and EGF may maintain the lung in the normal state of cell multiplication and differentiation once growth is complete. Studies on the unilateral transplanted rat lung suggest that this balance may be disturbed in the contralateral recipient lung. The findings suggest that growth factor production by one lung can affect the growth of the other, and therefore studies on the expression of lung growth factors in this experimental model may help elucidate the more general principles determining control of lung growth.

Following unilateral left lung transplantation in immature rats, the peripheral airways increased in size in both the transplanted and recipient native lung (26). Both lumen diameter and airway wall thickness were greater than normal. The individual components of the airway wall, epithelium, bronchial smooth muscle, and connective tissue increased in a proportional manner. These changes were not seen after pneumonectomy or denervation and were related to transplantation itself (46). Recent studies have shown that cold preservation and reimplantation of the rat lung causes an increase in the number of basal cells in the epithelium of the peripheral airways (33). This damage seemed irreversible since it was maintained for up to 6 months after transplantation. The role played by these basal cells in initiating and maintaining the increase in airway size is not clear. In vitro studies showed that cooling enhanced the proliferative response of the epithelial cells to media produced by cooled cultured fibroblasts, emphasizing that the trigger disturbing control of airway cell number was activated during cold preservation. These studies raise the possibility that damage incurred during preservation may be linked to the development of obliterative bronchiolitis, a disease of the peripheral airways, through the up-regulation of growth factors affecting epithelial cells and fibroblasts. Bleomycin injury in rats modulates EGF receptors and TGF-α production (40). Platelet-derived growth factor (PGDF) and fibroblast growth factor (FGF) have been implicated in the development of obliterative bronchiolitis in the human lung because they are increased in the bronchoalveolar lavage (BAL) fluid from patients with obliterative bronchiolitis (23). Once the airways are damaged it is possible that infection may provoke the development of obliterative bronchiolitis. Winter et al. (61) showed that infection with Sendai virus 6 months after transplantation caused obliterative bronchiolitis in rat lungs.

Restricted airflow as occurs in obliterative bronchiolitis may impair alveolar development, and infection by parainfluenza virus in young rats leads to reduced alveolar development and reduced airway size (10). The lungs of such infected rats did not show "catch-up" growth during recovery (11). Cyclosporin treatment may have an effect on lung growth. In experimental animals, high doses of cyclosporin suppress total body growth (56) and can also reduce the multiplication of aortic medial smooth and endothelial cells (18). However, another study has shown that low doses of cyclosporin do not affect somatic growth or the compensatory growth of the remaining kidney after single nephrectomy in the rat (42). Six months after allogeneic lung transplantation, the ultrastructure of the alveoli was normal in rats treated with cyclosporin (6). It seems unlikely that cyclosporin was responsible for the enhanced lung growth seen in the rat experimental studies, since we have found that syngeneic transplanted animals that were not treated with cyclosporin also had abnormally large native lungs. Treatment by artificial ventilation or steroids may also affect lung growth. High oxygen tensions reduce alveolar septation in newborn rats (21, 53) and increase airway smooth muscle and hyperresponsiveness (22). Hyperoxia and barotrauma for 48 h also led to a decrease in compliance and an increase in resistance in newborn piglets (1–2 days old) (15). This was associated with areas of inflammation and atelectasis likely to lead to impairment of alveolar multiplication. In infants, the use of glucocorticoids enhances the maturation of alveoli and prevents inflammatory damage (17, 62, 63), but when glucocorticoids were given to rats postnatally, alveolar multiplication was inhibited (58) and glucocorticoids given in the presence of a high oxygen tension had a greater inhibitory effect (52).

CONCLUSION

In conclusion, experimental studies show that an immature lung transplanted into either an immature or adult recipient can continue to grow. These data are encouraging and suggest that the transplanted lungs of young children may be able to fulfill their growth potential. But the human condition is complicated by rejection, infection, and treatment strategies that may compromise lung development to a much greater extent than transplantation itself.

REFERENCES

1. Backer, C.L., S. Ohtake ,V.R. Zales, J. LoCicero, L.L. Michaelis, and F.S. Idriss. Living-related lobar lung transplantation in beagle puppies. *J. Pediatr. Surg.* 26: 429–432, 1991.

1a. Balfour-Lynn, I.M., I. Martin, B.F. Whitehead, P.G. Rees, M.J. Elliott, and M.R. De Leval. Heart-lung transplantation for patients under 10 with cystic fibrosis. *Arch. Dis. Child* 76: 38–40, 1997.

2. Bridges, N.D., G.B. Mallory, C.B. Huddleston, C.E. Canter, and T.L. Spray. Lung transplantation in infancy and early childhood. *J. Heart Lung Transplant.* 15: 895–902, 1996.

3. Brody J.S. Time course of and stimuli to compensatory growth of the lung after pneumonectomy. *J. Clin. Invest.* 56: 897–904, 1975.

4. Brody, J.S., R. Burki, and N. Kaplan. Deoxyribonucleic acid synthesis in lung cells during compensatory lung growth after pneumonectomy. *Am. Rev. Respir. Dis.* 117: 307–316, 1978.

5. Buhain, W.J. and J.S. Brody. Compensatory growth of the lung following pneumonectomy. *J. Appl. Physiol.* 35: 898–902, 1973.

6. Bullard, A.G., A. Petersen, C.R.H. Wildevuur, J. Prop, and J.D. Crapo. Lung transplantation in the rat. *Transplantation* 53: 443–449, 1991.

7. Burnstock, G. Neurotransmitters and trophic factors in the autonomic nervous system. *J. Physiol.* 313: 1–35, 1981.

8. Burri, P.H. and S. Sehovic. The adaptive response of the rat lung after bilobectomy. *Am. Rev. Respir. Dis.* 119: 769–777, 1979.

9. Cagle, P.T., C. Langston, and M. Thurlbeck. The effect of age on post-pneumonectomy growth in rabbits. *Pediatr. Pulmonol.* 5: 92–95, 1988.

10. Castleman, W.L. Alterations in pulmonary ultrastructure and morphometric parameters induced by parainfluenza (sendai) virus in rats during postnatal growth. *Am. J. Pathol.* 114: 322–335, 1984.

11. Castleman, W.L., R.L. Sorkness, R.F. Lemanske, G. Grassee, and M.M. Suyemoto. Neonatal viral bronchiolitis and pneumonia induces bronchiolar hypoplasia and alveolar dysplasia in rats. *Lab. Invest.* 59: 387–396, 1988.

12. Crombleholme, T.M., N.S. Adzick, K. Hardy, M.T. Longaker, S.M. Bradley, B.W. Duncan, and E.D. Verrier. Pulmonary lobar transplantation in neonatal swine: a model for treatment of congenital diaphragmatic hernia. *J. Pediatr. Surg.* 25: 11–18, 1990.

13. Crombleholme, T.M., N.S. Adzick, M.T. Longaker, S. Bradley, B.W. Duncan, E.D. Verrier, and M.R. Harrison. Reduced-size lung transplantation in neonatal swine; technique and short-term physiological response. *Ann. Thorac. Surg.* 49: 55–60, 1990.

14. Davies, P., J. McBride, G.F. Murray, B.R. Wilcox, J.A. Shallal, and L. Reid. Structural changes in the canine lung and pulmonary arteries after pneumonectomy. *J. Appl. Physiol.* 53: 859–864, 1982.
15. Davis, J.M., B. Dickerson, L. Metlay, and D.P. Penney. Differential effects of oxygen and barotrauma on lung injury in the neonatal piglet. *Pediatr. Pulmonol.* 10: 157–163, 1991.
16. DiMari, S.J., A.M. Howe, and M.A. Haralson. Effect of transforming growth factor-β on collagen synthesis by fetal rat lung epithelial cells. *Am. J. Respir. Cell Mol. Biol.* 4: 455–462, 1991.
17. Fan, L.L. and C. Langston. Chronic interstitial lung disease in children. *Pediatr. Pulmonol.* 16: 184–196, 1993.
18. Ferns, G., M. Reidy, and R. Russell. Vascular effects of cyclosporin A in vivo and in vitro. *Am. J. Pathol.* 137: 403–413, 1990.
19. Guignon, I., M. Cassart, P.A. Genenois, C. Knoop, M. Antoine, J.C. Yernault, and M. Estenne. Persistent hyperinflation after heart-lung transplantation for cystic fibrosis. *Am. J. Respir. Crit. Care Med.* 151: 534–540, 1995.
20. Hammainen, P.T. Single lung transplantation in piglets. Technique and follow-up. *Scand. J. Thorac. Cardiovasc. Surg.* 27: 71–80, 1993.
21. Han, R.N.N., S. Buch, I. Tseu, J. Young, N.A. Christie, H. Frndova, S.J. Lye, M. Post, and A.K. Tanswell. Changes in structure, mechanics, and insulin-like growth factor-related gene expression in the lungs of newborn rats exposed to air or 60% oxygen. *Pediatr. Res.* 39: 921–929, 1996.
22. Hershenson, M.B., A. Garland, M.D. Kelleher, A. Zimmermann, C. Hernandez, and J. Solway. Hyperoxia-induced airway remodelling in immature rats. Correlation with airway responsiveness. *Am. Rev. Respir. Dis.* 146: 1294–1300, 1992.
23. Hertz, M.I., C.A. Henke, R.E. Nakhleh, K.R. Harmon, W.A. Marinelli, J.M. Fox, S.H. Kubo, S.J. Shumway, R.M Bolman., and P.B. Bitterman. Obliterative bronchiolitis after lung transplantation: a fibroproliferative disorder associated with platelet-derived growth factor. *Proc. Natl. Acad. Sci. USA* 89: 10385–10389, 1992.
24. Hislop, A.A. and S.G. Haworth. Airway size and structure in the normal fetal and infant lung and the effect of premature delivery and artificial ventilation. *Am. Rev. Respir. Dis.* 140: 1717–1726, 1989.
25. Hislop, A.A., R.J. Lee, C.G.A. MacGregor, and S.G. Haworth. Lung growth after transplantation of an adult lobe of lung into a juvenile rat. *J. Thorac. Cardiovasc. Surg.* 115: 644–651, 1998.
26. Hislop, A.A., N.J. Odom, C.G.A. McGregor, and S.G. Haworth. Growth potential of the immature transplanted lung—an experimental study. *J. Thorac. Cardiovasc. Surg.* 100: 360–370, 1990.
27. Hislop, A. and L. Reid. Intrapulmonary arterial development during fetal life—branching pattern and structure. *J. Anat.* 113: 35–48, 1972.
28. Hislop, A. and L. Reid. Pulmonary arterial development during childhood: branching pattern and structure. *Thorax* 28: 129–135, 1973.
29. Hislop, A.A., M. Rinaldi, R. Lee, C.G.A. McGregor, and S.G. Haworth. Growth of the immature lung transplanted into an adult recipient. *Am. J. Physiol.* 264: L60–L65, 1993.
30. Hislop, A., J.S. Wigglesworth, and R. Desai. Alveolar development in the human fetus and infant. *Early Hum. Dev.* 13: 1–11, 1986.
31. Holmes, C.W.M. and W.M. Thurlbeck. Normal lung growth and response after pneumonectomy in the rat at various ages. *Am. Rev. Respir. Dis.* 120: 1125–1136, 1979.

32. Hosenpud, J.D., L.E. Bennett, B.M. Keck, B. Fiol, M.M. Boucek and R.J. Novick. The Registry of the International Society for Heart and Lung Transplantation: Fifteenth official report—1998. *J. Heart Lung Transplant.* 17: 656–668, 1998.
33. Huntley, A.L., S.M. Hall, A.A. Hislop, N. Odom, C.G.A. McGregor, and S.G. Haworth. Airway structure following preservation and transplantation in the unilateral transplanted rat lung model. *Am. Rev. Respir. Dis.* 147: A261, 1993.
34. Jetten AM. Growth and differentiation factors in tracheobronchial epithelium. *Am. J. Physiol.* 260: L361–L373, 1991.
35. Jetten, A.M., J.E. Shirley, and G. Stoner. Regulation of proliferation and differentiation of respiratory tract epithelial cells by TGF-β. *Exp. Cell Res.* 147: 539–549, 1986.
36. Kern, J.A., I.L. Kron, T.L. Flanagan, O.A. Binns, W.W. Scott, B.B. Chan, J.G. Zografakis, and C.G. Tribble. Denervation of the immature porcine lung impairs normal airway development. *J. Heart Lung Transplant.* 12: 34–40, 1993.
37. Kern, J.A., C.G. Tribble, T.L. Flanagan, B.B. Chan, W.W. Scott, D.C. Cassada, and I.L. Kron. Growth potential of porcine reduced-size mature pulmonary lobar transplants. *J. Thorac. Cardiovasc. Surg.* 104: 1329–1332, 1992.
38. Langenburg, S.E., L.H. Blackbourne, S.A. Buchanan, M.C. Mauney, S.S. Kim, K.N. Sinclair, J.A. Kern, S.S. Teja, C.G. Tribble, and I.L. Kron. Compensatory growth of porcine right lungs after chronic rejection of transplanted left lungs. *Ann. Thorac. Surg.* 59: 28–32, 1995.
39. Lillehei, C.W., E. Everts, and R.C. Shamberger. Reduced-size lung transplantation from adult to neonatal sheep. *J. Pediatr. Surg.* 27: 1153–1156, 1992.
40. Madtes, D.K., H.K. Busby, T.P. Strandjord, and J.G. Clark. Expression of transforming growth factor-alpha and epidermal growth factor receptor is increased following bleomycin-induced lung injury in rats. *Am. J. Respir. Cell Mol. Biol.* 11: 540–551, 1994.
41. McGahren, E.D., W.G. Teague, T.L. Flanagan, B.J. White, G.W. Barone, A.M. Johnson, and I.L. Kron. Airway obstruction after autologous reimplantation of the porcine lobe. *J. Thorac. Cardiovasc. Surg.* 97: 587–592, 1989.
42. Myers A.K., S. Canale, J.C. Penhov, P.W. Ramwell, and M.L. Foegh. Preservation of renal compensatory growth in uninephrectomised rats by low-dose cyclosporin. *Transplantation* 49: 879–882, 1990.
43. Pasque, M.K., L.R. Kaiser, C.M. Dresler, E. Trulock, A.N. Triantifillou, and I.D. Cooper. Single lung transplant for pulmonary hypertension: technical aspects and immediate hemodynamic results. *J. Thorac. Cardiovasc. Surg.* 103: 475–482, 1992.
44. Pasque, M.K., E.P. Trulock, I.D. Cooper, A.N. Triantafillou, C.B. Huddleston, M. Rosenbloom, S. Sundaresan, J.L. Cox and G.A. Patterson. Single lung transplantation for pulmonary hypertension—single institution experience in 34 patients. *Circulation* 8: 2252–2258, 1992.
45. Radley-Smith, R.C., M. Burke, A. Pomerance, and M.H. Yacoub. Graft vessel disease and obliterative bronchiolitis after heart/lung transplantation in children. *Transplant. Proc.* 27: 2017–2018, 1995.
46. Rinaldi, M., A.A. Hislop, N.J. Odom, S.G. Haworth, and C.G.A. McGregor. Surgical factors affecting growth potential of the immature rat lung. *Eur. J. Cardiothorac. Surg.* 5: 218–222, 1991.
47. Spray, T.L., G.B. Mallory, C.B. Canter, and C.B. Huddleston. Pediatric lung transplantation. *J. Thorac. Cardiovasc. Surg.* 107: 990–1000, 1994.
48. Springall, D.R., J.M. Polak, L. Howard, R.F. Power, T. Krausz, S. Manickam, N.R. Banner,

A. Khapani, M. Rose, and M.H. Yacoub. Persistence of intrinsic neurone and possible phenotype changes after extrinsic denervation of human respiratory tract by heart lung transplantation. *Am. Rev. Respir. Dis.* 141: 1538–1546, 1990.

49. Starnes, V.A., M.L. Barr, and R.G. Cohen. Lobar transplantation. Indications, technique and outcome. *J. Thorac. Cardiovasc. Surg.* 108: 410–411, 1994.

50. Sundell, H.W., M.E. Grey, F.S. Serenius, M.B. Escobedo, and M.T. Stahlman. Effects of epidermal growth factor on lung malformation in fetal lambs. *Am. J. Pathol.* 100: 707–726, 1980.

51. Sweet, S.C., T.L. Spray, C.B. Huddleston, E. Mendeloff, C.E. Canter, D.T. Balzer, N.D. Bridges, A.H Cohen, and G.B. Mallory. Pediatric lung transplantation at St. Louis Children's Hospital, 1990–1995. *Am. J. Respir. Crit. Care Med.* 155: 1027–1035, 1997.

52. Thibault, D.W., B. Heimes, M. Rezaiekhaligh, and S. Mabry. Chronic modifications of lung and heart development in glucocorticoid-treated newborn rats exposed to hyperoxia or room air. *Pediatr. Pulmonol.* 16: 81–88, 1993.

53. Thibault, D.W., S. Mabry, and M. Rezaiekhaligh. Neonatal pulmonary oxygen toxicity in the rat and changes with aging. *Pediatr. Pulmonol.* 9: 96–108, 1990.

54. Thomas, D.D., T.A. Standaert, W.R. Anton, D.R. Jones, J.D. Godwin, G. Raghu, W.A. Hodson, and M.D. Allen. Growth potential of the transplanted lung in the infant primate. *Ann. Thorac. Surg.* 56: 1274–1278, 1993.

55. Thomassen, D.G., U. Saffiotti, and M.E. Kaighn. Clonal proliferation of rat tracheal epithelial cells in serum-free medium and their responses to hormones, growth factors and carcinogens. *Carcinogenesis* 7: 2033–2039, 1986.

56. Thomson, A.W., P.H. Whiting, J.T. Blair, R.J.L. Davidson, and J.G. Simpson. Pathological changes developing in the rat during a 3 weeks course of high dosage cyclosporin A and their reversal following drug withdrawal. *Transplantation* 32: 271–277, 1981.

57. Thurlbeck, W.M. Postnatal human lung growth. *Thorax* 37: 564–571, 1982.

58. Tschanz, S.A., E.M. Damke, and P.H. Burri. Influence of postnatally administered glucocorticoids on rat lung growth. *Biol. Neonate* 68: 229–245, 1995.

59. Van-Meurs, K.F., W.D. Rhine, E.W. Benitz, S.J. Shochat, G.E. Hartman, A.M. Sheehan, and V.A. Starnes. Lobar lung transplantation as a treatment for congenital diaphragmatic hernia. *J. Pediatr. Surg.* 29: 1557–1560, 1994.

60. Whitehead, B.R., R. Lane, R. Dinwiddie, S. Adwani, J. Fabre, P. Rees, M. Elliott, and M. De Leval. Pulmonary function in children with cystic fibrosis following heart-lung transplantation. *Pediatr. Pulmonol.* 18 (Suppl. 10): 272, 1994.

61. Winter, J.B., A.S. Gouw, M. Groen, C. Wildevuur, and J. Prop. Respiratory viral infections aggravate airway damage caused by chronic rejection in rat lung allografts. *Transplantation* 57: 418–422, 1994.

62. Yeh, T.F., J.A. Torre, A. Rastogi, M.A. Anyebuno, and R.S. Pildes. Early postnatal dexamethasone therapy in premature infants with severe respiratory distress syndrome: a double-blind, controlled study. *J. Pediatr.* 117: 273–282, 1990.

63. Yoder, M.C.J., R. Chua, and R. Tepper. Effect of dexamethasone on pulmonary inflammation and pulmonary function of ventilator-dependent infants with bronchopulmonary dysplasia. *Am. Rev. Respir. Dis.* 143: 1044–1048, 1991.

64. Zeltner, T.B., J.H. Caduff, P. Gehr, J. Pfenninger, and P.H. Burri. The postnatal development and growth of the human lung. I. Morphometry. *Respir. Physiol.* 67: 247–267, 1986.

Index